Clinical Skills

Second Edition

EDITED BY

T. A. Roper

Consultant Geriatrician
Leeds Community Healthcare NHS Trust
Leeds, UK

Illustrated by T. A. Roper

O
U...

OXFORD
UNIVERSITY PRESS

Great Clarendon Street, Oxford OX2 6DP,
United Kingdom

Oxford University Press is a department of the University of Oxford.
It furthers the University's objective of excellence in research, scholarship,
and education by publishing worldwide. Oxford is a registered trade mark
of Oxford University Press in the UK and in certain other countries

First Edition published in 2005

Second Edition published in 2014

Impression: 1

Published in the United States of America by Oxford University Press
198 Madison Avenue, New York, NY 10016, United States of America

British Library Cataloguing in Publication Data
Data available

Library of Congress Control Number: 2013943042

ISBN 978-0-19-957492-6

Printed in Great Britain by
Bell & Bain, Glasgow

We dedicate the book to our wives and children:
Donna Cox and Debbie Roper
Louis, Adam, Susannah, Anthony and Samuel Roper
And also to our God.

Preface

As a medical student entering the clinical years, you will find that talking to and examining patients is rather different from analysing the Krebs cycle (or whatever fancy biochemistry you get up to these days).

The purpose of this book is to allow you to make the transition from scholar to hands-on physician as smoothly as possible. It is about those techniques in history and examination that need to be practised and cannot be learned just by studying. These clinical skills are described in the style of a tutor teaching at the patient's bedside. Common difficulties encountered are faced head on, not just ignored, and solutions are suggested. Whether you are a veteran, albeit a neurotic one, about to take your Finals, or a fresh-faced third year (or possibly first year) starting your first clinical attachment, this book is on your side.

Good luck!

Niall Cox and T. A. Roper

Acknowledgements

All illustrations by Dr T. A. Roper, except the cartoons by Paul Brown, Medical Illustration Leeds.

Photography by Sian Jarvis-Colbeck, Stuart Pearson, and Timothy Zoltie, with thanks to Mark Hinchcliffe for organizing the photographers.

We acknowledge the following individuals for providing slides:

- Dr Andrew Catto, Consultant in Geriatric Medicine, Airedale Hospital (Figs. 4.7, 5.2, 6.15, 6.16, 6.17, 6.20, 6.85, 6.86, 7.2, 7.5, 7.7, 7.9, 7.11, 7.34, 7.37, 7.38, 11.13, 11.15a, 11.19, 12.4, 12.40, 13.7, 13.11, 13.14, 13.16)
- Dr Michael Darby, and Dr Rod Robertson, Consultant Radiologists at Leeds Teaching Hospitals, and Dr Hilary Moss, Consultant Radiologist at Harrogate District Hospital (Figs. 15.6, 15.7, 15.8, 15.14, 15.17, 15.20, 15.21, 15.22, 15.23, 15.24, 15.25, 15.26, 15.27, 15.28, 15.30, 15.32, 15.37)
- Mr Paul Finan, Consultant Surgeon in Colorectal Surgery at Leeds General Infirmary (Figs. 8.10, 8.11, 8.12, 8.13, 8.14, 12.9)
- Dr Douglas Chalmers, Consultant Physician in Gastroenterology (retired) (Figs. 5.7, 7.6, 7.10, 12.37, 12.38, 13.15a, 13.17)
- Dr Alexander Fraser, Consultant Physician in Rheumatology at Mid-Western Hospital, Limerick (Figs. 12.3c, 12.3d, 12.28, 12.39)
- Dr Mike Henry, Consultant Physician in Respiratory Medicine at Cork University Hospital (Fig. 15.29)
- Dr Martin Muers, Consultant Physician in Respiratory Medicine (retired) (Fig. 5.1)
- Dr Peter Sheridan, Consultant Physician in Endocrinology (Figs. 4.3, 6.20, 6.21, 7.3, 7.4, 7.8, 7.13, 7.19, 11.11, 11.14, 11.15b, 11.16, 11.17, 11.18, 12.5, 12.7, 13.1, 13.2, 13.3, 13.4, 13.5, 13.6, 13.9, 13.12, 13.13)

All other X-rays courtesy of the X-Ray museum at St James Hospital, Leeds.

Thanks to Dr Andy Brown for finding rheumatology slides and contributing the GALS assessment section in Chapter 12, as well as for further advice.

Thanks also to Dr George Fonfe, Consultant Paediatrician and Lead for Child Protection, Leeds Teaching Hospitals NHS Trust, for his contribution to the 'Child protection and safeguarding' section in Chapter 14.

And thanks to Ramsi Ajjan, Consultant Endocrinologist, for his advice on the presentation of thyroid symptoms in Chapter 11 and also Catherine Exley, Speech Therapist, for her advice on speech problems in Chapter 6.

We reserve a special thanks to Charlie Taylor and to his parents who gave us permission to use his pictures before and after surgery for cleft palate (Fig. 14.19).

Thanks to all our models: Kathryn Richardson, Debbie Roper, Tom Mwambingu, Namal Perera, Julie Forster, Joni Walker, Alistair Walling, Helen Parkinson, Holly Guy, Angela McGowan, Claristine Smith, and to our babies, Wilf Peacock and Maariyah Khan.

I would also like to thank Dr Dagmar Long for being a helpful and valued colleague while I was working on the book.

Thanks to Hannah Wilkinson and Katrina Watson for producing the OSCE examples at the end of each chapter (with the exception of Chapter 9 and Chapter 14). And thanks finally to the staff at Oxford University Press, especially Hannah Lloyd, Geraldine Jeffers, Caroline Davidson, Laura Quigley, Jonathon Crowe, Kathleen Lyle, and Abigail Stanley for bringing this second edition to fruition.

Contents

Contributors

Jan Clarke, Consultant Physician in Genitourinary Medicine, Centre for Sexual Health, Leeds General Infirmary

Niall Cox, Consultant Geriatrician, Dewsbury and District Hospitals

Harveer Dev, Academic Foundation Doctor, Cambridge University Hospitals NHS Foundation Trust

Chris Gale, NIHR Clinician Scientist Award Associate Professor of Cardiovascular Health Sciences, University of Leeds

Richard Gale, Consultant Ophthalmologist, Yorkshire, UK

Ruchi Gulati, Specialist Registrar Paediatric Neurodisability, Yorkshire and Humber Deanery

Nicola Jane Holme, Academic Clinical Fellow and Neonatal Registrar, Leeds General Infirmary

Kieran Horgan, Consultant Surgical Oncologist, Department of Surgery, Leeds General Infirmary

James Masters, Academic Foundation Doctor, University Hospitals Coventry and Warwickshire NHS Foundation Trust

Catriona McKeating, Academic Specialist Registrar in Paediatrics and Child Health, University Department of Paediatrics and Child Health, Leeds General Infirmary

Helen Parker-Bray, Specialty Registrar Genitourinary Medicine, Leeds Centre for Sexual Health, Leeds General Infirmary

Amanda Peacock, Paediatric Registrar in Endocrinology and Diabetes, Paediatric Endocrinology Department, Leeds General Infirmary

Anita Sainsbury, Consultant Gastroenterologist, St. James University Hospital, Leeds

Aravamuthan Sreedharan, Gastroenterology and Hepatology Services, Lincolnshire, UK

Siân Taylor, Clinical Research Fellow, Centre for Immunology and Infection, Department of Biology, University of York

Chakrapani Vasudevan, Clinical Research Fellow in Neonatal Medicine, University Department of Paediatrics, Leeds General Infirmary

Harriet E. Wallace, Specialty Registrar in Genitourinary Medicine, Leeds Centre for Sexual Health, Leeds General Infirmary

Abbreviations

ABC	Airway, breathing, circulation
ABCDE	Airway, breathing, circulation, disability, exposure
ABG	Arterial blood gases
ACE	Angiotensin-converting enzyme
ACTH	Adrenocorticotropic hormone
AF	Atrial fibrillation
AFP	Alpha-fetoprotein
ANCA	Anti-neutrophil cytoplasmic antibody
ANDI	Aberrations of normal development and involution
ARMD	Age-related macular degeneration
ASD	Autistic spectrum disorders
AVPU	Alert, verbal, pain, unresponsive
AVSD	Atrioventricular septal defect
BIH	Benign intracranial hypertension
BNF	British National Formulary
BPH	Benign prostatic hypertrophy
BPPV	Benign paroxysmal positional vertigo
BV	Bacterial vaginosis
CABG	Coronary artery bypass graft
CDGP	Constitutional delay in growth and puberty
CF	Cystic fibrosis
CFTR	Cystic fibrosis transmembrane regulator
CIN	Cervical intraepithelial neoplasia
CK	Creatinine kinase
CMC	Carpometacarpal
CMV	Cytomegalovirus
CNS	Central nervous system
COPD	Chronic obstructive pulmonary disease
CPK	Creatine phosphokinase
CRP	C-reactive protein
CSF	Cerebrospinal fluid
CXR	Chest radiograph
DDH	Developmental dysplasia of the hip
DEXA	Dual energy X-ray absorptiometry
DF	Difficulty factor (see Introduction)
DIP	Distal interphalangeal (joint)
DMD	Duchenne's muscular dystrophy
DMSA	Dimercaptosuccinic acid
DVT	Deep-vein thrombosis
ECG	Electrocardiograph
EEG	Electroencephalograph
ELISA	Enzyme-linked immunosorbent assay
EMG	Electromyography
EMI	Elderly mentally infirm
EMQ	Extended matching question
ENT	Ear, nose, and throat
ERCP	Endoscopic retrograde cholangiopancreatography
ESR	Erythrocyte sedimentation rate
FBC	Full blood count
FGM	Female genital mutilation
FISH	Fluorescent in situ hybridization
FSGS	Focal segmental glomerulosclerosis
FVC	Forced vital capacity
GALS	Gait, arms, legs, spine
GCS	Glasgow Coma Scale
GH	Growth hormone
GI	Gastrointestinal
GMC	General Medical Council
GORD	Gastro-oesophageal reflux disease
GTN	Glyceryl trinitrate
HCAI	Healthcare-acquired infection
HHT	Hereditary haemorrhagic telangiectasia
HPC	History of presenting complaint
HPV	Human papilloma virus
HSMN	Hereditary sensory motor neuropathy
HSP	Henoch–Schönlein purpura
HSV	Herpes simplex virus
Ig	Immunoglobulin
IHD	Ischaemic heart disease
IM	Intramuscular
INO	Internuclear ophthalmoplegia
IOP	Intraocular pressure
ITP	Immune-mediated thrombocytopenic purpura
ITU	Intensive care unit
IU	International unit

IUS	Intrauterine system		**PEEP**	Positive end-expiratory pressure
IVCO	Inferior vena caval obstruction		**PEFR**	Peak expiratory flow rate
JIA	Juvenile idiopathic arthritis		**PID**	Pelvic inflammatory disease
JVP	Jugular venous pressure		**PIP**	Proximal interphalangeal
KD	Kawasaki disease		**PKU**	Phenylketonuria
LACS	Lacunar syndrome		**POCS**	Posterior circulation syndrome
LGA	Large for gestational age		**PR**	Per rectum
LGV	Lymphogranuloma venereum		**PTH**	Parathormone
LH	Luteinizing hormone		**PUV**	Posterior urethral valves
LMN	Lower motor neuron		**PV**	Processus vaginalis
LogMAR	Logarithm of the minimum angle of resolution		**RA**	Rheumatoid arthritis
LPR	Laryngopharyngeal reflux		**RBS**	Random blood sugar
MCAD	Medium-chain acyl-CoA dehydrogenase		**RSV**	Respiratory syncytial virus
MCADD	Medium-chain acyl-CoA dehydrogenase deficiency		**SARA**	Sexually acquired reactive arthritis
			SCC	Semicircular canal
MCD	Minimal change disease		**SCD**	Sickle cell disorders
MCGN	Mesangiocapillary glomerulonephritis		**SGA**	Small for gestational age
MCP	Metacarpophalangeal (joint)		**SLE**	Systemic lupus erythmatosus
MCUG	Micturating cystourethrogram		**SNHL**	Sensorineural hearing loss
MI	Myocardial infarction		**SOB**	Shortness of breath
MMR	Measles, mumps, and rubella		**SOL**	Space-occupying lesion
MPH	Midparental height		**SSRI**	Selective serotonin reuptake inhibitors
MRSA	Meticillin-resistant *Staphylococcus aureus*		**STEMI**	ST-elevation myocardial infarction
MS	Multiple sclerosis		**STI**	Sexually transmitted infections
MSM	Men who have sex with men		**SVC**	Superior vena caval
MTP	Metatarsophalangeal (joint)		**SVT**	Supraventricular tachycardia
MUAC	Mid upper arm circumference		**TACS**	Total anterior circulation syndrome
NAAT	Nucleic acid amplification tests		**TB**	Tuberculosis
NGU	Non-gonococcal urethritis		**TCPP**	True central precocious puberty
NICE	National Institute for Health and Care Excellence		**TFT**	Thyroid function tests
NPA	Nasopharyngeal airway		**TRH**	Thyrotropin-releasing hormone
NSAID	Non-steroidal anti-inflammatory drug		**TSH**	Thyroid stimulating hormone
NSTEMI	Non-ST-elevation myocardial infarction		**TVF**	Tactile vocal fremitus
NSU	Non-specific urethritis		**U&E**	Urea and electrolytes
OME	Otitis media with effusion		**UMN**	Upper motor neuron
OSCE	Objective structured clinical examination		**UTI**	Urinary tract infection
PA	Posteroanterior		**VHD**	Valvular heart disease
PACS	Partial anterior circulation syndrome		**VR**	Vocal resonance
PAN	Polyarteritis nodosa		**VSD**	Ventricular septal defect
PCB	Postcoital bleeding		**WBC**	White blood cell
PCR	Polymerase chain reaction		**WHO**	World Health Organization
PE	Pulmonary embolism		**WSW**	Women who have sex with women

1 Introduction: about this book

Clinical skills—what are they?

Clinical skills are the skills needed to practice clinical medicine. So when a patient comes to the doctor with a problem, the doctor has two main tasks:

- to **make a diagnosis** by evaluating the patient's symptoms (taking a history), carrying out the relevant examination, and then performing or arranging investigations
- to organize **treatment** aimed at improving the patient's condition.

History, examination, investigation (these first three aimed at diagnosis), and treatment comprise the clinical skills.

The aim of this book

Clearly, the area of clinical skills represents a vast subject requiring a wealth of both factual knowledge and technical expertise.

This book focuses on those aspects of clinical skills that need to be practised and cannot be learned just by studying—particularly history and examination (the key diagnostic skills). It is a book for medical students and nurse practitioners who require these skills and the description of various techniques is aimed at someone who has not done them before. Common difficulties encountered are discussed and solutions suggested along with some useful practical tips. At the end of each chapter is a 'diseases and investigation' section which functions as a glossary of terms introduced earlier in the text. These descriptions are usually brief to allow you to understand the terms in their clinical context. (This is **not** a textbook of medicine.) Following this there is a 'Finals' section designed to demystify those stressful exit exams. There is still some reference to the traditional format of clinical exams as we recognize that some of our international readers may still experience this. However, we also realise that the standardized objective structured clinical examination (OSCE) format is rapidly displacing this style of exam globally and hence we have some OSCE tasters at the end of most chapters. This culminates in a finals chapter written by two recent OSCE veterans which is rich in practical, common-sense tips as well as describing what to expect.

This second edition is the result of constructive criticism from medical students and academic readers and has been pruned in parts to allow the inclusion of new material suggested by the students. This includes chapters on the examination of the breast and external genitalia, and the examination of children, as well as a more cohesive approach to the neurology chapter. **Ultimately this is a book designed by students, delivered by enthusiastic teachers, for students**.

Difficulty factor

Proficiency in clinical skills is hard won over many years. In the same way that we easily forget that we used stabilizers before we learned to ride a bicycle, doctors will not always remember the difficulties they encountered when they first dealt with patients. This may give you the impression that history and examination should be easy—and in turn may result in frustration and self-doubt if (and when) you find that they are not. In a sense, it is reassuring to know that **some skills are difficult and come only with practice**. Consider examination of the jugular venous pressure (JVP). As a student, I remember doctors waxing lyrical about the triple waveform—yet I could not see a single ripple. I spent hours scouring books for the answer, to no avail. If I had only known that the JVP can be very difficult to assess, then I would have known to put my difficulties down to inexperience and set about the business of examining JVPs until I became proficient.

In the major systems (cardiovascular, respiratory, neurological, and abdominal), clinical signs are given a mark out of 10 (a **difficulty factor**, DF) to give the student some idea of how much practice is needed to get it right. Thus, if difficulties are being experienced with a sign that we have given a DF of 4/10, it is likely that a basic error is being made, which should be easily corrected. If problems are being experienced with a sign given a DF of 9/10, there still may be a basic error but the chances are it is lack of practice that is the problem. Please note that DF is a subjective mark given by the authors and entirely arbitrary. It is not found in other books and teachers will not be familiar with it. Symptoms are not given DFs: here the difficulty depends very much on what is causing the symptom rather than the symptom itself.

2 Clinical settings

CHAPTER CONTENTS

Introduction

This chapter provides a brief overview of the system in which undergraduates work in the UK. Apologies are made to readers from other countries to whom some of this may not be applicable.

It is the aim of all medical schools that their students acquire an adequate knowledge of medicine and learn to apply this knowledge to help patients with their problems—to become good doctors. The best way to learn medicine is to talk to and examine as many patients in as many different situations as possible and to combine this with reading books about the relevant symptoms, signs, and conditions you have seen. You will spend most of your time in hospitals but hopefully a fair proportion with general practitioners as well.

Clinical settings

Your early clinical years will usually be spent in teaching or local hospitals (see Fig. 2.1) as this is where the greatest pool of patients is. This is where you will cut your teeth, learning the skill of history-taking and examination.

As your skills mature you will find your clinical horizons opening. Most undergraduate schemes will try to increase your exposure to many different specialties. This will include primary care with sessions in GP surgeries and community clinics. This will not only add to the variety of your experience but will give you a taste of specialties that you might not have considered for a future career.

There are too many specialties to list, but Table 2.1 lists some broad areas that you may be exposed to.

Clinical work

As you migrate around the health service you will usually be attached to a consultant and their team. In the UK for the last two decades there has been a redesign of training and the consultant's team structure. The consultant team may now consist of a foundation doctor, foundation year 1 (FY1) or foundation year 2 (FY2), and/or a specialist trainee, year 1 (ST1) through to year 5 (ST5), depending on local resources. These replace the old House Officer and Registrar grades respectively.

You may also find you may spend some time in primary care with a GP and their team.

There may be exposure to specialist community clinics such as diabetic clinics or continence clinics as well as community teams such as district nurses and other specialist nurses. On some occasions you may see patients in their own homes. In both primary and secondary care settings you may be exposed to clinics run by specialist

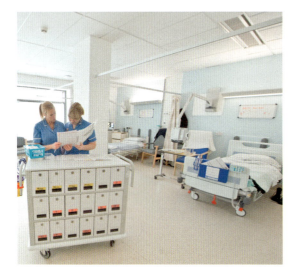

Figure 2.1 Hospital ward.

Table 2.1 Some clinical settings you may visit

Primary care[a]	Secondary care (in-patients and outpatients)[b]
GP surgery	Medical specialties
Community clinics	Surgical specialties
Home visit	Anaesthetics
	Mental health

[a] **Primary care** is the initial point of contact for a patient in the health service and includes GP surgeries, dental surgeries, pharmacies and other community services.
[b] **Secondary care** is the care provided by specialists and is usually accessed by referral from a primary care practitioner. As the majority of specialists are found in hospitals secondary care is often equated with hospitals.

nurses or nurse practitioners. Although the terminology can vary from country to country, and even within countries, these nurses usually have been trained in advanced clinical skills or have a good working knowledge of the specialist area they have chosen.

Clinical teaching may be timetabled or informal.

Timetabled clinical teaching

This can take three main forms:

1 **Group teaching**. This is where a doctor takes a group of between 2 and 10 students to a patient. One student is

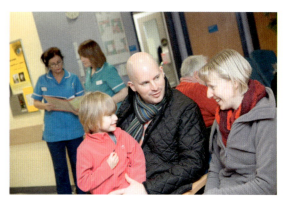

Figure 2.2 Outpatient clinic waiting area.

picked out (usually at random) to either take a history or perform an examination. Try not to avoid being picked out. You may be afraid and embarrassed by being put in the spotlight but your fear will only worsen if you continue to hide. These sessions (which may be infrequent) should not be missed as it is here that doctors most easily impart their hard-won knowledge.

2 **Outpatient teaching**. Here you will either sit in with a doctor while they do clinic (see Fig. 2.2) or see patients yourself and then tell (present) their story to the doctor.

3 **Ward rounds**. This is where the consultant and their team go round the ward evaluating their patients. Students are usually expected to attend but ward rounds are becoming increasingly business-like (due to pressure of time) and their vast teaching potential is often untapped.

Early in your student career you may find during timetabled teachings that you are present in an observational role only, particularly in the ward round setting, a GP's surgery or an outpatient clinic. What you get out of these settings can depend on the enthusiasm and teaching skills of the doctor/nurse practitioner that you are attached to. However, there are a few things you should observe to get the most out of these situations:

- Listen to the questions that are asked and the responses from the patient.
- Did the clinician put the patient at their ease?
- Did the practitioner gain consent to examine the patient?
- Observe the non-verbal communication between the doctor and the patient (see Chapter 3).

- Try to work out what went well with the encounter and what did not go so well.
- Do not be afraid to ask questions as to why something was said or done to the patient.
- Also ask what the plan (called the management) is for the patient.
- When you get time, read up about a case that has captured your interest.

Informal clinical teaching

Some of your time during a clinical attachment is unsupervised. Lingering around a ward wasting time or just staying at home may be tempting, but is clearly counterproductive. A systematic approach to this unsupervised time should be adopted: you will learn twice as much in half the time.

- To learn history-taking, take histories from patients on the ward and present them either verbally or in written form to a doctor for criticism.
- Once you have seen a patient, make sure you follow their progress; find out what tests they have undergone, what diagnoses are made, what treatment they receive, and whether it works.
- To learn examination technique, join a fellow student or students and visit patients in twos or threes (if you go alone you never quite get the critical atmosphere required).
- As finals approach, this self-teaching may escalate into an unsavoury game of 'patient hunting'. 'There's a spleen on ward 136B' will be a common whisper (Fig. 2.3). Sometimes, it is an important clinical skill to know when not to examine.
- The ward staff may be very busy; it is very easy to feel a bit like a spare part. Be enthusiastic—if you show willingness and are courteous to both the junior doctors and the nurses, you will soon be made very welcome.
- Simply 'shadowing' the junior doctor can be extremely rewarding. Be as helpful as you can; this will give them more time to discuss issues with you.

Patients' feelings

Patients vary in their responses to involvement in student teaching. Sometimes, medical students get themselves a bad reputation because of the 'patient hunting' just

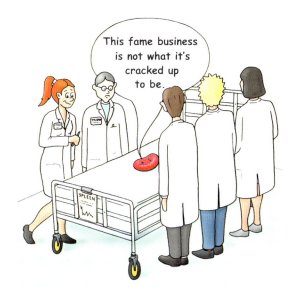

Figure 2.3 The price of fame.
© Paul Brown, Medical Illustrations Leeds

mentioned. However, most patients quite enjoy involvement with students. Not only does it relieve the boredom of hospital but often students are the only 'doctors' who have enough time to listen to **all** a patient's complaints and worries. Remember always to treat patients courteously and thank them when you have finished.

Infection control

This subject is high on the agenda in both primary and secondary care and as students you need to be aware of its importance. There has been a rise in healthcare-acquired infections (HCAI), which are infections given to patients as a result of healthcare interventions. The inference is that these infections should be avoidable if attention

CASE 2.1

Problem. I understand why we have to wear gloves but I have a latex allergy. What can I do?

Discussion. There are hypoallergenic alternatives to latex such as nitrile gloves. All healthcare providers will have local policies for infection control and have a responsibility for providing appropriate substitutes for staff with an allergy.

HAND CLEANING TECHNIQUES

How to handwash?
WITH SOAP AND WATER

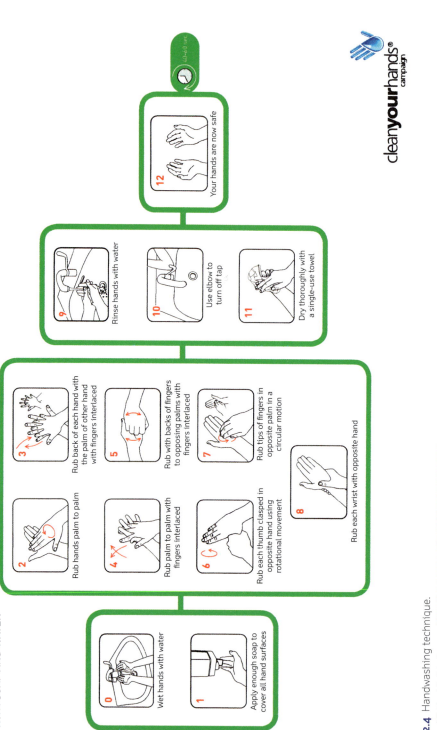

Figure 2.4 Handwashing technique.

© National Patient Safety Agency. http://www.npsa.nhs.uk/cleanyourhands/.

HAND CLEANING TECHNIQUES

How to handrub?
WITH ALCOHOL HANDRUB

1a
1b

Apply a small amount (about 3ml) of the product in a cupped hand, covering all surfaces

2

Rub hands palm to palm

3

Rub back of each hand with the palm of other hand with fingers interlaced

4

Rub palm to palm with fingers interlaced

5

Rub with backs of fingers to opposing palms with fingers interlaced

6

Rub each thumb clasped in opposite hand using rotational movement

7

Rub tips of fingers in opposite palm in a circular motion

8

Rub each wrist with opposite hand

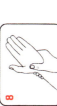

20–30 sec

9

Once dry, your hands are safe

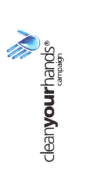

cleanyourhands® campaign

Figure 2.5 Technique of cleaning the hands with alcohol gel.

© National Patient Safety Agency. http://www.npsa.nhs.uk/cleanyourhands/.

to hygiene and proper aseptic techniques are used when dealing with patients. According to the National Institute for Health and Care Excellence (NICE) around 300 000 patients a year in England acquire a healthcare-associated infection as a result of care within the NHS. In 2007, meticillin-resistant *Staphylococcus aureus* (MRSA) bloodstream infections and *Clostridium difficile* (C diff) infections were recorded as the underlying cause of, or a contributory factor in, approximately 9000 deaths in hospital and primary care in England. This problem is seen in many healthcare systems around the world and is recognized by the World Health Organization (WHO).

As students there are some simple steps you can take to help in keeping HCAIs to a minimum:

- Wear shirts or blouses with short sleeves (or sleeves that are easily rolled up).
- Keep fingernails short and clean.
- Avoid jewellery and wristwatches.
- Wear gloves if there is the possibility of contact with bodily fluids such as blood, urine, faeces, etc. Also wear them if the patient has a known pathogen which can be transferred by contact. See Case 2.1.
- Wear a disposable apron if there is the risk of being splashed by bodily fluids as above. If you are dealing with a patient with a known pathogen such as MRSA, there should be ready access to the gloves and aprons just outside (or inside) the room. When you have finished you should dispose of the items in the special bin for infectious waste provided in the room so they can be disposed of safely. Do not walk out of the room with these items on.
- If you are going to a surgical attachment, the standard of hygiene required is extremely high if you are going into theatres. You will be shown how to scrub up properly and will have to wear gloves, gowns, special footwear, and masks.

Handwashing

Washing your hands is the single most important step in reducing the spread of infection in primary and secondary care. As a result we make no excuse for emphasizing this repeatedly in the examination routines provided in this book. The hope is that washing your hands will become second nature to you as you perform your clinical assessments.

WHO have tried to provide a unified approach to handwashing worldwide and have outlined five moments or instances when you should wash your hands:

1 Before patient contact
2 Before an aseptic procedure
3 After risk of/or exposure to bodily fluids
4 After patient contact
5 After contact with the patient's surroundings

The correct technique for handwashing is shown in Fig. 2.4.

Thorough drying with towels also reduces the burden of microorganisms, so do not be tempted to skimp on this. You should normally have access to appropriate handwashing facilities in hospitals and GP premises, but facilities may be more rudimentary in patient's own homes. In these circumstances community teams often take portable bottles of alcohol gel with them on visits. Alcohol gel has been shown to be an acceptable alternative to handwashing so long as the hands are not visibly dirty (see Fig. 2.5).

If your hands are dirty, or before any aseptic procedure, the hands must be washed with soap and water. See Cases 2.2 and 2.3.

Clinical skills centres

Many medical schools now have clinical skills centres where students can practise many techniques such as use of the stethoscope or ophthalmoscope or inserting intravenous cannulas. Videos, computers, and manikins (dummy

CASE 2.2

I have multiple allergies and I also have eczema of my hands. I am worried that all this handwashing and alcohol rubs will worsen my eczema or cause a rash.

This is a real concern because during a working day you can end up washing your hands repeatedly and this does have a drying effect which can aggravate your eczema. However, eczematous hands are also a good breeding ground for microorganisms so there is a need to keep your hands as clean as possible. There are hypoallergenic soap substitutes you can use if you are allergic to the perfume in soaps. Alcohol gel is an acceptable substitute so long as your hands are not soiled, and they are less drying than soap and water. Also alcohol is unlikely to cause an allergic response. Most healthcare providers will have moisturizing creams available to offset the drying properties of handwashing.

CASE 2.3

After washing my hands should I use an alcohol gel as well?

There is no need to do this and there is no evidence to support it, although there is a study which showed that an alcohol gel was superior to washing with soap and water in preventing the transmission of Gram-negative organisms to a urethral catheter. This raises the possibility that the two used together could be more effective, and you might use both before doing an invasive procedure such as urethral catheterization or venepuncture.

patients) are used. These are excellent for practising techniques, but do not fool yourself into thinking you can learn all you need without seeing real patients.

Non-clinical skills

Your training and working life, as in many other professions, will be rewarding but can be intense and all-consuming. There seems to be a bewildering number of sources telling you what to do; to read innumerable textbooks, to read research papers, pass your exams, practise skills, and when you have finished, to read more books.

Key points

- Unsupervised time can be frustrating, but be focused and enthusiastic and your time will be highly productive
- Be aware of the infection control procedures of the clinical environment you are attached to
- Learn to wash your hands effectively
- Alcohol gel is an effective substitute for handwashing so long as your hands are not dirty
- Try to maintain your non-clinical skills throughout your career

However, you need to pay attention to non-clinical matters too. Preserve your relationships with your family and friends (you will inevitably lose touch with some but you will make new ones too). All students have hobbies such as sport, music, art, or more esoteric activities such as morris dancing. Try to maintain these as much as possible. There will be times when exams and other requirements will squeeze everything out but once they have passed pick them up again. Put simply, do not be afraid to enjoy yourself from time to time. Not only will this make you more resistant to burn-out and depression, it can also help you connect with patients who also have interests such as sport, music, art, and even morris dancing. Striking a work/life balance and enjoying life are essential non-clinical skills.

3 Core aspects of history-taking and examination

Introduction

Congratulations! If you have made it this far, you have either secured a place in medical school or perhaps are a nurse practitioner learning advanced clinical skills. You will be united in wanting to do the best for patients, to try to cure them or to relieve suffering. History-taking and examination are crucial first steps in this process and this chapter is your introduction to these skills. Of the two, history-taking is the most important in leading you to the cause of illness (diagnosis). The role of examination is to provide supporting evidence for your suspicions. Of course medicine is not always that easy and sometimes you will have to revise your thinking in the light of new evidence gained from the patient or eyewitnesses at a later date or from your examination findings. Even if you remain unsure of the diagnosis a well-taken history should point you to what system of the body is affected so that you can arrange the most appropriate test. Not only will we endeavour to give you a structure to mastering history-taking and examination but we will shed some light on communication skills as well. Awareness of the essential components of communication is a precursor to developing your 'bedside manner' and establishing empathy with your patients. Succeed in this and you will maximize the success of your consultation. Finally, having completed your history and examination you need to be able to pass on your hard-earned fruits to others either through oral presentation or via a written record in the notes. Sections are devoted to these aims as well as tips on how to answer the supplementary questions that your supervising doctor may ask. We believe that these are the core aspects of history-taking and examination that you need to master.

An introduction to communication skills

Communication is the lifeblood of the medical profession. Information has to be coaxed from the patient, a potential diagnosis deduced from it and then that information translated into medical language so that this can be communicated to other members of the team or to other specialties if required. Once a management plan is worked out then this information has to be translated back to ordinary language so that the patient can understand and

CASE 3.1

Problem. Why must the medical profession produce such jargon? Could they not come up with simpler terms that everyone can understand?

   Discussion. It is interesting you use the term 'jargon' as it is a double-edged term. It can mean the specialized language of a profession or trade but can also mean meaningless drivel. Sometimes the media seem to emphasize the latter and portray the profession as deliberately engineering big words to elevate the status and mystique of doctors. The reality is that these terms bring precision to our profession so that when you communicate with other doctors they understand exactly what you mean. For example, atrial fibrillation, supraventricular tachycardia, and ventricular tachycardia all cause palpitations but the treatment in each case is different.

CASE 3.2

Problem. You have just stated that there are a number of models of consultations but you have not described any. Why?

   Discussion. The idea of this introduction is to raise your awareness of the importance of communication and to let you know that various models exist. However, we want this book to concentrate on the hard currency of how you diagnose through history-taking and examination. Once you begin to become fluent in these skills it will be useful to look at those models to refine your skills. Some models do not just focus on diagnosis but look at treatment, modifying behaviour, and even breaking bad news. All of this is important but we want you to walk before you can run. What we will do is draw attention to simple things you should consider before you get started such as the importance of non-verbal communication and how this affects your patient.

make informed decisions and participate successfully in their treatment. Clearly there is great scope for things to go wrong in this process. Case 3.1 discusses the need for medical jargon.

Why does communication matter?

Historically patients consulted their doctors and the doctors would dispense their wisdom and treatments and patients would accept this passively. This has become regarded as the 'medical model' (although many professions and trades behaved in similar ways). However, when it comes to health, research has shown that this approach is inadequate. Poor or incomplete communication creates dissatisfaction among patients as their concerns are not always heard; they may not understand their disease or fail to take their medication (called lack of concordance or lack of treatment adherence, and formerly lack of compliance). Furthermore, the patient's dissatisfaction can manifest as a complaint or even litigation.

   There is a growing realization that communication skills need much greater prominence in undergraduate education. Various models of consultations have been proposed to try to maximize the desired outcome of diagnosis and successful treatment while improving patient satisfaction (see Case 3.2). This has been driven particularly in primary care where GPs have to be focused and succinct in their consultations. The good news is that communication skills can be taught, and in the UK GPs have led the way in videoing consultations and giving feedback to their trainees.

The knowledge base around clinical communication has grown substantially and is beyond the remit of this book. We recommend *Clinical communication skills* by Peter Washer for a more detailed account of this subject.

Non-verbal communication

What is it?

Non-verbal communication is the unspoken messages that you or your patient transmit to each other through your appearance, facial expressions, body language, etc. Some key areas to consider include:

- appearance
- facial expression
- eyes
- personal space
- body language and posture
- gestures
- touch
- vocal tone, rhythm, and inflection.

Why does it matter?

Non-verbal communication matters because if used correctly it can help you create a rapport with your patient which will enable you to be more successful in your consultation. It also helps to emphasize any health or treatment messages that you give. The converse is also true if you do not pay sufficient attention to the non-verbal messages that you radiate. You can put off your patient and lose their cooperation and you may give contradictory messages, i.e. a mismatch between what your voice is saying and what your body is expressing, which can lead to you losing credibility with your patient.

What can be done?

The good news is that many of you will not be starting from scratch. In fact many of you may already be skilled in reading and influencing people. However, you will have to modify your abilities for a new clinical environment. Most of you will also have had some experience of being a patient at some time in your life and can readily empathize with patients who find themselves in a similar position.

Appearance

It goes without saying that you need to create a good first impression and to be smartly dressed. Avoid the two extremes of being either too casual or wearing outlandish fashion items. Otherwise wear what you are comfortable in, with the proviso that it needs to be practical (see 'Infection control' in Chapter 2): try to wear shirts/blouses with short sleeves. If you wear a tie, you need to ensure that it is either tucked in or secured with a tiepin to stop it trailing over the patient. See Case 3.3.

Facial expression

Facial expressions are a rich source of information that translates surprisingly well across many cultures. For example, a happy or sad face can be recognized universally despite a language barrier. So it is highly recommended that you supplement your initial contact with your patient with a relaxed smile. Also, remember communication is a two-way process. So use your skill at reading people to work out if they are in pain, look depressed, relaxed, irritable, etc.

Eyes

Although the eyes contribute to facial expression they are considered separately for two main reasons. The first is that eye contact with your patient is extremely important in generating trust and conveying interest to your patient. Too little eye contact can suggest to your patient that you are not interested in them. At the other extreme, beware of

CASE 3.3

Problem. I believe that when I qualify and have to work long and intense shifts that I should be able to wear something casual and comfortable. At the end of the day if I have a medical degree it should not matter what I wear and people should respect this.

Discussion. I used to think like you and I understand some of your argument. However, like it or not, appearance matters. I remember when I did weekend sessions on-call in the past; I would wear a comfortable rugby top underneath my white coat. One time I looked after a young girl with spina bifida who was very ill and needed a central line and close medical supervision. She had devoted parents who visited regularly over the weekend and I would give updates on her progress. Happily she recovered and I met her father by chance in the corridor a week later. He thanked me for all I had done for his daughter and then confessed that both he and his wife had experienced great anxiety because my appearance had made them unsure of my credibility as a doctor. They were just an ordinary couple who had no particular axe to grind and I felt bad realizing that I had caused them needless worry solely because of the way I had dressed. Since then I dress comfortably but smartly because I do not want to risk just one more patient or their relatives having a similar experience. Like it or not, all people make judgements on your appearance and remember that most of the patients you will look after will be older and perhaps more traditional than you (unless you do paediatrics).

staring too intensely because this may make the patient feel that you are domineering or just plain weird. The second reason is that your eyes are also expressive and sometimes even when you try to keep your face deadpan, your eyes can betray inner emotion, e.g. before breaking bad news.

Also try to read how your patient is feeling. If they are constantly averting their gaze, they may feel anxious, inferior, or embarrassed and may be hiding something. This could be your cue for more sensitive exploration, so be alert.

Personal space

Everyone has a virtual, unmarked zone around them which they feel is their territory. If anyone encroaches on this space they begin to feel threatened. Often, if this happens, the threatened individual will take a step back to maintain their comfort level. The difficulty you face is that peoples' personal space can vary from culture to culture and even within cultures, and many misunderstandings can occur. I can still remember vividly when I was younger, feeling extremely self-conscious when an African man stood next to me and held my hand (according to his custom).

Body language and posture

Body language and posture are important as it is easy to build unintentional barriers by the way you sit and stand. If you are taking a history, try to sit face-to-face or at a comfortable angle (no more than 90°) with your patient. Try to be at the same eye-level if you can because if you are much higher than your patient you may appear to threaten and dominate. Try not to cross your legs or your arms, as these can appear to be defensive. Try to lean gently towards your patient and show interest in them with the appropriate eye contact. At the same time, observe the posture of your patient and try to gauge if they are relaxed, or seem stiff and anxious, or even perched forward in an aggressive posture. Again these cues should prompt you to take the appropriate action, i.e. to reassure or maybe to de-escalate simmering tensions.

Gestures

Gestures are highly personal and some flamboyant individuals use a lot while others use very few if any. Do what feels comfortable to you, but beware that the overuse of gestures can be distracting. However, if used wisely they can underpin the message you are trying to give verbally. Again, some gestures like nodding can show interest in what your patient is saying.

Touch

This is also highly individual. Some people are more tactile than others. Some doctors will hold the hand of patients and this can be a very powerful way of connecting and demonstrating sympathy. The downside is that this can be a turn-off for those patients who do not like being touched, especially by strangers, so it is a matter of fine judgement.

Vocal tone, rhythm, and inflection

This is included in non-verbal communication because there are aspects of vocalization that can convey meaning apart from the words spoken. If your delivery is dull, laboured, and monotonous you could convey boredom. Too jolly a voice could suggest that you are not taking the situation seriously, or a hesitant voice could convey a lack of confidence. If you pay attention to your patient's vocalization there could actually be clues to a potential diagnosis lurking. If their delivery is dull, laboured, and monotonous this could indicate depression or even Parkinson's disease (see Chapter 6). If their voice is euphoric, with very fast speech that jumps from topic to topic, this could indicate the psychiatric state of hypomania. If their speech is hesitant they may be anxious or even have the speech of cerebellar dysfunction (see Chapter 6).

Cases 3.4 and 3.5 highlight some common frustrations with communication.

Introduction to history-taking and examination

When a patient consults their doctor about a problem, the doctor evaluates which conditions might be causing their symptoms. To do this they use three techniques:

CASE 3.4

Problem. I'm beginning to find all this confusing and you haven't even started teaching history and examination yet. You say make plenty of eye contact and then say too much is not good. You can touch some patients and not others. We mustn't invade their personal space and yet there is no sign saying that's far enough. How on earth are we expected to get it right?

Discussion. I appreciate that it can all seem exasperating but you must not forget that you may already be clued up on how to interact with people. All we are trying to do is to raise your awareness of where things could

go wrong—and they will! If, for example, you touched someone and they recoil, just apologize immediately and remember not to do it to that patient in future. Your whole consultation, verbal and non-verbal, is a series of negotiations. So if you unwittingly intrude into their personal space and they step back, they have informed you of your encroachment and you have to honour this. Think of all this in terms of attending a job interview. Much of what has been discussed is valid for the interview setting. You are trying to give the best possible impression so that all your hard-core knowledge can bear fruit.

CASE 3.5

Problem. I hear that doctors' communication skills are generally poor. Is this true?

Discussion. In such a large body of professionals there will be some excellent communicators and unfortunately some dire ones too. They basically reflect the general population they come from and you will find the same distribution wherever you choose to look. As this chapter has tried to demonstrate, no matter how good you are there are things you can do to improve your performance. However, like any type of performance it can vary according to your circumstances. For me the most pressing threat to communication is time. When I was a student like you, there seemed to be an unlimited amount of time to produce a really comprehensive clerking (except in exams). It was a real shock when I was introduced to the pressures of real-life working, where patients were tired of waiting in the emergency department or outpatients and beleaguered nurses would keep urging you on to clear the waiting areas. This tension can clearly intrude into the consultation. Other variables that can affect your performance include fatigue (so be wary of overdoing nights out before a difficult shift), missed meals, or personal tragedies in your life. Try to avoid some of the factors that can impair your performance if you can and don't forget the plea from the previous chapter to maintain your friendships and hobbies. Hopefully this will help you to maintain your performance even under great stress.

- they discuss the patient's complaints with them (history-taking)
- they do any relevant physical examination
- they perform or arrange appropriate investigations.

General aspects of the first two techniques—history and examination—are discussed in this chapter.

History-taking

What is a history?

The patient's history is the story of their problems. It has two main components:

- the patient's actual 'raw' complaint(s)
- further information gleaned by the doctor.

The aims are:

- to lead to a diagnosis—the doctor's fundamental objective;
- to evaluate the impact of the patient's symptoms on their lives.

Sometimes the history will produce a clear diagnosis but often there is a range of possibilities—this is known as differential diagnosis.

How to take a history

There are two main elements of history-taking:

- developing a rapport with the patient—the 'bedside manner'
- evaluating the patient's complaint(s) in detail.

The 'bedside manner'

A doctor's bedside manner is their approach or attitude to the patient and is important for several reasons:

- **Compassion**. When a patient sees any health professional, they are often at a low ebb psychologically. It is clearly important that they are made to feel at ease, for humanitarian reasons.
- **Confidence**. A good bedside manner tends to increase the patient's confidence that they are being cared for properly and so makes them feel more settled.
- **Doing your job**. The more at ease the patient is, the more likely they are to feel free to tell you all their problems. The more information the patient gives you, the more likely you are to get the right diagnosis—and the correct diagnosis provides the key to effective treatment.

How to adopt a good 'bedside manner'

The key to adopting a good bedside manner lies in your appreciation of non-verbal communication as well as the things you say. Many students try to be friendly, smiley, and jokey, and many patients like this—to a point. But patients will often interpret joviality as evidence that you do not know what you are doing; a few patients will take exception to any frivolity where their health is concerned.

CASE 3.6

Problem. I'm not sure about shaking hands. Is it not a bit old fashioned?

   Discussion. Shaking hands can be reassuring when visiting a teacher, car salesman, or doctor and is recommended. Just be careful with patients with arthritis or frail older patients that you do not squeeze hard and cause discomfort. If you see signs of reluctance, abort the handshake.

My own very personal belief is that the best style is confident with a tinge of authority, yet open to questions; kind and thoughtful; and reassuring but not misleading.

- Introduce yourself and offer to shake their hand (see Case 3.6). Say something like 'Hello, I'm Michaela Quinn, a third-year medical student. Do you mind if I have a few words with you about why you had to come into hospital?'

- Mostly your patient will be sitting down. Do not stand towering over them. Ask permission to sit down next to them at a sociable distance—not too far, not too near.

- Avoid appearing too busy to listen. Patients often imagine that doctors have a lot of more serious cases to deal with. If you appear rushed, they will hesitate to bother you with what they might feel are their 'trivial problems'.

Evaluating the patient's complaint(s) in detail

The aims are:

- to look for clues that will lead to a diagnosis—so that appropriate treatment can be started

- to determine the effects of symptoms on the patient's life—so that strategies can be put in place to support them; for example, an old person with joint pains may no longer be able to get to the shops and may need someone to help with their shopping.

A major part of the history involves asking questions directly relating to the patient's complaint(s). First of all, ascertain what the patient's basic complaint is (known as the **presenting complaint**). Then find out more details about this complaint; for example, when it started, how long have they had it for (this is known as the history of the presenting complaint).

   Other important information should be obtained:

- drug history
- family history
- social history
- any other symptoms.

   This is often a complicated business. Assessing even the simplest of complaints can be a major challenge and is the focus of the next few pages.

The presenting complaint

You need to define the problem that is troubling the patient and why they have come to see you. Ask 'What was the problem that brought you into hospital?' The patient may well answer with a diagnosis such as 'a heart attack'. If so, you need to focus on symptoms: ask questions like 'How did it affect you?' or 'What did it feel like?'

History of the presenting complaint

To evaluate the presenting complaint(s) further, you need to ask questions aimed at working out the cause and effects of the symptom(s). This is known as the history of the presenting complaint. An example is given in Table 3.1.

What to ask

1 Find out more about the symptom(s) themselves. Ask about:

- site
- duration/onset
- severity (if necessary, ask patient to rank pain out of 10)
- character
- precipitating factors
- relieving factors
- similar symptoms suffered previously.

   The importance of these features varies widely for different symptoms. It requires considerable experience and knowledge to know how much detail to go into for each symptom and which are the most useful questions for each symptom. Try to avoid 'leading questions'. There is a danger that suggestible patients may lead you up the wrong avenue in their attempts to be helpful: if the patient has chest pain and you suspect angina, you may wish to find out if the pain is brought on by exertion. Avoid the temptation to ask 'Does walking bring the pain on?' but instead say 'Does anything seem to bring the pain on?' Then, if the patient says 'yes', ask 'What brings on the pain?' This will guarantee an authentic answer. If, however, you find that your patient is vague or is having difficulty, then it is reasonable to be more direct and ask 'Does walking bring on the pain?' See Case 3.7 for a strategy for dealing with vague responses.

Table 3.1 History of presenting complaint: a patient with headache

Presenting complaint

Headache

Further details of main complaint

Duration: 3 h

Onset: sudden, at its worst within a minute

Site: back of head

Severity: 10 out of 10

Character: dull

Precipitating factors: came out of the blue while watching TV

Relieving factors: paracetamol no good, co-codamol partial relief

Previous similar symptoms: no previous headaches

Other symptoms in the affected system

Dizziness: no

Diplopia: no

Hearing loss: no

Weakness: no

Syncope: fell to the ground at some point early on, not sure if blacked out

Questions relevant to possible causes

Subarachnoid haemorrhage must be a possibility. This may also cause vomiting and is more common in people with high blood pressure, so check:

Vomiting: twice

High blood pressure: no

Effects of the symptoms on the patient's life

Not really relevant given short timescale

2 Find out about other symptoms in the affected system. Thus, if a patient complains of coughing up blood (haemoptysis, pronounced *he-mopped-a-sis*), this is a respiratory symptom, so also ask about cough, phlegm, breathlessness, wheeze, and chest pain.

CASE 3.7

Problem. I don't have any problem talking to patients. However, I do find that often the patient talks a lot without giving me the information I need but when I butt in to find out more about their main complaint, I can't help feeling very rude.

Discussion. Some, but by no means all, patients are bursting to tell you about all their problems. They will switch from one problem to another dipping in and out of the past, apparently at random, describing diagnoses that don't seem to fit to their symptoms. It is tempting to stop such patients at each turn and demand clear details. However, this can be a little unfriendly so early on in the interview. It may be best to give such a patient a free rein for 2–3 minutes. Don't ask them many questions. Just listen while you give them a chance to have their say. After that time, the patient's complaints can be summarized back to them and suggestions made as to how you're going to proceed. For example, 'So you're a diabetic on insulin but you've been quite well recently until 5 days ago. Then you started to feel sickly and off your food. This morning you've developed some pain in your tummy and vomited twice. Now, I need to ask you some more questions about your tummy pain . . .'

3 Ask questions about possible causes. In the patient with haemoptysis, you need to be thinking about what might cause this and also what other questions you should ask about these causes. So if you think of pulmonary embolism, you ask about recent operations, pleuritic chest pain, or leg swelling—or you may think of lung cancer and ask about weight loss and smoking.

4 Find out about the effects of the symptoms on the patient's life. Ask how the symptoms have affected their lifestyle; for example, whether they have had to miss work or give up hobbies or whether they are unable to do their shopping.

Tip

Asking about previous episodes is quite useful. For instance, a patient may present with a severe occipital headache—suggestive of a subarachnoid haemorrhage (bleeding into the brain). If he tells you he has had a similar headache seven times in the last year without major ill effect, this is less likely to represent sub-arachnoid haemorrhage than if he tells you he has no previous headaches.

Tip

It is useful to ask 'When were you last well?' and '. . . then, what happened?'

Past medical history

There are two main reasons for delving into the past:

- If the patient has a long-standing disease, there is a strong chance that any new symptom could relate to this.

- Past history is useful in deciding how active a patient (and their doctor) might want the doctors to be with their treat-ment. If, for example, you consider two different patients both with lung cancer and one has a long-standing severe disability due to stroke whereas the other has been previ-ously well, there may well be a difference in their attitudes to chemotherapy or radiotherapy.

What to ask

It is surprising how some patients can forget their past, so you may have to probe quite a bit to find out about previous problems. Ask 'Do you suffer from any long-term health problems?' and 'Have you been in hospital before?'

Ask specifically about these common important conditions:

- heart attack
- angina
- stroke
- high blood pressure
- rheumatic fever
- tuberculosis
- diabetes
- epilepsy
- jaundice
- chronic bronchitis/emphysema
- anaemia
- stomach ulcers
- operations
- allergies.

When the patient says 'yes' to any of these, you must try to verify the diagnosis. For example, if the patient admits to having previously suffered a stroke, ask 'How did the stroke affect you?'

Alcohol intake and smoking can be included in the past medical history (students usually include these in the social history). It is important to know the full history of alcohol intake and smoking: a patient may tell you he does not smoke or drink but may admit he smoked 40 a day until yes-terday and drank 40 pints of beer a week until 2 years ago.

Tip

It is better to ask about 'high blood pressure' than 'hypertension', which many patients understandably think is a nervous complaint.

Drug history

A drug history is very important because of the following:

- Drug side effects may cause all or part of the patient's problem. As an example, if a patient has recently devel-oped diarrhoea, it is important to know if they have recently had a course of antibiotics.

- Before adjusting treatment or starting any new treat-ments, you need to know what the patient is taking already:
  - In cases where a patient is already taking medica-tion for a condition, you need to know the current doses. Prescribing furosemide 80 mg for a patient's deteriorating heart failure will not help much if this is the dose they are already taking.
  - You need to make sure the old and new treatments will not cause problems when used together. So, if you want to start a patient on a non-steroidal anti-inflammatory drug such as diclofenac, it is important to know whether they are taking an anti-coagulant such as warfarin. If so, the risks of diclof-enac causing bleeding from the stomach are greatly increased.
  - The medication list also helps to give an idea of what diseases a patient is suffering from. So if the patient is taking mesalazine, this suggests that the patient has inflammatory bowel disease.

What to ask

Patients are often unsure about their medications and the more they take (polypharmacy) the more difficult it is for the patient to remember them. Equally, the more medications a patient takes, the more chance there is of adverse drug interactions—so you need to be thorough.

Ask the patient 'Are you taking any tablets, inhalers, or drops for anything?' If yes, ask if they've got their medication with them.

- If they have, go through the boxes or bottles individually reading the labels. These will usually give the name of the tablet, the dose, and how often the patient is taking them. Often the label is out of date, or the patient's adherence to their medication regime is imperfect, so check with the patient what they think they should be taking, the dose, and the frequency. Record their responses.
- If they have not, the patient may have a list of medications. Again, go through this with the patient checking each medication as you go.

Patients are often unsure of their current medication. This is especially so in hospital where drugs are often changed. The drugs will be written on a drug chart, which is usually at the end of the patient's bed. If the patient cannot give you a good drug history, look at the drug chart. The format of the drug chart varies from hospital to hospital. Ask one of the nurses or doctors on the ward how to interpret it. If you are not sure about any of the drugs, look them up in the *British national formulary*, which is an invaluable guide to drugs and usually available on the ward (and now online).

....

Tip

When asking patients about drugs, do not use the word 'drugs'. To many patients 'drugs' suggests cocaine, heroin, and so on. Instead, you should enquire about 'tablets', 'medicines', or 'inhalers'.

....

Family history

Family history may sometimes give a clue to the cause of the patient's problems. Ask the following.

- 'Has anyone in your family had similar problems?'
- 'Do any diseases run in the family?'
- 'Did anyone in your family die young—and if so, how?'

It can be difficult to decide how much detail to take. For instance, in a woman with haemoptysis, it may not be particularly helpful to know that her sister has a stomach ulcer.

Social history

This helps to build up a general picture of the patient: what they were like in the past and how the current illness is affecting them. Ask about the following.

- **Marital status and children**. Ask briefly about the family's state of health. It is particularly important in frail elderly patients to get an idea whether family will be able to care for the patient if needed.
- **Occupation (or previous occupation if unemployed or retired)**. Some occupations may bring increased risk of certain illnesses: shipbuilders may suffer from asbestos-related diseases. Some occupations may find particular problems more troublesome: lorry drivers with epilepsy must give up their job. If the patient has had multiple jobs, you may not have time to discuss the ins and outs of all of these. Focus on the current job and on any jobs that may have involved exposure to toxic materials.
- **Where they live**. Some people live in care homes, suggesting that they are no longer able to look after themselves. Some care homes employ carers who can help with personal care such as washing, dressing, meals, and medications. Others employ trained nurses for more disabled people. Some homes specialize in looking after people with a specific condition such as dementia.
- **How your patient's condition restricts them and what help they have in coping with any restrictions**. Who does the shopping? Who collects the pension? It is often said that if an old person is able to collect their own pension they are probably coping reasonably well. Who does the washing and cleaning? Do they have a home help, a warden, or meals-on-wheels?

Some patients may consider these questions intrusive. If so, it is best just to skip on to the systematic questions.

Systematic questions

It is often possible to miss important symptoms from the history because you forget to ask or the patient neglects to mention them. Systematic questioning is something of a dredging system but acts as a fail-safe mechanism to make sure you do not miss anything vital. Often you will only turn up minor things but occasionally it can be something important. For instance, in a patient with haemoptysis you may have forgotten to ask about breathlessness.

Ask about the following symptoms:

- general:
  - weight loss
  - anorexia
  - night sweats
  - itch
- cardiovascular:
  - oedema
  - palpitations
  - chest pain
  - breathlessness
  - orthopnoea
  - paroxysmal nocturnal dyspnoea
  - dizziness
  - syncope
- respiratory:
  - cough
  - phlegm
  - wheeze
  - haemoptysis
  - chest pain
  - breathlessness
- abdominal:
  - heartburn
  - nausea
  - vomiting
  - haematemesis
  - indigestion
  - abdominal pain
  - diarrhoea
  - constipation
  - rectal bleeding
  - jaundice
  - dysphagia
- genitourinary:
  - dysuria
  - haematuria
  - frequency
  - nocturia
  - incontinence
- locomotor:
  - joint pains
  - stiffness
- central nervous system:
  - dizziness
  - diplopia
  - hearing loss
  - weakness
  - syncope

- paraesthesia/numbness

You will learn more about these symptoms in the relevant chapters.

Your chances of working out the diagnosis depend on:

- your knowledge of possible causes of the symptom(s)
- your ability to ask relevant questions to establish which conditions are more likely
- the patient's ability to answer your questions
- whether the history is typical for the condition causing it
- whether the patient has a common condition.

Clearly, your knowledge of different symptoms and conditions will vary, as will the features of the conditions that individual patients demonstrate. Thus, your success in establishing a diagnosis will vary greatly from patient to patient. You will always do better with patients whose conditions you know about and who present with classical features.

Despite this, you can always approach each case in a systematic way evaluating duration, severity, precipitating factors, and so on even if you're not sure of the relevance of the answers. Cases 3.8, 3.9, 3.10, 3.11 and 3.12 offer advice when history taking becomes exasperating or difficult.

....

Tip

The aim is to get through the systematic questions quickly but without missing anything.

....

Tip

Before finishing your history it is always worth asking 'Is there anything else you think I might have missed out?' Just in case!

....

CASE 3.8

Problem. I thought I'd cracked history-taking yesterday when I saw a patient with chest pain. I got a really good history and diagnosed angina, which turned out to be correct. But today I was really disappointed. I didn't know where to start with my patient who complained of dizziness.

Discussion. When you start your clinical attachments, the doctors will likely send you off with the apparently casual instruction: 'Go and take a history from Mrs Smith'. This can lead you to expect history-taking to be easy. Don't become disheartened when you inevitably find it difficult.

CASE 3.9

Problem. I saw a patient with chest pain yesterday. I felt fairly confident that the pain was cardiac and knew that it was important to find out how long the pain lasted. But the patient couldn't tell me. Then I got criticized by the doctor for not finding out.

    Discussion. Although medical knowledge is clearly important in determining how good your history is, dogged perseverance is equally important. In this sort of situation, give the patient options: 'Does the pain last a few seconds, 5 minutes, half an hour, a few hours, a few days?' Usually the patient will get the idea and give you a rough duration.

    Note that, 'a long time' or 'not very long' means next to nothing.

CASE 3.10

Problem. My patient came in feeling sickly and vomiting but she has a multitude of other complaints and I realize I've ended up being side-tracked by these.

    Discussion. It is very easy to lose sight of your main objective—to establish the cause of the patient's most important complaints. Patients often like to dwell on the past and to be fair to them, we doctors like to ask them all sorts of questions not directly related to the presenting complaint. It's no wonder that sometimes we all miss the point.

    At all times, keep a focus on the patient's main problem.

Examination

Examining the patient often provides important information with regard to

- the diagnosis causing the patient's symptoms
- the severity of their condition.

In this chapter, it is not the intention to give an overview of examination technique. All the techniques used are different and are described individually throughout the book. Here the aim is to prepare students for the process by which they will be taught examination skills.

System routines

The most commonly used method of teaching and learning examination technique is visiting patients and examining a system such as the cardiovascular or respiratory system. These system routines have some advantages:

- They allow the teaching of examination techniques to be divided into logical, manageable chunks.
- They allow the doctor to assess a student's ability both to elicit a range of signs—normal and abnormal—and then to tie them together to make a rational diagnosis.

They are not without their faults See Case 3.13.

- They are somewhat artificial—for example, a patient suffering from breathlessness requires assessment of both the cardiovascular and respiratory systems.
- There is an unwritten rule that no history should be taken—mainly so that the patient does not spoil the learning opportunity by inadvertently giving you the answer. This is rather unrealistic. In their daily work, a doctor would be negligent not to take a history prior to examining the patient.

There are some general rules that apply when examining systems.

- **Be courteous at all times**. The patient is doing you a favour and you should treat them accordingly. Make all efforts not to hurt the patient—though it may be impossible to completely avoid inflicting pain, for example, when assessing for tenderness.
- **Introduce yourself**. Always introduce yourself to the patient and shake hands. Say something like 'Hello, I'm Leonard McCoy, a third-year medical student' (extend hand for shaking).
- **Ask permission**. You should ask the patient for permission to carry out whatever examination you are doing: 'Do you mind if I examine your heart and pulses?' Sometimes the patient will either not hear you or may misunderstand you. If so, do not just ignore this. Ask permission again until it is clearly given.
- **Left side of the bed**. Always examine from the left side of the bed (patient's right side). This is simply a matter of tradition. If the patient's bed is right up against the wall you will have to move it rather than examine from the right side of the bed (Fig. 3.1).
- **Correct positioning is essential**. For most systems the patient should be in a particular position, such as lying flat for the abdomen or sitting at 45° for the cardiovascular system. You should get the patient into the correct position before commencing examination.

CASE 3.11

Problem. I've been talking to an 81-year-old man for several minutes but I can't work out what he is complaining of. What might the problem be?

Discussion. The problem may simply be a lack of focus on either your or your patient's part. However, you must consider the alternative possibilities that the patient is confused or suffering from speech problems. As regards speech problems, the patient may be unable to express himself (expressive dysphasia) or unable to understand the spoken word (receptive dysphasia). Expressive and receptive dysphasia may coexist. They are caused by neurological disease, most commonly stroke. First, assess the patient's word-finding ability. Ask 'Do you mind if I ask you a few questions to test your speech?' Show the patient some common objects—such as a watch, a strap, a buckle, a tie, or a pen—and ask them to name them. Difficulty suggests expressive dysphasia. Next, assess the patient's ability to understand the spoken word. Ask him to follow some instructions. Start off simple: 'close your eyes, please . . . put out your tongue'. Move on to more complicated instructions: 'lift your right arm up in the air . . . touch your nose with your left index finger'. Resist the temptation to show the patient what you mean—the aim is to assess language abilities. Difficulty following instructions suggests receptive dysphasia.

If the patient's language skills seem reasonably preserved, move on to assess for confusion. It's best to use the same questions for all patients. Patients should be questioned about the following 10 items; their answers are used to calculate the abbreviated mental test score (see Hodkinson 1972):

- their age
- their birthday

- give the patient an address to remember and ask them to remember it for a few minutes ('42 West Street' is traditionally used)
- what year it is
- what month it is
- what time it is (to the nearest hour)
- where they are
- the date of the start of the First World War
- the monarch—ask 'Is there a king or queen in Britain these days?' and then check they've got the name right, 'What's her name?'
- count backwards from 20 to 1 (give the patient a start to show what you mean 20, 19, 18 . . .)
- ask if they can remember the address (42 West Street).

Give a mark for each correct answer. No half marks should be given for being close. The score out of 10 gives you some idea of the patient's ability to provide a relevant history.

A patient who scores 3 or less is very confused. History-taking is likely to be very difficult and you will need to rely on any third parties you can find such as relatives if available, nurses, the medical notes including the GP's letter, and casualty records.

If the patient scores between 4 and 6, much of the patient's history may be unreliable and you must bear this in mind, particularly if certain parts of the story seem difficult to put together. Again, it is wise to consult any third parties who may have knowledge of the patient's illness.

If the patient scores 7 or more, you should be able to obtain useful information from the patient. I suggest you quickly go through all the systematic questions for clues noting any positive symptoms. Once you have got all these, then go back over them in more detail.

Abbreviated Mental Test Score' reproduced from 'Evaluation of a Mental Test Score for Assessment of Mental Impairment in the Elderly' by H.M. Hodkinson in *Age and Ageing*, Vol. 1 1972, with permission from Oxford University Press.

If the patient misinterprets your instruction do not get flustered—just ask again! It is easy to feel you are wasting time but positioning is important. Get it right! (Sometimes, though, your patient will be confused or frail and unable to cooperate; then you will need to compromise.)

Tip
Learn how to adjust the headrest on hospital beds!

- **The general look**. There is much emphasis on taking a general look at the patient before examining them. The idea here is that students adopt a holistic approach to the patient and avoid tunnel vision, which it is all too easy to develop. Unfortunately many students waste time taking some kind of vague gormless look at the patient. The general look is the impression obtained prior to examining. So in the respiratory system the general look involves looking for cyanosis, tachypnoea, a sputum pot, and a nebulizer while you are introducing

CASE 3.12

Problem. I was taking a history from an 88-year-old woman who had recurrent falls. She seemed to be confused and drowsy and did not seem to be able to concentrate for long on what I was asking.

Discussion. This situation is worrying. Sometimes you are unable to get much or any history from a patient and you may have to go straight for examination. In this circumstance it is useful if you assess their conscious level using the Glasgow Coma Scale (GCS). This is a 15-point scale modified from the original devised by Teasdale and Jennett in 1974. It is based on the best responses a patient makes either spontaneously or incurred by verbal or painful stimuli. The responses that are observed are the best eye, verbal, and motor responses and a score is awarded for each of the three domains. See Table 3.2.

The lowest score is 3, representing deep unconsciousness, and the highest is 15, representing the normal conscious level. So if your patient is drifting in and out of sleep but opens their eyes when you call their name, they score 3. If they attempt to answer your questions but are clearly disorientated and confused they score 4. If they follow your commands to move a limb etc. they score 6. This can be represented as E3, V4, M6 with a total GCS of 13/15. Pain should only be applied if you are certain that the patient is not just sleeping, i.e. they do not respond to normal modes of arousal. This can be applied in the form of pressure to a fingernail bed or a sternal rub but this is best done only after you have seen experienced clinicians doing it.

Ideally you need an eyewitness account; if possible, ask a colleague to ring up a relative or next of kin while you examine the patient. With an elderly patient there could be a range of possibilities. She is exhibiting a delirium (a temporary state whereby the individual suffers with confusion, disorientation, and often visual hallucinations as a result of a disease process). This disease process could be an infection, medication toxicity, or a metabolic condition such as a diabetic coma. All these problems could lead to her falling. Your examination and investigations need to systematically rule out or identify what is causing the delirium. Another possibility that needs to be urgently investigated is the consequence of a fall and the possibility of head trauma. She has had recurrent falls and in one of these there could have been a blow to the head. In older people this can lead to a subdural haematoma (see Chapter 6) which is a medical emergency. Ultimately this patient may need a CT head scan to rule this possibility out.

---

yourself, positioning, and waiting for the patient to undress.

- **Always inspect**. No matter what you are examining, good inspection is essential. Students may worry about wasting time during inspection and rush it. Alternatively, they may look slow and ponderous because they are not sure what they are looking for.

- **The hands**. The cardiovascular, abdominal, and respiratory system examinations all begin with the hands. Get off to a good start by knowing what you are looking for in the hands when you start these examinations: cardiovascular—clubbing, splinters, and nicotine staining; respiratory—clubbing, cyanosis, flap, and nicotine staining; abdomen—leuconychia, palmar erythema, Dupuytren's, spiders, and flap.

- **Use easily identifiable signs to guide you with more difficult ones**. For instance, if you palpate an irregular pulse and a tapping apex beat and hear a loud first heart sound (all relatively easily identifiable signs of mitral stenosis), you should auscultate intently for the more difficult opening snap and mid-diastolic murmur of mitral stenosis. Think again about difficult signs you have found if easier signs contradict them. For instance, if you find chest expansion by palpation (a difficult sign) is reduced on one side but percussion and breath sounds (easier signs) are normal, you need to reconsider whether expansion really was reduced.

···

Tip

Experience normal as well as abnormal. Approach the fitter patients on your ward and ask for permission to examine them. Only by getting a feel for what is normal will you be able to identify abnormalities.

···

Tip

One step at a time. When practising unsupervised, take your time to examine for individual signs—pulse, jugular venous pressure, tendon reflexes, and so on. Once you are getting the hang of these, practise combining signs into systems examinations.

···

Table 3.2 Glasgow Coma Scale

Responses	Points
Eye opening	
Spontaneous—open with blinking	4
To verbal command or speech	3
To pain only, e.g. 'sternal rub'	2
No response	1
Verbal	
Speaks normally and is orientated	5
Confused conversation and attempts to answer questions	4
Inappropriate words	3
Incomprehensible grunts and groans	2
No response	1
Motor	
Obeys commands for movement	6
Purposeful movement to prevent painful stimulus	5
Withdraws in response to pain	4
Flexion in response to pain (decorticate posturing)	3
Extension response in response to pain (decerebrate posturing)	2
No response to any stimulus including pain	1

Reproduced from Teasdale G; and Jennett B. Assessment of coma and impaired consciousness: a practical scale; *The Lancet*; 1974; **2** (7872) 81–4, with permission from Elsevier.

Writing it down

Why write it down?

When working as a doctor, you should make a note in the patient's records every time you see them or receive some new medical information such as test results. This is for two main reasons.

- No matter how good your memory, you will not be able to remember the subtleties of the patient's clinical features in a week's time.

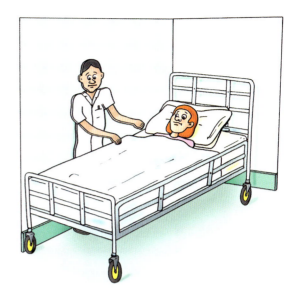

Figure 3.1 Examining from the left side.
© Paul Brown, Medical Illustrations Leeds.

The medical care of any individual patient is shared by a number of doctors who may all be called to attend the patient at different times and without the initial doctor being available. Thus, it is important that doctors record in the notes all their findings and what they believe to be the diagnosis so that the next doctor who sees the patient does not have to start from scratch.

It should not be forgotten that when patients make complaints or legal action against doctors, the written record in the notes carries great weight with the adjudicating parties.

How to write it down

- Write the history down in rough as you go along and fill in bits as the patient gives them. Structure your history in headings such as presenting complaint, history of presenting complaint, and so on (see Case 3.14), so people can follow your clerking more readily. Often it is best to let the patient have their say about the past medical history (which they may often dwell on more than the present problem) or social history before talking about the main complaint.

- There is no need to write down everything the patient says, as much will not be relevant to their medical condition.

- Often, when taking the history you will miss important facts about the main complaint. It is always wise to leave a space on your sheet of paper at the end of the history of

CASE 3.13

Problem. Yesterday, I examined for a collapsing pulse when examining the cardiovascular system and the consultant criticized me saying it was superfluous. So today, I omitted checking for a collapsing pulse from the examination and another doctor told me I was wrong. Can they not make their minds up?

Discussion. Often it is the order and content of the routines that are the source of most problems for the student. Every book and doctor suggests different orders—the student is never quite sure which is correct. For example, some doctors insist that you check for a collapsing pulse (see Chapter 4) every time you do the cardiovascular examination. Others feel this is wasting time unless you find other signs of aortic regurgitation—the condition that usually produces this sign.

Each system routine is an abbreviation of all the possible tests (there may be hundreds) that might be done for that system. There is no agreement on exactly how a particular routine should be abbreviated. Don't waste time scouring books for the perfect routine that will win honours with every examiner. What is really important is that you know **why** you are doing what you're doing. If you can justify why you have done something, no one can complain. In this book routines have been suggested for the various systems. While these routines may not satisfy all teachers all the time, they will always give you a strong pass.

the presenting complaint so that you can fill in additional features as you go along. You might not have thought of lung cancer as a cause of the haemoptysis but when you asked about smoking you realized it was a possibility. Indeed, many relevant parts of the history may not occur to you until you have examined the patient. It may be that in a woman with haemoptysis the diagnosis of lung carcinoma occurs to you only when you find clubbing and only then do you remember to ask about anorexia and weight loss.

Presentation

Why present?

As a doctor, you will never know everything about your patient's condition. Medical practice is a constant round of

CASE 3.14

Problem. When I look in the medical notes, there seem to be all sorts of abbreviations that I don't understand. What are they?

Discussion. Rightly or wrongly, it is traditional to use various abbreviations to demarcate different parts of the history:

PC	presenting complaint
HPC	history of presenting complaint
PMH	past medical history
DH	drug history
SH	social history
FH	family history
SQ	systematic questions
SE	systems enquiry

You will also notice various other abbreviations. Any abbreviations can cause confusion and in an ideal world should not be used but some are so commonplace that you should be familiar with them:

SOB	short of breath
PND	paroxysmal nocturnal dyspnoea
O/E—	on examination
°	no, as in °murmurs = no murmurs
a/c/j	anaemia/cyanosis/jaundice
club/ lymph	clubbing/lymphadenopathy
HS	heart sounds

od, once daily; bd, twice daily; tds, three times a day; qds, four times a day; nocte, at night.

second opinions. Whether as a junior doctor telling your consultant about a patient just admitted to hospital or a professor asking for ideas from a specialist in another field, you will need to be able to pass on the important facts about your patient to other health professionals. In your early years as a doctor, this is nearly always done by simple word of mouth. Thus presenting your findings on history and examination is an essential part of working as a medical student.

How to present

History

Your opening line is the presenting complaint. Give a brief statement describing the patient's name, age, occupation, and mode of admission and the main symptom and its duration. In one sentence, this gives an overview of the problem: 'Mrs Jones is a 62-year-old retired teacher, admitted via the GP with a 2-day history of coughing up blood.'

Next, you elaborate on the presenting complaint—this is the history of presenting complaint (HPC). The HPC is meant to be an account of how the patient's symptoms have developed over a period of time and should include anything you think relevant to the main complaint. 'Two days ago Mrs Jones coughed up around a teaspoonful of dark red blood. This has recurred six times over the last 2 days. It has never happened previously. She normally suffers from a cough with occasional white phlegm. She has felt breathless over the last 6 months and her exercise tolerance has fallen from being very active to 20 yards. She hardly ever gets out of the house now. She has no orthopnoea or wheeze and no chest pain—pleuritic or otherwise. She had a spontaneous deep vein thrombosis 4 years ago. She used to smoke 30 cigarettes a day until 2 years ago. She also admits to 2 stone weight loss and increasing anorexia over the last 6 months. She has been constipated in the last few weeks.'

Here, the following have been described:

- the main complaint—haemoptysis
- other respiratory symptoms and how they have affected the patient
- important negative symptoms such as no chest pain, or no wheeze
- risk factors for possible causes (previous deep vein thrombosis is a risk factor for pulmonary embolism and smoking is a risk factor for lung cancer)
- other symptoms that give a clue to the cause of the main complaint, i.e. weight loss and anorexia suggest lung cancer.

To do this, included are elements gleaned from the past medical history, the social history, and the systematic questions. This is an inexact science and different people will consider different features to be important. For example, here constipation has been mentioned in the HPC. This is probably not related to the main complaint and many people would not mention it here. But there is a chance that the constipation is related to hypercalcaemia secondary to a possible lung cancer—hence it can be considered reasonable to mention it in the HPC.

Having presented the HPC, run through the rest of the history: past medical, family, drug, and social histories and systematic questions. Mention negatives only where relevant. Keep it flowing. Use phrases such as 'In the past, Mrs Jones had a myocardial infarction . . . ' rather than 'Past medical history: Mrs Jones had a myocardial infarction . . . '.

It is said that you should always use the patient's own words—however, this may not be useful unless something very striking is said.

Examination

It is traditional that the student presents what they find on examination. Just as it is important to start the examination confidently, so it is essential to finish with a good presentation.

- **Leave presentation to the end**. It is often difficult to decide whether to present as you go along or to wait until you have finished. In general, I suggest that you save presentation until you have finished examining and have all the information together.
- **Use the end of your examination to think about your presentation**. As you come close to finishing examining the patient, focus your mind on what you have found, what you think the diagnosis is and what you're going to tell the examiner.
- **Do not wait to be asked**. Once you have finished examining, stand up straight and present your findings!
- **If you suspect a particular diagnosis, say so**. 'Mrs Smith has aortic stenosis as shown by a low volume pulse, a forceful but non-displaced apex beat, and an ejection systolic murmur radiating to the carotids. Jugular venous pressure was normal.'
- **Stick to your guns**. Teachers sometimes enjoy teasing students (they have got to get their fun somehow!) by querying findings even when they are correct. So it is important you stick to your guns if you are certain of your findings. You should back down only if you are shown something that convinces you that you are wrong.

Answering doctors' questions

After presenting a case to a doctor, they will often ask you questions. These tend to follow a couple of themes:

- questions relating to the cause of your individual findings;
- questions relating to how you might deal with a patient with a particular symptom, sign, or condition.

Clearly, a certain amount of factual knowledge is required but just as important is a good system. There are some useful general rules to help you make the most of your knowledge.

Questions relating to the cause of your individual findings

A reasonable classification and an emphasis on common pathology are more important than the exact answer. Thus, when asked 'What are the causes of a pleural effusion?' a student might give a very comprehensive list: 'pneumonia, pulmonary emboli, nephrotic syndrome, systemic lupus erythematosus, rheumatoid arthritis, cardiac failure, bronchial carcinoma, lymphoma, mesothelioma, subphrenic abscess, Meig's syndrome, and hepatic failure.' However, such an answer implies little understanding of how pleural effusion occurs and no understanding of which causes are more likely. However, such understanding is paramount when it comes to actually managing such a problem. A much more preferable, though less comprehensive, answer might be 'Pleural effusion may be classified into transudates and exudates. Transudates have protein content less than 30 g/litre and are often bilateral. Exudates have protein content more than 30 g/litre and tend to be unilateral. Transudates are commonly caused by cardiac failure. Exudates are commonly caused by lung malignancy, infection, or infarction.'

Questions relating to how you might deal with a patient with a particular symptom, sign, or condition

Here, the key is ABC (airway, breathing, circulation) for emergencies and history, examination, and investigation for non-emergencies. Thus, when asked 'How would you manage a patient having a myocardial infarction?' students are inclined to say 'thrombolysis . . . oxygen . . . analgesia . . . '. A better answer is 'First of all, I would ascertain that the patient was conscious and breathing, with a palpable pulse. Presuming this to be the case, I would immediately insert an intravenous cannula and give high-dose oxygen. Then, I would give intravenous analgesia (such as diamorphine) and an intravenous antiemetic (such as metoclopramide). Next, I would give aspirin, provided the patient was not allergic to it and intravenous streptokinase, provided there were no contraindications.'

When asked 'How would you manage a patient with jaundice?' students are inclined to say 'ultrasound scan . . . liver biopsy . . . blood count . . . '. A better answer is 'I would attempt to establish a diagnosis. First I would take a history—Does the patient drink alcohol? Have they had abdominal pain? Have they started new drugs recently? Next, I would examine the patient—Are the sclerae jaundiced? Are there signs of chronic liver disease? Is there an abdominal mass? Is there hepatomegaly? Then I would investigate—liver function tests, bilirubin, and ultrasound scan of abdomen.'

Reflection

We recommend that you get in the habit of reflecting on the cases you see and on your performance as this could be a way of introducing improvements into your working life. I tend to do an immediate reflection which is linked to the management of the case and a later one which tends to dwell on my performance although sometimes this distinction can be blurred.

Immediate reflection

I try to earmark 3–5 minutes of time where I allow my mind to think a little more laterally about a case. I have used this in examination situations and still use it in my

---

Key points

- The prime aim of history and examination is to arrive at a diagnosis or to produce possible differential diagnoses
- An awareness of communication skills is the precursor to developing a good bedside manner
- A good bedside manner allows patients to impart information to the doctor more easily and enhances patient satisfaction
- Knowledge, experience, and perseverance together are essential for a good history
- History-taking may produce a morass of information. In all this, it is absolutely vital you are clear what the patient's main problem is
- Always introduce yourself to the patient and gain consent for examination
- There is no perfect routine for examining systems
- Practise your presentation and note keeping as these are essential aspects of the communication process
- When managing emergencies, think 'airway, breathing, circulation'
- When managing non-emergencies, think 'history, examination, investigation'

working life. As well as the business focus of making a diagnosis, determining investigations and treatment, I will also ask myself what else could the diagnosis be, even if the diagnosis seems straightforward because the unexpected can always occur in medicine. I may try to consider what complications could arise and what I should do if the treatment does not work. I find this discipline allows me to be semi-prepared so that if these situations do arise I am already one step ahead. This may seem a little excessive but sometimes with the intensity of work you may never get another chance to think about the case until you are rung up about it (usually as you are trying to sort something else out).

Late reflection

This can be done as you are travelling home or when you are at home.

It is worth reflecting on some of your more difficult cases and evaluating what could have been done differently. Some things may be out of your control, e.g. patient's and colleague's personalities, overwhelming disease, etc. However, sometimes as you think you may realize that you could have approached a patient in a different way or that the processes you work with actually hinder rather than help you. These could be the first steps in making improvements to your performance or that of your department. Your observations could form the basis of a valuable departmental audit to inform your colleagues and even your hospital. Whatever you do, please do not spend too much time ruminating obsessively over every mishap you encounter or you will end up presenting your own history to a psychiatric colleague.

References and further reading

Hodkinson HM. Evaluation of a mental test score for assessment of mental impairment in the elderly. *Age and Ageing* 1972; **1**:233–7.

Teasdale G, Jennett B. Assessment of coma and impaired consciousness: a practical scale; *The Lancet* 1974; **2** (7872) 81–4.

Washer P. *Clinical communication skills*. Oxford University Press, Oxford, 2009.

4 Cardiovascular system

CHAPTER CONTENTS

Introduction

The cardiovascular system is made up of the heart and the vascular system—arteries, veins, and capillaries. It is of great importance because it is affected by several very common and potentially serious diseases, in particular coronary artery disease, which causes angina, myocardial infarction, and congestive cardiac failure. Furthermore, many non-cardiac diseases produce cardiovascular effects—fast heart rate, low blood pressure, and excess vascular fluid.

In this chapter, you will learn what questions to ask patients with cardiovascular diseases and how to examine the cardiovascular system. Two of the most important cardiovascular investigations are the chest radiograph and the electrocardiogram (ECG). The chest radiograph is discussed in Chapter 15.

Symptoms

Chest pain

Chest pain is a very common symptom. It is important for several reasons: it is common, it may signify unpredictable and dangerous diseases, and patients, understandably, can get very anxious about it. Thus, you should have a good idea how to assess it. Although discussed in this (cardiac) chapter, chest pain is not always due to heart problems. Common and important causes are given in Table 4.1 and this discussion is confined to these.

Stable angina, unstable angina, and myocardial infarction all occur mostly in patients with coronary artery disease. In coronary artery disease, lipid deposits (atherosclerosis) in the walls of the coronary arteries produce narrowing of the arteries. This results in reduced blood flow to and hence hypoxia of the heart—ischaemic heart disease. High-risk groups for coronary artery disease include smokers and ex-smokers and patients with hypertension (high blood pressure), diabetes mellitus, hyperlipidaemia (*high-per-lipid-ee-mia*), or a family history of coronary artery disease.

In stable angina, the narrowed coronary arteries can cope when the patient is resting, but when the heart needs more

Table 4.1 Common and important causes of chest pain

Common causes of chest pain	
Cardiac (coronary artery disease)	Stable angina, unstable angina, myocardial infarction, pericarditis
Respiratory	Infective pleurisy, pulmonary embolism
Upper gastrointestinal	Gastro-oesophageal reflux disease, oesophagitis
Musculoskeletal	Viral infection of muscles, muscle strain
No cause found	Very common
Other less common but important causes of chest pain	
Pneumothorax, aortic dissection	

oxygen, as when the patient is walking, it cannot get enough oxygen (this is called ischaemia [*iss-key-mia*]). This ischaemia is felt as pain (angina). Because the pain is predictable the angina is said to be 'stable'. Stable angina may also occur in other conditions such as anaemia (because of reduced oxygen-carrying capacity of the blood) or thyrotoxicosis (increased oxygen demand from the tissues). Unstable angina occurs when a thrombus forms on the diseased arterial wall but does not totally occlude (block) it. Such a thrombus may resolve or may go on to occlude the artery resulting in a myocardial infarction, hence 'unstable'. A myocardial infarction is usually due to a thrombus completely blocking off one of the coronary arteries so that an area of heart muscle actually dies—this is also known as a 'heart attack'.

Pericarditis (*perry-card-eye-tiss*) is an inflammation of the pericardial sac. It is commonly caused by viruses or occurs shortly after a myocardial infarction. Other rare causes are chronic kidney failure (uraemia), underactive thyroid (hypothyroidism), and tumours. Infective pleurisy (*ploor-issy*) occurs when pneumonia involves the pleural sac. Pulmonary embolism (*em-bo-liz-em*) is where a thrombus lodges in one of the pulmonary arteries often resulting in an area of pulmonary infarction. It commonly follows a thrombus in the leg veins (deep venous thrombosis) which detaches from the wall of the vein and reaches the pulmonary arteries via the right atrium and ventricle. Gastro-oesophageal reflux occurs when stomach acid refluxes back up from the stomach into the oesophagus. When this acid reflux causes mucosal damage, which is visible with an endoscope (camera test), this is called oesophagitis (*os-offer-jye-tiss*). Muscular pain may be due to muscular strain of the intercostal muscles or a viral infection of the muscles. Pneumothorax (*new-mo-thore-axe*) is where air gets into the pleural sac, usually resulting in a degree of lung collapse. Aortic dissection (*ay-or-tick dis-sex-shun* or *dye-sex-shun*) is where a tear occurs in the wall of the ascending aorta or the arch of the aorta. This split in the wall of the aorta may spread to involve other arteries.

What to ask

This can be broken down into three sections: (1) questions about the pain itself, (2) questions about potential causes of the pain, and (3) questions about other cardiac symptoms.

Questions about the pain itself

As with any symptom, your questions should initially be open, for example, 'tell me about this pain', but there are certain key facts you need to establish.

- Was this a single bout of pain or were there several?
- How long did it last? You need an answer in seconds, minutes, hours, and so on. 'Not long' or 'for ever' can mean anything. The patient may be reluctant to hazard what may be a misleading guess. Reassure them that you only need an estimate. If necessary (and it often is), give options: 'Did it last 2 seconds, 5 minutes, 1 hour, 5 hours . . . ?'
- Did anything bring it on? Ask specifically about exercise (such as walking) and breathing in. Pain worsened by inspiration is known as 'pleuritic pain'.
- Did anything make it better? Ask about the effect of rest and treatments. Ask specifically about whether the patient uses a tablet or spray under their tongue. This is glyceryl trinitrate (GTN); it usually relieves the pain of stable angina.

- Where was the pain? Ask specifically about radiation (spread) of the pain to arms, neck, and jaw.
- What kind (character) of pain was it? It may be easiest to give options: knife-like, tight, burning, heavy, or aching.

- Onset? Was this gradual with a slow build-up or was the worst pain at the start?

You may notice that severity does not come into this list of questions even though myocardial infarction pain is often very severe. However, severity is so subjective and so difficult to quantify it is really not worth spending too much time on. Furthermore, many myocardial infarction pains are quite mild—indeed, chest pain is absent in 25% of cases.

Questions about potential causes of the pain

The answers to your questions about the pain may lead you to suspect certain diagnoses. Ask about associated symptoms and risk factors relevant to the condition(s) you suspect. If these are present, it increases your index of suspicion.

Questions about other cardiac symptoms

You should always ask about the other cardiac symptoms—whether the patient also had breathlessness, palpitations, dizziness, or syncope around the time of the chest pain and also whether they have a tendency to ankle swelling.

Stable angina is suggested by a pain lasting 1–30 minutes brought on by exertion and relieved by rest or GTN within a minute or two. The pain is usually in the centre of the chest and may radiate into the arm(s), neck, or jaw. The character is usually tight or aching but it can be heavy or burning; knife-like pain is rare.

Associated symptoms are breathlessness, palpitations, and belching. Risk factors are family history, smoking, hypertension, diabetes mellitus, hyperlipidaemia, and previous cardiac history.

In unstable angina, two patterns are possible. The patient's stable angina deteriorates so that they have more severe angina after less and less exertion—with the character of the pain similar to their normal stable angina. This is also known as 'crescendo angina'. Alternatively, angina may occur at rest—often with the pain coming and going. It is unusual for pain to be present continuously for longer than half an hour but it may last several hours on and off. Associated symptoms are nausea and vomiting, belching, sweating, breathlessness, and palpitations. Risk factors are as for stable angina.

Tip

When taking a family history, younger relatives with cardiac histories are more important. If a younger sister died aged 40 from a myocardial infarction it is more significant than a grandfather dying aged 85. Ask about bypass operations. These are fairly hard second-hand evidence of cardiac disease.

The pain of myocardial infarction is traditionally said to be 'heavy and pressing' but it is just as often tight, burning, or aching. The pain quickly builds in severity and involves the central chest possibly radiating into the arm(s), neck, or jaw. The pain usually lasts for over half an hour. Associated symptoms are nausea and vomiting, belching, sweating, breathlessness, and palpitations. Risk factors are as for stable angina.

Tip

When a patient with chest pain is also suffering from nausea, vomiting, or sweatiness, these associated symptoms greatly increase the chance that the patient is having a myocardial infarction.

Tip

A very important risk factor in a patient with prolonged chest pain is a previous history suggestive of stable angina. Patients may tell you they have got angina. Do not just accept this. They may have been diagnosed by the plumber. You must go through the history and convince yourself.

Pericarditis produces a knife-like sternal pain, which is constant and may last for days. The pain may be eased by

sitting forward and worsened by breathing in. Associated symptoms depend on the cause. A viral cause is associated with influenza-like symptoms such as feeling hot and cold, sweating, musculoskeletal pains, a cough, phlegm, and a sore throat. If the cause is a recent myocardial infarct, associated symptoms will be as described previously.

Infective pleurisy typically produces a knife-like pain worsened by inspiration. It lasts for days and occurs anywhere on the chest especially the sides and back. Associated symptoms are a cough, phlegm, feeling hot and cold, sweating, and musculoskeletal pains. Risk factors are previous history, contacts, and history of chest disease.

Pulmonary embolism produces a sudden-onset knife-like pain, usually, but not always, worsened by inspiration and it may occur anywhere on the chest. The site may change from hour to hour. Duration may be minutes to days. Associated symptoms are breathlessness, haemoptysis (*hemop-ta-sis*), and leg swelling (suggestive of deep venous thrombosis in the leg). Risk factors are recent immobility or operation, previous history of pulmonary embolism, or deep venous thrombosis.

Tip

The patient may have more than one type of chest pain. Try to separate them out and analyse them individually.

Gastro-oesophageal reflux disease and oesophagitis tend to result in a pain that is retrosternal and burning, that is made worse by citrus fruits and spicy foods and sometimes by bending over, and that is eased by milk and antacids. It may last from a few minutes to several hours. It tends to be recurrent. It may occasionally be relieved by GTN, where this reduces oesophageal spasm through its muscle-relaxant properties. Associated symptoms are nausea, vomiting, and abdominal pain. Risk factors are smoking and alcohol consumption. See Case 4.1 to see how gastric pain and cardiac pain can be further confused.

Muscular pain tends to be knife-like, it may occur anywhere on the chest, and it may be increased by movement but this is very variable. It may come and go or it may last weeks. A risk factor is recent unusual physical activity.

Pneumothorax produces a sharp chest pain, which is worse on inspiration and usually localized to one area. Breathlessness is an associated symptom. Risk factors are previous pneumothorax and recent chest injury. See Cases 4.2 and 4.3 for very ill patients with chest pain.

Sometimes, an exact diagnosis of the cause of the chest pain is impossible. The history can never be 100%

CASE 4.1

Problem. Your patient is a 73-year-old woman. She has burning chest pain but somehow seems more unwell than you might expect for someone with heartburn or oesophagitis. Why might this be?

Discussion. The patient may be having a myocardial infarction! It is often said that angina pain is tight, myocardial infarct pain is heavy, and oesophageal pain is burning. This is true: 95% of burning chest pain is oesophageal and only 5% is cardiac. However, cardiac chest pain may be burning or aching so that perhaps 30% of patients with myocardial infarction describe their pain as burning.

CASE 4.2

Problem. You're seeing a 50-year-old man with chest pain just arrived in the emergency department. He doesn't look well, yet after several minutes you've only got the answers to a couple of questions and you're starting to panic.

Discussion. Your approach to the history should alter according to the situation. In this emergency situation, you must combine your history with examination (pulse and blood pressure especially), arranging an ECG, inserting an intravenous cannula (a little plastic tube inserted into the vein with help from a needle that allows treatment to be given), and giving treatment (oxygen, analgesia, aspirin, and thrombolytic drugs). Such a scenario makes precise detail in the history both less important and more difficult to achieve. The key questions should address (1) duration and character of the pain; (2) effect of inspiration; (3) presence of nausea and sweating; (4) smoking, diabetes, and hypertension; and (5) previous cardiac history. If you believe the patient is having a myocardial infarction, you will need to ask about possible reasons where treatment with aspirin or thrombolysis (*throm-bo-lie-sis or throm-bol-iss-iss*) might be dangerous—such as a recent gastrointestinal bleed. More commonly, the student will see the patient either a few days after this event or when they are describing less severe, more intermittent symptoms not currently present. Here a more comprehensive history is both achievable and expected.

CASE 4.3

Problem. Your patient is a 40-year-old man. He looks very unwell and is complaining of severe chest pain together with pain between the shoulder blades, yet the ECG shows no sign of myocardial infarction. Why might this be?

Discussion. Consider aortic dissection. This is where a tear occurs in the wall of the aorta. This often produces a sudden searing pain in the chest and between the shoulder blades. The pain of dissection is worst at onset as opposed to the more gradual build-up of pain in myocardial infarction. This split in the wall of the aorta may spread to involve other arteries. In around half of all cases, the left subclavian artery is involved but not the right—resulting in a reduced left radial pulse. The dissection may occasionally involve the aortic valve producing signs of aortic regurgitation (10%) and there may be evidence of a left pleural effusion (3%). Risk factors include hypertension, pregnancy, and Marfan's syndrome. In around 1% of cases, the dissection may involve the coronary arteries—producing signs of a myocardial infarction. This is important because thrombolysis (clot busting), which is used in the treatment of myocardial infarction, is dangerous in aortic dissection, where it makes the bleeding worse. **Thus, all patients with an apparent myocardial infarction should have their pulses compared before giving thrombolysis.**

conclusive. This is even more the case if the patient is vague or through anxiety exaggerates their symptoms (usually by lengthening them) so making them sound less cardiac. Therefore, doctors often confine themselves to confirming or excluding the more serious causes, such as cardiac ischaemia or infarction and pulmonary embolism or more treatable causes, such as infective pleurisy. This limited aim is not often explained well to the patient who can be understandably annoyed or worried to be sent home from hospital with no diagnosis for a chest pain deemed severe enough to require admission.

Breathlessness

Like chest pain, breathlessness (dyspnoea) (*dis-knee-a*) is a very common symptom. You should be confident in

Key points

- Chest pain has multiple causes, not just cardiac causes.
- The most important causes are cardiac causes, pulmonary embolism, and aortic dissection.
- Your approach to taking a chest pain history depends greatly on the urgency of the situation.
- Various features in the history of chest pain point to or away from certain diagnoses but no single feature or group of features can exclude or conclusively diagnose any chest pain.
- There are two main types of question: those about the pain itself and those about potential causes of the pain.
- Onset, duration, site, character, precipitating factors, and relieving factors are the most important features when asking about the pain itself.

- Duration is useful in deciding whether a particular cardiac pain represents angina or myocardial infarction.
- Pain lasting just a few seconds or continuously for longer than 24 hours is rarely cardiac.
- Cardiac pain is usually central, not left sided.
- Relief by rest or GTN and aggravation by exertion are probably the best ways of diagnosing stable angina.
- The character of myocardial infarction pain is quite non-specific.
- Associated symptoms such as sweating or nausea are important in deciding how likely it is for prolonged chest pain to be due to a myocardial infarction.

Table 4.2 Common and important causes of breathlessness

Cardiac	Cardiac failure which may be acute (associated with angina or myocardial infarction) or chronic; angina equivalent
Respiratory	Asthma, pneumothorax, pneumonia, bronchitis, bronchiectasis (*bron-key-eck-ta-sis*), COPD, pulmonary fibrosis, pulmonary embolism
Non-cardiorespiratory	Anaemia, hyperventilation including diabetic ketoacidosis, overweight

Tip

Be careful when using the terms 'heart failure' or 'cardiac failure' to patients. Take time to explain that the heart has not ground to a complete halt but rather it is not working as well as it should.

- Angina equivalent is caused by coronary artery disease in the same way as angina, the difference being that the primary symptom is breathlessness rather than pain.
- Asthma is where the bronchial airways are obstructed (usually reversible to some extent).
- For pneumothorax, see 'Respiratory diseases and investiagtions' and Fig. 15.32.
- Inflammation of the lungs is usually caused by infection. It may affect the bronchi alone (bronchitis) or may also affect the alveoli (pneumonia). In bronchiectasis, the primary problem is dilated bronchi; these are prone to infection.
- Chronic obstructive pulmonary disease (COPD) occurs when there is longstanding airways obstruction, which is mostly irreversible. It may be a sequela (*see-quill-a*) of either chronic bronchitis, emphysema (*em-fi-seem-a*), or both (most common). Chronic bronchitis is defined as sputum production for most days in 3 months of 2 successive years. Emphysema is defined on a histological basis as dilated air spaces but clinically is a disease of smokers associated with minimal previous sputum production.

evaluating patients with breathlessness. Common and important causes are listed in Table 4.2 and this discussion is confined to these. Breathlessness is a symptom of many conditions, not just cardiac conditions. It could equally be discussed under a respiratory system heading.

- Cardiac failure is where the heart is unable to pump enough blood to meet the demands of the body tissues. Fluid accumulates throughout the body. In the lungs, this results in pulmonary congestion and oedema (*ee-dee-ma*) so causing breathlessness.

- Patients with pulmonary fibrosis have widespread fibrosis of the lungs. It may be idiopathic (*id-ee-owe-path-ick*) or result from autoimmune disease, dust exposure (asbestos or coal), or drugs (such as amiodarone (*am-ee-owe-da-roan*)).
- For pulmonary embolism, see Figs. 15.33 and 15.34.
- Anaemia is where a patient's haemoglobin level is low. This may result in 'high-output' cardiac failure.
- Hyperventilation is where breathing is excessive, more than is necessary to maintain oxygen and carbon dioxide levels. It is usually a reaction to anxiety where hyperventilation results in a respiratory alkalosis but occasionally it is a response to metabolic acidosis as in renal failure or diabetic ketoacidosis (*key-toe-acid-owe-sis*).

What to ask

As with chest pain, your approach to the history depends greatly on the situation. If your patient has just come through the emergyency department doors and is in distress, your history need not be so comprehensive and you will need to combine it with examination (especially pulse, blood pressure, respiratory rate, chest, and temperature), inserting an intravenous cannula, arranging or doing tests (such as arterial blood gases, chest radiograph, ECG, and blood count), and giving treatment (oxygen, diuretic, steroids, and bronchodilator depending on the cause). The questions can be broken down into three sections: (1) questions about the breathlessness itself, (2) questions about other cardiac and respiratory symptoms, and (3) questions about potential causes of the breathlessness. See Cases 4.4 and 4.5 for an approach to the very breathless patient.

Questions about the breathlessness itself

Your questions should initially be open, for example, 'tell me about this breathlessness', but there are certain key facts you need to establish.

- When did the breathlessness start? Are we talking about a single bout or recurrent bouts of breathlessness (acute) or has the breathlessness been present for some time (months or years)?—chronic? If the latter, has there been a recent deterioration?—acute-on-chronic?
- How bad is it? How disabling is it? What can the patient not do that they used to be able to do? This may be obvious, the patient may be breathless at rest but if not,

it is best to ask how much exercise they can do. Get a specific answer—a flight of stairs, 10 yards, 100 yards, a mile—or their metric equivalents. Patients may find this difficult. Ask if they get out much. If so, do they walk to or around the shops, to the pub, and so on? Try to get a comparison with normal, say a few months ago.

- Do they get breathless lying flat (orthopnoea) (*or-thop-knee-a*)? If so, do they regularly prop themselves up in bed and how many pillows do they use? Orthopnoea suggests a more severe degree of breathlessness. It is more typical of cardiac breathlessness but also occurs in patients with respiratory causes.
- Does the patient suffer from paroxysmal nocturnal dyspnoea? This is where the patient wakes up at night feeling breathless. There may or may not be a story of the patient either sitting over the side, getting out of bed, or putting their head out of the window for a breath. Again, this is more suggestive of cardiac breathlessness but by no means an absolute rule.
- What treatment have they previously had for their breathlessness and did it work?

Questions about other cardiac and respiratory symptoms

Ask about chest pain, palpitations, dizziness or syncope, and ankle swelling. Also ask about the main respiratory symptoms—cough, phlegm, haemoptysis, and wheeze.

Questions about potential causes of the breathlessness

Hopefully, your previous questions will have given you some idea of what the diagnosis is, so obtain further information about what you think are the likely causes. Ask about associated symptoms and risk factors relevant to the condition(s) you suspect.

The answers to these questions should give you some idea of the cause. It is simplest to divide causes into acute, chronic, and acute-on-chronic.

Acute

- **Angina equivalent**. Breathing difficulties lasting 1–30 minutes brought on by exertion and relieved by rest or GTN within a minute or two. Associated symptoms are palpitations and belching. Risk factors are a family history, smoking, hypertension, diabetes mellitus, and hyperlipidaemia.
- **Stable angina with cardiac failure**. Breathlessness and chest pain lasting 1–30 minutes brought on by exertion and relieved by rest or GTN within

a minute or two. The pain is usually in the centre of the chest and may radiate into the arm(s), neck, or jaw. The pain is usually tight or aching but can be heavy or burning; knife-like pain is rare. Associated symptoms are palpitations and belching. Risk factors are as for angina equivalent.

- **Myocardial infarction with cardiac failure**. Sudden-onset acute breathlessness at rest, which may be severe. Associated symptoms are chest pain, nausea and vomiting, belching, sweating, and palpitations. Risk factors are as for angina equivalent.
- **Asthma**. Intermittent bouts of breathlessness, especially in young people, which may be severe. It responds to bronchodilators in either inhaler or nebulizer form. Associated symptoms are wheeze and a dry cough. Risk factors are a history of allergy and a family history.
- **Pneumothorax**. Sudden-onset breathlessness in (often young) people who were usually not breathless previously. An associated symptom is pleuritic chest pain. A risk factor is a history of chest disease.
- **Pneumonia and bronchitis**. Gradual-onset breathlessness but of short duration (days). Associated symptoms are a cough, phlegm, feeling hot and cold, and pleuritic chest pain. Risk factors are a previous history, contact with patients with a similar illness, and a history of chest disease.
- **Pulmonary embolism**. Sudden-onset breathlessness, which may be severe. May be eased by lying flat (see Case 4.6). Associated symptoms are pleuritic chest pain, breathlessness, haemoptysis, and leg swelling suggesting deep venous thrombosis. Risk factors are recent immobility or operation and a previous history of pulmonary embolism or deep venous thrombosis.
- **Hyperventilation**. Sudden-onset breathlessness. An associated symptom is anxiety. Risk factors are uncontrolled diabetes, acute renal failure, and anxiety.

Chronic

- **Cardiac failure**. Chronic breathlessness with orthopnoea, with or without paroxysmal nocturnal dyspnoea; responds to diuretics. An associated symptom is ankle swelling. Risk factors are ischaemic heart disease (myocardial infarction or angina), smoking, hypertension, and valvular heart disease.
- **COPD**. Long history of breathlessness with orthopnoea; may respond to bronchodilators, antibiotics, or steroids. Associated symptoms are a cough, phlegm, and wheeze. A risk factor is smoking.

- **Bronchiectasis**. Long history of breathlessness associated with producing large amounts of sputum. Associated symptoms are a cough and copious phlegm. Risk factors are childhood measles or whooping cough and smoking.
- **Pulmonary fibrosis**. Long history of breathlessness with orthopnoea. An associated symptom is a cough. Risk factors are smoking, coal mining, asbestos exposure, and amiodarone treatment.
- **Pulmonary embolism**. Occasionally multiple pulmonary emboli may cause chronic breathlessness. See previous list for associated symptoms and risk factors.
- **Anaemia**. Chronic breathlessness. An associated symptom is fatigue. Risk factors are chronic bleeding—overt or occult. Ask specifically about use of non-steroidal anti-inflammatory drugs.
- **Hyperventilation**. Gradual-onset breathlessness, especially in renal failure. An associated symptom is the tingling of fingers and toes. Risk factors are diabetes and kidney failure.

Acute-on-chronic

All the acute causes commonly occur in patients with chronic diseases causing breathlessness. Thus, in many patients with breathlessness the onset is 'acute-on-chronic'. Acute cardiac problems tend to occur in patients with chronic cardiac disease and acute respiratory problems tend to occur in patients with chronic respiratory disease. See Case 4.7.

Ankle or leg swelling

See also the text discussing examination of ankle oedema and examination of sacral oedema. Patients may

> **CASE 4.4**
>
> **Problem.** My patient is very breathless, so much so he can't answer my questions. What should I do?
>
> **Discussion.** Hopefully, the patient has a companion who can help with history. If not, use the history the patient can give you along with clues from any medication he may have with him and examination findings to come to a diagnosis. You may have to give treatments such as nebulizers and diuretics without being entirely sure they are appropriate. Do not delay.

CASE 4.5

Problem. A 23-year-old man arrives in the emergency department. He is so breathless he cannot speak; his friend tells you he has asthma. But when you listen to his chest with the stethoscope, he seems to be getting good amounts of air into and out of his lungs. What might be going on? What sign and which test will help you to decide?

Discussion. The patient may be hyperventilating. It is not surprising that some asthmatic patients may misinterpret their own symptoms and work themselves into a hyperventilation frenzy. Beware of making this diagnosis lightly: your patient's anxiety may be well founded and they could be having a severe asthmatic attack. The patient's heart rate may be helpful. If the patient's heart rate is above 120 beats/min, his symptoms are unlikely to just be caused by anxiety. Never diagnose hyperventilation without checking arterial blood gases. If Po_2 is greater than 10.6 kPa and pH is greater than 7.45, hyperventilation is likely. A low Pco_2 may occur in both asthma and hyperventilation.

CASE 4.6

Problem. I am a nurse practitioner and I have just seen a 75-year-old man who had a hip operation 10 days ago. He has a past history of cardiac failure. All was going well until today when he developed a sudden onset of breathlessness eased by lying flat. What might be happening?

Discussion. Although the patient has had cardiac failure in the past you should be thinking of pulmonary embolism. The breathlessness of pulmonary embolism may be unusual because sometimes it is eased by lying flat, which increases right ventricular filling and hence cardiac output. In this patient, the postoperative timing is typical of a pulmonary embolism. Ask about leg swelling (suggesting deep venous thrombosis).

CASE 4.7

Problem. Your patient is an 80-year-old man complaining of severe breathlessness on a background of chronic breathlessness. How do you decide whether he has chronic cardiac failure or chronic respiratory disease?

Discussion. This is a common problem and nowhere near as simple as it might sound. Ask about indicators of heart disease such as chest pain and previous history of angina or myocardial infarction. Ask about indicators of respiratory disease such as a cough and phlegm along with a previous history of chest disease. Oedema points slightly towards cardiac failure. Wheeze points slightly towards chest disease. Both groups tend to be smokers. Ask about medications. If the patient is mostly on bronchodilators, respiratory causes are more likely while diuretic therapy suggests cardiac failure. Physical examination and the chest radiograph are helpful. Often, though, the conditions may coexist or it is difficult to decide which condition is predominant—as demonstrated by the high number of patients on both types of treatment.

Key points

- Try to decide if breathlessness is acute, chronic, or acute-on-chronic.
- Get an idea of how disabling the breathlessness is.
- Orthopnoea and paroxysmal nocturnal dyspnoea are said to suggest cardiac causes but may also occur in respiratory causes.
- Response to diuretics suggests a cardiac cause.

the cause clear. However, when build-up of fluid occurs within the tissues, this can be quite rapid and hence noticeable to the patient.

Classification of peripheral oedema

Peripheral oedema may be generalized or localized (see Table 4.3). Generalized oedema is caused by fluid overload or hypoproteinaemia (where a reduction in plasma osmotic pressure causes leakage of fluid across the capillaries). In generalized oedema, gravity dictates where the fluid collects so in a normally ambulant patient, fluid tends to initially

complain of leg or ankle swelling. Leg or ankle swelling may be caused either by fat or by abnormal accumulation of fluid within the subcutaneous tissues (peripheral oedema). Patients do not tend to complain of leg swelling when the cause is fat as the onset is so gradual and

Table 4.3 Causes of peripheral oedema

Generalized (usually results in bilateral oedema)	
Fluid overload	Heart failure, oliguric renal failure, iatrogenic (*eye-at-roe-jen-ick*)[a]
Hypoproteinaemia	Gastrointestinal malabsorption, protein malnutrition, liver cirrhosis (*si-roe-sis*), nephrotic (*nef-rot-ick*) syndrome
Localized (often results in unilateral oedema)	
Chronic venous insufficiency (varicose veins)	Usually bilateral
Venous obstruction	Venous thrombosis, tumour
Increased capillary permeability	Injury, infection
Lymphatic obstruction	Lymphoedema (Milroy's[b] congenital hypoplasia of lymphatic vessels, tumour)
Postural	Standing for long periods

[a] Iatrogenic: caused by a doctor's intervention.
[b] William Forsyth Milroy (1855–1942), American physician.

collect around the ankles. The most common serious cause of ankle swelling is the generalized oedema of cardiac failure. However, ankle oedema is caused by many other conditions (Table 4.3), the most common being postural oedema exacerbated by incompetent venous valves. So be careful before diagnosing cardiac failure on the basis of ankle swelling alone.

What to ask

If the patient has bilateral ankle swelling, evaluate for a cardiac cause. Ask about chest pain, breathlessness,

Key points
- Bilateral ankle swelling is a feature of heart failure but also occurs in many other situations.
- Ask about other cardiac history and varicose veins.

previous angina, myocardial infarction, and smoking. Remember also to ask about varicose veins.

Palpitations

What are they?

Palpitations are an awareness of the patient's own heart beating.

What are they due to?

Palpitations may be due to sinus tachycardia (*tacky-card-ia*), ectopic beats (extrasystoles) (*extra-sis-toe-lees*), or arrhythmias (*ay-rith-me-as*).

Palpitations due to sinus tachycardia are a normal response to exercise and may occur in various conditions, particularly infections and stress. Ectopic beats are cardiac beats that do not originate from the sinoatrial (*sigh-no-ay-tree-al*) node. They are often one-off abnormal beats of minimal significance but may sometimes be caused by coronary ischaemia. Arrhythmias are abnormal heart rhythms lasting for more than a few beats. They are usually caused by electrical problems in the heart. Sometimes, the primary problem may be ischaemia, which damages the electrical pathways. They may be worsened by electrolyte imbalance.

You will come across palpitations in three main situations.

1 The patient has noticed occasional 'missed beats'. This is rarely important and is usually due to ectopic beats.

2 The palpitations are a minor part of a more serious situation such as when the patient is suffering a myocardial infarction.

3 The patient is suffering from intermittent bouts of prolonged palpitations, which are their main symptom.

It is this third scenario that I will now discuss. Common causes are shown in Table 4.4.

When taking a history you are aiming to decide the following.

What does the patient mean by palpitations

Some patients will use the term 'palpitations' in an apparently knowledgeable way but when you ask them you will find they are talking about a chest pain, indigestion, or even a shaking feeling. Ask 'Do you get a feeling of your heart beating in your chest?'

Table 4.4 Common causes of palpitations

Common types of palpitations	Features
Sinus tachycardia	Fast, regular, gradual onset and end
Atrial arrhythmias	
Atrial tachycardia	Fast, regular, abrupt onset and end
Supraventricular tachycardia	Fast, regular, abrupt onset and end
Atrial fibrillation	Fast, irregular, abrupt onset and end
Atrial flutter	Fast, regular or irregular, abrupt onset and end
Ventricular arrhythmias	
Ventricular tachycardia	Fast, regular, abrupt onset and end, tendency to black out
Multiple ectopic beats	
Atrial or ventricular	Slow, irregular

CASE 4.8

Problem. My patient complains of palpitations. Could this be due to her high coffee intake?

Discussion. Contrary to popular opinion, caffeine rarely causes a sinus tachycardia. In fact, most of the evidence points to a bradycardia. Caffeine does cause a sensation of tremulousness and this can be mistaken for palpitations.

Are the palpitations caused by sinus tachycardia or an arrhythmia? If it is an arrhythmia, is it ventricular tachycardia or atrial fibrillation or is it due to ischaemia?

Find out what the palpitations are like.

- Are the beats fast, slow, regular, or irregular?

Tip
Patients may find it difficult to describe the speed and regularity of palpitations. Ask them to tap the rhythm out on a desk or table. If necessary, give them a demonstration of what you mean.

- Was the onset of the palpitations sudden or gradual (see Table 4.4)?
- Ask about blackouts.
- Was there any chest pain? Did the pain precede the palpitations?
- Ask about potentially avoidable precipitating factors: exercise, stress, and alcohol. These can all cause sinus tachycardias or precipitate other arrhythmias.

A gradual onset suggests sinus tachycardia whereas an abrupt onset suggests an arrhythmia. However, patients often find it difficult to decide how suddenly the palpitations started. Irregular palpitations suggest atrial fibrillation (*fib-rill-ay-shun*). Ventricular tachycardia is important as it may be life threatening. Usually it results in a markedly reduced cardiac output so palpitations are not felt and blackout occurs instead. Sometimes, though, the patient may feel palpitations and there may be associated blackouts (dizziness may be associated with any type of palpitation). Arrhythmias may result in reduced cardiac output and so patients may develop cardiac ischaemia with angina. However, sometimes ischaemia is actually the primary problem. If the pain precedes the palpitations, then ischaemia is likely to be the primary problem. If the palpitations precede the pain, ischaemia is likely to be secondary. It has to be said that patients do not always find this differentiation easy.

How troublesome the palpitations are to the patient

Apart from ventricular tachycardia, atrial fibrillation, and arrhythmias due to ischaemia, most other types of arrhythmia are quite benign, more troublesome than life threatening (see Case 4.8). You should find out how much trouble they cause. Ask how often the palpitations happen, how long they last, and whether they stop the patient doing things they would otherwise like to?

Syncope

Syncope is discussed in Chapter 6.

The importance of examining the cardiovascular system

The clinical approach to examining the cardiovascular system has changed greatly in recent decades. First, rheumatic (*room-attic*) heart disease is now much rarer

Key points

- Make sure you and the patient are on the same wavelength when using the word 'palpitations'.
- Ask about speed of onset, rate, regularity, chest pain, blackouts, precipitants, and effects on quality of life.
- Gradual onset and ending suggests sinus tachycardia.
- Irregularity suggests atrial fibrillation.
- When palpitations are accompanied by blackouts, think about ventricular tachycardia.
- If chest pain occurs find out whether it precedes or follows the palpitations.

in Western countries. Rheumatic heart disease causes valvular heart disease, which in the past caused considerable illness and death in relatively young people. These valvular lesions produced specific physical signs so that, with good technique, the physician could make diagnoses using clinical examination. Valvular heart disease has not gone completely but it is rarer, especially the distinctive lesions produced by rheumatic heart disease. Second, the development of new investigations has meant that most, if not all, examination techniques can be equalled by 'tests'. For example, a cardiac monitor can be used to assess pulse rate and rhythm, a chest radiograph (Chapter 15) can be used to check for heart failure, and an echocardiogram (echo) can be used to evaluate heart valves.

Despite these changes, skill in cardiovascular system examination remains extremely important. Why? The ability to examine pulse rate and rhythm, blood pressure, jugular venous pressure, and basal lung crackles is absolutely essential in managing acutely unwell patients, while clinical assessment of valvular lesions remains an important part of medical work. And remember you may not always have access to technology when you really need it.

The key to examining the cardiovascular system is practice. By getting a feel for normality you can quickly tell when something is not quite right. As elsewhere in the book, a difficulty factor (DF) has been assigned to each sign. This gives some general idea of how difficult a test is and how much practice is needed. Examining the cardiovascular system may seem daunting initially but with practice becomes quite easy.

Many cardiac lesions produce signs that are best described in relation to the 'cardiac cycle', which will be briefly described (see Fig. 4.1). Do not waste time trying to learn this off by heart now. Use it as a reference for the rest of the chapter. The cardiac cycle can be divided into ventricular systole (*sis-toe-ly*) (contraction) and diastole

(*die-ass-toe-ly*) (relaxation). At the start of diastole, all heart valves (mitral, tricuspid (*try-cuss-pid*), aortic, and pulmonary) are closed. This is the period of isovolumetric (*ice-so-vol-you-metric*) relaxation. 'Isovolumetric' means that the volume of blood in the ventricles remains constant. Next, the mitral and tricuspid valves open and blood pours from the atria into the relaxed ventricles. Initially, this flow of blood is fast (period of rapid ventricular filling), then it slows down (period of reduced ventricular filling). Then the atria contract to force a further small bolus of blood into the ventricles (atrial systole). Now, the ventricles begin to contract and the mitral and tricuspid valves are forced shut. There is a short period of isovolumetric contraction before the aortic and pulmonary valves are forced open. Blood is now ejected from the ventricles. Initially this is fast (period of rapid ventricular ejection), then it slows down (period of reduced ejection). As the contraction ends, the aortic and pulmonary valves shut again and diastole begins with the period of isovolumetric relaxation.

As with all systems, a routine has been used to discuss the various physical signs. This has the advantage of simulating how students are taught and examined. Like all routines, it is an abbreviation of all the signs you might possibly look for. Routines are not perfect; for instance, rare tests such as inspection for splinter haemorrhages are included in this cardiovascular system routine while important tests such as blood pressure measurement are excluded.

Cardiovascular system examination summary

This summary contains many terms that you will not understand on first reading. These terms are explained in the next section 'Cardiovascular examination in detail'.

1 Introduce yourself to the patient and ask for permission to examine.

2 Wash your hands.

3 Ask the patient to get on to the bed (if not already on the bed). You may need to ask for help!

4 Ask the patient to remove all garments covering chest and arms. For female patients, offer to cover the chest with a sheet or towel.

Key point

- With practice, examining the cardiovascular system becomes easy.

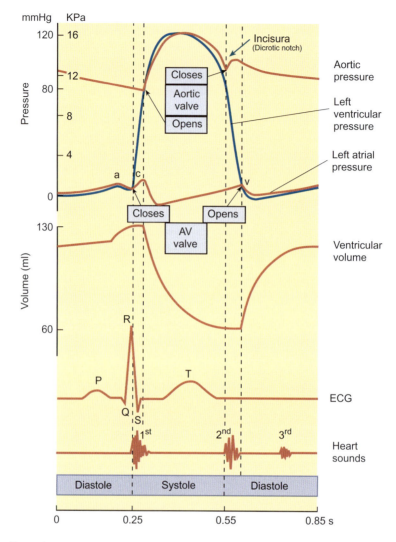

Figure 4.1 The cardiac cycle.

Reproduced by permission of Oxford University Press from Fig. 15.11 (p. 286), *Human Physiology: The Basis of Medicine*, by G. Pocock and C. Richards (1999).

5 Arrange the patient so that their chest is at 45°.

6 While doing 1–4, be having a 'general look'. Is the patient distressed, for example?

7 Inspect both hands and fingernails for splinter haemorrhages (DF 5/10), clubbing (DF 8/10), and tar staining (DF 1/10).

8 Palpate right radial pulse for pulse rate (DF 3/10) and rhythm (DF 6/10). Palpate right and left radial pulses together and compare (DF 8/10). Check for collapsing pulse (DF 6/10).

9 Inspect face for malar (*may-lar*) flush (DF 7/10) and xanthelasmata (*zan-the-laz-matta*) (DF 2/10). Inspect eyes for corneal arcus (*ark-us*) (DF 2/10). Inspect conjunctivae for anaemia (DF 9/10). Inspect tongue for cyanosis (*sigh-an-owe-sis*) (DF 9/10).

10 Palpate right carotid pulse for pulse character (DF 8/10).

11 Inspect right internal jugular vein for jugular venous pressure (DF 9/10). Check for hepatojugular reflux (DF 8/10).

12 Take sheet off chest (female patients). Inspect prae-cordium (*pre-cord-ee-yum*) in general and specifically for scars, cardiac impulse, and any other abnormal pulsations (DF 5/10).

13 Palpate at apex for apex beat, assessing position and character (DF 9/10). Palpate for left parasternal impulse (DF 9/10) and aortic and pulmonary thrills (DF 6/10).

14 Auscultate (DF 8/10)—while palpating carotid pulse to time any murmur. Listen with:

- diaphragm at mitral area (move to axilla if systolic murmur heard)
- bell at apex with patient lying on their left side
- bell at tricuspid area (normal patient position)
- diaphragm at tricuspid area
- diaphragm at pulmonary area
- diaphragm at aortic area
- diaphragm at right, then left carotid
- diaphragm over lower left sternal edge with patient sat forward with breath held in expiration
- diaphragm to auscultate over lung bases.

15 Palpate for ankle or shin oedema over lower anterior tibia (DF 3/10).

16 Consider looking for other signs, such as radiofemoral delay and pulsatile liver.

17 Wash your hands.

18 Now say 'I would like to check the blood pressure'. Pause briefly and then present findings.

Cardiovascular system examination in detail

Getting started

1 Introduce yourself to the patient and ask for permission to examine

- Put out your hand to shake the patient's hand.
- Say something like 'Hello, I'm William Osler, third-year medical student. Do you mind if I examine your heart and pulses?' Do not just say 'heart'! The patient will wonder what you are up to when you start looking at his hands!

2 Wash your hands

3 Ask the patient to get on to the bed (if not already there). You may need to ask for help!

Usually, this will be no problem, but if the patient is unable to get on to the bed, offer your assistance only if you have had moving and handling training. If not, ask for help from trained nurses or healthcare assistants. This is because some patients (particularly those with memory impairments) may overestimate their abilities and could fall or cause you injury.

4 Ask the patient to remove all garments covering chest and arms. For female patients, offer to cover the chest with a sheet or towel

The cardiovascular system is examined with the patient's chest bare (Fig. 4.2). It is best to get this sorted out at the start of the examination—and in female patients offer to cover the chest up with a sheet or towel untill you get to the examination of the chest itself (Case 4.9). At least one woman (such as a medical student or nurse) must be present to act as a chaperone.

5 Arrange the patient so that their chest is at 45°

The cardiovascular system is examined with the patient sitting so that the upper part of their body is at 45° to the horizontal; the patient's neck should be **relaxed** against the pillow (Fig. 4.2), primarily to facilitate examination of

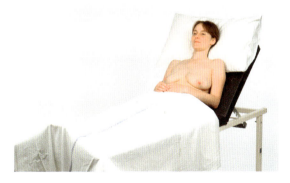

Figure 4.2 Patient exposure for cardiovascular system examination.

CASE 4.9

Problem. I don't feel quite right asking women to bare their chests especially when the first part of the cardiovascular examination doesn't involve the chest.

Discussion. Students, quite understandably, are often unsure if this is appropriate. Such doubt can create a confidence problem—not a good thing at this early stage of the cardiovascular examination. I suggest you say something like 'Ideally, it's best if I examine you with your chest bare. Is that all right? I can cover up your chest with a sheet for part of the examination.' Give the patient opportunity to refuse. If she refuses (unusual), do not take this as a slight, just get on with the examination as best you can.

the jugular venous pressure. You may need to adjust the bed's headrest to get the patient in the correct position.

....

Tip

Get to know how to work the headrests on hospital beds and try to become familiar with the controls of the electric profiling beds.

....

6 While doing 1–4, have a 'general look'. Is the patient distressed, for example?

- Patient distress suggests severe illness.
- An intravenous cannula suggests recent chest pain (the cannula is in case analgesia or resuscitation are required) or heart failure (requiring intravenous diuretics). Rarely, the cannula is being used to give intravenous antibiotics in patients with infective endocarditis.
- A monitor suggests recent chest pain or arrhythmia.
- A malar flush suggests mitral stenosis (*my-tral-sten-owe-sis*).
- Tachypnoea (*tack-kip-nia*) suggests heart failure.
- Cyanosis suggests hypoxia.
- Forceful neck pulsations may indicate aortic regurgitation.

See 'Cardiovascular diseases and investigations' for further information on specific conditions.

....

Tip

Always remember that the general look is something you do while sorting other things out. Do not stand back to have an aimless gawp.

....

Hands

7 Inspect both hands and fingernails for splinter haemorrhages (DF5/10), clubbing (DF8/10), and tar staining (DF1/10)

Splinter haemorrhages

What are they?

These are small haemorrhages within the nailbed under the nail.

Significance

Inspection for splinter haemorrhages is included in the cardiovascular system examination because they occur in patients with infective endocarditis, which is infection of the heart. Infective endocarditis affects the heart mainly by damaging the valves. It may also cause widespread inflammation of small vessels (vasculitis). Vasculitis in the nailbed may be followed by haemorrhage—producing splinter haemorrhages. However, 90% of patients with infective endocarditis do not have 'splinters'. Furthermore, they are more commonly caused by minor trauma to the nails. When due to trauma, they are much more common in fingers than in toes and occur particularly in manual workers.

How to examine

Splinter haemorrhages usually look like dark pen marks under the nail (Fig. 4.3), though occasionally they are bright red. They lie parallel to the long axis of the nail. Though they are small, they are relatively easy to see if you look carefully. Be careful, they may occur in just one nailbed. It is said that splinter haemorrhages due to endocarditis are more commonly seen in the proximal part of the nail, though hard evidence for this is lacking.

1 Take the patient's right hand.

2 Stoop down to inspect the nails.

3 Combining thoroughness and speed, carefully inspect all the nails of the right hand.

4 Do the same for the left hand.

The main trouble with finding splinter haemorrhages is that because they are rare, students may find themselves just going through the motions so that when they do occur, they miss them. Avoid complacency!

Clubbing

Clubbing is mainly seen in respiratory disease and is therefore discussed in detail in Chapter 5. However, it may be seen very rarely in cardiovascular disease—cyanotic congenital heart disease and infective endocarditis. Clubbing is a late

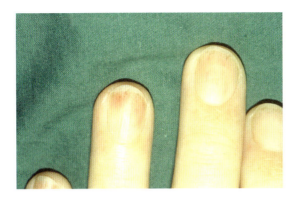

Figure 4.3 Splinter haemorrhages: small, dark, longitudinal marks in nailbed.

feature of infective endocarditis, so if clubbing is due to this, there will be other more convincing features of infective endocarditis present.

Tar staining

Tar staining is easily recognizable as a yellowish discolouration of the fingers caused by cigarettes. It raises the possibility of coronary artery disease, which may cause angina, myocardial infarction, arrhythmias, and heart failure (nicotine is colourless).

> **Key point**
> - Splinter haemorrhages are usually caused by trauma but also occur in 10% of patients with infective endocarditis.

Radial pulse

8 Palpate right radial pulse for pulse rate (DF 3/10) and rhythm (DF 6/10). Palpate right and left radial pulses together and compare (DF 8/10). Check for collapsing pulse (DF 6/10)

Palpate right radial pulse for pulse rate and rhythm

The right radial pulse is used to assess pulse rate and rhythm. These are both extremely important signs. Pulse character is better assessed at the carotid pulse though you may get a sense of it at the radial pulse.

Rate

Normal pulse rate is 60–100 beats/min. A slow pulse rate (<60 beats/min) is known as bradycardia (*braddy-card-ia*).

Table 4.5 Major causes of bradycardia

Common	Normal finding in fit young people, β-blocker drugs
Less common	Heart block, hypothyroidism

Table 4.6 Major causes of tachycardia

Exercise
Anxiety
Pyrexial illness
Hyperthyroidism
Drugs (β₂ agonists—salbutamol, etc.)
Hypovolaemic (*high-poe-vole-ee-mick*) shock (as in gastrointestinal bleeding)
Arrhythmias

For causes, see Table 4.5. A fast pulse rate (>100 beats/min) is known as tachycardia. For causes, see Table 4.6. Tachycardia in resting patients is always abnormal.

Rhythm

Pulse rhythm is either regular or irregular. The normal rhythm of the heart is known as sinus rhythm because it is controlled by the sinoatrial node. Normally, the heart speeds up during inspiration and slows down in expiration. This is because during inspiration the normal tone of the vagus nerve (which slows the heart) is inhibited, leading to an increase in heart rate. During expiration, vagal tone returns, slowing the heart. In most patients over 40 years, this 'irregularity' is subtle and the pulse feels regular. In younger patients, the pulse may feel irregular—known as 'sinus arrhythmia'. This is a misleading term as an arrhythmia is defined as an abnormality of cardiac rhythm of any type—whereas sinus arrhythmia is quite normal.

Causes of an irregular pulse are shown in Table 4.7. An irregular pulse may be 'regularly irregular' or 'irregularly irregular'. With the former, there is some consistency to the irregularity such as every fourth beat is missed or the rate varies with respiration in a consistent fashion. With the latter, there is no pattern. It is difficult to differentiate between the different causes of an irregularly irregular pulse clinically. An ECG is required. However, the effect of exercise may be helpful. Often (but not always), ventricular ectopic beats may be abolished by exercise so

Table 4.7 Causes of an irregular pulse

Regularly irregular pulse
Sinus arrhythmia
Wenckebach (*when-key-back*) second-degree heart block[a]
Irregularly irregular pulse
Atrial fibrillation (most common)
Multiple ventricular ectopic beats
Atrial flutter with variable block

[a] Karel Frederik Wenckebach (1864–1940), Dutch physician.

that the pulse becomes regular. If the irregular pulse is due to atrial fibrillation, then exercise will not make the pulse regular.

What is the pulse deficit?

This is a term you may hear mentioned. In atrial fibrillation, not only is the rhythm irregular, but the strength of the pulse is irregular too. This is because the ventricle contracts randomly and may not always be completely filled when ejection occurs. Sometimes, the amount of blood the left ventricle ejects (stroke volume) is so low that no pulse is felt at the radial artery. Thus, if you listen to the heart with a stethoscope while feeling the pulse, the rate on auscultation may be faster than at the radial pulse. For example, the rate might be 126 beats/min at the apex compared to 116 beats/min at the wrist. This difference is termed a 'pulse deficit'—in this case 10 beats/min.

How to examine

The radial pulse is felt on the radial side of the flexor surface of the forearm just a few centimetres proximal to the wrist (Fig. 4.4).

1 Hold the patient's right hand with your right hand.
2 Then, use the tips of both the index and middle fingers of your left hand to palpate the pulse. See Case 4.10.
3 Once you have found the radial pulse you must time it; use your watch and count the beats over 20 seconds. Then multiply by 3 to give beats/min.
4 While counting the rate, you should also be concentrating on the pulse rhythm. Is it regular or irregular? If it is irregular, is it irregularly irregular or regularly irregular (see Case 4.11)?

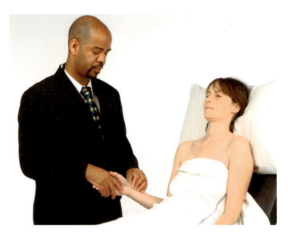

Figure 4.4 Palpation of the radial pulse.

CASE 4.10

Problem. I've examined a well-looking 25-year-old man but couldn't palpate the radial pulse.

Discussion. Perhaps, it isn't there (congenital anomaly)—but usually this is because you've missed the pulse. Occasionally, the student puts their fingers down on the patient's wrist in the right place but then moves them—away from the pulse—when they do not feel the pulse immediately. When you feel for the radial pulse, wait for at least 10 seconds in any one position before palpating somewhere else. Usually, you will feel the pulse if you just wait. Then, if you want, you can move your fingers to where you sense the pulse is stronger.

Palpate right and left radial pulses together and compare

Significance

The right and left radial pulses may differ in the following circumstances:

- in acute aortic dissection
- in proximal arterial disease such as atherosclerosis of the axillary artery or stricture of the axillary artery following angiography.

How to examine

Keep your fingers on the right radial pulse and simultaneously feel the left radial pulse with your right hand (Fig. 4.5). Compare the strength of both sides. See Case 4.12.

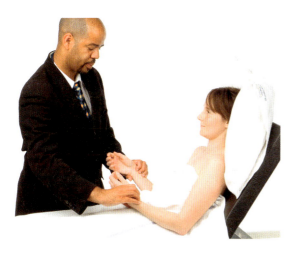

Figure 4.5 Comparing pulses.

Check for collapsing pulse

Pulse character is normally best assessed at the carotid pulse (or the brachial (*brake-key-al*) pulse in children). However, the radial pulse can be used to assess for a collapsing pulse.

Significance

A collapsing pulse is a sign of aortic regurgitation. (In the context of valvular lesions, 'regurgitation' and 'incompetence' mean the same thing.)

How to examine

1 Ask the patient if they have any pain in the shoulder.
2 If not, use your left hand to raise the patient's right arm while holding their wrist with your fingers (do not keep your fingers specifically on the pulse) (see Fig. 4.6).
3 If you feel the pulse vibrating back down your fingers, this is a collapsing pulse.

Face, eyes, and tongue

9 Inspect face for malar flush (DF 7/10) and xanthelasmata (DF 2/10). Inspect eyes for corneal arcus (DF 2/10). Inspect conjunctivae for anaemia (DF 9/10). Inspect tongue for cyanosis (DF 9/10)

Malar flush

Malar flush, also known as mitral facies (*face-ease*), is found in mitral stenosis. It refers to rosy cheeks with something of a bluish tinge. It is caused by dilation of the

---

CASE 4.11

Problem. The rhythm seems generally regular but you have noticed one slight irregularity.

   Discussion. This is either a ventricular or atrial ectopic beat—so the rhythm is 'sinus rhythm with occasional ectopic beats'.

CASE 4.12

Problem. I always think the pulses are asymmetrical!

   Discussion. It is more awkward to feel the left pulse and this may produce an (incorrect) impression of asymmetry. **Take your time**. Make sure you are happy with how you are palpating before moving on.

capillaries of the cheek, which in turn is secondary to pulmonary hypertension. Most patients with rosy cheeks do not have mitral stenosis!

Xanthelasmata and corneal arcus

Xanthelasmata and corneal arcus are both signs of hyperlipidaemia. Xanthelasmata are little yellowish papules (fatty deposits), usually around the eyes. They nearly always suggest hyperlipidaemia.

   Corneal arcus (sometimes known as arcus senilis (*sen-ill-iss*)) is a grey ring around the outer margin of the iris (again due to fat deposits) (see Fig. 4.7). This is usually a normal finding in the elderly. In patients less than 50 years of age, though, it is suggestive of hyperlipidaemia.

> **Key points**
> - Bradycardia may be normal.
> - Tachycardia has multiple causes and is often not due to cardiac pathology.
> - While counting pulse rate, concentrate also on rhythm.
> - Sinus arrhythmia becomes less marked with age.
> - Atrial fibrillation is the most common cause of an irregularly irregular pulse but an ECG is required to decide the cause.
> - Never forget to compare right and left radial pulses; always consider aortic dissection in patients with apparent myocardial infarction.
> - When testing for a collapsing pulse, hold the whole wrist—not just the pulse.

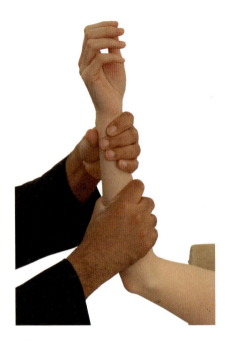

Figure 4.6 Palpating for collapsing pulse. Hold up the patient's left arm with your right, holding the flexor surface of the wrist with your fingers.

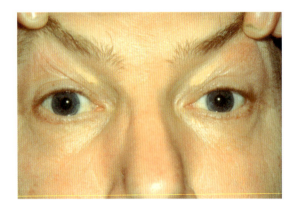

Figure 4.7 Corneal arcus.

Anaemia

Significance

Anaemia may be a cause of heart failure or angina and hence is included in the cardiovascular examination. Skin colour is a poor reflection of the haemoglobin level. Anaemia is best looked for in the conjunctivae of the lower eyelid. Even then, this is quite a crude test and experienced physicians are often wrong.

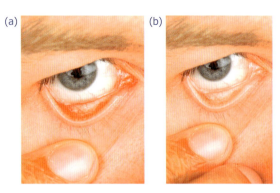

Figure 4.8 Examining for anaemia in (a) normal patient, (b) anaemic patient.

How to examine

1 Ask the patient's permission: 'Can I pull down your eyelid?'
2 Use your right index finger to gently pull down the right lower eyelid to expose the conjunctiva and inspect (Fig. 4.8a).
3 Normally, the anterior part of the conjunctiva is a brighter red compared to the posterior portion. In anaemic patients, this distinction is lost (Fig. 4.8b).

Cyanosis

See Chapter 5.

Causes

When examining the cardiovascular system, you are looking for central cyanosis. The most common cardiovascular cause is pulmonary oedema. Pulmonary oedema may come on suddenly usually due to coronary ischaemia or myocardial infarction or may be chronic due to valvular lesions or left ventricular systolic dysfunction. Right-to-left cardiac shunts are a very rare cause of cyanosis.

How to look for central cyanosis

See Chapter 5.

> **Key point**
> ● Skin colour is a poor reflection of anaemia; examine the conjunctivae but even this is not always reliable.

Problem. I can't see the internal jugular vein. Why might this be?

Discussion. Of course you may just have missed it but there are other possible reasons.

- It is not actually visible. Often, the venous pressure is not high enough for the jugular vein to be visible in the neck with the patient lying at 45°.
- The internal jugular vein cannot be seen if the neck is not relaxed. The main problem with technique is that at various points in the procedure the patient's neck may not be relaxed in the correct position:

(1) if the head is not against the pillow at any time, (2) when you ask the patient to turn to the left, or (3) when you ask the patient about abdominal tenderness and they turn their head to answer you. A relaxed sternocleidomastoid should just blend into the neck. If the muscle is prominent (Fig. 4.16) it is not relaxed. If the patient is not relaxed, ask them to rest their head back against the pillow and 'sink into the bed'. You may have to say this several times at different stages of the examination (telling patients to relax rarely has the desired effect).

Carotid pulse

10 Palpate right carotid pulse for pulse character (DF 8/10)

What is pulse character?

You may have heard the terms 'volume' and 'character' interchanged. There is a subtle difference between the two. When you feel a pulse, you get a sensation of the power of the pulse. This is pulse 'volume', which depends on the cardiac stroke volume. Pulse volume may be altered not only by cardiac lesions but also by other states, especially low blood pressure (hypotension). Students usually find assessment of volume quite simple but assessment of character is trickier. Character relates not only to the power of the pulse but also to how slowly or quickly it achieves its power. Abnormal pulse character is more indicative of a valvular lesion. Because it is often subtle, character is best assessed at the carotid pulse—the nearest accessible artery to the heart.

Significance

Abnormal pulse character is a characteristic feature of aortic valve disease (see Fig. 4.9):

- **aortic stenosis**: slow rising, plateau pulse;
- **aortic regurgitation**: fast rising (waterhammer), fast falling (collapsing) pulse;
- **mixed aortic valve disease**: 'bisfiriens' (*biss-firi-enz*) pulse—double impulse pulse;
- other conditions may occasionally affect the pulse character, one rare example being **hypertrophic obstructive cardiomyopathy**—jerky pulse.

How to examine

See Fig. 4.10. The carotid pulse is not always easy to find.

1 Ask the patient to turn their head to the left. Make sure the patient's head is lying back against the pillow so that their neck is relaxed. If the neck is not relaxed, ask your patient to 'sink down into the bed' (just asking the patient to relax usually makes them go rigid).

2 Next, warn your patient: 'I am going to feel the pulse in your neck and it will be slightly uncomfortable.'

3 Use your left thumb and place it **gently** against the thyroid cartilage (Adam's apple).

4 Gently move the thumb laterally and posteriorly until you no longer feel the cartilage. Usually the carotid pulse is palpable just here.

5 Decide on pulse volume and how quickly it rises and falls.

Practise feeling normal pulses; only then will you be confident in diagnosing an abnormality. If unsure about the character, consider whether there are other signs of aortic valve disease. If so, the likelihood of pulse abnormality is increased.

Jugular venous pressure

11 Inspect right internal jugular vein for jugular venous pressure (DF 9/10). Check for hepatojugular reflux (DF 8/10)

The right atrial pressure is an important indicator of cardiac or pulmonary disease but clearly it cannot be measured directly at the bedside. However, the right atrium communicates with the right internal jugular vein, so that the pressure within the right internal jugular vein gives an accurate indication of right atrial

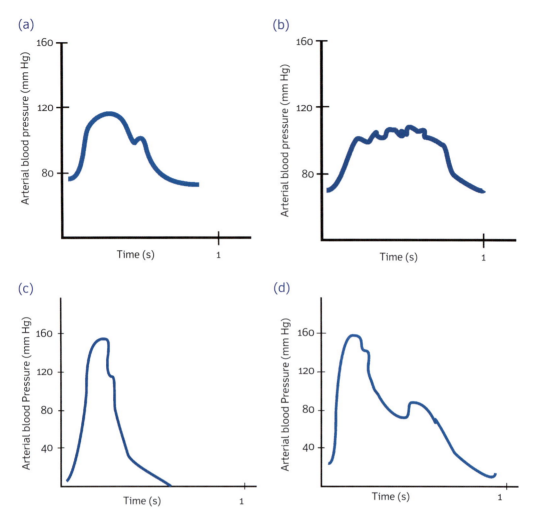

Figure 4.9 Pulse waveforms: (a) normal, (b) aortic stenosis, (c) aortic regurgitation, and (d) mixed aortic valve disease.

pressure. Thus, assessment of jugular venous pressure is an essential part of routine medical practice.

Unfortunately, the internal jugular vein can be very difficult to examine and this can be very frustrating for the student. Do not be alarmed! Everyone experiences difficulties in assessing the jugular venous pressure. **Practice is everything!**

In the next few pages, jugular venous examination will be reviewed, with a focus on anatomy, physiology, significance, and examination technique.

Anatomy

The internal jugular vein lies quite deep in the root of the neck between the sternal and clavicular heads of the sternocleidomastoid (*stern-owe-clyde-owe-mast-oid*). It travels deep underneath the medial aspect of the sternocleidomastoid

towards the ear; see Fig. 4.11 and Case 4.13. The external jugular vein lies lateral to the sternocleidomastoid muscle and is more superficial so it is much easier to see. See Case 4.14.

Key points

- Abnormal pulse volume may occur in non-cardiac disease.
- Pulse character abnormalities are important indicators of cardiac disease—usually aortic valve disease.
- Pulse character is a tricky sign; students' most common mistake is to say character is abnormal when it is not—usually because they are describing volume, not character.

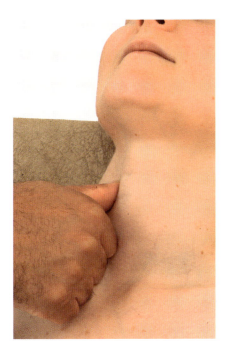

Figure 4.10 Palpation of the carotid pulse: neck relaxed, use left thumb.

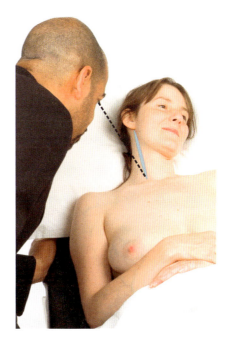

Figure 4.11 Inspection of the jugular venous pressure waveform. Patient at 45°. Neck relaxed against pillow and turned to the left. Delineate internal and external jugular veins and root of neck.

Physiology

The right atrial pressure (and so jugular venous pressure) varies through the cardiac cycle. It is worth revising how:

- in ventricular systole the tricuspid valve is closed and the right atrium fills passively;
- as the ventricle relaxes in diastole, the tricuspid valve opens and blood flows passively from the atrium into the ventricle;
- the right atrium then contracts and squeezes further blood into the ventricle;
- the right atrium then relaxes, the tricuspid valve closes and ventricular systole starts again.

The jugular venous waveform is shown in Fig. 4.12. There are three stages at which pressure increases (known as A, C, and V waves) and two stages at which pressure decreases (known as X and Y descent).

- The A wave is caused by right atrial contraction.
- The X descent is due to right atrial relaxation.
- There is a slight blip in the X descent, known as the C wave. The exact cause of this is unclear. It may be due to the tricuspid valve flicking back into the right atrium

CASE 4.14

Problem. I can't see the deep pulsation you're talking about but I can see the external jugular vein. Is this not just as good?

Discussion. This is a contentious point. The external jugular vein lies lateral to the sternocleidomastoid muscle and is more superficial so it is much easier to see. Traditionally, it is taught that it **should not be used** because it has valves—so its height is an unreliable index of the right atrial pressure. However, it is now accepted that the internal jugular also has valves and these do not cause any problems. It is probably also true that the external jugular is prone to kinking. Experience shows, though, that the internal and external jugulars generally give the same result. So if you cannot see the internal jugular, the external jugular is a reasonable substitute.

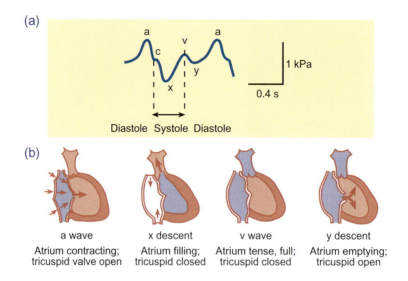

Figure 4.12 The jugular venous pressure waveform.
Reproduced by permission of Oxford University Press from Fig. 15.13 (p. 306), *Human Physiology: The Basis of Medicine* (2nd edn), by G. Pocock and C. Richards (2004).

at the start of the systole or may possibly be caused by the carotid artery pulsation.

- The V wave follows. This is due to passive atrial filling (with the tricuspid valve closed).
- The Y descent occurs during ventricular diastole when the tricuspid valve opens and blood flows passively from the atrium to the ventricle.
- The A wave then represents atrial contraction again.
- The normal right atrial pressure at the top of the A wave is 7 cm water.

Significance

An elevated jugular venous pressure is most commonly due to right heart failure. This is usually secondary to left heart failure, which in turn is caused by ischaemic heart disease or occasionally mitral valve disease. Right heart failure may also be secondary to pulmonary disease—cor pulmonale (*core-pull-ma-nail-ee*). In the case of pulmonary emboli, cor pulmonale may present acutely. Other important causes of elevated jugular venous pressure are given below.

- **Fluid overload**. This may be due to kidney failure or excess intravenous fluids.
- **Tricuspid regurgitation**. The tricuspid valve does not shut properly so the internal jugular pressure reflects

the right ventricular pressure; when the right ventricle contracts, the jugular venous pressure is very high (giant V wave).

- **Complete heart block**. Here, there is atrioventricular dissociation so that the atrial and ventricular contractions are not related in time. Atrial contraction may occur when the tricuspid valve is shut, so producing a large venous pulsation, known as a 'cannon A' wave. These are irregular, reflecting the fact that sometimes the tricuspid valve is shut and sometimes it is open when the right atrium contracts.
- **Superior vena caval obstruction**. See Fig. 5.7. The jugular vein is distended and elevated without pulsating. This is usually due to mediastinal lymphadenopathy (*media-sty-nal-limf-adder-nop-path-ee*) secondary to lung carcinoma (*car-sin-owe-ma*). Hepatojugular reflux is negative (because of the obstruction).
- **Atrial fibrillation**. Here, there is no atrial systole so consequently the jugular venous waveform has no A wave.

How to examine

The vein is usually examined with the patient at 45°, for the following reasons:

- The normal maximum right atrial pressure is 7 cm water.
- With the patient sitting straight up, the venous pulsations are normally too deep in the chest to be seen (Fig. 4.13).

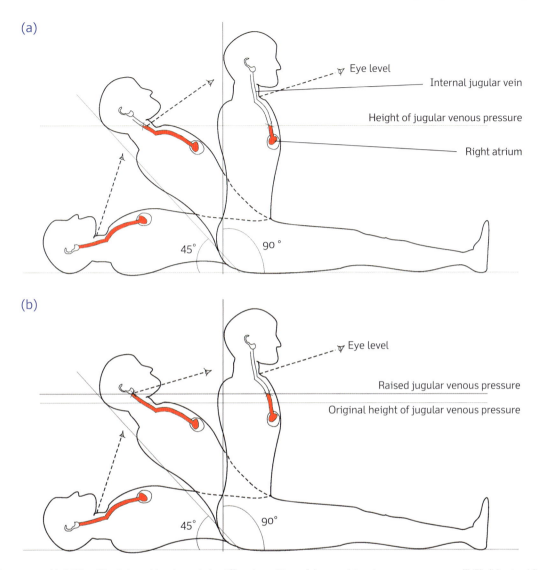

Figure 4.13 Visibility of the internal jugular vein in different positions: (a) normal jugular venous pressure (JVP), (b) raised JVP.

- With the patient lying flat, the vein is always full and there is no visible pulsation.
- With the patient at 45°, the venous pulsations are normally at the level of the clavicle between the heads of sternocleidomastoid. They may or may not be visible here. In a patient with elevated venous pressure, the pulsation is seen higher up in the neck.

If the jugular venous pressure is extremely elevated, the top of the pulsation may be above the neck and so not visible. In such patients, the internal jugular vein is better observed with the patient sitting up straight.

Initial inspection

See Fig. 4.11.

1 Ensure the patient is at 45°, with head and neck relaxed back against a pillow.

2 Ask the patient to turn their head slightly (perhaps 30°) to the left, keeping the neck relaxed (see Case 4.15).

3 If lighting is poor, switch on the patient's bedside lamp and focus it on the neck.

4 The internal jugular vein is best seen tangentially, so lean slightly across the patient.

CASE 4.15

Problem. The patient can't turn their neck to the left. Should I examine the left internal jugular vein?

Discussion. Yes. However, it is not ideal as veins from the left side of the neck reach the heart by traversing the mediastinum and may be compressed by the aorta, occasionally resulting in distortion of the pressure level.

5 Inspect between the heads of sternocleidomastoid just above the clavicle. This is where the jugular vein may be seen in normal patients.

6 Look slightly higher in the neck along the medial aspect of sternocleidomastoid for a pulsation. If you see a pulsation here, this suggests an increased JVP.

7 If none is seen, look also at the earlobe in case this is pulsating.

8 Next assess for hepatojugular reflux (sometimes called abdominojugular reflux). This is helpful in two ways: (1) in deciding if a particular pulsation is venous and (2) in making the diagnosis of right heart failure.

On initial inspection, you may see a pulsation but not be sure whether it is venous or arterial (see Case 4.16). Pressing on the abdomen increases venous pressure transiently so the internal jugular vein becomes more prominent for a few seconds. This is known as hepatojugular reflux (see Case 4.17). Usually, the venous pulsation quickly returns to normal (even while pressure is maintained on the abdomen). If it persists at its new level for longer than a few seconds, this is suggestive of right heart failure. Arterial pulsations, on the other hand, are not affected by pressing in the abdomen. The following points should be noted.

1 Patient should stay in the same position with neck relaxed against the pillow and turned to the left.

2 Ask the patient if their 'tummy' is tender, pointing to the right upper quadrant.

3 Ask permission to press on the 'tummy', being especially considerate if the patient admits to having some discomfort. Proceed if permission is given.

4 If you have previously seen what you think is a venous pulsation, you should concentrate on it throughout the procedure. If not, keep focused on the root of the neck (between the heads of sternocleidomastoid just above the clavicle).

5 Press gently in the right upper quadrant of the abdomen for 10 seconds (Fig. 4.14) and be aware that this may be uncomfortable for the patient. If discomfort is a problem, stop.

6 If you have seen a pulsation on initial inspection, check if it alters when you press on the abdomen. If so, it is venous. If not, it is arterial. If venous, decide how high it is above the clavicle. Also, decide if it stays at its new level for more than 5 seconds. If so, this suggests right heart failure.

7 If you did not see a pulsation on initial inspection, look carefully at the root of the neck. The jugular vein pulsation may just become visible here as you press in the abdomen.

By the end of this examination you should have decided whether the jugular vein is visible. If it is, you should be able to state whether the pressure is elevated and by how much (in terms of centimetres above the clavicle). In normal patients, the internal jugular vein is often not visible with the

CASE 4.16

Problem. Are there any other ways of assessing whether pulsations in the neck are venous or arterial?

Discussion. There are many ways of distinguishing arterial from venous pulsations. The best is checking for **hepatojugular reflux**. Sometimes, you will still not be sure. A good alternative is to apply pressure in the root of the neck. Gently press between the two heads of sternocleidomastoid just above the clavicle. If the pulsation alters, particularly if it becomes less visible, then it is venous. Other ways are as follows.

- Venous pulsations, unlike arterial pulsations, vary with posture. Sitting the patient up or lying them flat will alter a venous but not an arterial pulsation.
- Venous pulsations, unlike arterial pulsations, vary with respiration. This is quite subtle, not least because of movement of the neck during respiration.
- Venous pulsations are not usually palpable, whereas arterial pulsations are. However, when the venous pressure is very high, the venous pulsation may be palpable.

Problem. I see a pulsation but I'm not sure whether hepatojugular reflux is positive or not.

Discussion. This happens when you're not watching the pulsation before as well as when you press on the abdomen. Always make sure that you are focused on any possible pulsation in the neck **just before** you press in the abdomen. That way, you will be able to follow it clearly and so decide whether hepatojugular reflux is present.

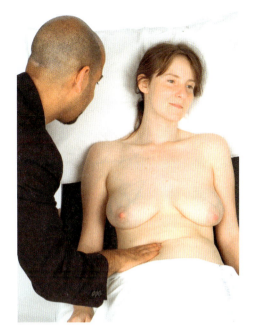

Figure 4.14 Assessing for hepatojugular reflux.

patient sitting at 45° and may not even appear when you press on the abdomen. However, seeing it in the root of the neck is reassuring in that it means you have not missed a vein with elevated pressure. See Fig. 4.15. Cases 4.18, 4.19, and 4.20 discuss further difficulties with the JVP.

....

Tip
Practise with the patient (or your friend) lying at 30°. This makes it easier to see the internal jugular vein in patients with normal right atrial pressure.

....

Key points

- The pressure in the internal jugular vein is a reflection of right atrial pressure.
- It is an important sign because the JVP is elevated in right heart failure.
- The internal jugular vein is often not visible.
- To see the internal jugular vein, it is essential that the patient's neck is relaxed.
- Deciding whether a neck pulsation is arterial or venous is never easy; assessing for hepatojugular reflux can be very helpful.

Inspection of praecordium

12 Take sheet off chest (female patients). Inspect praecordium in general and specifically for scars, cardiac impulse, and any other abnormal pulsations (DF 5/10).

The praecordium

The praecordium is the front of the chest over the heart. Various areas on the praecordium are of particular importance (Fig. 4.17).

- **Apex/mitral area**. The area around the left fifth intercostal space in the mid-clavicular line is the area where the apex beat is normally felt and mitral valve sounds are best heard. Hence, it is known either as the 'apex' or the 'mitral area'.

- **Tricuspid area**. The area around the left fourth intercostal space just lateral to the sternum is where tricuspid valve sounds are best heard and is known as the 'tricuspid area'.

- **Pulmonary area**. The area around the left second intercostal space just lateral to the sternum is where pulmonary valve sounds are best heard and is known as the 'pulmonary area'.

- **Left sternal edge**. The area just to the left of the sternum is known as the 'left sternal edge'—significant because the murmur of aortic regurgitation is best heard here.

- **Aortic area/base**. The area around the right second intercostal space just lateral to the sternum is where aortic valve sounds are best heard and is known as the 'aortic area'. The aortic area may also be referred to as the 'base' or the 'base of the heart'.

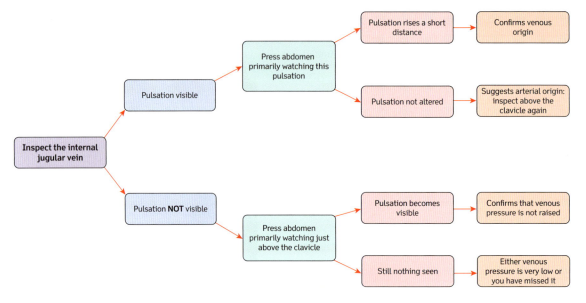

Figure 4.15 Assessing the jugular venous pressure.

CASE 4.18

Problem. I've been told to use the manubriosternal angle as the reference point for the JVP.

 Discussion. Potentially, the manubriosternal angle is a useful reference point (and widely described) because the right atrium is around 5 cm inferior to the manubriosternal angle no matter what angle the patient is lying at. The right atrial pressure is around 7 cm of blood. So normally the internal jugular vein pulsation should be no higher than 2 cm above the manubriosternal angle no matter what position the patient is in. This can be considered unnecessarily complicated. If you see the internal jugular vein around the level of the clavicle with the patient lying at 45°, this is normal. If the pulsation is higher up in the neck, the JVP is elevated by that amount.

CASE 4.19

Problem. I can't see the triple waveform and if I'm honest I can't see the double waveform.

 Discussion. The triple waveform A, C, and V is not visible. However, with time (a lot of time, perhaps) it is possible to see that the venous pulsation has a double peak. These are the A and V waves. Picking up the giant V wave of tricuspid regurgitation or the cannon A wave of complete heart block can be very difficult—it can be simply seen that the venous pressure is elevated. Similarly, the absent A wave of atrial fibrillation is a tricky sign to identify. If you do see a double pulsation and wish to identify the A and V waves, the heart sounds are useful. The A wave tends to be in time with the first heart sound and the V wave with the second heart sound.

The areas do not relate to the surface markings of the appropriate valve because sounds produced by the valves radiate from their point of origin (the surface marking is the point on the skin underneath which the valve is sited). Further important markings are the **midclavicular line**, the **anterior axillary line**, and the **midaxillary line**. These are imaginary vertical lines usually used to define apex beat position.

What you are looking for on inspection

Scars

The most useful finding on inspection of the praecordium is the presence of a scar, suggesting previous surgery. Scars are of two main types:

- **Midline sternotomy (*stern-not-tummy*) scar**. This is a vertical scar over the sternum. The usual reason is coronary artery bypass grafting (commonly known as

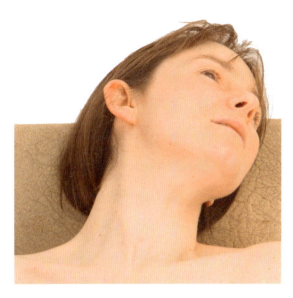

Figure 4.16 Non-relaxed sternocleidomastoid. Note how clearly visible the muscle is. It should blend into the neck.

CABG and pronounced *cabbage*). Aortic and mitral valve replacements also require a midline sternotomy scar so such a scar should alert you to the possibility of prosthetic valves.

- **Left thoracotomy (*thor-ack-cot-tummy*) scar**. Here the scar lies in a diagonal from underneath the left breast to the left axilla. The most common reason is mitral valvotomy surgery. Mitral valvotomy was used in the past as a treatment for mitral stenosis; here an object (dilator) is passed through the narrowed mitral valve to open it up. Patients who have had mitral valvotomy may have signs of mitral regurgitation (which may be caused by the operation) or mitral stenosis (as this tends to recur around 10 years after the operation).

Chest deformity

Sternal depression, scoliosis, and kyphosis may all result in an ejection systolic murmur or a displaced apex beat. So if you find no other cause for these, chest deformities may be the explanation.

Cardiac impulse

This may be seen at the apex—and often is easier to see than to palpate. If it is seen lower or more lateral, it is displaced. For causes of a displaced apex beat, see the 'Palpation of praecordium' section.

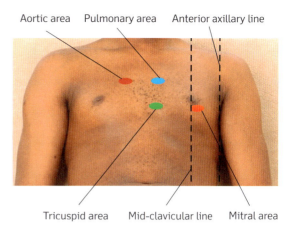

Figure 4.17 The praecordium.

Pacemaker

A permanent pacemaker may lie under the skin, just inferior to the left clavicle (occasionally on the right).

How to inspect the praecordium

If this is part of a general cardiovascular system examination, you will just have finished assessing the JVP. If the patient is female, she may have a sheet covering her chest.

1 At this stage, you should ask the woman's permission to remove the sheet from her chest and if given, then do so.

2 Make a brief (seconds only) general inspection for chest deformity, abnormal pulsations, pacemaker, and scars.

3 Inspect the midline for midline sternotomy scar—usually easy to see, but be careful in men with a lot of chest hair.

4 Now inspect under the left breast for cardiac pulsation and possible left thoracotomy scar.

5 With women, you will usually need to lift the left breast to see this area properly. Ask permission first, 'Do you mind if I lift up your breast?' and if granted, proceed to lift breast with your left hand and inspect (Fig. 4.18).

6 Decide (1) whether you can see the cardiac pulsation and make a subjective decision on its position (this will be quantified when you palpate) and (2) whether there is a left thoracotomy scar; keep the left breast held up so that any skin creases (which may hide the scar—surgeons prided themselves on this) are smoothed out and look very carefully under the breast and in the axilla.

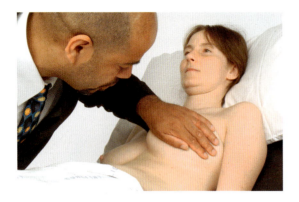

Figure 4.18 Inspection of the cardiac impulse.

Palpation of praecordium

13 Palpate at apex for apex beat, assessing position and character (DF 9/10). Palpate for left parasternal impulse (DF 9/10) and aortic and pulmonary thrills (DF 6/10).

Why palpate?

The cardiac impulse

This is a brisk but light movement felt against the hand just after the start of systole, which retracts before the end of systole. Its exact origin is unclear. The apex beat is the cardiac impulse at the most lateral and inferior position at which it can be felt. Normally, the apex beat is felt around the fifth intercostal space in the region of the midclavicular line.

Cardiac impulse abnormalities

The cardiac impulse beat may either be displaced or have an abnormal character. A displaced cardiac impulse is not always due to cardiac pathology; pulmonary conditions and skeletal abnormalities may also displace the cardiac

impulse. The character of the cardiac impulse is usually only altered in cardiac disease.

- In mitral stenosis, the cardiac impulse is tapping in character but not displaced. The tapping character is due to a palpable first heart sound (i.e. the noise made by closure of the mitral and tricuspid valves).

- Aortic stenosis and hypertension both cause obstruction to outflow. This high 'pressure load' causes left ventricular hypertrophy (*high-purr-tra-fee*), which in turn produces a sustained, heaving, minimally displaced (down and out) cardiac impulse.

- In both mitral regurgitation and aortic regurgitation there is increased filling of the left ventricle to compensate for the retrograde flow associated with these conditions. The resultant 'volume overload' of the left ventricle results in a forceful, thrusting, and displaced (down and out) cardiac impulse. Because there is no obstruction to outflow, the cardiac impulse is not unusually sustained.

- Left ventricular dilation (as in heart failure) produces a displaced (down and out) cardiac impulse. The cardiac pulsation is diffuse and may be felt from the apex to the left parasternal area.

- Left ventricular aneurysms produce a dyskinetic (*dis-kye-net-tick*) cardiac impulse—where the impulse appears to have several different components.

Left parasternal impulse

A left parasternal impulse is produced by left atrial hypertrophy (as in mitral stenosis or regurgitation) or right ventricular hypertrophy (which may be secondary to right or left heart disease or lung disease—cor pulmonale).

Key points

- The aortic area is on the right side of the chest.
- Left thoracotomy scars may be well hidden; you may have to lift the patient's breast to see one. Such a scar should alert you to the possibility of mitral regurgitation and/or stenosis.
- It may be easier to see the cardiac pulsation at the apex than to palpate it.

(a)   (b)

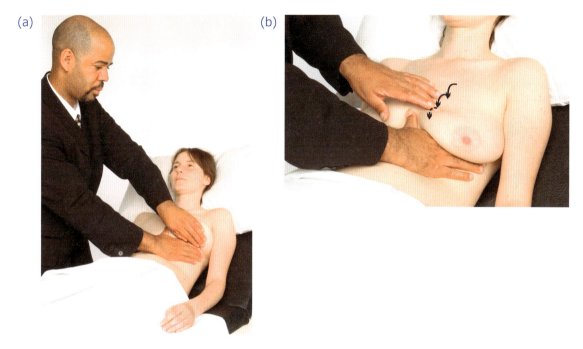

Figure 4.19 Palpating for the cardiac impulse: (a) locating the apex beat; (b) counting down the ribs.

Thrills

Rarely, murmurs are palpable producing a vibrating sensation a bit like a cat purring. A thrill nearly always indicates a significant lesion. Aortic stenosis, which may produce a thrill in the aortic area, is the only common cause.

How to examine

1 **Palpate the cardiac impulse**. If you have seen a pulsation during inspection, palpate for this first with the index, middle, ring, and little fingers of your right hand. If you did not see anything on inspection, palpate around the fifth intercostal space, in the midclavicular line (Fig. 4.19). Always wait at least 10 seconds before deciding you cannot feel it and trying elsewhere. See Case 4.21.

2 **Find the apex beat**. Once you have found an apical pulsation, feel a little further down and out to see if it is still palpable. Continue until it is no longer palpable. Go back to the furthest point down and out at which you felt the cardiac impulse. This is the apex beat.

3 **Decide on the character of the cardiac impulse**. While doing this you should also be deciding if the cardiac impulse character is normal or abnormal. If abnormal

> ### CASE 4.21
>
> **Problem**. I can't feel the cardiac impulse. Why might this be?
>
> **Discussion**. In 50% of patients, the cardiac impulse is not detectable—so don't panic. There are a number of reasons for this (the first two are the most common):
>
> - **Obesity**. The subcutaneous fat masks the cardiac impulse.
> - **Emphysema**. In this condition the lungs overinflate, increasing the barrier between the hand and the heart.
> - **Pericardial effusion**. Fluid in the pericardial sac.
> - **Dextrocardia**. Occasionally the heart develops on the right side of the chest. Suspect this if when auscultating the heart, sounds get louder as you move away from the apex to the left sternal edge.

is it tapping, heaving, or thrusting? Does it last longer than normal (sustained)?

4 **Ascertain apex beat position**. First, decide on how lateral the apex beat is—whether the position you have found coincides with the midclavicular line (normal), the anterior axillary line, or the midaxillary line (both displaced). Next decide on the vertical level. This is done (in rather undignified fashion) by 'counting down the ribs'. Keep the fingers of your right hand over the apex. Using your left hand, palpate for the manubriosternal (*man-oo-brio-stern-al*) angle. Palpate the intercostal space next to this. This is the second intercostal space. Now, by palpating the ribs, count down the intercostal spaces. When you reach the fifth space palpate laterally along it and so decide if the apex beat coincides with this or another intercostal space. This may feel very clumsy, particularly in women, but keep practising. However, many experienced physicians have made their minds up on the apex beat position before they have counted down the ribs. When you have palpated enough normal apex beats, you will get a feel for when its position is abnormal—without counting down.

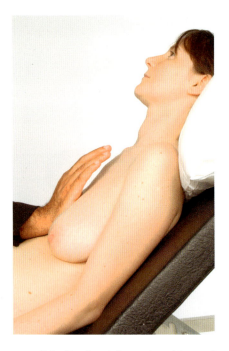

Figure 4.20 Palpating for a left parasternal heave. Press the heel of your right hand on the chest to the left of the sternum.

Tip
A tapping apex beat represents a palpable first heart sound. If you do not hear a loud first heart sound on auscultation, reconsider whether you really felt a tapping apex. Similarly, decisions on whether the cardiac impulse is sustained or whether it is heaving or thrusting are quite subtle. Consider your other signs before deciding on these nuances. Thus, if you have found other signs of aortic regurgitation, you are likely to be correct if you felt the cardiac impulse was thrusting and non-sustained.

5 **Palpate for left parasternal impulse**. Next, place the heel of your hand (fingers pointing upwards) over the praecordium, just to the left of the sternum (Fig. 4.20). Normally, you will feel the movement of respiration. If a left parasternal impulse is present the heel of your hand is lifted with each heartbeat (this is sometimes described as a left parasternal heave).

6 **Palpate for thrills**. Now, palpate the pulmonary area with the index, middle, and ring fingers of your right hand, then the aortic area in the same way. Any thrill will be felt as a vibration like a cat purring.

Tip
A thrill represents a palpable murmur. If you do not hear a loud murmur on auscultation, reconsider whether you really felt a thrill.

Percussion
You may have noticed that percussion has been omitted from this cardiovascular system routine. In the past, percussing out 'cardiac dullness' was used as a method of determining heart size. This was unreliable and has been superseded by the chest radiograph. Hence it is no longer used.

Key point
● Do not percuss over the heart.

Auscultation of the heart

14 Auscultate (DF 8/10) while palpating carotid pulse to time any murmur.

Initially, auscultation (*os-cull-tay-shun*) of the heart will seem like a new language. This is not helped by the myriad rare or trivial abnormalities described—e.g. split heart sounds and the like—which may be heard on auscultation. However, with practice, auscultation becomes one of the easier parts of clinical examination. In the pages that follow, the most important abnormalities are highlighted. Four areas are discussed:

- a description of the normal heart sounds;
- a description of various abnormal noises that may occur;
- a routine for auscultating the heart;
- an action plan on how to decide what you are hearing.

The stethoscope was invented by the French physician Rene Laennac in 1816. Before its introduction, physicians placed their ears directly on the chest to auscultate the heart. Your stethoscope has two settings: a 'bell' and a 'diaphragm' (Fig. 4.21). The bell is better for listening to very low-pitched sounds. It should be pressed only very lightly on the skin—otherwise it actually acts like a diaphragm. The diaphragm is for listening to higher-pitched sounds—though even these are usually quite low pitched.

Normality

There are normally two heart sounds, called the first and second heart sounds. The first heart sound results from the closure of the mitral and tricuspid valves (which happen at about the same time). The second heart sound results from the closure of the aortic and pulmonary valves (which again happen at about the same time).

There are various ways of denoting the heart sounds. The first heart sound may be written HS1, S1, or I. The second heart sound may be written HS2, S2, or II. The time after S1 until S2 is in time with systole. From S2 to S1 is in time with diastole.

Which heart sound is which?

- The heart sounds come in pairs, with S1 first and S2 second. This is because systole is normally shorter than diastole (Fig. 4.22). During a tachycardia, diastole shortens and it becomes more difficult to detect the pairings.

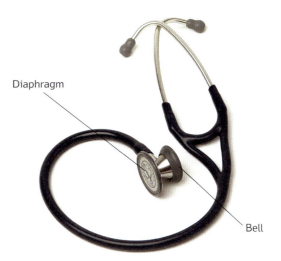

Figure 4.21 A stethoscope. New stethoscopes have just one ending which functions as either bell or diaphragm depending on pressure applied.

- S1 is lower pitched than S2. S1 gives a 'lubb' sound and S2 gives a 'dup' sound: 'lubb–dup'.

Splitting of S2

This is a normal finding. You should understand what it is about, but hearing it is difficult and not essential. Both heart sounds result from the shutting of two separate valves. Very rarely—and to the skilled ear only—it may be possible to detect splitting of S1. Splitting of S2, though still a difficult finding, may be easier to hear, especially when the patient is breathing in. Inspiration decreases intra-thoracic pressure and so increases peripheral venous return. The right side of the heart takes longer to fill and thus longer to contract—so that pulmonary valve closure is delayed. Thus in inspiration it may be possible to hear a split S2. This is best heard in the pulmonary area. This 'extra' sound after S2 is sometimes known as P2.

Abnormal ausculatory findings

Altered heart sounds

- **Loud S1**. Occurs in mitral stenosis. Although the mitral valve is narrowed, when it shuts, it does so suddenly, producing a loud first heart sound. It shuts suddenly because the valve is stiff and does not close at the end of diastole as it should. As the ventricle contracts, the chordae tendinae tense and force it suddenly shut.

```
S1 ------ S2 ----------- S1 ------- S2 ------------ S1 ------ S2 ------------ S1 ------- S2
   systole    diastole      systole    diastole      systole    diastole      systole
```

Figure 4.22 The first and second heart sounds.

- **Soft S1**. Occurs in mitral regurgitation, because the mitral valve does not close completely.
- **Soft S2**. Occurs in calcific aortic stenosis because of reduced valve movement.
- **Wide fixed splitting of S2**. Occurs in atrial septal defect. The left-to-right shunt increases right heart work so right ventricular filling is delayed—resulting in a wide split. It is 'fixed' in that the split does not vary with respiration—unlike the normal splitting of S2. This is because the two atria communicate, equalizing pressure in both throughout respiration.
- **Prosthetic heart sounds**. Metallic artificial valves produce clicking heart sounds, which are often audible without the stethoscope. Prostheses vary, but metallic mitral valves usually produce a loud S1 and a loud 'opening snap' (which occurs after S2.) Metallic aortic valves usually produce a loud S2 and an 'ejection click' after S1 (as well as an ejection systolic murmur). Artificial tissue valves produce relatively normal heart sounds.

Extra heart sounds

- **Third heart sound (S3)**. This is a low-pitched sound best heard with the bell at the mitral area. It comes just after S2, giving the impression of a double-beat S2. The exact mechanism of the third heart sound is unclear. It occurs in the early period of diastole when diastolic filling is most rapid. Two factors seem to be important in its production: unusually rapid diastolic flow and a non-compliant ventricle. S3 is often a normal physiological finding in healthy young people and pregnant women who have a large stroke volume resulting in particularly rapid diastolic flow. The most important pathological cause is left ventricular failure. Here S3 occurs despite a reduced stroke volume. The left ventricle is stiff and in some way this results in S3 at the time of rapid diastolic flow. Other causes include mitral regurgitation and aortic regurgitation—in these, increased stroke volume is the cause.
- **Fourth heart sound (S4)**. This is also a low-pitched sound and like S3 is best heard with the bell at the mitral area. It occurs just before S1, giving the impression of a double-beat S1. S4 is produced at the time of atrial contraction when a sudden bolus of blood contacts the stiff ventricle. It is never normal—occurring in conditions with a non-compliant ventricle—aortic stenosis, systemic hypertension, congestive cardiac failure, and hypertrophic obstructive cardiomyopathy.

The addition of either S3 or S4 to the normal heart sounds results in a 'triple rhythm'. This is also known as a gallop rhythm if in combination with the tachycardia of heart failure. If both occur together, as in cardiac failure, this may be called a summation gallop. It should be noted that both S3 and S4 are difficult to hear. Research studies have shown that even cardiologists often disagree on their presence.

Additional noises

- **Opening snap**. Opening of the mitral valve is normally not audible. In mitral stenosis there is elevated left atrial pressure, which causes forceful opening of the mitral valve. This results in a high-pitched 'opening snap' after the second heart sound, best heard at the mitral area or tricuspid area with the diaphragm (as the mitral stenosis progresses and the valve stiffens and calcifies, the opening snap may become quieter and disappear).
- **Aortic ejection click**. Similarly, opening of the aortic valve is normally not audible. However, if the cusps are abnormal, as occurs in congenital bicuspid aortic stenosis, aortic valve opening may be audible as an 'ejection click' just after the first heart sound; this is best heard in the aortic area. The 'click' precedes the aortic stenosis murmur.
- **Midsystolic click**. This occurs in mitral valve prolapse. Mitral valve prolapse involves a 'floppy' mitral valve prolapsing into the atrium during systole. If the prolapse is severe, there is also an element of regurgitation. The 'midsystolic click' arises at the point when the prolapsing mitral valve leaflet has reached the full extent of its prolapse. Interestingly, a midsystolic click may also occur in left-sided pneumothorax. The cause is unclear but it may result from contact and separation of the pleural surfaces in synchrony with the heartbeat.

Murmurs

Murmurs result from turbulent flow in the heart. Such turbulent flow may be due to rapid flow in a normal heart (innocent flow murmur) or turbulent flow in an abnormal heart. Murmurs have a blowing quality and are quite prolonged compared to the short-lived banging qualities of heart sounds. Murmurs are normally classified according to their timing in the cardiac cycle, so there are two main categories—systolic and diastolic.

The murmur may be described further by

- its exact timing
- the site at which it is best heard
- where else it radiates to
- any procedures which accentuate it
- its pitch
- its loudness.

Loudness is graded as:

- grade 1—just audible with patient's breath held
- grade 2—quiet
- grade 3—quite loud
- grade 4—loud enough to have accompanying thrill
- grade 5—very loud
- grade 6—can be heard without a stethoscope.

It is important to point out, though, that the loudness often does not relate to the severity of the lesion. Thus, a small ventricular septal defect (VSD) causes much more turbulence than a large VSD and so produces a much louder sound. Similarly, as aortic stenosis worsens, left ventricular failure develops and cardiac output is reduced. This results in decreased flow across the damaged valve so the murmur gets quieter. However, in mitral and aortic regurgitation, the intensity of the murmur usually increases with the severity of the pathology.

Systolic murmurs are of three main types: pansystolic, ejection systolic, and late systolic. Below, their individual characteristics are discussed, though in practice, distinction can be very difficult.

- **Pansystolic murmurs**. These are heard throughout systole. They are more or less uniform in intensity throughout systole—thus usually producing a gentle, blowing quality. The most common cause is mitral regurgitation where the mitral valve cannot close fully. It remains open during systole so blood flows backwards across the mitral valve when the left ventricle contracts. The murmur of mitral regurgitation is best heard at the mitral area but may radiate all over the praecordium. It may radiate to the axilla.

- **Ejection systolic murmurs**. Here the murmur does not start immediately after S1. When it does begin, it builds up intensity before reducing—described as 'crescendo–decrescendo'. This tends to result in a harsher quality. The most important cause is aortic stenosis. Here, there is turbulent flow across the stenosed aortic valve during left ventricular ejection. Left ventricular ejection starts after the aortic valve opens—just after S1. Thus the murmur does not start immediately after S1. The murmur of aortic stenosis is usually best heard in the aortic area though in patients with calcific aortic stenosis, the murmur may be loudest at the mitral area. Either way, the murmur may be heard all over the praecordium and sometimes radiates to the carotids in the neck. If you hear a murmur-like sound over the carotids but no heart murmur, you should consider a 'carotid bruit' as an alternative. This is a very similar sound but is often caused by narrowing of the carotid artery. Such a narrowing is an important cause of stroke disease. Other common causes of ejection systolic murmurs are innocent flow murmur and aortic sclerosis. Innocent flow murmurs are not pathological. They are due to rapid flow through normal valves and occur especially in children and young adults. They are quiet and often have a musical tone. Aortic sclerosis is a condition seen in older people; the aortic valve is thickened but not stenosed. The murmur is similar to aortic stenosis, but it does not usually radiate to the carotids.

- **Late systolic murmurs**. These begin late in systole. The most common cause is mitral valve prolapse. If the prolapse is severe, there is also an element of regurgitation, so resulting in a late systolic murmur. Hypertrophic obstructive cardiomyopathy may cause damage to the papillary muscle and consequent mitral regurgitation, resulting in a late systolic murmur.

Diastolic murmurs are of two main types: early and mid-diastolic. Diastolic murmurs are always abnormal.

- **Early diastolic murmurs**. An early diastolic murmur has a high-pitched quality. It begins loudly and quickly gets quieter. The most common cause is aortic regurgitation. Here, the murmur occurs because of retrograde leakage of blood through the regurgitant aortic valve. The pressure in the aorta is highest at the beginning of diastole and then falls, resulting in a murmur that is initially loud but then becomes quieter. The murmur of aortic regurgitation is best heard at the left sternal edge with the patient sitting up and breath held in expiration (this is how the aortic valve is brought closest to the stethoscope).

- **Mid-diastolic murmurs**. A mid-diastolic murmur starts later in diastole. It has a low-pitched 'rumbling' quality and is best heard with the bell. The key cause is mitral stenosis. Blood normally flows across the mitral valve during filling of the left ventricle in diastole. This starts after the mitral valve opens shortly after S2. Thus the turbulent flow of mitral stenosis begins in the middle period of diastole. In theory, when atrial contraction occurs near the end of diastole, flow across the mitral valve will increase, resulting in a louder murmur—so-called 'presystolic accentuation'. Almost always, though, mitral stenosis is associated with atrial fibrillation so there is no atrial contraction—and no presystolic accentuation. The murmur of mitral stenosis is best heard at the mitral area with the patient lying slightly on their left side to bring the mitral valve closest to the stethoscope. It is rare to hear it other than at the mitral area.

Pericardial friction rub

This is a sign of acute pericarditis. It is a scratching sound that may be heard in systole or diastole. It is best heard at the left sternal edge with the patient sitting up and holding their breath in expiration. Like the pain of pericarditis, it may vary from hour to hour. The rub is thought to be due to the inflamed visceral and parietal pericardial sacs rubbing against each another—and so should not occur in the presence of a pericardial effusion. However, one study has shown that a rub is just as likely to occur in the presence of a pericardial effusion.

The auscultation routine

There is no consensus on what constitutes the correct auscultation routine. Any routine should take account of the fact that while a loud sound may be heard all over the praecordium, a quiet sound may be heard only at particular places using particular techniques. The routine on the next page achieves this in a quick but thorough way. Throughout this routine, if you hear what you think are abnormal sounds you should time them by feeling the carotid pulse—which is synchronous with the onset of systole.

Tip

Overall auscultation should take no more than 2 minutes. Spend 40 seconds on the mitral area and the rest elsewhere.

Tip

Sometimes breath sounds may make it very difficult for you to hear the heart: if need be, ask the patient to hold their breath for a few seconds.

1 Listen over the mitral area with the diaphragm. If you hear a systolic murmur, move the stethoscope to the axilla and listen there too. Systolic murmurs of all types may be heard here, so hearing a murmur in this area does not clinch a diagnosis. However, the pansystolic murmur of mitral regurgitation is usually louder here than in the aortic area. The opposite applies to the ejection systolic murmur of aortic stenosis. The opening snap of mitral stenosis may also be heard here. The pansystolic murmur of mitral regurgitation may radiate into the axilla (ejection systolic murmur does not usually), so if you hear a systolic murmur here, then edge your way with the diaphragm into the axilla, listening to see if it radiates there.

2 Next, ask the patient to roll over slightly on to their left side and listen over the mitral area with the bell at the apex (Fig. 4.23). This is the ideal method for auscultating the low-pitched mid-diastolic murmur of mitral stenosis. S3 and S4 are also best heard here with the bell.

3 Ask the patient to roll back to a straight position. Listen over the tricuspid area with the bell. This is the position for the mid-diastolic murmur of tricuspid stenosis.

4 Listen over the tricuspid area with the diaphragm. This is the best position for the pansystolic murmurs of tricuspid regurgitation, pericardial friction rubs, and innocent flow murmurs. The opening snap of mitral stenosis may also be heard here.

5 Listen over the pulmonary area with the diaphragm (best place for pulmonary murmurs). Note that there is no specific role for listening with the bell at the pulmonary area.

6 Listen over the aortic area with the diaphragm (Fig. 4.24). This is the best place for ejection systolic murmurs of aortic stenosis and aortic sclerosis—although occasionally these are better heard at the mitral area). Note that there is no specific role for listening with the bell at the aortic area.

7 Listen over the right, then the left carotid with the diaphragm (listening for (1) radiation of a murmur to the carotids, a feature of aortic stenosis (not sclerosis) and (2) carotid bruits).

8 Ask the patient to sit forward, breathe in, breathe out, and then hold their breath (without taking another breath in) and listen with the diaphragm at the lower left sternal edge (Fig. 4.25). This accentuates the murmur

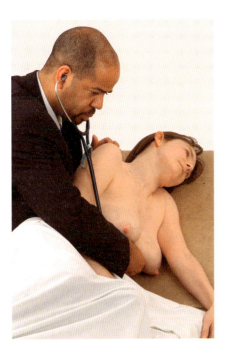

Figure 4.23 Auscultating for the murmur of mitral stenosis.

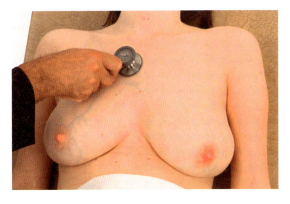

Figure 4.24 Auscultating over the aortic area with the diaphragm.

of aortic regurgitation. Let the patient know they can breathe again before moving on.

Tip

Do not listen too long here or the patient will collapse.

9 With the patient still sitting up, listen with the diaphragm at the lung bases at the back. Here you are

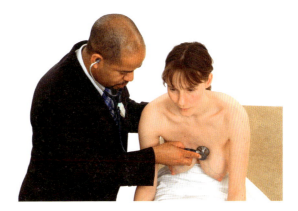

Figure 4.25 Auscultating for the murmur of aortic regurgitation. Listen with the breath held in expiration.

listening for the fine, late inspiratory crackles of left ventricular failure.

Tip

Most valvular lesions can produce murmurs audible all over the praecordium. Thus a murmur at the pulmonary area does not guarantee pulmonary valve pathology. However, if this is the only place it is heard, it makes the pulmonary valve the likely candidate.

An action plan for auscultation

Initially, auscultation may seem like a new language, but do not be put off! Your first priority should be to get to grips with normal heart sounds. Then, learn how to recognize a loud first heart sound and the murmurs of aortic stenosis, aortic regurgitation, mitral stenosis, and mitral regurgitation. Thankfully, these abnormalities are not only the most important findings, they are also the easiest. Ideally, you should also be able to hear an opening snap and third and fourth heart sounds.

You should have a reasonable stethoscope costing around £40–60. The £10 stethoscopes are clearly inferior. The £120+ 'cardiology' stethoscopes are only slightly better than the £40 ones—but much more annoying to lose.

The two normal heart sounds, S1 and S2, are best heard at the mitral and tricuspid areas with the diaphragm. Note that they may be very quiet, particularly in the aortic and pulmonary areas and particularly in patients with hyperinflated chests, as in emphysema. Furthermore, the heart sounds become quieter with age. To distinguish S1 from S2 remember that because systole is normally shorter than diastole, the heart sounds seem to come in pairs with S1 first and S2 second. Also, S1 is a lower-pitched sound—'lubb' than S2—'dupp'.

Having mastered the normal, your next test is to unravel the abnormal.

1 **Detecting an abnormality**. First, you need to hear that something is wrong. How easy this is depends on the actual abnormality:

- loud or soft S1 or S2 (DF 3/10)
- extra 'bumps'—S3, S4, opening snap, clicks (DF 8/10)
- systolic murmur (DF 4/10)
- diastolic murmur (DF 9/10).

('Bump' is the author's own term, not to be repeated in front of experts.)

Your other physical findings should put you on the alert for particular auscultatory findings. For example, if you have found a collapsing pulse you should listen very carefully for the early diastolic murmur of aortic regurgitation.

2 **If there is an abnormality, take a moment to decide if S1 and S2 are normal**. This is normally quite easy (DF 3/10) but may be more difficult if there is a loud murmur.

For each abnormality you must decide 3–6.

3 **Is the abnormality a 'bump' or a murmur? (DF 2/10)**. The various 'bumps'—heart sounds, clicks, and snaps—all have a short, banging quality, as opposed to the prolonged blowing quality of murmurs, making this an easy decision.

4 **If it is a 'bump', what is it? (DF 6/10)**. To decide, you need to make up your mind

- which area you hear the 'bump'
- whether it is best heard with the bell or diaphragm
- whether it is high or low pitched
- most importantly, what is its timing in the cycle.

So, having decided on these factors, does your abnormal sound fit with any of the common 'bumps'?

- S3—low pitched, heard with bell at the mitral area or left sternal edge, just after S2—making S2 sound like a double beat
- S4—low pitched, heard with bell at the mitral area or left sternal edge, just before S1—making S1 sound like a double beat

- opening snap—high-pitched, heard with diaphragm at mitral or tricuspid areas, just after S2.

5 **If it is a murmur, is it systolic or diastolic? (DF 6/10)**. Because murmurs can make S1 and S2 difficult to hear, this is best decided by timing the murmur against the carotid pulse (DF 8/10). Less scientific but helpful are the facts that systolic murmurs are much more common and are usually easier to hear than diastolic murmurs and that diastolic murmurs are often heard only when using one specific method.

6 **If it is a diastolic murmur, is it mitral stenosis or aortic regurgitation? (DF 4/10)**. There are only two important diastolic murmurs and because one of them, the mid-diastolic murmur of mitral stenosis, is so specific in its site and pitch, it is easy to differentiate this from the other—the early diastolic murmur of aortic regurgitation. The mid-diastolic murmur of mitral stenosis is heard only at the mitral area; it is a low-pitched 'rumbling' sound, best heard with the bell and with the patient lying on their left side. The early diastolic murmur of aortic regurgitation is best heard with the diaphragm at the left sternal edge with the patient sitting up and breath held in expiration. If you hear it in other areas, it will always be audible at the left sternal edge too.

7 **If it is a systolic murmur, what are its characteristics? (DF 9/10)**

- Where does it occur in systole? Is it ejection systolic, pansystolic or late systolic? (DF 9/10)
- Where on the praecordium is it heard best? (DF 3/10)
- Does it radiate? (DF 4/10)
- Do any procedures accentuate it?
- What is its pitch?
- How loud is it?

It is usually easy to say where a murmur is best heard and where it radiates to. It is more difficult to decide its exact timing. To ascertain this, you have to decide the following: Is there a gap between S1 and the murmur? Is the murmur uniform or 'crescendo–decrescendo'? Using 1–6, you should be able to describe the murmur.

8 **Presenting your findings**. Always start by mentioning the heart sounds, whether they are abnormal or normal, and then describe any extra sounds: 'first and second heart sounds are normal, there were no other abnormal sounds' or 'the first heart sound was loud with a normal second heart sound, followed by an opening snap and there was a quiet, low-pitched, mid-diastolic

murmur heard with the bell at the mitral area and with the patient on their left side'.

Peripheral oedema

15 Palpate for ankle or shin oedema over lower anterior tibia (DF 3/10).

Why test for ankle oedema in cardiovascular examination?

Peripheral oedema is a common symptom and sign of heart failure, hence its inclusion in the cardiovascular routine. However, it is caused by many other conditions—the most common being postural oedema exacerbated by incompetent venous valves (Table 4.3).

Pathogenesis of peripheral oedema in heart failure

For many years it was thought that increased venous pressure in heart failure caused increased capillary pressure and consequent leakage across the capillary. Thus, it was said that if the JVP was not raised, then any oedema present was not cardiac. However, it is now clear that the degree of cardiac oedema does not correlate with the venous pressure: cardiac oedema need not be associated with a raised JVP.

Instead, it is fluid overload that is the cause of cardiac oedema—but what causes this? The full answer to this is complex and beyond the scope of this book. However, fluid overload is at least partly related to changes in renal blood flow in cardiac failure, which result in increased renin (*ree-nin*), aldosterone (*al-dough-steer-own*), and vasopressin (*vay-zo-press-in*) production. The consequent sodium and water retention results in fluid overload.

Key points

- Practise to get a sense of normality.
- The normal heart sounds come in pairs: S1 and S2.
- Hearing S3 and S4 is tricky.
- Know the basic murmurs: pansystolic murmur in mitral regurgitation; ejection systolic murmur in aortic stenosis; early diastolic murmur in aortic regurgitation; mid-diastolic murmur in mitral stenosis.
- Do not waste time looking for the perfect routine that will satisfy everyone—it does not exist!
- The key to auscultation is timing; this is best done by palpating the carotid pulse, which is in time with the onset of systole.
- Your other physical findings prior to auscultation may point towards certain diagnoses, the murmur of which you should listen particularly attentively for.
- Systolic murmurs are easy to hear but it is more difficult to decide exactly which type they are.
- 'Bumps' and diastolic murmurs are more difficult to hear but once heard it is usually quite easy to say which type they are.

What is pitting oedema?

Oedema caused by fluid with low protein content (as in heart failure) will indent quickly on pressing (within 2–3 seconds) producing a pit within the subcutaneous tissues—pitting oedema. It is sometimes taught that oedema caused by more proteinaceous fluid as in lymphatic obstruction by a tumour does not indent—non-pitting oedema. However, when such lymphoedema is new, it will usually indent if pressed on for a longer period. As the lymphoedema becomes chronic, it fibroses and hardens and will no longer pit. See Case 4.22 for another cause of non-pitting swelling of the legs.

How to examine (DF 4/10)

Although usually described as 'ankle' oedema it is actually the shin that is examined. Palpating for oedema may be

CASE 4.22

Problem. My patient is overweight. Could her leg swelling simply be due to fat?

Discussion. Certain factors point towards leg swelling being due to fat: (1) the foot is relatively spared from swelling; (2) the swelling does not pit.

painful, so be careful and watch the patient's face while doing so.

1 Ask permission to examine the patient's legs. You may also have to remove bedclothes to get at the shin.

2 Press your thumb down on the medial aspect of the patient's shin **gently** for 5 seconds. Watch the patient's face as you press—swollen legs can be tender.

3 Lift your thumb: does the indentation persist (pit) for a few seconds (Fig. 4.26)? If so, there is oedema and it is likely due to low-protein fluid. If not, press again for 30 seconds. Lift your thumb again. Does the indentation now persist? If so, the oedema is likely due to fluid with higher protein content.

4 If oedema is present, you should find the level at which the oedema stops. This may be above the knee and the oedema may even progress to the skin of the abdominal wall.

....

Tip

In a patient known to have heart failure, the degree of oedema gives useful information on the progress of treatment. Thus, in hospitals, patients with peripheral oedema secondary to heart failure often have their weight recorded regularly to monitor progress.

....

Key points

- Ankle oedema is tested for over the shin.
- Ankle oedema is a sign of heart failure but also occurs in many other situations.

Other cardiovascular signs

16 Consider looking for other signs such as radiofemoral delay and pulsatile liver.

As mentioned previously, the cardiovascular system routine is an abbreviation of all possible cardiovascular signs. Some cardiovascular signs normally omitted from the routine are discussed in the next pages.

Blood pressure measurement

The most important of these other cardiovascular signs is blood pressure measurement—and I do not understand why this is not routinely required when examining the cardiovascular system.

What is blood pressure?

Blood pressure is the pressure exerted by the flow of blood in the main arteries. It varies through the cardiac cycle, being highest in systole and lowest in diastole (Fig. 4.1). Until recently blood pressure was usually measured with a machine that used mercury and so it is usually expressed in terms of millimetres of mercury (mmHg).

The systolic blood pressure is normally given first, followed by the diastolic blood pressure. If a patient has a systolic blood pressure of 120 mmHg and a diastolic blood pressure of 80 mmHg, this is written as 120/80 mmHg and expressed as '120 over 80'. Although expressed as a fraction, the reading is not used as a fraction. The difference between the two (120 − 80 = 40 mmHg) is known as the pulse pressure.

What is a normal blood pressure?

There is no easy answer to this question. What represents low blood pressure (hypotension) for an individual

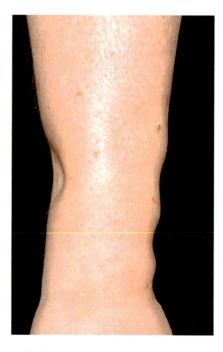

Figure 4.26 Testing for ankle oedema. Press on medial aspect of lower shin.

depends on their normal blood pressure. Thus, a blood pressure of 110/70 is hypotensive in a patient with a normal blood pressure of 180/110. However, a systolic blood pressure less than 80 mmHg is rarely normal and usually indicates serious hypotension.

Hypertension (high blood pressure) is commonly defined as a blood pressure **persistently** greater than 140/90 mmHg. Hypertension is a diagnosis, therefore, that can only be made after several consultations and blood pressure measurements.

Significance

Blood pressure measurement is an absolutely essential part of examining acutely unwell patients in whom low blood pressure is a critical finding. Hypotension may be caused by many illnesses but the most common are myocardial ischaemia/infarction, sepsis, and hypovolaemia secondary to bleeding. High blood pressure (hypertension) is an important risk factor for ischaemic heart disease and cerebrovascular disease.

The principle of blood pressure measurement

To measure arterial blood pressure directly would require an intra-arterial catheter connected to a pressure-measuring device! A more convenient indirect method makes use of a sphygmomanometer (*sfig-mow-man-om-meter*) (Fig. 4.27). This consists of a tourniquet (*tour-knee-kay*) with an inflatable cuff connected to a balloon (to inflate the tourniquet) and a pressure-measuring device. In the past the pressure was measured using a column of mercury. Because of concern with mercury toxicity, mercury sphygmomanometers are being replaced by aneroid sphygmomanometers.

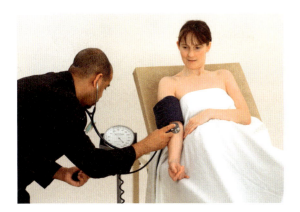

Figure 4.27 Checking blood pressure by auscultation. Tourniquet inflated, diaphragm over the brachial artery.

The tourniquet with inflatable cuff is tied around the upper arm and inflated. Once the pressure in the tourniquet is higher than that in the brachial artery, arterial blood flow is occluded. Then, as the pressure in the cuff is reduced, brachial artery flow returns, but initially this occurs only momentarily at the point at which arterial blood pressure is at its highest. As the cuff pressure is further reduced, blood flow occurs throughout more and more of the cardiac cycle—until cuff pressure is less than the lowest diastolic pressure and blood flow is continuous throughout the cardiac cycle.

If you auscultate with the stethoscope over the brachial artery during this procedure, you will hear various noises, known as Korotkoff (*core-rot-cough*) sounds (*Nikolai Sergeievichj Korotkoff (1874–1920), Russian surgeon*). These are divided into five phases as the cuff pressure is reduced. In phase I, there is a thudding sound in time with the heartbeat. The thud is due to the short-lived flow of blood at the height of systole. Phase I signifies the systolic blood pressure. As the cuff pressure reduces, the sounds first increase in intensity (phase II), before gradually reducing (phase III) (phases II and III are of no practical significance). When the cuff pressure is less than the diastolic pressure and blood flow occurs throughout the whole cardiac cycle, the sounds quieten quite suddenly (phase IV) before stopping completely (phase V). Sometimes, though, the sounds never stop completely—there is no phase V. There is some debate over whether phase IV or phase V should be used as the diastolic pressure. Although phase IV is a more accurate estimation of diastolic blood pressure, phase V produces more consistent readings when taken by different individuals (less interobserver variation) and is therefore preferred. If the sounds never stop completely, phase IV is used.

A less accurate method for measuring the systolic blood pressure is to palpate the radial pulse during cuff inflation and deflation. The point at which the pulse disappears and reappears is roughly the systolic pressure (the diastolic pressure cannot be gauged by palpation).

How to measure blood pressure

1 Patient should be relaxed, laid down for 5 minutes (see Case 4.23 for exception). The patient's arm should be straight, uncovered, and relaxed, either lying on the bed or held by you. It is reasonable to roll the patient's sleeve up but only if this does not impinge on the tourniquet. Otherwise, the shirt sleeve must be removed.

CASE 4.23

Problem. My patient looks unwell. Can I afford to wait 5 minutes to take their blood pressure (allowing the patient to relax)?

Solution. No, in such a patient your main concern is hypotension. Waiting 5 minutes is only important when assessing for high blood pressure.

CASE 4.24

Problem. My patient's blood pressure is very high but I'm not sure if the cuff is working properly. He's a very big man.

Discussion. The pressure exerted by the inflatable cuff on the brachial artery depends not only on the amount of air in it but also on the size of the patient's arm. Thus, a normal adult cuff will exert an excessively high pressure on a child's brachial artery, producing an artificially low reading—the converse applies to overweight patients. So there are a variety of cuff sizes to suit different patients—neonate, child, normal adult, and obese adult.

2 Tie the tourniquet around the arm with its lower border 2 cm from the antecubital fossa and with the centre of the inflatable cuff over the brachial artery. There is often an arrow at the centre of the cuff. The brachial artery is positioned roughly one-third of the way across the antecubital fossa on the medial side. The cuff should be roughly at the patient's heart level—it usually is.

3 First, check the blood pressure by palpation:
- palpate the radial pulse;
- inflate the cuff by squeezing the balloon—watch the sphygmomanometer dial rising, indicating the cuff pressure;
- feel the point at which the radial pulse disappears—this is the blood pressure by palpation.

4 Now, check blood pressure by auscultation (Fig. 4.27):
- deflate the cuff (to allow the patient's arm to recover)
- then, reinflate the cuff to a pressure 20 mmHg higher than the blood pressure by palpation

CASE 4.25

Problem. I hear a phase I sound but, on further listening, it disappears. Why might this happen?

Discussion. This may be because the patient is in atrial fibrillation. Here the systolic blood pressure varies with each beat.

CASE 4.26

Problem. I keep hearing a rustling noise, which doesn't seem to relate to the point at which the radial pulse disappears. Why is this?

Discussion. This is likely to be caused by you inadvertently moving your stethoscope. Keep it still!

CASE 4.27

Problem. My patient looks very unwell, the nurses are looking worried, and my blood pressure skills have deserted me. I can't hear the blood pressure. What's going on? What else could I try?

Discussion. The patient's blood pressure is probably very low (less than 80 mmHg). In such situations, taking the blood pressure is difficult and it is often easier to palpate using the radial pulse than to auscultate.

- place the diaphragm of the stethoscope on the brachial artery and auscultate
- now deflate the cuff 5 mmHg at a time
- ascertain the points at which you first hear heart sounds (phase I), at which the sounds become muffled (phase IV), and at which the sounds disappear (phase V).

5 The blood pressure is described to the nearest 5 mmHg as phase I over phase V, such as 120/85 mmHg—'120 over 85 millimetres of mercury'. Phase IV is used if there is no phase V. See Cases 4.24, 4.25, 4.26, and 4.27 for issues concerning blood pressure measurement.

Tip

Measuring blood pressure can hurt, especially in frail patients. Do not dither too long deciding exactly what the systolic blood pressure is with the tourniquet at high pressure.

Tip

Ask the patient if they felt dizzy when they stood up. In some patients with postural hypotension, the fall in blood pressure is very brief and you may have missed it by the time you get a reading. If the patient admits to transient dizziness on standing it is worth trying again and rechecking lying and standing blood pressures.

Postural blood pressure measurement

Normally, when a person stands up, their blood pressure alters a little: the systolic blood pressure falls by around 3 mmHg while the diastolic blood pressure rises by around 5 mmHg. A fall in systolic blood pressure greater than 20 mmHg on standing is arbitrarily defined as postural hypotension. Such a blood pressure reduction occurs in 25% of patients over 75 years and is often asymptomatic. However, some patients may be symptomatic, that is, become dizzy on standing. Causes depend on whether this is a recurrent or a one-off phenomenon. Recurrent postural hypotension is most commonly caused by drugs, particularly diuretics (causing chronic hypovolaemia) and vasodilators such as nitrates. Acute postural hypotension has the same causes as hypotension itself.

How to measure

1 Take blood pressure with patient lying down as normal.

2 Reduce cuff pressure to zero, but keep cuff on.

3 Stand the patient up and make sure they are steady.

4 Immediately, reinflate cuff to 5 mmHg above the lying systolic pressure and gradually reduce cuff pressure listening for the standing blood pressure.

5 Ask the patient to stay standing and repeat again in 2 minutes.

Key points

- Blood pressure measurement is an absolutely essential part of examining acutely unwell patients.
- The diagnosis of hypertension (high blood pressure) should only be made after a series of blood pressure checks on different days.
- Blood pressure measurement is easy (DF 6/10) in patients with normal or high blood pressure, but difficult (DF 8/10) in those with very low blood pressure (systolic <80).
- Phase IV is a more accurate measure of diastolic pressure but phase V produces more consistent readings when taken by different people.
- Cuff size should vary depending on the individual.

Peripheral pulses

Significance

Both chronic ischaemia due to atherosclerosis (peripheral vascular disease) and acute ischaemia due to thrombosis or embolism are common conditions that need early identification, so it is important that you can palpate the peripheral pulses.

How to examine

Brachial artery (DF 6/10)

1 Use your thumb.

2 Locate the artery in the antecubital fossa about one-third of the way across on the medial (ulnar) side—just medial to biceps tendon.

Femoral (fem-uh-ral) artery (DF 7/10—more difficult in overweight patients)

1 The patient should be lying flat or almost flat.

2 Use your index and middle fingers together—pointing upwards and slightly medially.

3 Locate the femoral artery in the groin area, half way between the pubic tubercle and anterior superior iliac (eye-lee-yak or ill-lee-yak) crest.

Popliteal (pop-lit-tea-al) artery (DF 9/10)

1 Use both hands; the patient should be lying flat or almost flat.

2 Bend the patient's knee to 120°.

3 Put thumbs on either side of front of knee with fingers in the popliteal fossa palpating for the pulse.

Posterior tibial (tibby-al) artery (DF 6/10)

1 Use your index finger.

2 Inspect for pulsation behind the medial malleolus (it is often visible here).

3 Feel for pulsation behind the medial malleolus.

Dorsalis pedis (door-sallis-pee-diss)
artery (DF 9/10)

1 Use index and middle finger.

2 Locate dorsalis pedis, just lateral to the extensor hallucis tendon—about one-third of the way down the dorsum of the foot. Press down against the tarsal bones here (Fig. 4.28).

Radiofemoral delay (DF 9/10)

What is it?

This is a subtle sign only rarely seen. The femoral pulse is felt half way between the pubic tubercle and the anterior superior iliac spine. Normally, the radial and femoral pulses coincide in time; if the femoral pulse is delayed and appears to come after the radial pulse, this is 'radiofemoral delay'.

Significance

Radiofemoral delay is a sign of coarctation (*co-ark-tay-shun*) of the aorta. In this condition there is a stricture in the aortic arch distal to the left subclavian artery, so that blood flow to the arms is good, but flow to the legs is reduced. As well as radiofemoral delay, the femoral pulse is weaker than the radial pulse. Blood pressure is usually elevated. There is often a systolic murmur at the left sternal edge and a continuous (systolic and diastolic) murmur over the scapula.

How to examine

1 The femoral pulse is best located with the patient lying flat.

2 Palpate the right femoral pulse as above (with your right hand.)

3 Now palpate the right radial pulse with your left hand. Decide if the two pulses coincide in time, and if the femoral pulse is weak compared to the radial.

Your teacher may query why you have not included this in the routine. This is a moot point. It can be considered best to exclude it from the routine because it is so rarely present and because it requires poking in the patient's groin early on in the examination (a bit confusing for the patient, who expects you to listen to the heart). It is advised to check it in all patients with hypertension or in any patient in whom other features point to coarctation.

> ### Key points
> - Radiofemoral delay is a subtle sign.
> - It is seen in coarctation of the aorta—and should be checked for in all patients with hypertension.

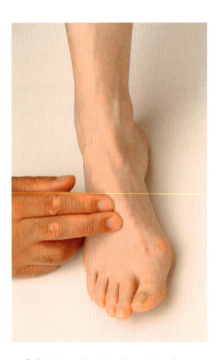

Figure 4.28 Palpating the dorsalis pedis pulse.

Sacral oedema (DF4/10.)

Generalized oedema collects in the lowest dependent site due to gravity. Normally, this site is the feet and ankles but in bed-bound patients the oedema collects around the sacrum. If present, sacral oedema is a more useful sign of generalized fluid overload than ankle oedema. This is because there are multiple causes of ankle oedema such as venous damage—whereas sacral oedema has fewer causes.

1 Ask permission.

2 Sit patient forward.

3 Press over sacrum for 10 seconds (be aware of any tenderness).

4 Lift your thumb and observe for any indentation in the skin.

> ### Key point
> - Sacral oedema may occur in bed-bound patients; when present it is a more specific sign of heart failure than ankle oedema.

Pulsatile liver

This occurs in tricuspid regurgitation. Here, the tricuspid valve cannot shut fully so when the right ventricle contracts, blood refluxes into the superior vena cava into the jugular veins producing the giant V wave. Similarly, blood refluxes into the inferior vena cava and then into the hepatic vein—so causing the liver to pulsate. Also, because it is engorged with blood, the liver is enlarged. The pulsatile liver is examined for in the same way as the liver is normally examined (see Chapter 7).

1 The patient should be lying flat.
2 Palpate superficially over the right upper quadrant for a pulsation.
3 Then, assess for an enlarged liver: perform deep palpation starting in the right iliac fossa, moving superiorly to the right upper quadrant.

Wash your hands

17 Wash your hands.

Once you have finished your examination you must wash your hands. This simple measure will reduce the spread of infections among your patients, yet it is so easy to forget when you are learning new techniques or are trying hard to make sense of a case.

Presentation of findings

18 Now say 'I would like to check the blood pressure'. Pause briefly and then present findings.

Having felt for ankle oedema (and checked other signs as appropriate), stand up straight and say 'I would like to check the blood pressure'. The examiner will usually indicate that this is not necessary.

Then, start the presentation. The exact style of presentation depends on your findings. If your findings are compatible with a condition then start off by mentioning it:

'This woman has aortic stenosis as shown by a slow rising pulse, a heaving, sustained, non-displaced apex beat, and an ejection systolic murmur heard throughout the praecordium, loudest at the mitral area, radiating to both carotids. She is comfortable at rest, there is no clubbing or splinter haemorrhages, pulse was 62 per minute and regular, JVP was not raised, there were no abnormal heaves or thrills in the praecordium, and heart sounds were normal. There was no evidence of heart failure.'

If your findings are inconclusive, detail them, give a differential diagnosis and if this includes a valvular lesion, suggest an echocardiogram. The following presentation refers to the same patient:

'This woman is comfortable at rest, there is no clubbing or splinter haemorrhages. Pulse was 62 per minute and there was a regular sinus rhythm with a normal character. JVP was not elevated. There were no heaves or thrills. The apex beat is heaving and non-displaced. There is an ejection systolic murmur radiating to the carotids. The most likely diagnoses are aortic stenosis and aortic sclerosis and I feel an echocardiogram would be useful to decide.'

Here, the student has not identified the slow rising pulse but has made a highly acceptable presentation.

Tip
Do not forget to mention the blood pressure.

Key point
- If you are fairly sure of the diagnosis, mention it early in your presentation.

Cardiovascular diseases and investigations

In the earlier parts of this chapter, various medical conditions and investigations have been mentioned. In this section I now describe these. In general these descriptions are brief though certain selected topics are discussed in more detail.

Echocardiography

This is a 'heart scan'. It uses an ultrasound technique. An echo is especially useful for assessing valves and left ventricular systolic function.

Exercise test

This is used to diagnose and assess the severity of coronary artery disease. The patient is exercised, usually on a treadmill. They are monitored for symptoms of angina and ischaemia on the ECG.

Coronary angiogram

A coronary angiogram (*ann-jee-owe-gram*) is used to assess the coronary arteries for evidence of coronary artery disease. A cannula is inserted, usually into the femoral artery, and passed to the coronary arteries where dye is released to delineate the arteries.

Cardiac catheter

This involves direct assessment of the heart valves and pressures. Again, a cannula is inserted, usually into the femoral artery and passed to the heart.

Rheumatic fever

This is an acute illness resulting from an immunological reaction to group A β-haemolytic streptococcus (also known as *Streptococcus pyogenes* (*pie-oj-en-knees*)). Typically, the patient develops pharyngitis from which they recover. Then, around a month later, the patient develops various problems including fever, sweats, arthritis, and carditis. Although cardiac function is usually normal initially, there is healing with scarring, which may affect the valves. Around 25% of patients suffer long-term damage to their heart valves—the condition is then known as rheumatic heart disease. The mitral valve is most commonly affected (75%), followed by the aortic valve (50%), the tricuspid valve (10%), and the pulmonary valve (2%). Sydenham's chorea (*sid-en-ams-core-ear*) (St Vitus (*vie-tuss*) dance) is characterized by jerky, purposeless movements. It may occur as part of rheumatic fever or on its own. In either case, it may later result in rheumatic heart disease (*Thomas Sydenham (1642–1689), English physician*).

Infective endocarditis

This is infection of the heart valves or adjacent endocardium—usually resulting in valvular regurgitation. Previously infective endocarditis was divided into subacute bacterial endocarditis and acute bacterial endocarditis but in recent decades the distinction has become blurred. Furthermore, non-bacterial organisms have been implicated. Hence the simple term 'infective endocarditis'. The most common infecting organism is *Streptococcus viridans* (*viri-dans*), which is responsible for around 50% of cases.

Key points
- Rheumatic fever is an immunological reaction to infection by group A β-haemolytic streptococcus (*Streptococcus pyogenes*).
- 25% of patients suffer long-term damage to heart valves.
- Infective endocarditis is a direct infection of the heart—the most common infecting organism is *Streptococcus viridans* (α-haemolytic strep).

Streptococcus viridans refers to a group of α-haemolytic streptococci including *Streptococcus mitis* (*my-tiss*), *Streptococcus sanguis* (*sang-wiss*), *Streptococcus mutans* (*mute-anns*), and *Streptococcus millieri* (*milly-air-ee*).

Mitral stenosis

This is narrowing of the mitral valve.

Cause

Rheumatic heart disease is the only significant cause.

Pathophysiology

Narrowing of the mitral valve results in reduced left ventricular filling during diastole. The normal mitral valve area is 5 cm^2. If this reduces to 2.5 cm^2 or less, symptoms start to occur.

Features

See Fig. 4.29.

How do you measure the severity of mitral stenosis?

- Severity of symptoms.
- Length of murmur (reflects degree of left atrial hypertrophy). The longer the murmur, the more severe the stenosis.

Key point
- Signs of mitral stenosis: irregularly irregular pulse, malar flush, tapping cardiac impulse, loud first heart sound, mid-diastolic murmur, opening snap.

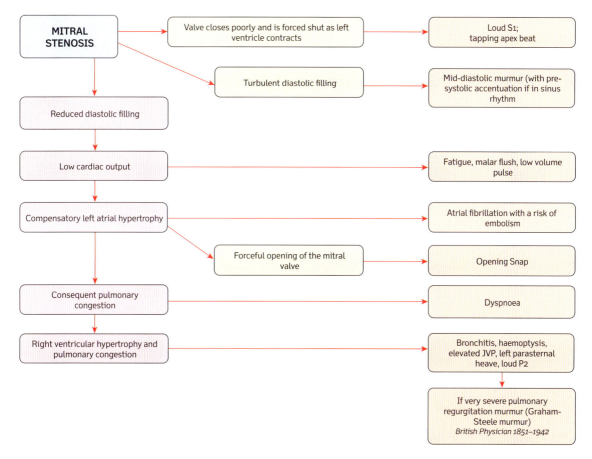

Figure 4.29 Features of mitral stenosis. Note that if the valve is calcified, as occurs with more severe disease, it becomes immobile. Thus S1 may not be loud and there is no opening snap.

- The time between S2 and opening snap (reflects degree of left atrial hypertrophy). The shorter the time, the more severe the stenosis.
- Signs of pulmonary hypertension (see Fig. 4.29).
- Area of valve on echocardiogram. A small area indicates severe stenosis.

Mitral regurgitation

This is where the valve cannot shut completely.

Causes

The main causes are rheumatic heart disease, mitral valve prolapse, and 'functional', where left ventricular dilation caused by, say, ischaemic heart disease produces dilation of the valve—the valve itself is not actually abnormal.

Pathophysiology

The mitral valve cannot shut completely so when the left ventricle contracts to eject blood during systole, some blood flows backwards to the left atrium rather than forward to the tissues.

Features

See Fig. 4.30. Mitral regurgitation may occur acutely as a result of (1) myocardial infarction, producing dysfunction or rupture of papillary muscles or (2) infective endocarditis.

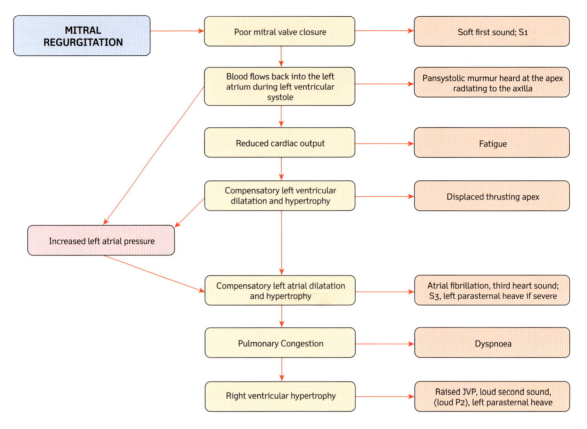

Figure 4.30 Features of mitral regurgitation.

When acute, it presents with pulmonary oedema. The left atrium is not dilated.

Mixed mitral valve disease

Mitral stenosis and mitral regurgitation may coexist—this is mixed mitral valve disease. It is usually due to rheumatic heart disease but may also result from endocarditis of a stenotic valve. The systolic murmur of mitral regurgitation is easy to hear, the diastolic murmur of stenosis more difficult. It may be possible to say which is more significant using clinical signs. The key to this is the apex beat. If mitral stenosis predominates, this will be tapping and not displaced; if mitral regurgitation predominates, this will be thrusting and displaced. The heart sounds may also be helpful. S1 is soft in mitral regurgitation and loud in mitral stenosis (this is not so clear cut as a calcified stenotic valve does not produce loud S1). Furthermore, S3 may be present in mitral regurgitation but not in mitral stenosis.

Tip

S1 should be soft in isolated mitral regurgitation. If it is not or if it is loud, listen carefully for the opening snap and murmur of mitral stenosis.

Key point

- Key signs of mitral regurgitation: displaced, thrusting cardiac impulse, soft S1, pansystolic murmur.

Key point

- In mixed mitral valve disease, the apex beat and S1 help to decide whether the regurgitation or stenosis is more important.

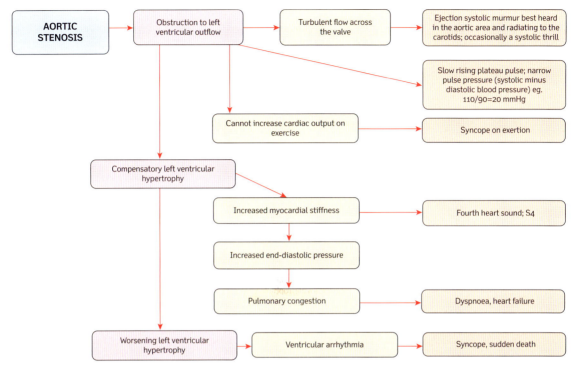

Figure 4.31 Features of aortic stenosis.

Aortic stenosis

This is narrowing of the aortic valve. Normal aortic valve area is 2 cm². Narrowing to less than 1 cm² causes significant aortic stenosis.

Causes

Rheumatic fever, calcific degeneration (elderly patients), congenital bicuspid valve (presenting in adults), and congenital aortic stenosis (presenting in childhood).

Pathophysiology

Aortic stenosis makes it difficult for the left ventricle to eject blood to the tissues when it contracts.

Features

See Fig. 4.31. The murmur tends to get louder with increasing severity of stenosis, but then becomes quieter as left ventricular failure supersedes. A thrill—suggesting a loud murmur—indicates quite severe stenosis.

Aortic sclerosis

This is a degenerative condition of older people. The aortic valve thickens and there is a consequent ejection systolic murmur. Because of this, it can be mixed up with aortic stenosis. However, there are no haemodynamic problems and it is asymptomatic. Signs of aortic sclerosis differ from aortic stenosis in that the pulse character is normal, there is no thrill, and there is only slight radiation to the carotids. However, these signs are not always present in aortic stenosis so in practice, an echocardiogram is often required to differentiate the two.

Aortic regurgitation

This is when the aortic valve cannot shut completely.

Causes

Congenital or acquired (rheumatic fever, infective endocarditis, trauma, dilation of aorta—syphilis, ankylosing spondylitis, Marfan's syndrome, and atherosclerosis).

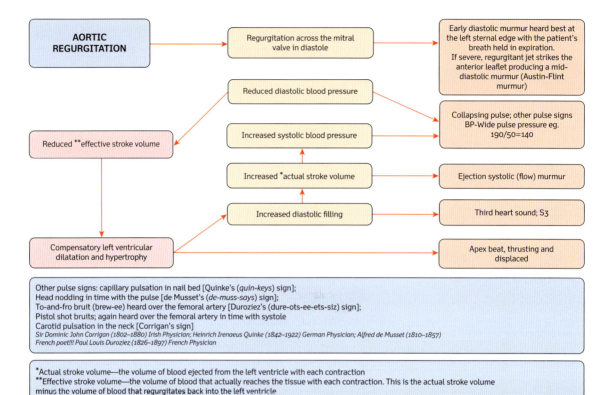

Figure 4.32 Features of aortic regurgitation.

Pathophysiology

During diastole the pressure in the aorta is much higher than that in the left ventricle. The closed aortic valve prevents blood flowing backwards into the left ventricle. In aortic regurgitation, the aortic valve cannot shut completely so some blood flows back into the left ventricle during diastole.

Features

See Fig. 4.32.

Mixed aortic valve disease

Aortic stenosis and aortic regurgitation may coexist—this is mixed aortic valve disease. It is nearly always caused by rheumatic heart disease but may also result

from endocarditis affecting a stenotic valve. A characteristic sign of mixed aortic valve disease is a bisfiriens pulse (Fig. 4.9d)—this refers to the character of the pulse, which gives an impression of a double pulse. The features in Table 4.8 are helpful in deciding clinically whether the stenosis or regurgitation is more important (though echo is best used).

Note that in a patient with aortic regurgitation, a systolic murmur does not necessarily indicate aortic stenosis. It may simply be a flow murmur.

Heart failure

'Heart failure' is not an ideal term but it is the one that is used. 'Heart weakness' would be more accurate. Avoid using the term 'heart failure' in front of patients—it invariably increases anxiety levels. Heart failure is where the heart cannot maintain adequate cardiac

Table 4.8 Aortic regurgitation versus aortic stenosis

	Aortic regurgitation	**Aortic stenosis**
Pulse	Collapsing	Slow rising
Pulse pressure	Wide	Narrow
Cardiac impulse	Thrusting, displaced	Heaving, minimal displacement
Systolic murmur	Not loud or harsh Loud and harsh	
Systolic thrill	No	Yes

Table 4.9 Causes of heart failure

Left heart failure

Generalized myocardial disease, producing left ventricular systolic dysfunction (due to ischaemic heart disease, alcohol consumption, idiopathic cardiomyopathy[a])

Segmental myocardial dysfunction (due to myocardial infarction)

Valvular lesions (such as aortic stenosis and regurgitation, mitral stenosis, and regurgitation)

Hypertension

Right heart failure

Secondary to left heart failure (congestive heart failure)

Segmental myocardial dysfunction (due to right ventricular myocardial infarction)

Valvular lesions (such as tricuspid, pulmonary valve lesions)

Pulmonary vascular hypertension (idiopathic (primary), secondary to lung disease (cor pulmonale) as in COPD, secondary to pulmonary emboli)

Non-cardiac (increased demand)

Anaemia

Thyrotoxicosis

[a] Cardiomyopathy: a disease of the myocardium where no cause is identified.

output or does so only by maintaining elevated filling pressure.

Elevated filling pressure

The heart works better (initially at least) when it dilates to increase filling pressure (the Starling mechanism) (*Ernest Henry Starling (1866–1927), English physiologist*). Thus, one of the first responses of the heart to reduced function is to dilate in order to increase filling pressure and cardiac output.

Classification

There are several different ways of classifying heart failure:

- right or left
- acute or chronic
- high output or low output.

The simplest classification divides heart failure by causes into left-sided heart failure, right-sided heart failure, and non-cardiac heart failure. Table 4.9 is by no means exhaustive, but gives the main causes. The most common type of heart failure is where right and left heart failure coexist—this is known as congestive heart failure.

Features

In most cases of heart failure, it is the compensatory mechanisms producing increased backward pressures that cause the predominant features. So in left heart failure, pulmonary congestion predominates and in right heart failure it is peripheral tissue congestion that predominates. In Tables 4.10 and 4.11, the features are divided into right- and left-sided; however, as already mentioned, these most commonly coexist in congestive heart failure.

Signs of fluid retention

The old idea that fluid retention relates purely to increased venous pressure is losing sway. It is now thought that it is abnormal renal flow and the consequent compensatory mechanisms that produce fluid retention. All the same signs of fluid retention are common in right heart failure, particularly ankle and sacral oedema. If severe, hepatic congestion producing tender hepatomegaly, ascites, and pleural effusion may also occur.

Investigations

The key signs of heart failure on chest radiograph are enlarged heart (>50% of thoracic diameter), upper lobe venous diversion, lymphatic congestion producing Kerley A and more particularly Kerley B lines, and pleural effusion. For details on chest radiograph, see Chapter 15 and Figs. 15.26 and 15.27. Echocardiography is useful in assessing left ventricular systolic and valvular function. Left ventricular systolic function is probably best assessed subjectively as good, poor, or very poor. However, computer-generated measurements of left ventricular size and the so-called 'ejection fraction' are often preferred—probably because they produce a handy number. Ejection fraction is the proportion of blood in the ventricle that is ejected with each systolic contraction. Normally this is greater than 45%.

Acute heart failure

This may be provoked by acute myocardial ischaemia or infarction, arrhythmias, chest infection, pulmonary emboli, and reduction of therapy for chronic heart failure.

Table 4.10 Features of left heart failure

Produces pulmonary congestion leading to pulmonary oedema	
Symptoms	Breathlessness, orthopnoea, paroxysmal nocturnal dyspnoea
Signs	Tachypnoea, tachycardia (due to increased sympathetic tone), fine late inspiratory basal crepitations (due to pulmonary congestion), third heart sound (poorly compliant left ventricle), fourth heart sound (poorly compliant left ventricle)
If severe, dilation of left ventricle also causes dilation of the mitral valve, which cannot shut completely, resulting in mitral regurgitation (known as functional mitral regurgitation). Such mitral regurgitation may produce signs of its own	

Table 4.11 Features of right heart failure

Produces peripheral congestion and consequent tiredness, ankle swelling, abdominal discomfort, and anorexia	
Signs	Raised JVP, left parasternal heave, right ventricular S3 (poorly compliant right ventricle), ankle or sacral oedema
If severe, signs of 'functional' tricuspid regurgitation may occur because of dilation of right ventricle involving the tricuspid valve	

Finals section

In this section, some specific issues dealing with Finals will be discussed. This is not a summary section. For revision, it is suggested that you read the examination summary and the key points throughout the chapter. The emphasis of this section is on the short cases, as this format usually causes the most uncertainty and is still used in some UK medical schools and in many worldwide. The Objective Structured Clinical Examination (OSCE) usually has more straightforward and standardized instructions. Despite the different formats, the clinical approach remains the same.

The cardiovascular system is at the centre of general medicine. Because of this and because it is well suited to the format of the formal examination routine, the cardiovascular system is the single most important system for medicine short cases. In your Finals examination, it is very likely you will be asked to examine the cardiovascular system. Do well and you will be on your way. **Thus, if you know nothing else, know how to examine the cardiovascular system**.

The most common serious cardiovascular pathology is ischaemic heart disease. However, this does not produce consistent physical signs and so is unsuitable for Finals short cases. Most Finals short cases will be a lesion affecting the heart valves producing a heart murmur. Valvular lesions have become increasingly rare with the reduced incidence and severity of rheumatic fever in the last 30 years. However, they continue to represent a good challenge in tying together more than one abnormal cardiovascular system sign. So medical schools make an effort to recruit patients with valvular lesions for the Finals examination.

Most patients with valvular lesions will have single lesions. You will be a bit unlucky to get mixed valve lesions and very unlucky to get a mixture of aortic and mitral valve problems. If the patient does have multiple valvular lesions, the examiner will not expect you to get the correct answer. So, if there seem to be multiple different contradictory signs, do not panic! As long as you perform a reasonable examination and give a sensible description of what you have found, you will be all right. Common Finals cases are given in Table 4.12.

In day-to-day ward teaching, patients with systolic murmurs with no other accompanying cardiovascular system signs are most common. These may be non-pathological 'innocent' murmurs, as occur in a minority of normal people, or may represent early valvular disease. So, do not be alarmed if you have found no abnormality by the time you reach auscultation (and do not feel the need to invent an abnormality). Common day-to-day cases are given in Table 4.13.

Key diagnostic clues

In day-to-day clinical practice, the key signs are those pointing to arrhythmia or cardiac failure, such as pulse rate and rhythm, blood pressure, JVP, and basal lung crepitations. However, as regards short cases—where diagnosis of valvular lesions is most important—it is **carotid pulse character** and **auscultation of the heart** that provide the most important clues.

Key signs of the most important valvular lesions

- **Mitral stenosis**. Pulse irregularly irregular, malar flush, cardiac impulse tapping, loud first heart sound, mid-diastolic murmur heard, opening snap.
- **Aortic stenosis**. Pulse character slow rising, sustained, heaving, slightly displaced cardiac impulse, ejection systolic murmur heard all over praecordium and radiating into the carotids.

Table 4.12 Common Finals cases

Mitral stenosis
Aortic stenosis
Aortic regurgitation
Mitral regurgitation
Mixed mitral valve disease
Mixed aortic valve disease

Table 4.13 Common day-to-day cases

Systolic murmur with no other accompanying cardiovascular system signs
Any of the Finals cases
Cardiac failure

- **Aortic regurgitation**. Collapsing pulse, thrusting, displaced cardiac impulse, early diastolic murmur best heard at lower left sternal edge with patient sitting forward and breath held in expiration.
- **Mitral regurgitation**. Displaced, thrusting cardiac impulse, soft S1, pansystolic murmur.
- **Aortic sclerosis**. Ejection systolic murmur heard all over the praecordium but little radiation to carotids and normal character pulse.

If you know no other facts about the cardiovascular system, you should know those few signs.

Some advice relating to examination problems

General

Do not waste time looking for the cardiovascular system examination routine that will completely satisfy all examiners. It does not exist! Use the one given in this chapter.

The instruction

The examiner will usually ask you to 'examine the cardiovascular system'. Occasionally, they will say instead 'examine the heart'. These both mean the same thing. However, if the examiner gives a more specific instruction, such as 'examine the praecordium' or 'examine the radial pulse and auscultate the heart', you must do just as they request. With such requests, the possibility of confusion here is in how to fit in the 'general look'. This should be done, as always, while preparing the patient for examination.

Moving infirm patients

Always proceed with the aim of carrying out a full examination, asking the patient's permission as you go. If the examiner feels moving such a patient is inappropriate, they will stop you.

Positioning

Even if the patient is already sitting in bed at around 45°, you should alter their position, albeit minimally, to make it clear to the doctor/teacher that you know the patient should be at that angle.

CASE 4.28

Problem. Some examiners may ask you why you have not looked for anaemia or peripheral cyanosis in the hands.

 Discussion. The skin creases of the palms may be paler than usual in anaemic patients—but anaemia is better assessed at the conjunctivae (see Fig. 4.8). Peripheral cyanosis is either a sign of general hypoxia, in which case examination for central cyanosis in the mouth is more appropriate, or simply a sign of being cold. Strictly speaking, it may also occur in peripheral arterial problems such as brachial artery blockage, but such a problem would not be the subject of a medical short case. Therefore, these two signs are not routinely included in the cardiovascular system examination.

Hands

Tar staining in the short case context is very often a red herring. However, it may be an indicator of ischaemic heart disease, which may produce signs of heart failure or cause myocardial infarction complicated by pericarditis or VSD with resultant signs. Case 4.28 explains why some hand signs are not routinely assessed.

Radial pulse

Pulse character is better assessed at the carotid pulse, so although you may get a sense of it at the radial pulse, it is traditional that you do not comment on it. In the short case context, pulse rate and rhythm are often unremarkable. The most important finding is an irregularly irregular pulse, suggesting atrial fibrillation, which may be present in mitral valve disease.

Face

Not all rosy-cheeked patients will have mitral stenosis. All the same, if your short case patient has rosy cheeks always think of a malar flush and be on the alert for mitral stenosis.

Inspecting praecordium

It is often easier to see the cardiac impulse at the apex than feel it, so always inspect before palpating. See Case 4.29 for the further value of inspection.

CASE 4.29

Problem. While inspecting, you may feel an intense urge to get on with the 'real' examination.

Solution. Do not cut short your inspection! Your examiner expects you to be thorough. Look carefully for a left thoracotomy scar—this may involve asking the permission of female patients to lift the breast. If you find a left thoracotomy scar, be thinking of mitral stenosis or mitral regurgitation.

Palpating praecordium

- Potentially, palpation provides important information about valvular lesions. Unfortunately, though, signs such as the apex beat are not always reliable, thus limiting their usefulness. However, the presence of a tapping apex beat, a displaced apex beat, a left parasternal heave, or any thrills are all fairly reliable clinical signs.

- A tapping cardiac impulse represents a palpable first heart sound. If you do not hear a loud first heart sound, reconsider whether the cardiac impulse really was tapping.

- A thrill represents a palpable murmur. If you do not hear a loud murmur on auscultation, reconsider whether you really felt a thrill.

- Decisions on whether the apex beat is sustained or not, heaving, or thrusting are quite subtle. Consider your other signs before deciding. So, if you have found other signs of aortic regurgitation, you are likely to be correct if you felt the apex beat was thrusting and non-sustained.

- If you have been asked to examine the apex beat only, you should start with inspection of the apex.

- In many patients the apex beat is not palpable. During the short cases, do not spend longer than 20 seconds if you cannot find it. Know the causes of an impalpable apex. Although you may well have 'just missed it', you should always say 'the apex beat is impalpable' and then be prepared to answer the question 'Why do you think that is?' with one or all of the reasons given in the 'Palpation of praecordium' section.

- Counting down ribs is cumbersome but expected.

Auscultation

- You will not be expected to hear every click and squeak; the main thing is that you listen to the different areas of the heart in a professional way.

- Your cardiovascular system examination prior to auscultation should have given you a good idea what to listen for before starting auscultation. So, if you have seen a malar flush, palpated atrial fibrillation, and a tapping apex beat, you should be listening hard for the mid-diastolic murmur of mitral stenosis.

- By the time you lift the stethoscope off the patient's chest, you should have decided what you are going to say about the case as a whole. While listening to the chest at the back, you should be thinking as much as listening.

- Mitral stenosis is one of the most common short cases and you should know it well.

- The first heart sound should be soft in isolated mitral regurgitation. If it is not or if it is loud, listen carefully for the opening snap and murmur of mitral stenosis.

Other signs

If you feel any other sign might yield useful information, by all means test for it after you have checked for ankle oedema.

Wash your hands

It may not be normal practice to wash your hands prior to presentation at your medical school. However, it is good practice and also gives you time to get your thoughts together.

Presentation

Always offer to check the blood pressure. Try to be confident—avoid the words 'seems' or 'might'.

Good luck!

OSCE examples

History-taking scenario

You are an FY1 working in the emergency department. A 70-year-old man presents with a 1-hour history of shortness of breath, chest pain and nausea. Please take a history from this patient and present your findings and a differential diagnosis at the end. You have 10 minutes.

Remember:

- Introduce yourself to the patient.

- Take a pain history—remember the SOCRATES mnemonic.

- Ask in detail exactly what the pain is like, what associated symptoms are experienced, the onset and progress of the pain, and anything that makes the pain worse or better.

- Obtain a past medical history, a medication history including allergies and particularly consider cardiac medications such as beta-blockers and angiotensin-converting-enzyme (ACE) inhibitors.

- Social history and family history should not be overlooked. Cardiovascular risk factors are covered in these. Risk factors may be modifiable such as smoking, alcohol, obesity, sedentary lifestyle, stress; or non-modifiable such as age, gender, previous cardiovascular disease and family history.

- Key differentials in this case include ST-elevation myocardial infarction (STEMI), non-ST-elevation myocardial infarction (NSTEMI), and unstable angina.

- Non-cardiac causes of chest pain should also be considered, e.g. respiratory causes such as pulmonary embolism (PE), pneumonia and pneumothorax, and gastrointestinal (GI) causes such as gastro-oesophageal reflux disease (GORD) and peptic ulcer disease.

- Thank your patient.

- Present a concise summary of the history, and offer some differentials. Aim to list the most likely differentials first.

Examination scenario

You are an FY1 working in the cardiology department. A 67-year-old woman presents with shortness of breath and a new murmur. Perform a thorough cardiovascular examination on this patient and present your findings. This is a 15-minute station.
Remember:

- Politely approach the patient, introduce yourself, explain the examination and gain consent.

- Wash your hands/use the alcohol gel provided.

- Expose the patient's chest and inspect the patient from the end of the bed, look for bedside clues, e.g. GTN spray.

- Perform a thorough and systematic examination of the cardiovascular system, including the hands, face, neck and chest, looking for evidence of cardiac disease. Do not forget to look for a raised JVP.

- Carefully inspect the chest wall for any scars, e.g. valve replacements and pacemakers. Then proceed to palpate for the apex beat, a parasternal heave, and thrills.

- Ensure that you auscultate all four areas of the heart. If a murmur is heard, attempt to time it with the carotid

pulse to determine whether it is systolic or diastolic. Comment on intensity, added heart sounds and radiation of murmurs.

- Sit the patient forward and auscultate the lungs for pulmonary oedema, feel for sacral and ankle oedema and evidence of peripheral vascular disease.

- Thank your patient and wash your hands/use alcohol gel provided.

- State that you would also perform an ECG and chest radiograph (CXR), urine dipstick and check their general observations (pulse, BP, etc.)

- Summarize the salient points of the examination. Suggest a cause for any positive findings.

- Suggest a management plan if necessary.

Questions

1 What are the murmurs of mitral stenosis, mitral regurgitation, aortic stenosis, and aortic regurgitation?

2 Describe three reasons for an irregularly irregular pulse.

3 What is a collapsing pulse? In which condition does it occur?

4 What is the significance of phase I, IV, V Korotkoff sounds?

5 How do you differentiate arterial and venous pulsations in the neck?

6 Give three ways of determining the severity of mitral stenosis.

7 In mixed mitral valve disease, how can you say which lesion predominates clinically?

8 What are the key signs of aortic regurgitation?

9 How do you tell clinically which condition predominates in mixed aortic valve disease?

10 What are the signs of left heart failure?

References and further reading

Anonymous. Abdominojugular test. *Lancet* 1989; **i**:419–20.

Brugada P, Gursey S, Brugada J, Andries E. Investigation of palpitations. *Lancet* 1993; **341**:1254–8.

Butt Z, Ashfaq U, Sherazi SF. Diagnostic accuracy of 'pallor' for detecting mild and severe anaemia in hospitalized patients. *Journal of the Pakistan Medical Association* 2010; **60**(9):762–5.

Cook DJ, Simel DL. The rational clinical examination: does this patient have abnormal jugular venous pressure? *JAMA* 1996; **275**:630–4.

Crossland S, Berkin L. Problem based review: the patient with 'palpitations'. *Acute Medicine* 2012; **11**(3):169–71.

Davison R, Cannon R. Estimation of central venous pressure by examination of jugular veins. *American Heart Journal* 1974; **87**:279–82.

Desjardins VA, Enriquez-Sareno M, Tajik AJ, Bailey KR, Seward JB. Intensity of murmurs correlates with severity of valvular regurgitation. *American Journal of Medicine* 1996; **100**:149–56.

Fisher J. Jugular venous valves and physical signs. *Chest* 1984; **85**:685–6.

Ishmail AA, Wing S, Ferguson J, Hutchinson TA, Magder S, Flegel KM. Inter-observer agreement by auscultation in the presence of a third heart sound in patients with congestive heart failure. *Chest* 1987; **91**:870–3.

Jordan MD, Taylor CR, Nyhuis AW, Tavel ME. Audibility of the fourth heart sound. Relationships to the presence of disease and examiner experience. *Archives of Internal Medicine* 1987; **147**:721–6.

March SK, Bedynek JL Jr, Chizner MA. Teaching cardiac auscultation: effectiveness of a patient-centered teaching conference on improving cardiac auscultatory skills. *Mayo Clinic Proceedings* 2005; **80**(11):1443–8.

Markiewicz W, Brik A, Brook G. Pericardial rub in pericardial effusion lack of correlation with amount of fluid. *Chest* 1980; **77**:643–6.

McGee S, Abernethy WB, Simel DL. Is this patient hypovolaemic? *JAMA* 1999; **281**:1022–9.

NICE. *Hypertension: clinical management of primary hypertension in adults (CG 127)*, August 2011 http://www.nice.org.uk/CG127

O'Brien E. Ave atque vale: the centenary of clinical sphygmomanometry. *Lancet* 1996; **348**:1569–70.

Richardson TR, Moody JM Jr. Bedside cardiac examination: constancy in a sea of change. *Current Problems in Cardiology* 2000; **25**(11):783–825.

Sheth TN. The relationship of conjunctival pallor to the presence of anaemia. *Journal of General Internal Medicine* 1997; **12**:102–6.

Slater EE, DeSanctis RW. The clinical recognition of dissecting aortic aneurysm. *American Journal of Medicine* 1976; **60**:625–33.

Spitell PC, Spittell JA, Joyce JW, Tajik AJ, Edwards WD, Schaff HV, et al. Clinical features and differential diagnosis of aortic dissection: experience with 236 cases (1980 through 1990). *Mayo Clinic Proceedings* 1993; **68**:642–51.

Vinayak AG, Levitt J, Gehlbach B, et al. Usefulness of the external jugular vein examination in detecting abnormal central venous pressure in critically ill patients. *Archives of Internal Medicine* 2006; **166**(19):2132–7.

Young JB, Will EJ, Mulley GP. Splinter haemorrhages: facts and fiction. *Journal of the Royal College of Physicians of London* 1988; **22**:240–3.

5 Respiratory system

CHAPTER CONTENTS

Introduction

Chest disease is a common cause of morbidity and mortality in Western countries. Episodes of illness associated with acute increases in breathlessness are one of the commonest causes of hospital admission, and lung cancer remains the number one killer of all cancers.

In this chapter, you will learn what questions to ask patients with respiratory diseases and how to examine the respiratory system.

Symptoms

The key symptoms of the respiratory system are cough, phlegm, haemoptysis, wheeze, breathlessness, and chest pain. Breathlessness and chest pain have been dealt with in the cardiovascular chapter (Chapter 4) so they will not be discussed in any detail here.

Cough

It is normal for the respiratory mucosa to produce a small amount of secretions. These are removed by mucociliary (*mew-co-silla-ree*) action. When there is an abnormal amount of secretions or other foreign material, the normal mucociliary action is unable to cope and a cough is used to remove the material. Involuntary coughing always indicates an abnormality but the causes form a wide spectrum from minor, transient problems to serious, life-threatening disease.

When a patient complains of cough, the first question to ask about is duration. Cough may be categorized crudely, according to duration: less than 2 months is acute and more than 2 months is chronic. The two categories have different patterns of causation.

Acute cough

Causes

- Infection affecting any part of the respiratory tree—nasopharyngitis (*nay-so-fa-rinj-eye-tiss*) to laryngotracheobronchitis (*la-ring-owe-tray-key-owe-bronk-eye-tiss*) to pneumonia.
- Allergic reactions.
- Reaction to irritant.
- Any of the causes of chronic cough at their onset.

How to decide what the cause is

- **Infections.** Associated fever and chills; sputum, often but not necessarily mucopurulent (thick yellow or green); hoarseness if laryngitis; pain related to affected site—throat pain for pharyngitis or laryngitis, chest pain with tracheitis.
- **Allergic.** Associated sneezing; watery secretions.
- **Reaction to irritant.** Recent inhalation of irritant; no sputum.

As regards infections, it is very difficult to distinguish viral from bacterial infections clinically. Two points may help.

- Viral infections, particularly the common cold, are much more common.
- Streptococcal pneumonia tends to produce respiratory symptoms, especially pain, early on in its course—within hours of the onset of fever and chills—whereas viral pneumonias tend to have a prodrome of general symptoms before the more obvious respiratory symptoms develop.

Chronic cough

Causes

See Table 5.1. Note that several important causes (post-nasal drip, gastro-oesophageal reflux disease, and angiotensin-converting enzyme (ACE) inhibitors) are not chest diseases.

How to decide what the cause is

See Table 5.2. Ask about:

- timing—?nocturnal, ?morning
- exacerbating factors—?exercise ?cold weather ?meals
- sputum
- associated symptoms—breathlessness, heartburn, weight loss, anorexia, and night sweats
- smoking
- recent ACE inhibitors.

Key points

- Cough may be classified according to duration: less than 2 months is acute and more than 2 months is chronic
- If less than 2 months, think of infections (usually upper respiratory) and allergies
- If more than 2 months, think more of intrinsic lung disease but also consider sinonasal, gastrointestinal, and cardiac problems
- In patients with chronic cough ask about timing, exacerbating factors, sputum, associated symptoms, and smoking
- Do not forget to ask about ACE inhibitors
- The cough of lung cancer may be unremarkable (see Case 5.1)

Table 5.1 Causes of chronic cough

Common
Postnasal drip[a]
Asthma
Gastro-oesophageal reflux disease[b]
Chronic obstructive pulmonary disease
Smokers' cough (due to chronic irritation)
Less common
Bronchiectasis
Lung cancer
Tuberculosis
ACE-i
Heart failure

ACE-i, angiotensin-converting enzyme inhibitor
[a] Postnasal drip is due to pathology in the nasal mucosa or sinuses. It has multiple causes including allergic reactions and irritant reactions and it may be postinfective.
[b] Gastro-oesophageal reflux disease: it is now well recognized that acid refluxing into the larynx may cause a chronic cough.

Sputum

Sputum production accompanying cough is a feature of many conditions (Table 5.3). Sometimes sputum has a particular character that points to certain conditions:

- **foul smelling and tasting**—anaerobic infections
- **copious and mucopurulent**—bronchiectasis
- **foamy and pink tinged**—pulmonary oedema
- **rusty**—pneumococcal pneumonia
- **copious, frothy, and saliva like**—bronchoalveolar carcinoma
- **bloody**—see haemoptysis.

Sputum can be divided into serous (runny, clear), mucoid (viscous, clear), and mucopurulent or purulent (viscous, yellow/green). This classification can provide limited assistance in guiding antibiotic treatment. While mucoid or mucopurulent sputum may be either viral or bacterial, serous sputum is rarely bacterial.

Haemoptysis

Haemoptysis is the coughing up of blood or blood-tinged sputum. It has multiple causes, the most important of

> **Key point**
> - Acute onset mucoid or mucopurulent sputum may be either viral or bacterial; serous sputum is rarely bacterial

which are detailed in Table 5.4. In Hippocrates' day (*Hippocrates c.460–370 BC, Ancient Greek physician, often called 'father of medicine'*), the chief cause was tuberculosis. While tuberculosis remains an important cause of haemoptysis, bronchitis, bronchiectasis, and lung cancer are now the most common causes in the West.

Causes

The commonest causes of haemoptysis are bronchitis, bronchiectasis, and lung cancer. The following are helpful in making the diagnosis.

- Heart failure may cause frothy, pink sputum.
- Large quantities (>200 mL) of haemoptysis occur more typically with tuberculosis, pulmonary infarction, bronchiectasis, and bleeding diatheses.
- The colour of the blood does not usually help. Generally bright red blood represents fresh bleeding whereas darker blood is caused by blood that has oozed from the bleeding site and has had time to be metabolized before being coughed up.

So clinical evaluation of haemoptysis mainly relies on:

- assessing other symptoms or signs that might suggest other causes
- identifying causes needing urgent treatment
- evaluating patients for lung cancer.

Assessing other symptoms or signs that might suggest other causes

See 'Respiratory diseases and investigations' for lung cancer, bronchiectasis, acute bronchitis, chronic bronchitis, pulmonary infarction, tuberculosis, and lung abscess, and 'Cardiovascular diseases and investigations' for heart failure. As regards bleeding diatheses and anticoagulation, heparin or warfarin therapy, bleeding from other sites including purpura and bruises, or profuse bleeding should prompt you to do a clotting screen.

Identifying causes requiring urgent treatment

Certain conditions require urgent action:

Table 5.2 Analysis of causes of chronic cough

	Timing of cough	Exacerbating	Sputum	Associated symptoms	Other factors
Postnasal drip	Worst first thing in the morning		Yes		
Asthma	During the night	Exercise, cold weather	No	Paroxysmal breathlessness	
Gastro-oesophageal reflux disease		Meals	No	Heartburn	
COPD	On first going to bed and first thing in the morning but not much during the night		Often[a]	Chronic breathlessness	Usually smoker or ex-smoker
Smoker's cough	As for COPD		As for COPD		Smoker or ex-smoker
Bronchiectasis		Postural changes	Copious, may be blood streaked		
Angiotensin-converting enzyme inhibitor			No		May develop any time in the first year of treatment
Heart failure	During the night		May be frothy, sometimes bloody		
Lung cancer			Initially dry, later purulent sputum due to secondary infection or bloody sputum may develop[b]	Anorexia, weight loss	Usually smoker or ex-smoker
Tuberculosis			May be bloody	Anorexia, weight loss, night sweats	

COPD, chronic obstructive pulmonary disease.
[a] Chronic bronchitis is defined as cough productive of sputum on most days of 3 months in 2 consecutive years.
[b] A rare form of lung cancer—bronchoalveolar carcinoma—may cause production of copious amounts of watery sputum.

- If there is any suggestion of pulmonary embolism, anticoagulation should be initiated and investigations such as a 'spiral' CT lung scan arranged.
- If there is evidence of infection, antibiotics should be started.
- If heart failure appears a possibility, diuretics should be commenced.

Evaluating patients for lung cancer

Once this initial assessment has been carried out, there will be a group of patients with unexplained haemoptysis. Many of these will eventually be shown to have bronchitis or bleeding from the nasopharynx. However, a significant minority will be due to lung cancer. All patients with unexplained haemoptysis should have a chest radiograph,

Problem. What cough features point towards lung cancer?

Discussion. Although lung cancer is a rare cause of chronic cough, the serious nature of the diagnosis means that the cough of lung cancer warrants particular attention. The difficulty is that there are no clear characteristic features. Initially, the cough can be mild and the characteristic bloodstained sputum may not be present. The associated symptoms mentioned in Table 5.2 may also be absent. The diagnosis should be borne in mind in patients presenting with a new, **persistent** cough or in patients with a chronic cough who present with a change in cough pattern. All such patients should have a chest radiograph. If normal this makes the diagnosis of lung cancer unlikely. However, even if the radiograph is normal, the presence of weight loss, anorexia, or haemoptysis necessitates referral to a respiratory expert for consideration of bronchoscopy. If the patient is or has been a smoker, the index of suspicion should be higher.

Table 5.3 Causes of sputum production

Acute
Infection affecting any part of the respiratory tree—nasopharyngitis to laryngotracheobronchitis to pneumonia
Chronic
Common
Postnasal drip
COPD
Less common
Bronchiectasis (*bron-key-eck-ta-sis*)
Lung cancer
Tuberculosis
Heart failure

COPD, chronic obstructive pulmonary disease.

Table 5.4 Causes of haemoptysis

Common
Lung cancer
Bronchiectasis
Acute or chronic bronchitis
Pulmonary infarction
Less common
Tuberculosis
Lung abscess
Heart failure
Bleeding diatheses (*die-ath-ee-seize*)[a] and anticoagulation

[a] Bleeding diatheses are conditions such as haemophilia where patients have a propensity to bleed.

Key points

- Bronchitis, bronchiectasis, and lung cancer are the commonest causes
- Always consider causes needing urgent intervention such as pulmonary embolism, infection, and heart failure
- All patients with unexplained haemoptysis should have a chest radiograph (chest CT, and bronchoscopy as necessary to exclude lung cancer)

chest CT, and bronchoscopy as necessary to exclude lung cancer. See Cases 5.2 and 5.3.

Tip

Haemoptysis due to chronic bronchitis normally settles down within a couple of days. If it persists longer, think of lung cancer. If the cause is lung cancer, the haemoptysis is often preceded by weight loss.

Wheeze

When patients complain of wheeze, the first thing to do is to establish what exactly they mean by this. Wheeze should have a musical quality to it—more than just noisy

CASE 5.2

Problem. My patient has chronic bronchitis. Four months ago, she had a small amount of haemoptysis. Chest radiograph, CT scan, and bronchoscopy at that time were clear. Now, the patient has had another bout of haemoptysis. Do we need to do the tests all over again?

Discussion. Patients with chronic bronchitis are prone to recurrent bouts of haemoptysis. Clearly, common sense is needed when considering investigation. So, provided the amount of haemoptysis is similar, there are no new symptoms such as weight loss, and the tests were recent, it is reasonable not to repeat them.

CASE 5.3

Problem. My patient isn't sure whether he vomited or coughed up the blood. Do I have to investigate for both?

Discussion. You will usually be able to differentiate the two with a careful history going through the circumstances of the blood production. Failing this, a short period of inpatient observation may reveal the source. Occasionally it will remain unclear whether the blood was coughed up or vomited. In such circumstances, you will need to consider gastroscopy as well as the respiratory tests.

breathing—and is usually more prominent in expiration. Wheeze nearly always suggests small airways obstruction, as in asthma or chronic obstructive pulmonary disease (COPD). Patients with asthma will sometimes notice that the wheeze is increased during exercise or in cold weather.

There are a couple of other causes of wheeze:

- Occasionally wheeze is a feature of pulmonary oedema.
- Rarely the inspiratory noise of stridor (*stry-door*) may be mistaken for a wheeze, but it lacks the musical quality of a wheeze. See Table 5.5.

Other issues to discuss in the respiratory history

Many respiratory conditions have their roots in (1) exposure to noxious substances, (2) previous illnesses or treatments, or (3) contact with other people

Key points

- Wheeze should have a musical quality and is usually more prominent in expiration
- Wheeze usually suggests asthma or COPD
- However, do not automatically assume wheeze is due to small airways obstruction: always consider the possibility of pulmonary oedema or stridor

or animals. Thus, when a patient complains of respiratory symptoms, you need to broaden your enquiry.

Exposure to noxious substances

Smoking history

This is the most important, being a powerful risk factor for COPD and lung cancer; 90% of lung cancers are thought to be due to smoking. You need to get a clear history: roughly how many cigarettes are smoked, how long the patient has smoked, and when they stopped if relevant. When asked 'Do you smoke?', patients are inclined to answer 'no', carelessly omitting the fact that they stopped the previous day. Always ask, 'Did you ever smoke?', 'When did you stop?', 'How many did you smoke—2 a day, 20 a day, 60 a day?' See Case 5.4. If the patient smoked a pipe, try to get them to quantify tobacco use in ounces per week.

Occupational exposure

Always ask patients about current or previous exposures to dusts, fumes, and chemicals at work. The substances that can cause respiratory problems are many, ranging from mouldy hay (farmers' lung) to titanium. If the patient is currently working in such an atmosphere, try to establish if symptoms are worse when at work and better when on holiday. In the UK, you should specifically enquire about coal and asbestos and enquire about any noxious substances produced locally.

- Coal can cause a form of lung fibrosis—coal-miners' pneumoconiosis.
- Asbestos also causes fibrosis (asbestosis) and is also a risk factor for lung cancer and mesothelioma (*me-so-thee-lee-owe-ma*).

Previous illnesses or treatments

- Measles and whooping cough in childhood are risk factors for bronchiectasis.

CASE 5.4

Problem. I've heard smoking quantified in terms of pack years. What does this mean?

Discussion. You may find it helpful to quantify the tobacco exposure in terms of 'pack years'. So a patient who smoked 10 a day (half a pack) for 30 years has smoked 0.5 × 30 = 15 pack years. A patient who has smoked 40 a day for 15 years has smoked 30 pack years.

Key points

- Virtually any substance that can be inhaled can cause respiratory problems
- Take a detailed smoking history
- If you are considering tuberculosis, always ask about family contacts and foreign travel
- If you are considering pneumonia, always ask about birds as psittacosis is managed differently

- Rheumatoid arthritis may be complicated by lung fibrosis.
- Amiodarone—a cardiac drug—can cause fibrosis.
- Another type of cardiac medication—β-blockers—can worsen airways obstruction.

Contact with other humans or animals

If tuberculosis is a possibility, always enquire about family contacts. Ask specifically about foreign travel—many UK patients have their origins in India and Pakistan and may contract tuberculosis when they visit their relatives in Asia.

Animals may cause respiratory disease in two ways: (1) by passing on infection, or (2) through hypersensitivity reactions. So in patients with pneumonia, always enquire about exposure to birds. Any species of bird can transmit *Chlamydia psittaci* (*cla-mid-ia-sit-ak-eye*). This may cause psittacosis (*sit-ak-owe-sis*), which is a form of pneumonia. Psittacosis responds better to tetracyclines than penicillins. Your suspicions should be particularly aroused if the patient's parrot, budgie, or canary died recently after a brief illness. In patients with chronic breathlessness, enquire about exposure to pigeons. This can result in a hypersensitivity pneumonitis—pigeon-fanciers' lung. Pets, particularly cats and dogs, can exacerbate asthma.

The importance of examining the respiratory system

As in many other branches of medicine, modern investigations have reduced reliance on respiratory system examination findings. Tests such as the chest radiograph, lung function tests, and increasingly sophisticated scanning techniques provide much useful information about respiratory disease. Examination is far from being infallible and small pulmonary lesions may not produce any abnormal clinical signs.

That said, examination of the respiratory system remains a very important part of the doctor's assessment of chest problems. In the acutely unwell patient, examination findings may often yield very important and immediate information with regards to the severity and the source of the illness. Furthermore, in patients complaining of long-term breathlessness or symptoms suggestive of malignancy, examination findings are often extremely helpful in analysing the cause of the patient's problem. Examination involves assessing not just the chest but also looking at other areas, particularly the hands, pulses, and face, to glean further information as to the cause and severity of chest symptoms. While the scope of respiratory examination is far reaching, there are some general themes, which recur over and over again:

- signs pointing towards malignancy
- signs of unilateral pleural effusion (fluid collection), raising the possibility of malignancy, infection, or more rarely autoimmune disease
- signs of unilateral consolidation (solidification), usually suggesting infection but occasionally being due to immune or toxic effects.

Less common but important are:

- signs of unilateral lung collapse, raising the possibility of malignancy or alternatively a mucus plug, either in an asthmatic patient or postoperatively
- signs of lung fibrosis.

Respiratory system examination summary

This summary contains many terms that you will not understand on first reading. These terms are explained in the next section 'Respiratory examination in detail'.

1 Introduce yourself to the patient and ask for permission to examine.

2 Wash your hands.

3 Ask the patient to get on to the bed (if not already on the bed). You may need to get skilled help from a nurse or healthcare assistant! Ask the patient to remove all garments covering chest and arms. For female patients, ensure a chaperone is present and offer to cover the chest with a sheet or towel. Arrange the patient so that their chest is at 45° to the horizontal.

4 While doing 1 and 3, be having a general look and listen.

5 Inspect both hands for clubbing (DF8/10), peripheral cyanosis, tremor, muscle wasting, and tar staining.

6 Palpate right radial pulse for pulse rate (DF 3/10) and rhythm (DF 6/10) and consider if bounding (DF 6/10). Then, check respiratory rate (DF 4/10).

7 Check for flapping tremor (DF 8/10).

8 Inspect face for swelling (DF 8/10), eyes for Horner's (DF 7/10), and underneath tongue for cyanosis (DF 9/10).

9 Inspect right internal jugular vein for jugular venous pressure (DF 9/10). Check for hepatojugular reflux (DF 8/10).

10 Inspect front of chest from end of bed, assessing breathing pattern (DF 4/10), chest shape (DF 4/10), and movement (DF 8/10).

11 Inspect front of chest and neck close up (DF 5/10).

12 Palpate trachea (DF 9/10).

13 Palpate the praecordium for apex beat position (DF 9/10), axillary lymph nodes (DF 8/10), and if suspected, tender areas (DF 8/10).

14 Palpate for chest expansion anteriorly, comparing both sides (DF 9/10).

15 Percuss front of chest and in the axillae, comparing the two sides (DF 9/10).

16 Assess tactile vocal fremitus (*frem-it-us*) at the front of the chest and in the axillae, comparing the two sides (DF 9/10).

17 Auscultate over the front of the chest and in the axillae, comparing the two sides (DF 8/10).

18 Assess vocal resonance at the front of the chest and in the axillae, comparing the two sides (DF 9/10).

19 Change the patient's position to facilitate examination of the neck and the back of the chest (DF 6/10).

20 Examine the neck for enlarged lymph nodes (DF 8/10).

21 Inspect the back of chest assessing movement (DF 8/10), chest shape (DF 4/10), and other visible abnormalities (DF 4/10).

22 If appropriate, palpate the posterior aspect of the chest for possible rib fractures (DF 8/10).

23 Palpate for chest expansion posteriorly, comparing both sides (DF 8/10).

24 Percuss the back of chest comparing the two sides (DF 9/10).

25 Assess tactile vocal fremitus over the posterior aspect of the chest, comparing the two sides (DF 9/10).

26 Auscultate over the back of the chest, comparing the two sides (DF 8/10).

27 Assess vocal resonance over the back of the chest, comparing the two sides (DF 9/10).

28 Look for other signs such as whispering pectoriloquy or peripheral oedema if appropriate.

29 Wash your hands.

30 Pause briefly and then present findings.

Respiratory system examination in detail

Getting started

1 Introduce yourself to the patient and ask for permission to examine

Put out your hand to shake the patient's hand. Say something like 'Hello, I'm Russell Brock, a third-year medical exchange student. Do you mind if I examine your chest and hands?' Don't just say 'chest'! The patient will wonder what you are up to when you start looking at his hands!

2 Wash your hands

3 Ask the patient to get on to the bed (if not already there)

Ask the patient to remove all garments covering chest and arms. For female patients, ensure a chaperone is present and offer to cover the chest with a sheet or towel. Arrange the patient so that their chest is at 45° to the horizontal.

If the patient is unable to get on to the bed or undress himself, ask for help from the nurses or healthcare assistants. The respiratory system can only be examined properly with the patient's chest bare. Students, quite understandably, are often unsure if this is appropriate, particularly for women patients. Such doubt can create a confidence problem—not a good thing at this early stage of the examination. For a man, simply say something like 'It's best if I examine you with your chest bare. Could you take off your shirt and vest, please.' For a woman, say something like 'Ideally, it's best if I examine you with your chest bare. Is that all right? I can cover up your chest with a sheet for part of the examination.' Give the patient good opportunity to refuse. If she refuses, do not take this as a slight—just get on with the examination as best you can. If she's happy to undress, give her time to do so. Then, if requested, cover the chest up with a sheet or towel until you get to the examination of the chest itself. And remember, for a male doctor, a woman—medical student or nurse—should be present to act as a chaperone.

The best position for examining the respiratory system is not universally agreed. The two main options are sitting upright or lying at 45° as for the cardiovascular system. It is suggested that the examination is started with the patient at 45° as this is comfortable for most patients and good for examining the jugular venous pulse. Later in the examination, the patient can sit forward so that the back of the chest can be examined (see Fig. 5.14). However, if the patient is very breathless, they may be more comfortable sitting fully upright either in a chair or with their feet over the side of the bed from the start. See Case 5.5.

4 While doing 1 and 3, be having a general look and listen

Consider respiratory effort and pattern, stridor and hoarseness, cyanosis, nebulizer, oxygen, and sputum pot.

Moderate or severe respiratory distress may be suggested by (1) noisy or laboured breathing, which may be brought on or worsened by the effort of undressing and positioning, (2) a need to sit upright, or (3) the presence of an oxygen mask or a nebulizer machine (Fig. 5.1) by the bed. A nebulizer machine is used to supply high-dose bronchodilators and normally implies either asthma or COPD. See Case 5.6.

A rasping noise prominent in inspiration is suggestive of 'stridor'. This implies obstruction of the upper airways (Table 5.5) and requires expert attention. If the onset is sudden, immediate action is required to relieve the obstruction. Although rare, stridor is a particularly important sign

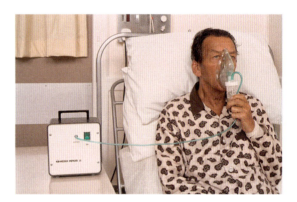

Figure 5.1 Using a nebulizer machine.

CASE 5.5

Problem. My patient is very breathless, needing to sit up. Do I insist on him lying at 45°?

Discussion. Definitely not. Common sense must prevail—examine the patient sitting up.

CASE 5.6

Problem. The patient is using a nebulizer, which is making considerable noise during your examination.

Discussion. Like any other complicated task, a physical examination is best performed with the minimum of distractions. As a doctor you will have to decide for yourself whether the potential longer-term benefit from a clearer analysis of symptoms and signs outweighs the immediate benefit to the patient of the nebulizer. As a student, you need to ask the patient's doctor or simply wait till the nebulizer treatment is finished—it usually takes around 10 minutes.

because the standard basic respiratory tests—chest radiograph, blood gases, and spirometry—will rarely identify this as the source of breathing difficulties.

The patient may sound hoarse. This is most commonly due to laryngitis but there are more serious causes: (1) lung cancer causing laryngeal nerve palsy or (2) laryngeal cancer.

If you see a sputum pot by the bed, open it up and have a look. Large volumes of yellow/green sputum suggest bronchiectasis, foul-smelling sputum may point to an anaerobic lung abscess, and blood in the sputum (haemoptysis) needs to be thoroughly evaluated (see 'Haemoptysis').

Hands

5 Inspect both hands for clubbing (DF8/10), peripheral cyanosis, tremor, muscle wasting, and tar staining

Clubbing

What is it?

Clubbing is a painless enlargement of connective tissue in the terminal phalanges of the digits. When severe, the ends of the digits look like clubs (Fig. 5.2). It is usually symmetrical and affects fingers more than toes. Clubbing was first described by Hippocrates and the term 'hippocratic fingers' is occasionally used. Initially, the soft tissue swelling causes tenseness within the skin and alters the 'nailbed angle'.

What is the nailbed angle?

The contour of the fingernail and the skin on the back of the finger do not run seamlessly together. The nailbed angle is the angle formed at the junction between the

skin of the finger and the nail (Fig. 5.3). When the soft tissue of the terminal phalanx enlarges, it pushes the nail upwards and the nailbed angle is gradually lost. At this stage clubbing is present (even if the fingers do not look like clubs). Later the nail becomes increasingly curved, especially in the long axis until finally swelling of the terminal phalanx leads to the classical appearance of the fingers, which resemble clubs (Fig. 5.2).

Significance

Clubbing is associated with a variety of diseases (Table 5.6), most of them respiratory in origin. It is not associated with asthma or COPD. Table 5.6 does not give the full story. Although it is true to say that patients with cyanotic congenital heart disease with clubbing are uncommon, 95% of patients with cyanotic congenital heart disease

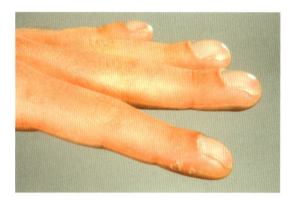

Figure 5.2 Severe clubbing.

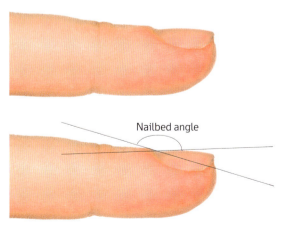

Figure 5.3 The normal nailbed angle.

Table 5.5 Causes of stridor

Sudden
Inhaled foreign body
Anaphylactic reaction
Gradual
Tumours of pharynx, larynx, or trachea
External compression of the trachea by enlarged lymph nodes or goitre

Table 5.6 Causes of clubbing

Common	
Bronchiectasis	
Lung cancer	
Idiopathic pulmonary fibrosis	
Rare	
Respiratory	Lung abscess, empyema, asbestosis, mesothelioma
Cardiac	Congenital heart disease with right-to-left shunt, infective endocarditis
Gastrointestinal	Cirrhosis, inflammatory bowel disease, coeliac disease

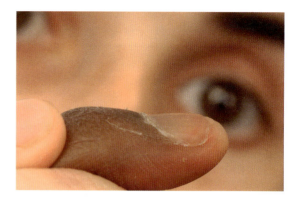

Figure 5.4 Inspecting the nailbed angle.

will have clubbing compared to 75% of patients with idiopathic pulmonary fibrosis, 30% of patients with bronchiectasis, and 25% of patients with lung cancer.

How does clubbing happen?

This question remains unanswered. The theory currently most favoured implicates megakaryocytes (*mega-carry-owe-sites*). Normally megakaryocytes (the precursors of platelets) are trapped in the pulmonary capillaries and do not appear in the systemic circulation. In the presence of lung disease, damage to the pulmonary capillaries results in megakaryocytes gaining access to the systemic circulation. They are then trapped in the capillaries of the fingers where they release growth factors into the surrounding tissue. This theory is supported by the fact that patients suffering from congenital heart disease with right-to-left shunt (bypassing pulmonary capillaries) are highly likely to have clubbing.

How to examine

1 Say to the patient, 'Do you mind if I examine your hands and fingers?'
2 Lift the patient's right hand up a few inches.
3 Bend down so that your eyes are at the same level as the patient's hand and look at the patient's fingers from the side (Fig. 5.4).
4 Focus on one finger, the right middle is best, and look at the nailbed angle.

> **Key points**
> - Clubbing is a painless enlargement of connective tissue in the terminal phalanges of the digits
> - Clubbing is a clue to many illnesses, the most common being idiopathic pulmonary fibrosis, lung cancer, and bronchiectasis
> - Clubbing is not associated with COPD
> - Clubbing is best examined by assessing for loss of the nailbed angle

5 Decide if the angle is lost or preserved. See Cases 5.7 and 5.8.
6 Next, examine other fingers on the right hand and then the left hand.

Case 5.9 explores other techniques for examining the nailbed angle.

Hypertrophic pulmonary osteoarthropathy

What is it?

This is rare. It is an inflammation of the periosteum (*perry-os-tea-um*) at the ends of long bones and may cause tenderness and swelling over the fingers and wrists. It has been described as a late manifestation of clubbing though this is probably not true: it may occur without clubbing and has different causes (80% associated with lung cancer, 10% with mesothelioma) implying a different pathological process altogether.

While examining for clubbing, other clinical features may provide clues to respiratory disease.

- Fine tremor may be a side effect of bronchodilator therapy for COPD or asthma.

CASE 5.7

Problem. I think the nailbed angle is lost but the patient's fingers don't look clubbed.

Discussion. This is the most common appearance of clubbing (Fig. 5.4). The club-like appearance is a late development. It can be difficult to be sure and this is one reason to look at several fingers on both hands—the loss of angle tends to vary a little from finger to finger so you may see a clearer example on another finger. It's also worth knowing that in Coury's original paper describing 350 cases of clubbing, 20% are classified as borderline or possible clubbing—so clearly, it is not always easy.

CASE 5.8

Problem. The patient's fingers look clubbed but there is no loss of nailbed angle.

Discussion. This appearance is thought to be normal. If the angle is not lost, it's not clubbing. Soft tissue swelling sufficient to make fingers look clubbed should be more than sufficient to obliterate the nailbed angle.

- Wasting of intrinsic muscles of the hand (T1 distribution) may be due to brachial plexus damage caused by an apical lung cancer.
- A bluish discoloration of the fingers may be part of a central cyanosis (see 'Cyanosis' in Chapter 4).
- The yellowish tinge of tar staining on the fingers suggests smoking-related disease such as lung cancer or COPD. The degree of staining does not predict the amount of tobacco smoked.

Radial pulse, respiratory rate, and flap

6 Palpate right radial pulse for pulse rate (DF 3/10) and rhythm (DF 6/10) and consider if bounding (DF 6/10). Then, check respiratory rate (DF 4/10)

Pulse rate and rhythm

Significance

The pulse rate and rhythm may be altered in respiratory disease.

CASE 5.9

Problem. I find the nailbed angle technique difficult. Are there any other ways of examining for clubbing?

Discussion. The nailbed angle technique may seem difficult initially but it is the most reliable. However, there are a couple of other techniques.

The first method is based on the fact that the increased soft tissue in the terminal digit makes it more fluctuant—and involves assessing the fluctuancy of the nailbed (Fig. 5.5):

1 Take the patient's right middle finger.
2 Position both your thumbs underneath the pulp of the finger.
3 Hold the proximal interphalangeal joint steady with the tips of your middle fingers.
4 Now palpate the nail with the tips of your index fingers.
5 Normally, there should only be very slight fluctuation. With clubbing, the nailbed may feel very spongy. This distinction between normal and abnormal fluctuation is very tricky and not one I have found convincing.

The second method was first proposed by *Leo Schamroth (1924–1988, South African cardiologist)*, who developed clubbing himself while suffering from endocarditis. Schamroth's sign is based on the finding that if a normal person places the terminal phalanges of corresponding fingers of both hands back to back, it produces a small diamond-shaped aperture between both nail beds. When clubbing is present, this window is abolished. I like this method although it is not well studied.

- Chest infections or pneumonias may cause a tachycardia or may be complicated by atrial fibrillation (irregularly irregular pulse), or atrial flutter with 2:1 block (Case 5.10).
- In the context of an asthma attack, a pulse rate >110/min indicates a severe attack. On the other hand, bradycardia in the asthmatic patient may be an indicator of life-threatening cardiac insufficiency in asthma. Case 5.11 illustrates another presentation of bradycardia in asthma. Case 5.12 describes a blood pressure phenomenon in severe asthma.
- A large-volume 'bounding' pulse may be a sign of carbon dioxide retention suggesting respiratory failure.

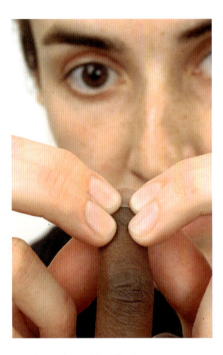

Figure 5.5 Assessing nailbed fluctuancy.

CASE 5.10

Problem. My patient has symptoms of a chest infection and is somewhat breathless but otherwise comfortable. I'm worried, though, because her pulse is 150/min and regular, suggesting a worrying development.

 Discussion. You're quite right to be worried. Normally a tachycardia of this degree suggests your patient is approaching a critical juncture. However, your observation that the patient looks well suggests this is much more likely to be atrial flutter with 2:1 block.

How to examine

Palpation of the right radial pulse is described in Chapter 4. In the respiratory system, the aim is to assess rate and rhythm and consider whether the pulse is large volume ('bounding').

Respiratory rate

What is the respiratory rate?

The respiratory rate is the number of breaths per minute.

CASE 5.11

Problem. My friend is a keen sportsman but suffers with asthma. I've checked his pulse and it's bradycardic (50/min). Does this mean his asthma is badly controlled even though he's well and not breathless?

 Discussion. When evaluating the pulse in the respiratory system, it should be used in the context of the patient's condition. This man simply has a resting bradycardia because he is physically fit.

CASE 5.12

Problem. I was seeing a patient with severe asthma today and the consultant asked me if there was evidence of pulsus paradoxus. What's that?

 Discussion. This is a difficult sign to elicit and as a result is rarely performed. Normally, the blood pressure falls slightly during inspiration. With pulsus paradoxus this is exaggerated and systolic blood pressure falls by more than 10 mmHg. It may occur in severe acute asthma, constrictive pericarditis, or cardiac tamponade. It can normally only be elicited by sphygmomanometry, but in tamponade it may be possible to palpate a reduced radial pulse volume on inspiration.

What is the normal rate?

There is some disagreement over the normal rate. A rate around 14 breaths per minute is commonly quoted. However, at least one study (see 'Further reading') suggests that the normal rate averages 20 breaths per minute with a normal range of 16–25 per minute. The author's experience is that the normal respiratory rate averages around 18 per minute.

What is abnormal?

Clearly, given the lack of clarity over what the normal rate is, it is a little difficult to say what is abnormal. However, it is generally agreed that the respiratory rate increases (tachypnoea) (*tack-kip-knee-a*) in patients with chest conditions such as pneumonia, pleurisy, and asthma/COPD. It may also be increased in patients with fever or any source or anxiety.

 British Thoracic Society guidelines use respiratory rate as an important indicator of severity in patients with acute asthma. In such patients, a respiratory rate >25/

Key points

- Check pulse rate and rhythm and consider whether it is bounding in nature
- In the context of an asthma attack, a pulse rate >110/min indicates a severe attack
- Continue to palpate the pulse while checking the respiratory rate
- The respiratory rate needs to be measured over at least 30 seconds
- Respiratory rate >30/min in the context of community-acquired pneumonia suggests severe pneumonia
- In the context of an asthma attack, a respiratory rate >25/min indicates a severe attack

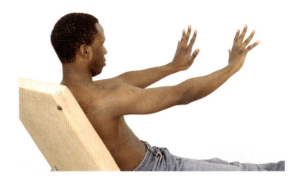

Figure 5.6 Assessing for flap.

Key points

- A flapping tremor may be a sign of respiratory failure (but unreliable)
- Show the patient what to do
- A flapping tremor is also found in liver failure and rarely kidney failure

min indicates that the attack is severe. In patients with community-acquired pneumonia, a respiratory rate >30/min has been shown to be one of the three key indicators (along with blood urea >7 mmol/L and diastolic blood pressure <60 mmHg) that predict a worse outcome. The respiratory rate is reduced (bradypnoea) in cases of opiate overdose or neurological conditions such as stroke or raised intracranial pressure. In such circumstances, there may also be Cheyne–Stokes (*chain-stokes*) breathing.

How to examine

The respiratory rate is one of the few signs that can be altered voluntarily. If patients realize you are watching their chest closely, they find it very difficult to ignore and tend to breathe self-consciously. Thus a little duplicity is required.

1 Having assessed the patient's pulse, continue to give the impression that you are examining it.
2 While doing this, inspect the patient's breaths in and out and count them over 30 seconds (10 seconds is too short).

Flapping tremor

6. Check for flapping tremor (DF 8/10)

What is a flapping tremor?

This is an irregular, coarse, jerky movement of the wrist.

Significance

In the context of respiratory disease this is a sign of carbon dioxide retention due to respiratory failure (usually in COPD). It is said to indicate the patient is in a critical condition, but this is unreliable. It can occasionally be present

in mild illness and is often absent in severe illness. It may also be found in liver failure or kidney failure.

How to examine

1 The tremor may be difficult to observe at rest. It is maximized by getting the patient to hold their arms outstretched, with wrists cocked and fingers spread slightly while showing them what you mean (Fig. 5.6). It may be easier to demonstrate the position you want for your patient. See Case 5.13.
2 Look for a coarse, irregular flapping movement at the wrists. Make sure you observe for at least 15 seconds before deciding that a flapping tremor is absent. Case 5.14 gives an alternative cause for a tremor.

Face, eyes, and tongue

8 Inspect face for swelling (DF 8/10), eyes for Horner's (DF 7/10), and underneath tongue for cyanosis (DF 9/10)

Facial swelling

Significance

Lung cancer may cause blockage of the superior vena cava either by direct tumour invasion or by thrombosis. This is known as superior vena caval (SVC) obstruction (Fig. 5.7). The SVC receives blood from the head, neck, and arms.

Problem. I've tried to test for flapping tremor but the patient won't cooperate.

Discussion. Carbon dioxide retention also causes drowsiness and confusion so testing for a flap can be difficult. Make sure you demonstrate clearly to your patient what you mean. Sometimes, the patient simply cannot cooperate. If so, think about performing a blood gas test to resolve the issue.

Problem. The patient seems shaky but is it a flap?

Discussion. A flapping tremor means what it says—a flap. It is quite different from the tremor due to β-agonist treatment seen in many patients being treated for respiratory disease.

When the SVC is blocked, the head and neck veins become engorged and there is a loss of the normal jugular pulsations (that is, a raised non-pulsatile jugular venous pressure (JVP). The face and neck also become oedematous but the arms tend to be less swollen as they are able to use an alternative collateral circulation involving the inferior vena cava. There may be visible distended veins on the chest wall providing this collateral circulation from the arms.

How to examine

1 Briefly look at the patient's face. Is it abnormally swollen? Is it plethoric or cyanosed?

2 If you think the face might be swollen, then look at external jugular vein. Is it distended and is it pulsating? Look at the chest wall. Are there distended veins?

The combination of a swollen face with a distended non-pulsatile external jugular vein suggests SVC obstruction and prominent chest wall veins lend support to the diagnosis. See Case 5.15.

Horner's syndrome (*Johann Horner (1831–1886), Swiss ophthalmogist*)

What is it?

This is a syndrome characterized by a small pupil (miosis) accompanied by drooping of the eyelid (partial ptosis) on the same side with reduced sweating (anhidrosis) on the same side of the face.

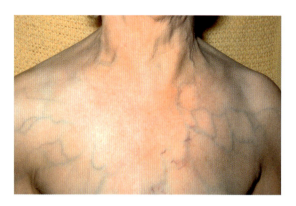

Figure 5.7 Superior vena caval obstruction.

Problem. The patient's face is a bit puffy but he's a bit overweight so maybe that's the cause.

Discussion. SVC obstruction is rare and most 'swollen' faces will be due to fatty tissue. What is important is that any sort of facial swelling prompts you to briefly check the external jugular and chest wall veins for evidence of SVC obstruction. If you don't think of it, you won't find it.

How does it happen?

Horner's syndrome is caused by damage to the sympathetic nerves to the eye and face. The sympathetic pathway to the eye takes a roundabout route:

1 First-order neurons travel from the hypothalamus to the spinal cord between levels C8 and T2.

2 Second-order neurons pass from the spinal cord over the apex of the lung and then up along the carotid artery to the superior cervical ganglion.

3 Third-order neurons emerge from the superior cervical ganglion and then diverge into two separate pathways, one going via the cavernous sinus to the eye—where it innervates the pupillary muscle and the eyelid—the other travelling alongside the external carotid artery to innervate the facial sweat glands.

Significance

A lung tumour situated in the apex of the lung may damage second-order neurons, causing Horner's. Other causes are listed in Table 5.7.

Table 5.7 Causes of Horner's syndrome

First-order neuron damage	Stroke
Second-order neuron damage	Lung tumour—usually squamous cell, thyroid tumour, neck or chest trauma
Third-order neuron damage	Skull fracture, cavernous sinus thrombosis

CASE 5.16

Problem. I'm sure I've been told that there's a fourth feature of Horner's, that is, the eye looks to be more sunken within the orbit (enophthalmos). Why haven't you mentioned this?

Discussion. Enophthalmos is often described as a feature of Horner's. It's difficult to be sure if the eye is truly indrawn or whether the ptosis simply makes it look indrawn. Either way, I don't think it helps very much in deciding whether Horner's is present.

How to examine

See Chapters 6 and 13, and Fig. 13.14. Cases 5.16, 5.17, and 5.18 discuss Horner's syndrome and other pupillary findings.

Cyanosis

What is it?

Haemoglobin that has not been oxygenated (deoxygenated haemoglobin) gives blood a blue colour. Cyanosis is a bluish discoloration of the skin and mucous membranes due to excess deoxygenated haemoglobin (usually >2.5 g/100 mL). Cyanosis may be peripheral or central. In peripheral cyanosis, only the blood supply to the extremities such as the fingers is reduced. Because of the reduced blood flow, the tissues remove more oxygen from the blood so resulting in an increase in deoxygenated haemoglobin and hence a blue discoloration (see Cases 5.19 and 5.20). In central cyanosis, all arterial blood is poorly oxygenated, so even tissues such as the tongue, with a good blood supply, go blue. Cyanosis is a crude estimate of arterial oxygenation and doctors vary greatly in their ability to pick out this subtle hue.

CASE 5.17

Problem. The patient appears to have Horner's but when I shine a light into the pupil it constricts normally. Should this happen?

Discussion. The size of the pupil depends on the relative influence of the sympathetic nerves (which dilate) and parasympathetic nerves (which constrict). In Horner's, the parasympathetic nerves are undamaged so pupillary constriction to light still occurs.

CASE 5.18

Problem. I've noticed that patients' pupils are often slightly different in size but there doesn't seem to be ptosis. Any advice?

Discussion. In normal individuals, the pupils are often slightly different in size. The difference is usually less than 1 mm in contrast to the size difference in patients with Horner's where it is usually more than 1 mm.

Significance

Any condition that reduces oxygen levels may cause cyanosis. Cyanosis may come on suddenly in patients with chest infections, pneumonia, or pulmonary emboli. Patients with chronic lung disease such as COPD or pulmonary fibrosis are particularly prone to develop cyanosis when such acute problems develop. Some patients with severe COPD or more rarely fibrosis may have chronic cyanosis. Pulmonary oedema due to cardiac pathology may also cause cyanosis.

How to look for central cyanosis

It is blood in the superficial venules and capillaries that gives the skin and mucous membranes their colour. Cyanosis is best seen where the epidermis is thin and these subepidermal blood vessels predominate—places such as lips, nose, ears, and oral mucous membranes. However, it is usual to evaluate cyanosis by inspecting the mucous membranes under the tongue because unlike the other extremities above, it is not affected by peripheral cyanosis.

1 Ask the patient to put out their tongue and inspect underneath the tongue.

2 Do not expect a bright blue discoloration; cyanosis has more of a purplish hue.

Key points

- SVC obstruction may occur in patients with lung cancer
- When examining the respiratory system, stop for a second to think whether the face is swollen
- Horner's is characterized by miosis, partial ptosis, and anhidrosis of the same side of the face
- Horner's is due to damage of the sympathetic nerve supply to the eye and face
- Cyanosis is due to an excess of deoxygenated haemoglobin
- Cyanosis can provide a crude estimate of arterial oxygenation
- Cyanosis usually represents severe hypoxia
- The blue hue of cyanosis can be difficult to spot
- Cyanosis occurs very late in anaemic patients (and early in polycythaemic patients)

CASE 5.19

Problem. Surely you're making things overcomplicated by talking about deoxygenated haemoglobin. Is cyanosis not simply a sign of hypoxia?

Discussion. True, hypoxia and cyanosis go together. But there is another important variable—the haemoglobin level. In a patient with a haemoglobin of 16 g/100 mL, oxygen saturation needs to fall to 85% (P_{O_2} 7 kPa) to produce deoxygenated haemoglobin greater than 2.5 g/100 mL (and so cyanosis). In an anaemic patient with a haemoglobin of 6 g/100 mL, oxygen saturation needs to be 60% (P_{O_2} is 4 kPa) for enough deoxygenated haemoglobin to be present to produce cyanosis. Either way, though, it is quite clear that patients need to be severely hypoxic before cyanosis is visible.

Jugular venous pressure

9 Inspect right internal jugular vein for jugular venous pressure (DF 9/10). Check for hepatojugular reflux (DF 8/10)

Why examine?

Advanced pulmonary disease may cause right heart failure (cor pulmonale) (*cor-pull-ma-nail-ee* or *cor pull-ma-narly*) and hence an elevated JVP. Two mechanisms

CASE 5.20

Problem. Is deoxygenated haemoglobin the only substance that makes the skin go blue?

Discussion. Blue discoloured skin may also occur in certain conditions characterized by abnormal haemoglobin such as methaemoglobinaemia. Methaemoglobin has a bluish colour. It is the same as haemoglobin except that the iron ion is in the ferric (Fe^{3+}) form rather than the ferrous (Fe^{2+}) form. There is normally a small component of methaemoglobin in the blood but enzyme deficiencies can result in increased levels especially in the presence of certain drugs (methaemoglobinaemia). In contrast to hypoxic cyanosis, oxygen treatment has no effect on the skin colour and the P_{O_2} is not reduced.

Key points

- In the absence of cardiac failure, an elevated JVP in the context of respiratory disease suggests cor pulmonale
- Cor pulmonale indicates advanced respiratory disease

are thought to be responsible for the right heart failure: (1) alveolar hypoxia or arterial hypoxaemia causing vasoconstriction and hence pulmonary hypertension and (2) lung disease causing direct damage to the pulmonary vessels so increasing vascular resistance. The JVP may also be elevated but non-pulsatile in SVC obstruction (see Fig. 5.7).

How to examine

See Chapter 4, 'Jugular venous pressure'.

Inspection of praecordium including chest expansion

The chest itself

It is now time to move on to examination of the chest itself. First, the front of the chest and the axillae are assessed. The examination is carried out in a sequence of inspection, palpation, percussion, tactile vocal fremitus (TVF), and auscultation, comparing the right and left sides. Then the back of the chest is examined in the same

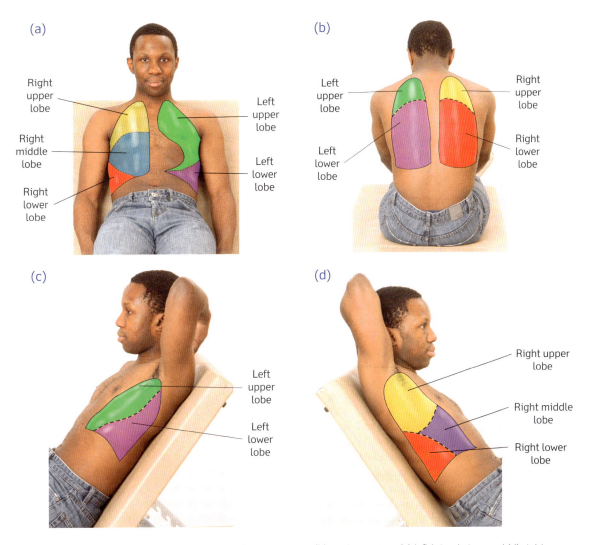

(a)

Right upper lobe

Left upper lobe

Right middle lobe

Left lower lobe

Right lower lobe

(b)

Left upper lobe

Right upper lobe

Left lower lobe

Right lower lobe

(c)

Left upper lobe

Left lower lobe

(d)

Right upper lobe

Right middle lobe

Right lower lobe

Figure 5.8 Surface markings of the lung lobes: (a) anterior view, (b) posterior view, (c) left lateral view, and (d) right lateral view.

way. It is helpful to know the surface markings of the lobes of the lungs (Fig. 5.8) so that you can correlate signs with lung anatomy. (Case 5.21 explains the difference between 'lobes' and 'zones' in case you are confused.) If right middle lobe pathology is present, you might expect to detect abnormal signs over the lower part of the right chest at the front and over the right axilla inferiorly and anteriorly but would not expect to detect any abnormality over the back. Disease in the upper lobes produces signs mainly in the upper chest at the front and back of the chest: sometimes signs may be found in the axillae. Disease in the lower lobes produces signs mainly over the lower back of the chest, sometimes in the axilla, and less often over the front of the chest.

10 Inspect front of chest from end of bed, assessing breathing pattern (DF 4/10), chest shape (DF 4/10), and movement (DF 8/10)

The aim now is to take a concentrated look at the overall chest shape as well as the breathing pattern and chest movement. These features are best assessed by stepping back a little and viewing the chest from the end of the bed.

CASE 5.21

Problem. I've heard doctors talking about lung zones. What's the difference between zones and lobes?

Discussion. Lung zone is a term best reserved for analysis of chest radiographs. When a lung abnormality appears on a standard chest radiograph, it is often difficult to say which lobe it is in based on the radiograph alone. Thus a shadow in the middle of the left lung on the radiograph may represent pathology either in the left upper or lower lobes. Which lobe the lesion is in depends on how close to the front or the back of the chest the lesion is—and this is information the chest radiograph doesn't provide. Thus, when assessing chest radiographs, it is more logical to divide the lungs into thirds (zones—upper, middle, and lower) to describe the radiological situation of any lung abnormality.

Breathing pattern

- **Pursed lips.** Patients with COPD sometimes purse their lips when they breathe out. This happens particularly during exacerbations. In such patients, there is good evidence that this improves ventilation and oxygenation.

- **Accessory muscle use.** Normally, the diaphragm is the only muscle that plays a part in breathing—and even then, it is only involved in inspiration; expiration is a passive process. However, in patients with respiratory muscle fatigue or COPD, particularly during an exacerbation, additional muscles may become involved. To aid inspiration, the sternocleidomastoids (*stern-owe-clyde-owe-mast-oids*) (anterior superficial neck muscles), the scalene (*scay-lean*) muscles (deep neck muscles), and the trapezius (posterior neck and back muscles) lift the rib cage. Expiration may be supplemented by the external oblique muscles (anterolateral abdominal muscles).

- **Leaning forward with hands on knees.** Patients with exacerbations of COPD often adopt this position.

- **Cheyne–Stokes (or 'periodic') breathing.** Here patients' breaths become gradually deeper and deeper and then more and more shallow. As the breathing becomes more and more shallow, it slows down and there may be apnoeic pauses for several seconds before the cycle resumes. Cheyne–Stokes breathing (*John Cheyne (1777–1836), Scottish physician and William Stokes (1804–1878), Irish physician*) may occur in patients with heart failure or in patients with a reduced level of consciousness due to neurological causes such as opiate overdose, stroke, or head injury.

- **Fast, deep breathing.** Usually, when patients are breathless, their respiration is fast but shallow. Sometimes, though, you may notice that the patient is breathing not just fast but also deep. This suggests hyperventilation. Hyperventilation is said to occur when the rate of ventilation is excessive for the level of carbon dioxide. Therefore it can only be properly diagnosed by finding a low carbon dioxide level in blood gases. Various conditions may cause hyperventilation: hypoxia, heart failure, asthma, fever, pain, and anxiety to name a few. Hyperventilation causes a metabolic alkalosis. This in turn reduces the level of ionized calcium in the blood. The resultant hypocalcaemia may be symptomatic with tingling of the fingers or around the mouth. Hyperventilation may be a compensatory response to metabolic acidosis as occurs in diabetic ketoacidosis and renal failure—in which case it is known as Kussmaul's (*kus-malls*) breathing (*Adolf Kussmaul (1822–1902), German physician*). Here, there is no alkalosis and so no hypocalcaemia or tingling.

Chest appearance

- **'Barrel chest'.** Normally, the lateral diameter of the chest is greater than the anterior-posterior (A–P) diameter (4:3 approximately). In patients with barrel chest, the A–P diameter is increased so that the proportion approaches 1:1. Barrel chest is a feature of COPD and is thought to be due to the accessory muscles pulling the ribs upwards. The presence of barrel chest usually suggests quite advanced COPD, though the degree of chest deformity is not a reliable indicator of disease severity.

- **Other abnormalities of chest shape.** The chest shape may be deformed in various ways, although these are becoming less common (see Table 5.8):

  - if the patient's sternum is depressed (pectus excavatum) (*peck-tus-ex-ca-vay-tum*), this puts them at risk of breathing difficulties (see Fig. 14.8a)

  - a prominent sternum (pectus carinatum) (*peck-tus-carry-nar-tum*) suggests the patient may have suffered from chest disease in childhood (see Fig. 14.8b)

  - a severely deformed spine (kyphoscoliosis) puts patients at considerably increased risk of breathing difficulties in later life

  - a severe deformity of one side of the chest raises the possibility of a thoracoplasty for tuberculosis in the past.

Table 5.8 Chest deformities

Funnel chest (pectus excavatum)

What is it?	A depressed sternum
How does it happen?	It is congenital; usually idiopathic but may be associated with connective tissue disorders such as Marfan's (*mar-fans*) syndrome
Effects	Cosmetic; effects on lung function usually minor but in some cases, it may cause breathlessness

Pigeon chest (pectus carinatum)

What is it?	A prominent sternum
How does it happen?	Develops in childhood in patients with rickets or severe chest disease. In those with chest disease, it is thought to be due to repeated strong contractions of the diaphragm while the ribcage is still pliable
Effects	Cosmetic; little additional effect on lung function beyond the causative condition

Kyphoscoliosis

What is it?	Spinal deformity resulting in increased A–P curvature (kyphosis) and lateral curvature (scoliosis) of the spine. It affects 1 in 1000 people with 1 in 10 000 affected severely. The patient's posture may look abnormal
How does it happen?	Mostly idiopathic, first noticed in childhood, but may be due to bone or connective tissue disease affecting the spine (osteoporosis, Ehlers–Danlos (*er-luz-dan-loss*) syndrome)
Effects	Cosmetic; may have quite severe effects on lung capacity resulting in breathlessness presenting in middle age

Thoracoplasty

What is it?	Thoracoplasty was an operation used in the past to treat tuberculosis. It involved removing several ribs and so can result in the treated side of the chest looking very deformed
Effects	Reduces lung capacity, which becomes more important with advancing years resulting in an increased propensity to breathing difficulties

Other features you may observe from the end of the bed

- **Chest drains for pneumothorax (*new-mow-thor-axe*) or pleural effusion.** For a pneumothorax, the chest drain is normally inserted in the front of the chest (second intercostal space in the midclavicular line) or in the axilla, whereas for a pleural effusion, the drain is usually inserted posteriorly. Thus a tube coming out of the front of the chest or armpit suggests recent pneumothorax whereas a tube coming out of the back suggests recent pleural effusion.

- **A general swelling of the neck and supraclavicular regions.** This may be due to air in the subcutaneous tissues (subcutaneous emphysema). It is usually diagnosed much more easily on palpation. It is a complication that can follow the insertion of a chest drain for a pneumothorax. Some air escapes through the hole created in the chest wall tissues rather than through the tube and tracks upwards resulting in swelling of the neck. This looks worse than it is. Subcutaneous emphysema may also be a result of air in the mediastinum (pneumomediastinum), the discussion of which is beyond the scope of this book.

- **Evidence of previous radiotherapy.** Sharply demarcated patches of erythematous or thickened skin raise the possibility of cancer, particularly lung cancer and lymphoma.
- **Prominent chest wall veins**. These suggest SVC obstruction (see Fig. 5.7).

Chest movement

Why examine?

Many chest conditions reduce chest movement. Most diseases are bilateral and so result in reduced chest movement on both sides. However, some important conditions (consolidation, effusion, collapse, fibrosis, and pneumothorax) may affect just one lung so resulting in reduced movement on that side. The consequent asymmetry of movement makes detection easier. Both inspection and palpation are used to assess chest movement.

How to examine

1 Walk confidently to the end of the bed.

2 Explain to the patient 'I now want to have a thorough look at your chest.' For female patients, if appropriate add, 'Could you please remove the towel?'

3 Stand and look carefully at the patient's chest.

4 Certain abnormalities will be obvious such as pursed-lip breathing, the presence of a chest drain, a depressed or prominent sternum, kyphoscoliosis, or previous thoracoplasty.

5 Go through a checklist in your mind.

- Is the patient's breathing pattern normal? If not, decide what is abnormal. Is the patient's breathing becoming deeper and deeper before ceasing for a period (suggesting Cheyne–Stokes respiration)?
- Are they using their accessory muscles? Sometimes, pursed-lip breathing and accessory muscle usage will go together.
- Is the chest shape normal? If not, does the chest look barrel shaped?
- Are there prominent chest wall veins (suggesting SVC obstruction)?
- Look at the neck. Is there swelling of the neck (suggesting subcutaneous emphysema)?

6 Next, ask the patient to take a deep breath in and then out through the mouth. Show the patient what you want them to do: 'Please take a deep breath in and out . . . like this.'

7 As the patient breathes, watch the chest carefully and concentrate on whether one side is moving more than the other. Force yourself to decide whether both sides move equally or if there is a difference.

8 Then, ask the patient to repeat their deep breath in and out. If your opinion remains unchanged, this part of the examination is complete. If not, ask the patient to breathe in and out again until your findings are consistent (see Case 5.22).

11 Inspect front of chest and neck close up (DF 5/10)

Why examine?

Having taken a look at the chest from the distance it is now time to look more closely at the chest. The aim is to (1) examine more closely any abnormalities seen from the end of the bed and (2) identify smaller pathology not easily visible from the end of the bed.

How to examine

1 Go back to the left-hand side of the patient's bed.

2 If there were any possible radiotherapy patches, inspect for small tattoo marks, which are often over the irradiated skin.

Key points

- Chest shape and movement are best assessed by standing at the foot of the bed
- Accessory muscle use and pursed-lip breathing suggest a deterioration in chest condition, most commonly an exacerbation of COPD
- Barrel chest is a sign of COPD
- Inspection of chest movement is a useful way of detecting unilateral chest pathology
- When inspecting chest movement, demonstrate to the patient how you would like them to breathe

---

CASE 5.22

Problem. I can't decide if my patient has asymmetrical chest movement and now he says he's dizzy.

Discussion. You have to be a little careful during the chest examination not to make your patient hyperventilate. Overbreathing can result in tingling, dizziness, and even collapse. I suggest a maximum of four deep breaths in and out at any one point in the examination.

3 Inspect for prominent chest wall veins suggesting SVC obstruction.

4 Look for a chest drain scar over the second intercostal spaces in the midclavicular line.

5 Ask the patient to lift up their right arm and look in the axilla for a chest drain scar—in the fourth, fifth, or sixth intercostal spaces in the mid-axillary line. Do the same for the left axilla. See Case 5.23 for the significance of a mid-line scar.

Palpation of trachea and praecordium

12 Palpate trachea (DF 9/10)

The trachea can normally be felt in the neck. It lies in the midline between the suprasternal notch and the cricoid (*cry-coid*) cartilage.

Why examine?

Examination of the trachea is somewhat uncomfortable for the patient but it is important to do it because displacement of the trachea to one side is an important sign. The trachea may be pulled to the side by unilateral upper lobe fibrosis or collapse. Upper lobe fibrosis usually suggests tuberculosis in the past. Lung cancer causing blockage of a main bronchus is usually responsible for upper lobe collapse. Furthermore, if the lung cancer has been treated surgically by removal of lung (pneumonectomy), the trachea will be pulled to that side. Rarely, the trachea may also be displaced by a tension pneumothorax or by a large pleural effusion—both of which push the trachea towards the opposite side. Case 5.26 describes 'tracheal tug' in the context of COPD.

How to examine

1 Keep the patient positioned at 45° with their neck relaxed against the pillow.

2 Say to the patient something like, 'I need to feel your windpipe. It's a little uncomfortable but I'll try to be gentle.'

CASE 5.23

Problem. On close inspection of the chest I've noticed a long vertical scar over the front of the sternum. Does this give a clue to respiratory disease?

Discussion. Big scars on the front of the chest usually represent cardiac operations. See Chapter 4 for more information.

3 Then, using your right middle finger, gently palpate the patient's neck about 2 cm superior to the suprasternal notch in the midline (Fig. 5.9).

4 You will feel a resistance there. If you move your finger 0.5 cm to the right or left, the resistance is more difficult to palpate. This resistance is the trachea. See Case 5.24 for a common difficulty in appreciating the trachea.

5 Palpate the space either side to get a feel for whether the trachea is central.

6 Decide whether the trachea is central or is it displaced to one side. See Case 5.25.

Key points

- Examining the trachea is somewhat uncomfortable for the patient—be gentle
- Tracheal deviation usually suggests unilateral upper lobe pathology

CASE 5.24

Problem. I thought I had got the hang of finding the trachea but I'm having great difficulty palpating this patient's.

Discussion. The usual reason for increased difficulty is excess adipose tissue in patients who are overweight—this can make it very difficult to identify the trachea.

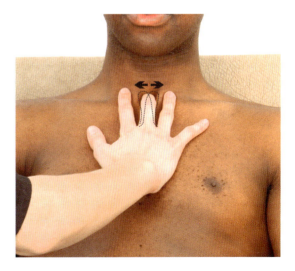

Figure 5.9 Palpation of the trachea.

CASE 5.25

Problem. The patient's trachea seems to be slightly deviated to the right but when I've examined the chest I've found nothing (collapse, fibrosis, and so on) to suggest a cause.

   Discussion. Very slight deviation to the right can be a normal variant.

Tip

Practise palpation of the trachea on your (consenting) friends; patients will not thank you for poking around unnecessarily in their necks.

13 Palpate the praecordium for apex beat position (DF 9/10), axillary lymph nodes (DF 8/10), and if suspected, tender areas (DF 8/10)

Why examine?

Palpation of the praecordium often provides only limited information about the respiratory system—but occasionally there may be positive findings.

- **Rib fracture.** The presence of an exquisitely tender area on the chest may suggest a rib fracture. This may be associated with a grinding/crunching sensation called crepitus (*crep-it-us*) where the broken ends of bone rub against each other. Rib fractures are usually due to trauma and may be complicated by a pneumothorax or haemothorax. Rarely this may be a pathological fracture where secondary spread of a cancer to the bones may cause the ribs to break from trivial trauma.

- **Subcutaneous emphysema.** General swelling of the upper chest and neck may suggest subcutaneous emphysema. When palpated this produces a very characteristic crackling sensation under the hand.

- **Apex beat.** The apex beat is defined as the most lateral and inferior position at which the cardiac impulse is felt. Its normal position is the fifth intercostal interspace in the midclavicular line. The apex beat position may give a clue to unilateral lower lung lobe pathology in the same way that the tracheal position gives clues to upper lobe pathology. Thus right lower lobe collapse (often due to lung cancer) or fibrosis (often after pneumonia) may result in slight movement of the apex beat to the right

CASE 5.26

Problem. I've heard of a sign called 'tracheal tug'. What's this?

   Discussion. Tracheal tug is said to be a sign of COPD. I have never found it helpful. It is said that in COPD, if you palpate the trachea during inspiration, it seems to move downwards—tracheal tug.

CASE 5.27

Problem. The apex beat is displaced laterally. But on further examination I've found nothing such as left lower lobe collapse or fibrosis or right pleural effusion to suggest a cause. Why might this be?

   Discussion. The apex beat is primarily a sign of cardiac disease and displacement of the apex is usually due to cardiac pathology—so it's usual not to find any explanatory respiratory pathology to explain a change in its position.

so it is felt more medially than the midclavicular line. Left lower lobe collapse or fibrosis may cause the apex beat to be displaced laterally. As with the trachea, a large pleural effusion or a tension pneumothorax will push the apex beat away from the side of the pathology. See Case 5.27 for a discussion of a displaced apex beat.

- **Axillary lymph nodes.** The lymphatic drainage of the lung is primarily through the neck nodes, which are discussed in more detail in the section 'Palpation for lymph nodes in neck'. The axillary nodes drain the breasts and the pleurae. In normal patients, it is often possible to palpate small axillary lymph nodes (<0.5 cm). A large (>1 cm) lump is nearly always pathological. If it is hard, this is suspicious of breast cancer (see Chapter 10)—or rarely mesothelioma. If firm rather than hard, any of the causes of generalized lymph node enlargement detailed in 'Palpation for lymph nodes in neck' may be responsible.

How to examine?

See Fig 5.10.

1 Ask the patient, 'Is the front of your chest painful or tender?'

2 If the answer is yes, ask for permission to examine: 'Do you mind if I examine the painful or tender areas?' If permission is granted gently palpate the painful spots.

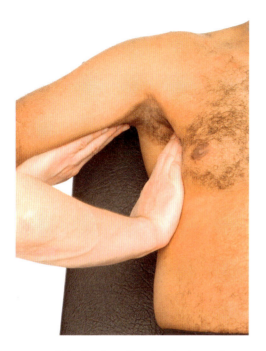

Figure 5.10 Palpating for axillary lymphadenopathy.

Can you elicit tenderness? Is the painful or tender spot within a hard bony area, suggesting rib injury?

3 If you have previously observed chest or neck swelling suggestive of subcutaneous emphysemas, gently palpate the area. If subcutaneous emphysema is present you will feel a continuous crackling sensation under the hand.

4 Palpate the apex beat position. See Cases 5.28 and 5.29.

5 To examine for axillary lymph nodes, the patient needs to abduct their arms: 'Please lift your right arm out to the side . . . Do you mind if I check in your armpit for glands?'

6 If the muscles and tendons around the axilla are tense, it is very difficult to palpate nodes so take the weight of the patient's right arm by holding it at the elbow with your left arm (to allow the shoulder muscles to relax) (Figs. 5.10 and 10.10).

7 Using the palmar aspect of the fingers of your right hand, palpate in sequence the medial, anterior, lateral, posterior, and apical aspects of the axilla. Do you feel any rounded masses?

8 If so, palpate these specifically with the tips of your fingers to get a clearer idea of size and consistency.

9 Then, do the same for the left axilla—this time using your right arm to support the patient's arm and your left hand to palpate for nodes (see Case 5.30).

CASE 5.28

Problem. I can't palpate the apex beat. Why might this be?

Discussion. The apex beat is impalpable in around 50% of patients. One common cause relating to the respiratory system is hyperinflation of the lung associated with COPD.

CASE 5.29

Problem. When examining the cardiovascular system, I've been taught to assess the apex beat character. Is this useful in the respiratory system?

Discussion. No, respiratory disease does not affect the character of the apex beat.

CASE 5.30

Problem. When examining the axilla for nodes, I tend to feel prominent areas but they don't feel like nodes.

Discussion. The tendons in the axilla, especially if they are tense, may feel hard and lumpy and may mimic nodes—but if you palpate carefully you will note that they have a linear character rather than the lumpiness of a node.

Key points
- Apex beat displacement may suggest unilateral lower lobe pathology
- To examine for axillary lymph nodes, make sure the muscles and tendons are as relaxed as possible

Tip
Avoid wiggling your fingers in the patient's armpit; this is tickling!

The remainder of the chest examination is dominated by a sequence of testing for expansion, percussion, TVF, auscultation, and vocal resonance (VR). This is done first over the front of the chest and the axillae and then over the back. As the principles are the same front and back, each technique will be described in one section rather than in separate sections for front and back.

Palpation of chest expansion

14 Palpate for chest expansion anteriorly, comparing both sides (DF 9/10)

Why examine?

Palpating for chest expansion is a comparative technique. The aim is to compare the two sides and detect any reduction in expansion on one side. Unilateral reduction in expansion at the front of the chest may be due to pathology of any lobe. Unilateral reduction in expansion low down the chest posteriorly suggests lower lobe pathology. The lower lobe is the most common site for important pulmonary conditions such as consolidation, effusion, fibrosis, and collapse. Unilateral reduction in expansion high up the chest posteriorly suggests upper lobe pathology.

Front of the chest

How to examine

1 Your examination of the praecordium should have identified any areas of tenderness—be careful around these.

2 Ask the patient to breathe in and then out and to hold their breath in expiration (so that the subsequent expansion will be maximal).

3 Then, having warned the patient, place your hands firmly on the chest wall with fingers gripping the patient's sides (the lower ribcage).

4 Bring your thumbs together to meet in the midline around the inferior part of the sternum but not touching the chest (Fig. 5.11a). Exactly where you grip the patient's side will vary according to the patient's size but essentially you grip in the position that allows you to bring you thumbs together to meet in the midline. See Case 5.31.

5 Ask the patient to take a deep breath in and watch your thumbs (Fig. 5.11b). If one thumb moves less than the other, this indicates reduced expansion on that side. See Case 5.32.

Back of the chest

How to examine

First concentrate on the lower lobes. The same procedure is followed as for the front of the chest, this time with the doctor standing behind the patient.

1 Ask the patient to breathe in and then out and to hold their breath in expiration.

Key points
- The main aim is to compare the two sides
- Grip the patient's ribcage with your fingers and bring your thumbs together in the midline
- Reduced expansion on one side of the chest anteriorly may be due to pathology in any lung lobe
- Reduced expansion on one side of the **lower** chest posteriorly suggests either pathology overlying the lower lobe (such as effusion) or pathology within the lower lobe (such as fibrosis, collapse, or consolidation)

2 To assess lower lobes:

- place your hands firmly on the chest wall with fingers gripping their sides (the lower ribcage) and bring your thumbs together to meet in the midline around the lower thoracic spine but not touching the chest (Fig. 5.12a)

- ask the patient to take a deep breath in and watch your thumbs (Fig. 5.12b), assessing if one thumb moves less than the other—indicating reduced expansion on that side.

3 To assess upper lobes:

- do the same again this time higher up with thumbs meeting around T3 level.

Cases 5.33, 5.34, 5.35 and 5.36 explore some of the questions you might have about this examination.

Chest percussion

15 Percuss front of chest and in the axillae, comparing the two sides (DF 9/10)

Chest percussion is one of the great arts of medicine. It requires considerable practice to achieve proficiency but once mastered it provides useful clues to chest disease. Percussion was first described in 1761 by *Josef Leopold Auenbrugger (1722–1809, Austrian physician)*. As with many great discoveries, Auenbrugger's ideas were pretty much ignored for 50 years, until they were adopted by *Rene Laennac (1781–1826, French physician, the inventor of the stethoscope)* and colleagues. At that time, percussion was a major diagnostic advance because it provided the first way to distinguish between pleural effusions and consolidations. Since the discovery of X-rays in 1895, percussion's importance has somewhat diminished but it remains an extremely useful tool for evaluating chest diseases when they first present.

(a) 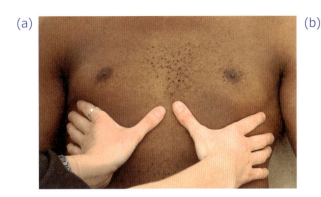 (b)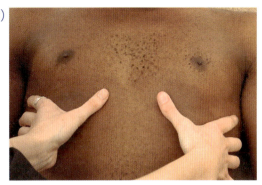

Figure 5.11 Palpation of chest expansion anteriorly.

(a) 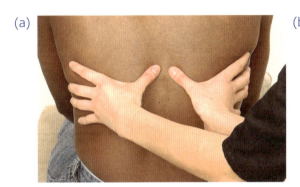 (b)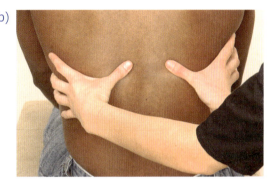

Figure 5.12 Palpation of chest expansion posteriorly—lower lobes.

Problem. When testing for expansion at the front, do my hands go over or under the breasts?

Discussion. Under. You may have to lift the patient's left breast up with your left hand (ask permission) so that you can grip the left ribcage properly with your right hand. Then, slide your left hand under the patient's right breast so that you can grip the right ribcage and bring your thumbs together in the midline.

How to examine: basic technique

There are two different techniques—a normal technique for percussing over the chest wall in general and a modified technique for over the clavicle.

Percussion over the chest wall

See Fig. 5.13.

1 Place your left hand palm down on the chest wall.

Problem. I've checked expansion but wasn't sure if the two sides were equal. When I tried again, it didn't seem to work very well.

Discussion. When repeating expansion, the temptation is just to ask the patient to breathe in again and see what happens to your thumbs. This never works—your thumbs will be separated by this stage. You have to release your grip and start again.

2 Align your fingers with the ribs so that your middle finger is between ribs.

3 Spread your fingers slightly apart (Fig. 5.13a).

4 Press your left middle finger firmly against the chest wall.

5 Now, hold your right hand extended at the wrist with the middle metacarpophalangeal (MCP) joint slightly flexed, so that the distal phalanx is roughly at right angles to the hand (Fig. 5.13b).

CASE 5.33

Problem. Is there any benefit in measuring actual chest expansion overall (as opposed to simply comparing the two sides)?

Discussion. This is not recommended as a routine test, but chest expansion overall can be measured.

1 Wrap a tape measure around the patient's chest (under each axillae).
2 Ask the patient to breathe out and hold it.
3 Tighten the tape measure round the chest and measure.
4 Loosen your grip.
5 Ask the patient to breathe in and hold it.
6 Tighten the tape measure again and measure.

The difference between the two measurements is the patient's chest expansion. Normally, this is >5 cm. A measure <2 cm is clearly abnormal and indicative of lung or chest wall disease. However, this measure does not correlate well with lung capacity.

CASE 5.34

Problem. I've noticed senior doctors sometimes lean over from the front to examine expansion at the back of the chest. Is this a better way?

Discussion. This method involves the same principle, that is, grip at the sides and compare how much the thumbs move in the centre. Some doctors find this more cumbersome and the line of sight can make it difficult to compare the movement of both sides of the chest satisfactorily.

CASE 5.35

Problem. I feel a little awkward when leaning across to examine expansion at the back of the chest. Is it all right to sit down on the bed behind the patient while checking expansion?

Discussion. This can be more comfortable for the examiner but it can also be more awkward. However, it is not unreasonable to sit down to check expansion posteriorly if you personally find it more comfortable.

CASE 5.36

Problem. Both inspection from the end of the bed and palpation are used to assess chest movement—which is better?

Discussion. This is a matter of personal preference. Some doctors find inspection from the end of the bed more informative but others prefer the palpation method. So experiment and find out what suits you.

6 Now hyperextend the wrist further in preparation to strike your left middle finger (Fig. 5.13c).
7 Then, briskly flex the wrist and use the pad of your right middle finger to strike the dorsum of the middle phalanx of the left middle finger (Fig. 5.13d).
8 Remove the percussing finger immediately.
9 With the same motion of the right hand, strike the left middle finger for a second time, again removing the percussing finger quickly (this second strike is non-essential and merely provides confirmation of your first attempt; if you are confident striking once, this is acceptable).
10 While doing step 7, listen to the noise made and sense the feeling of the two fingers meeting—the percussion note is both heard and felt.

Tip
Make sure the left middle finger is placed firmly against the chest wall. Lifting it even slightly makes the percussion note much duller.

Tip
Keep the fingernail of your right middle finger very short.

Percussion over the clavicle

For percussing the clavicle, only the right hand is used. The same technique is applied except that the pad of the right middle finger strikes the clavicle directly rather than the left middle finger. This can be painful for the patient, so be gentle.

Tip
Practice is essential to achieve the consistent action and force required. Particularly in the learning stages, percussion can be awkward (and uncomfortable at the clavicles) so it is helpful if students practise on each other first.

(a)

(b)

(c)

(d)

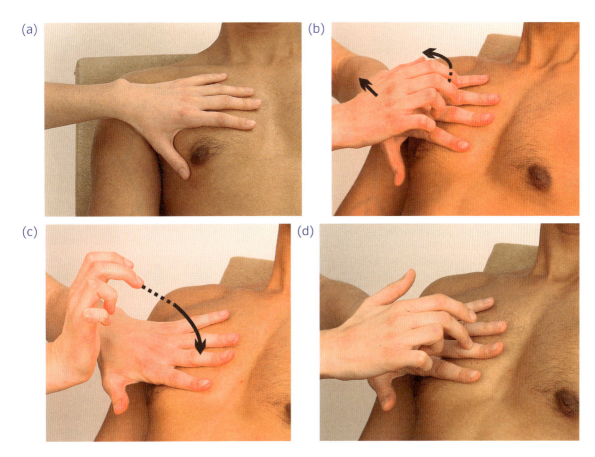

Figure 5.13 Percussion over the chest wall.

Tip

Initially your percussion action may be feeble and you will have to devote time to producing a stronger strike. However, as you improve, it can be easy to get carried away and use too much force—avoid this. The aim is to produce a consistent, audible note without hurting the patient.

How to examine: normality

The aim of chest percussion is to compare the right and left sides of the chest. There are three normal percussion sounds/sensations, which you can check on yourself using the chest wall two-hand technique:

- **dull**—occurs over solid organs such as the liver
- **resonant**—occurs over the lung
- **tympanic**—occurs over the abdomen.

The resonance over the lung is present to approximately the sixth rib anteriorly, the eighth rib in the axilla, and the tenth rib posteriorly. There is usually a dull area over the liver and heart anteriorly.

Why examine?

The percussion note is altered if lung tissue becomes airless, as in consolidation or collapse, or if lung tissue is pushed away from the chest wall by fluid, air, or pleural thickening (Table 5.9). Pleural effusion, consolidation, and lung collapse commonly produce signs over the lower lobes. It should be noted that the percussion note is normal in many patients with important lung disease (notably lung cancer) and can also be normal in minor degrees of the conditions in Table 5.9.

How to examine: a system

Front of the chest and axillae

The patient should remain at 45°, supported by pillows.

1 First, percuss the patient's right clavicle over its medial third (only the medial third overlies lung tissue).

Table 5.9 Types of abnormal percussion

Pleural effusion	Very (stony) dull
Consolidation	Dull
Collapse	Dull

2 Next percuss the left clavicle using the same force, comparing the noise and the sensation—is one side duller than the other?

3 Now percuss the chest wall anteriorly: upper right, upper left, middle right, middle left, lower right, lower left always using the same force and comparing the sides as you go. In women patients, the breasts may make the percussion note dull and percussion more difficult.

4 Ask the patient to abduct their right arm and then percuss the right upper axilla and compare with the left upper axilla; next percuss the right and then left lower axillae.

5 If at any point you think there might be a difference but are unsure, repeat the percussion in that area.

Tip

With the axilla it is perfectly acceptable to percuss down each intercostal space on one side before comparing it with the other axilla. This avoids the need to abduct each arm with consecutive percussion.

Back of the chest

1 The patient should be sitting up and percussion performed with the doctor standing slightly behind the patient (Fig. 5.14).

2 Percuss the chest wall posteriorly: upper right, upper left, middle right, middle left, lower right, lower left, always using the same force and comparing the sides as you go.

Cases 5.37, 5.38, 5.39 and 5.40 explore some of the challenges you may face with this examination.

Tactile vocal fremitus

16 Assess tactile vocal fremitus at the front of the chest and in the axillae, comparing the two sides (DF 9/10)

Traditionally, medical examination is performed according to a sequence: inspection, palpation, percussion, and

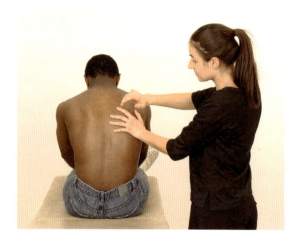

Figure 5.14 Percussion of the posterior chest.

Key points

- Use one hand when percussing over the clavicle, two hands elsewhere
- Make sure the left middle finger is placed firmly against the chest wall
- The percussion note is both heard and felt
- The aim is to compare the right and left sides of the chest using consistent force to produce an audible note without hurting the patient
- The dull side is usually the abnormal side (the exception is pneumothorax)
- Pleural effusion produces a very (stony) dull note, consolidation and collapse produce a dull note, while pneumothorax produces a hyper-resonant note
- The percussion note can be normal in many patients with serious lung disease
- Cardiac dullness makes useful comparisons of percussion note at the front of the chest difficult

expansion—so strictly speaking TVF would be done before percussion. However, TVF is most effective at evaluating areas that have been found to be dull to percussion—in particular differentiating between effusion and consolidation. Therefore, although a form of palpation, the author's view is that TVF is best done following percussion.

Why examine?

Low-frequency vibrations (100–200 Hz) can be detected at the chest wall by a palpating hand. Most speech contains low-frequency harmonics (<300 Hz) so when we

CASE 5.37

Problem. The patient seems perfectly well but there seems to be a large area of dullness over the left side of the chest at the front.

Discussion. This is the patient's heart and so is completely normal. Normal cardiac dullness does make comparison of the percussion note on the front of the chest difficult. However, if the right side of the chest is duller than the left, this does suggest pathology.

CASE 5.38

Problem. The right lung seems dull to percussion yet it appears to be expanding better than the left. Can you explain why?

Discussion. We tend to automatically assume that the side with the dull percussion note contains the pathology. This is usually but not always true. It is the lung that is not expanding that **is** always the one with the pathology. The likelihood is that this patient has a pneumothorax—so rather than the right chest being dull, the left chest is hyper-resonant, making the right side appear dull.

CASE 5.39

Problem. I'm a bit disappointed. I found no abnormality on percussion but the chest radiograph shows large bilateral pleural effusions. Yet I thought I percussed the patient's chest fairly competently.

Discussion. Percussion is essentially a comparative technique, which relies on you identifying differences between the two sides. When there is bilateral pathology, this difference is abolished, making detection of any abnormality more difficult. As you become more familiar with the percussion technique, you will start to get a sense of dullness even when it occurs bilaterally. However, even in the most experienced hands errors can still be made.

CASE 5.40

Problem. So consolidation produces a dull note, pleural effusions are stony dull. Am I really supposed to be able to tell the difference?

Discussion. You're right, it isn't easy. But the differentiation between effusion and consolidation was one of percussion's original benefits. Nowadays, TVF, VR, and the breath sounds provide supplementary information to help distinguish between effusions and consolidation clinically.

speak, low-frequency vibrations are transmitted through the lungs to the chest wall and can be detected by the palpating hand as TVF. The degree of TVF is affected by the thickness of the chest wall, being reduced in overweight patients. It is easier to detect TVF in men than in women because the vibrations created by their deeper (lower-frequency) voices are easier to palpate and are better transmitted through normal lung. When assessing TVF, the aim is to detect differences between the two sides: consolidation increases transmission of speech vibrations so TVF is increased, whereas effusion, collapse and pneumothorax result in reduced transmission and TVF.

How to examine

You should already have established if there are any tender areas—if so, you may need to modify your examination to avoid these areas.

Front of the chest and axillae

- Assess TVF at the apices:
  1 The vibrations over the clavicle are used to assess apical TVF.

  2 Place the ulnar border of your right hand on the patient's right clavicle.

  3 Ask the patient to say 'ninety-nine'. While they are speaking, concentrate on the vibration transmitted to your right hand.

  4 Next, place the ulnar border of your right hand on the patient's left clavicle, ask the patient to say 'ninety-nine', and again assess the vibration transmitted to your right hand. Is the vibration the same on both sides? It should be.

  5 If you are not sure, recheck.

- Assess TVF of the upper lobes:
  1 Place the flat of your right hand over the top of the right side of the patient's chest.

  2 Ask the patient to say 'ninety-nine', concentrating on the vibration transmitted to your right hand.

  3 Do the same on the patient's left side and consider if the two sides are equal.

  4 If you are not sure, recheck.

- Assess TVF of lateral aspects of the lungs:

  1 Ask the patient to abduct their right arm: 'Please lift your right arm out to the side . . . Do you mind if I feel in your armpit (again).'

  2 Place the flat of your right hand on the medial aspect of the patient's right axilla.

  3 Ask the patient to say 'ninety-nine', concentrating on the vibration transmitted to your hand.

  4 Do the same for the left axilla, again comparing the two sides.

Back of the chest

You should be standing behind the patient.

1 Assess TVF of the upper lobes:

- Place the flat of your right hand (see Case 5.41) over the top of the right side of the patient's chest and repeat as for the front, comparing both sides.

2 Assess TVF of lower lobes:

- Place the flat of your right hand over the lower aspect of the right side of the patient's chest and repeat as above, comparing both sides

Cases 5.42, 5.43, and 5.44 answer some questions you may have about assessing TVF.

Key points

- TVF is most effective at evaluating areas that have been found to be dull to percussion
- Consolidation increases TVF
- Effusion, collapse, and pneumothorax reduce TVF
- Assess TVF at apices, upper chest, and axillae anteriorly and over the upper and lower lobes posteriorly

Chest auscultation

17 Auscultate over the front of the chest and in the axillae, comparing the two sides (DF 8/10)

Like chest percussion, auscultation of the chest remains one of the great arts of medicine.

CASE 5.41

Problem. I find it easier to use my left hand when detecting TVF over the right side of the patient's chest—is that alright?

Discussion. There are no hard and fast rules. Use whichever hand gives you the most consistent results. The advantage of using the right hand (or left hand) throughout is that the same hand is sensing the vibration consistently. However, using the right hand throughout does result in a slightly awkward asymmetry in the way your hand contacts the patient's chest. Using your left hand on the patient's right side and your right hand on the patient's left side avoids this asymmetry. Another option is to use both hands together. This can be more difficult and a little embarrassing when examining women.

CASE 5.42

Problem. Why don't you assess TVF on the lower chest anteriorly?

Discussion. The heart causes a normal asymmetry in TVF between the right and left lower chest so there is little value in comparing TVF there.

CASE 5.43

Problem. Can I ask the patient to use phrases other than 'ninety-nine'?

Discussion. TVF was first demonstrated by German physicians who used 'neunzig und neun'. The English translation 'ninety-nine' conveniently produces the same resonances. There's little reason why ninety-nine is better than other phrases sometimes used, such as 'one-hundred-and-one', 'one, two, three', or 'one, one, one'.

How to examine: basic technique

Chest auscultation is performed with the stethoscope. There is no consensus on whether the bell or the diaphragm should be used. The case for the bell is strong: in theory it should be better for hearing breath sounds as these are mostly low pitched; skin or hairs being stretched under the diaphragm may create unwanted artefacts. However, these issues seem

CASE 5.44

Problem. What happens if the patient changes the volume of their voice as they repeat 'ninety-nine'?

Discussion. The louder the patient's voice, the greater the TVF. If the patient varies the volume, explain to them that they need to keep the volume even and try again.

to be of little practical importance and it is common practice to auscultate using the diaphragm apart from the lung apices where good contact with the diaphragm is difficult and the bell is used.

1 Place the diaphragm on the chest wall.

2 Ask the patient to breathe in and out through their mouth deeply and quite fast—respiratory rate about 30 breaths per minute.

3 Listen to the sounds generated.

Bear in mind that too much deep breathing may make the patient dizzy or even collapse (hyperventilation).

Tip

It may be helpful to spend a few seconds showing the patient how to breathe in the manner that you wish.

Tip

It may be best to keep saying 'In . . . out . . . in . . . out . . .' so that the patient is continually prompted.

How to examine: normality

The normal breath sounds over the chest wall are called 'vesicular' (*vee-sick-you-lar*). The quality of these sounds is soft. The French physician and inventor of the stethoscope, René Laennac compared them to leaves gently rustling. Their origin is not completely understood. The inspiratory sound is thought to be due to air turbulence within the small airways and alveoli (*al-vee-owe-lie*). Thus, the intensity of the sound gradually increases through inspiration as more and more air reaches the alveoli. The initial part of the expiratory sound is initially due to air flowing out of the alveoli. Once these have emptied, the sound heard originates in the large airways—further away from the stethoscope—so that the noise becomes quieter in the second half of expiration, fading away to become inaudible.

Why examine: abnormalities

Two types of abnormality may occur: abnormal breath sounds and added sounds.

Abnormal breath sounds

As most of the sound produced in normal breath sounds originates in the small airways and alveoli, diseases that damage these may alter the breath sounds.

- Small airway and alveolar damage is most severe when areas of the lung become consolidated, collapsed, or fibrosed. In such conditions, the breath sounds do not have the soft rustling component produced by turbulence within the alveoli. Instead, noises from the larger airways predominate producing a harsher sound—known as 'bronchial breath sounds' (DF 9/10). In bronchial breathing, the sounds gradually increase through inspiration but stop near the end of inspiration (when air would normally be flowing round the alveoli) and restart after a gap when air flows back through the larger airways during expiration. The expiratory sounds tend to be louder and longer than the inspiratory sounds. Detecting such areas of bronchial breathing can be surprisingly difficult (DF 9/10). However, in the case of consolidated lung, the solidified lung conducts sounds very well so that the bronchial breathing is easier to identify. The features of bronchial breathing are compared with those of vesicular breathing in Table 5.10. See also Case 5.45.

- If just some of the alveoli are damaged, again through consolidation, collapse, or fibrosis, the normal vesicular lung sounds may be reduced in intensity. This may also happen in COPD or asthma. A similar reduction in intensity may also occur where fluid (pleural effusion) or air (pneumothorax) have pushed the alveoli away from the chest wall (and consequently, the stethoscope).

- The expiratory component of the breath sounds may be prolonged in airways obstruction—as air takes longer to leave the alveoli.

Occasionally, in very thin patients, the vesicular breath sounds are louder than normal.

Tip

Because bronchial breath sounds are harsher and tend to sound louder than vesicular sounds, there is a tendency to overdiagnose any loud breath sounds as bronchial sounds. Before diagnosing bronchial breath sounds make sure that the expiratory sound is louder and longer than the inspiratory sound and that there is a gap between inspiration and expiration.

Table 5.10 A comparison of vesicular and bronchial breath sounds

	Vesicular	Bronchial
Quality	Soft, rustling	Harsh, blowing
Inspiratory sound: origin	Small airways and alveoli	Large airways
Expiratory sound: origin	Alveoli and small airways, then large airways	Large airways
Louder component	Inspiratory	Expiratory
Longer component	Inspiratory	Expiratory
Gap	Between expiration and inspiration	Between inspiration and expiration

CASE 5.45

Problem. I'm listening over the upper chest anteriorly and it's difficult to say if the breath sounds are bronchial or vesicular. Can you explain why?

Discussion. Over certain parts of the chest wall overlying the large airways, sounds from these airways dominate so that the normal breath sounds are not vesicular. Over the manubrium, the breath sounds may be bronchial. Close to the manubrium, over the first and second intercostal spaces, the breath sounds may be 'bronchovesicular'. Bronchovesicular sounds are half way between vesicular and bronchial sounds with inspiration and expiration of similar length and intensity and only a short gap between the two.

Tip

Sounds similar to but louder than bronchial breathing can be heard over the trachea normally. Listen to your own breath sounds over your chest and trachea and compare what you hear.

Added sounds

There are three types of added sounds (also known as 'adventitial' (*ad-vent-tish-al*) sounds): crackles (DF 5/10), wheeze (DF 2/10), and friction rub (DF 9/10).

- **Crackles.** Sometimes referred to as crepitations (*crep-it-ay-shuns*) ('creps') or rales (*rahls*), these are short crackly sounds similar to that heard when pulling apart strips of Velcro. They are predominantly (90%) inspiratory. In the past, it was thought that crackles were always due to air bubbling through fluid within the small airways and alveoli. This is clearly the case for patients with left ventricular failure, but it does not explain the marked crackles often heard in pulmonary fibrosis. In such patients, the crackles are thought to be due to changes in gas pressure causing sudden opening of small airways that had collapsed during the previous expiration. Crackles in different conditions have different origins and characteristics (Table 5.11). While crackles may occur in all these conditions, they are not always present, especially early in the disease process. Crackles can be described as fine, medium, or coarse. Fine crackles tend to be high pitched, scratchy sounds like rubbing your hair between your fingers or opening Velcro. Coarse crackles are lower pitch, wet bubbly noises, and medium crackles are in between the two. You will pick these sounds up with experience. See Case 5.46 for advice on distinguishing a crackle from a friction rub.

- **Wheeze**. Also known as rhonchi (*ronk-eye*), wheeze is a continuous whistling sound due to the vibration of opposing walls of narrowed airways as air passes through them. The term used to be restricted to the noise that could only be heard with the unaided ear. However, the sound is similar when heard with the stethoscope and hence the term 'wheeze' has been adopted to embrace all such noises (doctors will often talk of 'wheezes heard on auscultation' to avoid confusion with its traditional definition). They are usually due to small airway obstruction as in COPD or asthma. In such cases the following should be noted:

  - Wheezes are either confined to expiration (40% of patients) or heard throughout inspiration and expiration (60% of patients).

  - The pitch and duration of the wheeze is related to the degree of obstruction (and not its loudness). With severe asthma, so little air moves through

Table 5.11 Features of crackles

	Origin: site	Origin: pathology	Timing	Character	Coughing effects
Fibrosis	Alveoli	Pressure effects	Inspiratory[a]	Fine	No
COPD	Small airways	Pressure effects	Early inspiration	Medium	No
Left ventricular failure	Alveoli	Fluid	Inspiratory[a]	Medium (variable)	No
Bronchiectasis	Alveoli	Fluid and pressure effects	Inspiratory[a]	Coarse	Reduces, sometimes completely
Resolving pneumonia	Alveoli	Fluid and pressure effects	Inspiratory[a]	Coarse	Reduces, sometimes completely

COPD, chronic obstructive pulmonary disease.
[a] Throughout inspiration or second half.

the airways that the chest is effectively silent. The wheeze of asthma tends to be of higher pitch than that of COPD.

- The wheezes are widespread throughout the lungs and tend to have variable pitch (polyphonic) (*polly-fon-ic*).

There are other causes of wheeze. Heart failure may cause wheeze due to associated bronchospasm. The old-fashioned term 'cardiac asthma' sums this up succinctly. Features tend to be similar to asthma or COPD with polyphonic wheezes, either confined to expiration or heard throughout inspiration and expiration. An obstructing lesion within a lung due to a tumour or a foreign body produces wheezes with similar features except that they are monophonic (the same pitch) and localized to one area of the lung. An obstruction proximal to the extrathoracic trachea produces a monophonic rhonchus, which is confined to inspiration and is louder over the neck than over the chest (stridor).

- **Friction rub.** Also known as a pleural rub, this is a grating sound like creaking leather due to rough, thickened pleural surfaces rubbing together as the lungs expand and contract. Such pleural inflammation may be due to pneumonia, pulmonary infarction, or occasionally malignancy. In contrast to crackles, a friction rub tends to predominate in expiration and around two-thirds are confined to expiration. The patient usually complains of pain in the area, when it is known as pleurisy. You have to be very thorough and patient to hear a rub as it may be very localized.

How to examine: a system

Front of the chest and axillae

1 Place the diaphragm of your stethoscope over the patient's chest starting just below the right clavicle.

2 Ask the patient to breathe in deep and fast through the mouth. Demonstrate this to the patient.

3 After each breath move your stethoscope to the next site, comparing both sides. You may need to encourage the patient to keep breathing by saying 'In . . . out . . . in . . . out . . .'.

4 Decide on the intensity and character of the breath sounds and the presence or absence of added sounds as you go.

5 If you suspect an abnormality, listen longer in that area and confirm whether this is true; if so determine its nature (abnormalities may be quite localized so the abnormal sounds are heard only over a small area).

6 Finally, use your bell to listen to the right and left apices in turn.

Back of the chest

1 Stand behind the patient.

2 Use the diaphragm.

3 Auscultate over the chest: upper right, upper left, middle right, middle left, lower right, lower left.

Key points

- Normal vesicular breath sounds originate primarily from small airways or alveoli
- Vesicular breath sounds have a rustling quality, the inspiratory component predominates, and there is a gap between expiration and inspiration
- Breath sounds are reduced in intensity in many common conditions such as COPD and asthma, as well as pulmonary fibrosis, pleural effusion, pneumothorax, and lung collapse
- Bronchial breathing occurs when the small airways or alveoli have been damaged. They are best heard in consolidation but also occur in lung collapse or fibrosis
- Bronchial breath sounds are harsh and blowing, the expiratory component predominates, and there is a gap between inspiration and expiration
- Crackles are due to air bubbling through fluid or pressure effects in damaged small airways or alveoli
- Wheezes are due to small airways narrowing
- The pitch and duration (but not loudness) of wheezes correlate with the severity of obstruction
- When auscultating, compare both sides as you go for the intensity of breath sounds and to ascertain whether they are bronchial or vesicular and note any added sounds
- If you think there may be an abnormality, listen longer, confirm its presence, then determine its nature

Tip

If the patient has severe pain on inspiration (as in pleurisy), it is kinder to reduce the auscultation procedure and rely on radiographic investigation.

Tip

Keep away from the midline where the breath sounds may tend to be dominated by upper airways noise.

Vocal resonance

18 Assess vocal resonance at the front of the chest and in the axillae, comparing the two sides (DF 9/10)

Why examine?

This is a very similar test to TVF and indeed Cases 5.42, 5.43, and 5.44 apply equally to VR. Normally, if you listen

---

CASE 5.46

Problem. I've heard a crackling sound but I'm not sure if it's a friction rub or crackles.

  Discussion. The following points may be helpful: (1) crackles tend to be more prominent in inspiration whereas a rub is usually more prominent in expiration; (2) crackles may be altered by coughing whereas a rub never is; (3) pain over the area on inspiration or on coughing makes a rub more likely.

---

over a patient's chest with a stethoscope while they speak, you will hear muffled indistinct sounds. This is known as VR. The sounds seem to come from the chest piece of the stethoscope. Normal lung conducts lower-frequency sounds better so VR is greater in men than in women. As for TVF, the degree of VR is also affected by the thickness of the chest wall and so is reduced in overweight patients. See Case 5.47 for the relative merits of TVF vs VR.

Abnormalities

- Over an area of consolidation, sound transmission is increased. Words appear more resonant (though not necessarily intelligible) through the stethoscope and appear to be generated closer to the earpiece.
- Effusion, collapse, and pneumothorax result in reduced transmission and VR.

  When assessing VR, the aim is to detect differences between the two sides.

How to examine

Front of the chest and axillae

- Assess VR at the apices:
  1 Place the bell of the stethoscope over the patient's right supraclavicular fossa (Fig. 5.15).
  2 Ask the patient to say 'ninety-nine'.
  3 While they're speaking, concentrate on the sound coming through the stethoscope. Next, place the bell of the stethoscope over the patient's left supraclavicular fossa.
  4 Ask the patient to say 'ninety-nine' and again assess the sound coming through the stethoscope.
  5 Is the sound the same on both sides—it should be?
  6 If you are not sure, recheck.
- Assess VR of the upper lobes:

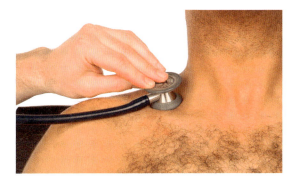

Figure 5.15 Assessing vocal resonance over the apices.

CASE 5.47

Problem. Which is better, TVF or VR? Do I really need to do both?

Discussion. There is no definite answer. They are both testing the same thing—sound transmission through the lungs. TVF is more cumbersome but does have an advantage in that you can more readily notice any variations in the patient's voice intensity that may be producing bogus results. The author finds both tests difficult but useful so prefers to do both using them to confirm or refute findings suspected with the other. Thus, if an area where TVF is suspected to be increased is found but this is not certain, it is useful to be able to test VR over that area: if TVF was truly abnormal, VR should be too. However, if you are very confident in your TVF findings, it is not unreasonable to omit VR (or vice versa).

1 Place the diaphragm of the stethoscope over the top of the right side of the patient's chest.

2 Ask the patient to say 'ninety-nine', concentrating on the sound transmitted through the stethoscope.

3 Do the same on the patient's left side and consider if the two sides are equal.

4 If you are not sure, recheck.

● Assess VR of the lateral aspects of lungs:

1 Ask the patient to abduct their right arm: 'Please lift your right arm out to the side . . . Do you mind if I listen in your armpit?'

2 Place the diaphragm of the stethoscope on the medial aspect of the patient's right axilla.

3 Ask the patient to say 'ninety-nine', concentrating on the sound transmitted through the stethoscope.

4 Do the same for the left axilla, again comparing the two sides.

Key points

● VR tests the same phenomenon as TVF
● Consolidation increases VR; effusion, collapse, and pneumothorax reduce it
● Assess VR at apices, upper chest, and axillae anteriorly and over the upper, middle, and lower chest posteriorly

Back of the chest

1 Stand behind the patient.

2 Use the diaphragm.

3 Assess VR over the chest: upper right, upper left, middle right, middle left, lower right, lower left.

Sitting forward

19 Change the patient's position to facilitate examination of the neck and the back of the chest (DF 6/10)

Now it is time to get the patient to sit forward. This allows examination of the neck and the posterior aspect of the chest. Examination of the anterior aspect of the chest and axillae has allowed a thorough examination over the upper and middle lobes of the lungs, but only a minor portion of the lower lobes. Examination of the back of the chest is particularly important as it allows the evaluation of the lower lobes (Fig. 5.8) where many pulmonary conditions tend to be prominent. The upper third of the posterior aspect of the chest overlies the upper lung lobes while the lower two-thirds overlies the lower lobes.

How?

1 Ask the patient to sit forward. The ideal position is arms crossed—so that the scapulae are rotated laterally. However, patients may have difficulty maintaining this position. A more comfortable alternative is for the patient to sit with their hands on their knees. See Case 5.48 for advice on positions to use for patients who cannot sit forward.

2 Explain that you now wish to examine their neck and the back of their chest.

3 Remove pillows and let down the headrest of the bed to allow easy access to the patient's back.

Key points

- Examination of the back of the chest allows thorough evaluation of the lower lobes of the lungs
- Make sure the patient is comfortable
- You may need to adopt a different position and approach if the patient is weak

4 If need be, ask the patient to shuffle down the bed to give you more room behind him.

5 Check that the patient is comfortable—he will need to stay in this position for a few minutes.

Palpation for lymph nodes in neck

20 Examine the neck for enlarged lymph nodes (DF 8/10)

Why examine?

Enlarged lymph nodes at any site may be due to either generalized or local disease (Table 5.12). When lung disease spreads via the lymphatics, it tends to involve the nodes of the neck, particularly the supraclavicular nodes. Thus, enlarged nodes in the neck may be an important sign of lung disease. About one in five patients with lung cancer have enlarged lymph nodes in the neck. The nodes tend to be hard. They may be very small initially but later may fuse together to form a mass that is fixed to structures underneath. The nodes tend to develop in the supraclavicular area especially deep between the sternal and clavicular heads of sternocleidomastoid. Other common causes of enlarged lymph nodes in the supraclavicular region are lymphoma, tuberculosis, and sarcoidosis. In these cases, the enlarged nodes are firm, rubbery (not hard), and discrete and do not attach to underlying structures. The exception is advanced tuberculosis, which can produce matted nodes that fuse together. Rarely, enlarged supraclavicular nodes are due to other cancers, such as those affecting the head or neck. Cancer affecting the stomach or pancreas may cause an enlarged node in the left supraclavicular region, known as Virchow's node (*Rudolf Virchow (1821–1902), German pathologist and politician*). Higher up the neck, enlarged nodes are most commonly due to local infections particularly throat infections, which usually produce tender, enlarged submandibular nodes.

How to examine

Also see Chapter 11. Just like the axillary nodes, it is important for the muscles to be as relaxed as possible to facilitate palpation of any neck nodes. Also, it is better

CASE 5.48

Problem. The patient can't sit forward.
   Discussion. Common sense is necessary. Depending on the patient's condition various solutions are possible.

- If the patient is slightly weak, help him to sit forward and then stabilize in the above position.
- If the patient is moderately weak, help him to sit over the side of the bed leaning on a table.
- If the patient is severely weak, it may not be appropriate to sit him up and you may have to confine yourself to auscultating from the front over posterior aspect of the axilla.
- With modern profiling beds the head rest can elevate and help to bring the patient forward.
- If you can get help, your assistant can support the patient for you.

For weak patients, you may need to abbreviate the subsequent examination to the most useful tests: percussion and auscultation at the bases of the lungs.

Table 5.12 Causes of enlarged lymph nodes

Generalized	
Malignant	Lymphoma, acute and chronic lymphatic leukaemia
Viral	Infectious mononucleosis, cytomegalovirus, HIV
Bacterial	Tuberculosis, syphilis, brucellosis
Toxoplasmosis	
Sarcoidosis	
Local	
Acute or chronic infection	

(less painful) if in general you use the flats of the palmar aspects of your fingers and only use the tips of your fingers where necessary to get a better feel.

1 Stand behind the patient.

2 Ask the patient to flex their head slightly (so that the neck muscles are relaxed).

3 If you palpate any lumps, ascertain their approximate size, consistency (firm or hard), whether they are discrete or fused together, and whether they are attached to underlying structures.

4 Supraclavicular:

   ● Using your index, middle, and ring fingers together, gently palpate both supraclavicular fossae (Fig. 5.16).

   ● Use the tips of your index fingers to palpate the space between the two heads of sternocleidomastoid (Fig. 5.17).

5 Sternocleidomastoids:

   ● It is best to examine the two sides separately—avoiding potential bilateral palpation of the carotid sinus, which may cause fainting.

   ● Use your right index, middle, and ring fingers together to slowly palpate up the right sterno-cleidomastoid to the angle of the jaw.

   ● Use your left hand to do the same on the patient's left side.

6 Submandibular:

   ● Here, you really have to use the tips of your fingers. Use index, middle, and ring fingers together to palpate both sides simultaneously.

   ● Palpate under the angle of the jaw.

   ● Work your way forwards on both sides to meet at the chin.

Posterior chest inspection and palpation

21 Inspect the back of chest assessing movement (DF 8/10), chest shape (DF 4/10), and other visible abnormalities (DF 4/10)

See also 'Inspection of praecordium including chest expansion'.

Why examine?

The aim is to examine for abnormalities of the back of the chest including:

● kyphoscoliosis

● thoracotomy scar—operations on the lungs especially for lung cancer often require a long, diagonal incision usually near the base of one lung

● chest drains, indicating pleural effusion

● sequelae of investigation or treatment of pleural effusions (large bandage or 0.5–1 cm scar indicating

Key points

● When lung disease spreads via the lymphatics, it may involve the nodes of the neck

● Lung cancer tends to produce hard nodes, which may fuse together to form a mass fixed to structures underneath

● Nodes due to lung cancer usually develop in the supraclavicular area especially deep between the sternal and clavicular heads of sternocleidomastoid

● Other causes of enlarged lymph nodes tend to result in firm, rubbery, discrete nodes, which do not fix to underlying structures

● To examine for lymph nodes, make sure the muscles and tendons are as relaxed as possible

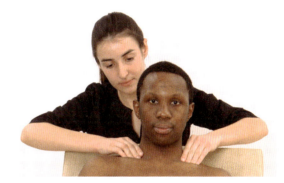

Figure 5.16 Palpating for lymph nodes in the supraclavicular fossae.

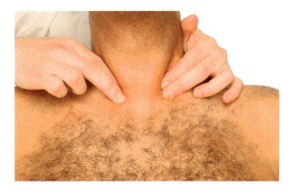

Figure 5.17 Palpating for lymph nodes between the two heads of sternocleidomastoid.

recent chest drain, 1 mm mark or small plaster indicating recent pleural aspiration).

How to examine

1 Stand behind the patient and inspect the back of the chest.

2 Certain abnormalities will be obvious such as kyphoscoliosis, thoracotomy scar, or a plaster over a chest drain or aspirate site.

3 Inspect carefully for marks at the base of the lungs suggesting recent chest drain or aspiration.

4 Next, ask the patient to take a deep breath in and then out through their mouth.

5 As the patient breathes, watch the chest carefully and concentrate on whether one side is moving more than the other—asymmetrical expansion suggests unilateral disease.

6 Then, ask the patient to repeat their deep breath in and out. If your opinion remains unchanged, this part of the examination is complete. If you are unsure get your patient to continue breathing until you are.

22 If appropriate, palpate the posterior aspect of the chest for possible rib fractures (DF 8/10)

See also 'Palpation of trachea and praecordium'.

How to examine

1 Ask the patient 'Is the back of your chest painful or tender?'

2 If the answer is yes, ask for permission to examine: 'Do you mind if I examine the painful or tender spots?'

3 If your patient consents, gently palpate the painful area. Can you elicit tenderness? Is the painful or tender spot within a hard bony area suggesting rib injury or tumour?

23 Palpate for chest expansion posteriorly, comparing both sides (DF 8/10)

See 'Palpation of chest expansion'.

24 Percuss the back of chest, comparing the two sides (DF 9/10)

See 'Chest percussion'.

Key points
- The principles are the same as for the front of the chest
- Look carefully for thoracotomy scars and sequelae of pleural effusions

25 Assess tactile vocal fremitus over the posterior aspect of the chest, comparing the two sides (DF 9/10)

See 'Tactile vocal fremitus'.

26 Auscultate over the back of the chest, comparing the two sides (DF 8/10)

See 'Chest auscultation'.

27 Assess vocal resonance over the back of the chest, comparing the two sides (DF 7/10)

See 'Vocal resonance'.

Other respiratory signs

28 Look for other signs such as whispering pectoriloquy or peripheral oedema if appropriate

As mentioned in Case 3.7, the respiratory routine is an abbreviated version of all possible respiratory signs. Some respiratory signs normally omitted from the routine are discussed in the next pages.

Whispering pectoriloquy (DF 8/10)

This is a very similar test to VR. Instead of the patient saying 'ninety-nine', they whisper the words. Compared to normal speech, whispering produces higher-frequency sounds (well over 400 Hz). Normally, whispered words are muffled when auscultated with the stethoscope and are not often heard. Consolidated lung conducts high frequencies even better than low frequencies so that in some cases of consolidation the whisper is heard well: this is whispering pectoriloquy. Whispering pectoriloquy can sometimes be heard at the top of large pleural effusions where some collapse or consolidated lung may be found.

Key points

- Whispering adds confirmatory evidence in the presence of increased VR
- Whispering pectoriloquy can sometimes be heard at the top of large pleural effusions if there is consolidation above the effusion

Various

Peripheral oedema

Peripheral oedema has many causes. However, if combined with an elevated JVP in a respiratory context it may indicate cor pulmonale. Cor pulmonale occurs when respiratory disease causes chronic hypoxia, which in turn results in pulmonary hypertension and right heart failure. Cor pulmonale indicates that the respiratory system is under considerable strain and as such represents a serious development in a patient with respiratory disease. So you should always check for peripheral oedema if you have found an elevated JVP suggesting cor pulmonale or if there are signs of chronic chest disease such as COPD or fibrosis.

....

Tip
Beware the trap of assuming all patients with respiratory disease with a raised JVP and peripheral oedema have cor pulmonale. As ischaemic heart disease is also common, your patient may have COPD and concurrent congestive heart failure.
....

Temperature

Fever (pyrexia) is defined as a temperature higher than the 99th percentile of temperature found in normal individuals. In healthy people between the ages of 18 and 40 years, this has been found to be an oral temperature >37.2 °C in the morning and an oral temperature >37.7 °C in the evening. The different cut-offs in morning and evening reflect the diurnal variation in temperature (mean temperature is 36.4 °C in the morning and 36.9 °C in the evening). Chest infections commonly (though not always) produce a pyrexia.

Sputum pot

If the patient has symptoms or signs suggestive of infection, you should ask if there is a sputum pot and if so request to inspect the sputum. Yellow/green sputum will

point you towards an infection. Copious amounts produced in one day should make you consider bronchiectasis. Also look out for signs of blood. Although blood can be found in infections, it does raise the spectre of cancer or tuberculosis. Your suspicions may deepen if other worrying symptoms such as weight loss or a persistent hoarse voice are present.

Wash your hands

29 Wash your hands

Do not forget this important infection control measure.

Presentation of findings

30 Pause briefly and then present findings

The aim is to describe your findings emphasizing any abnormality. Because you will have examined so many different areas, it is reasonable to omit certain signs if they are normal. However, certain findings must always be commented on whether normal or abnormal:

- general appearance
- presence or absence of cyanosis
- presence or absence of clubbing
- pulse rate
- respiratory rate
- signs of carbon dioxide retention
- signs of cor pulmonale
- tracheal position
- chest expansion, percussion, TVF, breath sounds (bronchial or vesicular, added sounds), and VR.

As regards carbon dioxide retention, a flapping tremor or bounding pulse need not be specifically mentioned if not present. Similarly if there is no evidence of elevated JVP or peripheral oedema, these need not be specifically mentioned. When describing expansion, percussion, TVF, breath sounds, and VR, it is not necessary to detail your findings over each area of the lungs. It is more important to emphasize any abnormal findings. An example might be as follows.

This woman looks generally well and is not cyanosed. However, she is tachycardic with a pulse rate of 110/min though has a normal respiratory rate at 14/min. She shows no signs of cor pulmonale or carbon dioxide retention. The trachea

is not deviated. Percussion note, TVF, and VR are normal over most of the chest with vesicular breath sounds. However, expansion is reduced on the right side and there is an area of dullness over the right lower lobe with bronchial breath sounds and increased TVF and VR. There are no added sounds. This is consistent with an area of consolidation in the right lower lobe.

Notice that many features that were examined for have not been mentioned, such as the face, eyes, tremor, and tar staining.

Case 5.49 gives advice when faced with conflicting findings.

CASE 5.49

Problem. My findings don't add up. I think I heard bronchial breathing at the right base but found no other abnormality on auscultation or percussion and no change in TVF or VR.

Discussion. You must have got something wrong. The findings should add up. If there really is bronchial breathing, there should be other signs of lung consolidation, collapse, or fibrosis. Check again. The other possibility is that the breath sounds are really vesicular (normal).

Key points
- Emphasize any abnormality
- If your findings don't add up, think again

Respiratory diseases and investigations

In the earlier parts of this chapter, various medical conditions and investigations have been mentioned. In this section I now describe these. In general these descriptions are brief though certain selected topics are discussed in more detail.

Clinical signs associated with important clinical conditions

See Table 5.13.

Pleural effusion

Pleural effusion refers to abnormal fluid in the pleural space.

What is the pleural space?

The visceral pleura is closely applied to the underlying parietal pleura, which in turn is adherent to the thoracic wall. The pleural space is the potential space between the visceral and parietal pleurae. This space is normally filled by a thin layer of lubricating fluid, which ensures friction-free movement of the pleural surfaces.

Causes

There are multiple causes of pleural effusion (Table 5.14). These are usefully categorized into transudates and exudates according to the protein content of the fluid. For this reason it is common to evaluate pleural effusions by aspirating a small amount of pleural fluid through a needle. The most important part of the diagnostic evaluation is to decide whether there is evidence of malignancy.

In general, transudates are bilateral though they may occasionally be unilateral (in which case they are usually right sided). Exudates are usually unilateral, though in the case of collagen vascular disease can be bilateral. Pulmonary emboli without infarction causes a transudate; if infarction is present, the fluid is an exudate.

Symptoms

Breathlessness.

Signs

- Expansion is reduced.
- Percussion is very (stony) dull.
- VR and TVF are reduced.
- Breath sounds are vesicular but of reduced intensity (often absent).
- If the effusion is large the trachea and apex beat may be displaced away from it.

Other types of fluid

The term 'pleural effusion' is usually reserved for serous fluid (though it may be bloodstained) within the pleural space. Other types of fluid are given specific names:

Table 5.13 Summary of clinical signs associated with important clinical conditions

Clinical condition	Position of trachea	Expansion	Percussion	Vocal resonance and tactile vocal fremitus	Whispering pectoriloquy	Auscultation
Normal	Central	Symmetrical	Resonant	Normal	Absent	Vesicular
Consolidation	Central	Decreased	Dull	Increased	May be present	Breath sounds bronchial with coarse crackles
Lobar collapse	Towards the lesion[a]	Decreased	Normal or dull	Decreased	May be present	Decreased breath sounds, may be bronchial breathing
Unilateral fibrosis	Towards the lesion[a]	Decreased on side of fibrosis	Normal	Increased	Absent	Fine crackles. Breath sounds usually vesicular but may be bronchial if fibrosis severe
Interstitial lung fibrosis	Central	Symmetrically decreased	Resonant	Increased	Absent	Fine crackles. Breath sounds usually vesicular but may be bronchial if fibrosis severe
Pleural effusion	Away from the fluid[a]	Decreased	Very (stony) dull	Decreased	Absent but may be present above a large effusion	Breath sounds vesicular but decreased
Pneumothorax	Central	Decreased	Hyper-resonant	Decreased	Absent	Breath sounds vesicular but reduced
Tension or large pneumothorax	Away from the pneumothorax[a]	Decreased	Hyper-resonant	Decreased	Absent	Absent breath sounds (may hear breath sounds from opposite lung)
Asthma or COPD	Central	Symmetrically decreased	Resonant	Normal	Absent	Breath sounds vesicular with chronic prolonged expiration and wheeze (either inspiratory or expiratory or both). Sometimes coarse crackles with added infection

COPD, chronic obstructive pulmonary disease.
[a] Any condition with the potential to shift the trachea (and hence the mediastinum) will only achieve this if it is of sufficient magnitude. Minor examples of these conditions will not cause a mediastinal shift.

Table 5.14 Causes of pleural effusion

Transudate (protein content <30 g/L)
Heart failure***
Hypoalbuminaemia due to chronic liver failure** or nephrotic syndrome*
Meig's syndrome (associated with an ovarian fibroma)* (*Joe Vincent Meig (1892–1913), professor of gynaecology*)
Pulmonary emboli**
Hypoalbuminaemia of other causes
Exudate (protein content >30 g/L)
Pneumonia***
Tuberculosis**
Tumour (effusion may be bloody)—bronchial carcinoma**, breast cancer*, lymphoma **, mesothelioma*
Collagen vascular disease (RA* and SLE*)
Pulmonary infarction (may be bloody)**
Asbestos exposure*
Abdominal pathology (subphrenic abscess, pancreatitis)**

RA, rheumatoid arthritis; SLE, systemic lupus erythematosus.
Ranging from * (uncommon) to *** (common).

- **haemothorax**—blood in the pleural space
- **chylothorax**—chyle in the pleural space
- **empyema**—pus in the pleural space.

Lung consolidation

Consolidation is where an area of lung is filled with fluid or solid matter. This classically occurs in infective pneumonia but may also be a feature of pulmonary haemorrhage or pneumonitis (lung inflammation due to non-infective causes such as drugs and autoimmune reactions). In the latter conditions, the consolidation is usually patchy and the signs variable. It is in infective pneumonia that enough lung is consolidated to give the classical signs of consolidation:

- Expansion is reduced.
- Percussion is dull.
- VR and TVF are increased.
- Breath sounds are bronchial breathing.

Lung collapse

If a bronchus is blocked off, the air in the part of the lung distal to the blockage is gradually reabsorbed leaving a portion of collapsed lung.

Causes

- **Pathology within the lumen.** Secretions—postoperative, asthma, cystic fibrosis, foreign body (classically a peanut).
- **Pathology in the wall.** Bronchial carcinoma.
- **Pathology compressing the wall from outside.** Enlarged lymph nodes usually due to bronchial carcinoma or lymphoma.

Symptom

Breathlessness.

Signs (may be minimal)

- Expansion is reduced.
- Percussion is dull.
- VR and TVF are reduced.
- Breath sounds are usually vesicular but of reduced intensity; there may be an area of bronchial breathing.
- If the area of collapsed lung is large, the trachea (especially with upper lobe collapse) or the apex beat (especially with lower lobe collapse) may be displaced towards it.

Lung cancer

Lung cancer, variously known as cancer of the bronchus, lung carcinoma, or bronchial carcinoma, continues to be the commonest cause of cancer death in the UK. The major risk factor is smoking, though one form of lung cancer (adenocarcinoma) appears not to be smoking related. Lung cancer may present with no symptoms or signs (when it has been identified by chance on a chest radiograph), otherwise it can cause a variety of symptoms and signs. Some of the more common features are described here.

- Local damage within the lung, producing
  - cough, haemoptysis, breathlessness, chest pain, and wheeze (symptoms)
  - inspiratory wheezes, signs of lung collapse or pleural effusion, and clubbing (signs).
- Direct spread within the thorax,
  - affecting the recurrent laryngeal nerve causing hoarseness
  - affecting the sympathetic nerve chain causing Horner's syndrome
  - affecting the phrenic nerve causing paralysis of the diaphragm (the paralysed diaphragm elevates, pushing the lung upwards; thus the part of the chest wall that normally overlies the lower lung overlies solid tissue such as liver instead (producing signs similar to a pleural effusion)
  - invading the superior vena cava causing SVC obstruction.
- Metastatic spread to:
  - supraclavicular lymph nodes
  - liver producing hepatomegaly
  - bones producing tender spots and pathological fractures
  - brain with signs of hemiparesis.
- Non-metastatic extrapulmonary manifestations:
  - anorexia, weight loss, and fever
  - hypercalcaemia
  - neuropathy
  - hypertrophic pulmonary osteoarthropathy
  - myasthenia-like syndrome.

Mesothelioma

Mesothelioma is a malignant tumour of the pleura due to previous asbestos exposure. It is much less common than bronchial carcinoma.

Symptoms

- Pain (sometimes but not usually pleuritic).
- Breathlessness.
- Tiredness.
- Weight loss.

Signs

- Clubbing.
- Hypertrophic pulmonary osteoarthropathy.
- Signs of a pleural effusion.
- Enlarged supraclavicular or axillary lymph nodes.

Lung infections

Various infections may occur:

- **Tracheitis.** Affects the trachea; usually viral; causes chest pain, cough, and sputum; no specific lung signs.
- **Bronchitis.** Affects the main bronchi; usually viral; causes chest pain, cough, and sputum; no specific lung signs.
- **Infective exacerbation of COPD.** Affects small bronchioles; usually due to viral infection, *Haemophilus influenzae*, or *Streptococcus pneumoniae* (pneumococcus); causes increased breathlessness, chest pain, increased cough and sputum, and wheeze; signs of carbon dioxide retention (flapping tremor, bounding pulse) may occur; lung signs—reduced intensity of breath sounds and increased wheezes; chest radiograph shows no new changes.
- **Bronchopneumonia.** Affects the lung parenchyma (mainly alveoli) in a patchy fashion; usually caused by bacteria of low virulence such as *Haemophilus influenzae*; causes breathlessness, chest pain, cough, and sputum; lung signs—crackles; chest radiograph shows patchy shadowing.
- **Lobar pneumonia.** Affects the lung parenchyma such that whole areas of lung are solidified due to the inflammation; usually due to more virulent organisms such as pneumococcus; causes breathlessness, chest pain, cough, and sputum; lung signs—signs of consolidation, may sometimes be complicated by pleural effusion or empyema producing mixed signs; as the consolidation resolves crackles develop; chest radiograph shows a distinct area of shadowing (Fig. 15.21).
- **Pleurisy.** Affects the pleurae; usually a consequence of lobar pneumonia; causes pleuritic chest pain and pleural rub.
- **Lung abscess.** Occurs when there is a localized collection of pus within the lung; may complicate pneumonia (especially that due to staphylococcus or klebsiella), aspiration of food into the lung, or bronchial obstruction by a foreign body; causes

production of large amounts of foul-smelling sputum; produces clubbing and signs of consolidation or crackles; chest radiograph shows one distinct area of shadowing, typically with a fluid level within it (see Fig. 15.25) (lung abscess can be multiple).

- **Empyema.** Occurs when there is a localized collection of pus within the pleural space; may complicate pneumonia but may also follow a subphrenic abscess or penetrating chest wound including surgery; produces clubbing and signs consistent with a pleural effusion; chest radiograph shows pleural effusion.

- **Tuberculosis.** The tubercle bacillus deserves particular mention. Its various stages can cause lung collapse, fibrosis, consolidation, and effusion or empyema. Clubbing is not a feature of tuberculosis.

There are a few points to add:

- Strictly speaking, tracheitis, bronchitis, pneumonia, and pleurisy are all defined as inflammation of the specific part of the respiratory tract. So they may result from physical, chemical, or allergic processes as well as infections. In the case of pneumonia, it is common parlance to use the term 'pneumonia' purely for infective processes. The term 'pneumonitis' is commonly used to describe non-infective processes.

- All these conditions may produce generalized symptoms and signs such as fever, lethargy, anorexia, weight loss, and sweats. The severity of these systemic symptoms (and the disease in general) tends to be greater for bacteria than viruses, for distal disease (such as pneumonia) than proximal disease (such as tracheitis), and where there are collections of pus as in empyema or lung abscess.

- The term 'chest infection' is often used. This is a vague, poorly defined term usually used to describe lung infections that do not produce shadowing on the radiograph, such as tracheitis, bronchitis, and infective exacerbations of COPD.

- Bronchiectasis is a condition which results in dilated bronchi and is often a sequelae of childhood infections. It is characterized by regular production of large amounts of purulent sputum. There may be associated breathlessness. Signs include clubbing and coarse crackles.

Small airways obstruction

There are two conditions characterized by small airways obstruction—asthma and COPD. Small airways obstruction primarily causes difficulty with expiration.

Asthma

Asthma is a clinical syndrome of unknown aetiology characterized by three components:

- Recurrent episodes of small airways obstruction that resolve spontaneously or with treatment.
- Airway hyper-responsiveness. This is an exaggerated tendency to bronchoconstrict to stimuli that have little effect on normal individuals.
- Inflammation of the airways.

Asthma can be a life-threatening condition and is a common cause of hospital admission. The characteristic symptoms are breathlessness and wheeze. On examination, the characteristic findings are increased respiratory rate and heart rate and on auscultation reduced breath sound intensity with prolonged expiration and expiratory wheezes (though there may also be inspiratory wheezes). The British Thoracic Society have produced guidelines that use clinical features to recognize severe or life-threatening attacks.

Severe acute asthma is indicated by the presence of **any** of the following:

- unable to complete sentences because of breathlessness
- respiratory rate ≥25 breaths/min
- heart rate persistently ≥110 beats/min
- peak expiratory flow rate (PEFR) <40% of normal
- a drop in systolic blood pressure on inspiration ≥10 mmHg (pulsus paradoxus).

A life-threatening attack of asthma is indicated by the presence of **any** of the following:

- silent chest on auscultation
- cyanosis
- bradycardia
- exhaustion, confusion, and unconsciousness.

Chronic obstructive pulmonary disease

COPD is characterized by airway obstruction due to chronic bronchitis or emphysema. This obstruction may vary but never returns to normal: there is an irreversible component. Chronic bronchitis is defined as the presence of cough productive of sputum on most days of at least 3 months of at least 2 successive years. The diagnosis of emphysema is pathological: destruction of air spaces distal to the terminal bronchioles due to destruction of their walls (mostly alveolar destruction). Both emphysema and chronic bronchitis are usually due to tobacco consumption and tend to occur together.

Effects

The characteristic symptoms of COPD are cough, sputum, breathlessness, and wheeze. Examination may reveal the following:

- increased antero-posterior chest diameter (barrel chest)
- pursed-lip breathing
- use of accessory muscles of respiration
- reduced expansion bilaterally
- percussion note may be a little hyper-resonant
- VR and TVF may be reduced bilaterally
- breath sounds are vesicular, but of reduced intensity, prolonged expiration, wheezes that may be confined to expiration or occur both in inspiration and expiration and crackles
- as the disease progresses, chronic hypoxia may produce cyanosis and signs of cor pulmonale (elevated JVP, ankle oedema, and right ventricular heave).

There are three points to add:

- Many patients have combinations of asthma and COPD where there is some reversibility. It may be difficult to say which is the more important component in such cases. Table 5.15 gives some differences, albeit stereotypical, which may help to decide which is more important.
- β_2-Agonist drugs such as salbutamol are one of the mainstays of treatment for both asthma and COPD treatment. They themselves may produce clinical signs; for example, tremor and tachycardia.
- Clubbing is not a feature of COPD.

Pulmonary fibrosis

Fibrosis of lung tissue is the reaction of the lung tissue to a variety of insults (Table 5.16). Different conditions tend to affect different parts of the lung to greater or lesser extents. Fibrosis can also be localized or generalized in distribution. Localized fibrosis may be caused by infection (especially tuberculosis), infarction, or previous radiotherapy. Generalized fibrosis may be caused by the inhalation of irritants, autoimmune disorders, or drugs. An immune response leads to a diffuse infiltrate in the lungs, which can lead to thickening and fibrosis around alveolar walls (called fibrosing alveolitis). The fibrosing alveolitis is called idiopathic or cryptogenic when the cause cannot be identified. More recently different histopathological groups have been identified with different natural histories and therefore prognoses. The term 'idiopathic interstitial pneumonia' has become the all-embracing term for these different groups and idiopathic fibrosing alveolitis has become one of the subgroups (and is

Table 5.15 Asthma compared with chronic obstructive pulmonary disease

	Asthma	Chronic obstructive pulmonary disease
Age group	Young	Old
Smoker for more than 10 years	No	Yes
Breathless between attacks	No	Yes

Table 5.16 Causes of pulmonary fibrosis

Autoimmune	
Idiopathic (= cryptogenic) pulmonary fibrosis	L
Scleroderma	L
Sarcoidosis	U
Rheumatoid arthritis	L
Inhalation of irritants	
Asbestosis	L
Coal-miners' pneumoconioisis	U
Silicosis	U
Extrinsic allergic alveolitis	U
Drugs (amiodarone, methotrexate)	L
Post infection or tuberculosis	U

U, predisposition to upper lobes; L, predisposition to lower lobes.

also known as usual interstitial fibrosis) (see Fig. 5.18). Whatever the cause, pulmonary fibrosis tends to cause breathlessness and a dry cough. The main signs are clubbing and crackles over the affected lobes. Breath sounds are usually vesicular but if the fibrosis is severe may be bronchial. Clubbing is a particular feature of idiopathic pulmonary fibrosis and asbestosis. It is rare in scleroderma, silicosis, sarcoidosis, tuberculosis, and drug-induced fibrosis.

Pulmonary embolism

This is where part of the pulmonary arterial circulation is blocked off by a thrombus that originated from the venous

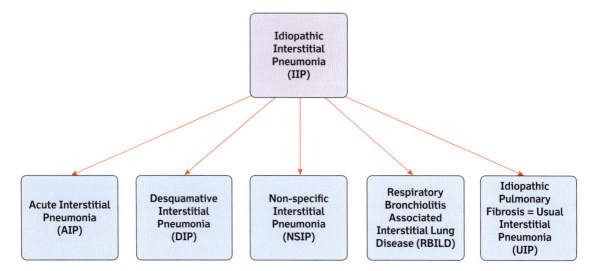

Figure 5.18 Classification of idiopathic interstitial pneumonia.

system. It is sometimes complicated by pulmonary infarction (where a portion of lung tissue infarcts).

Effects

The effects depend on the size of thrombus, whether the embolism is persistent, and whether it causes pulmonary infarction:

- **small embolism, one-off**—no clinical features
- **small emboli due to persistent embolism (chronic thromboembolic disease)**—breathlessness and signs of pulmonary hypertension—elevated JVP, right ventricular heave, and tricuspid regurgitation murmur
- **medium embolism, no infarction**—breathlessness and tachypnoea
- **medium embolism with associated pulmonary infarction**—breathlessness, pleuritic chest pain, tachypnoea, pleural rub, and pleural effusion
- **major embolism**—breathlessness, central chest pain, hypotension, cyanosis, elevated jugular venous pulse, and sudden death.

The clinical features of pulmonary embolism are neither sensitive nor specific in making the diagnosis.

- The diagnosis is best confirmed with a spiral CT lung scan (or isotope ventilation/perfusion scan). However, because of the potential seriousness of the diagnosis, anticoagulant treatment should be started as soon as the diagnosis is suspected—do not wait for the scan result.

- Patients with medium embolism and no infarction produce very non-specific clinical features. So always consider pulmonary embolism in patients with unexplained breathlessness.

....

Tip

Always check the legs for signs of a deep venous thrombosis: unilateral leg swelling, stiffness of the calf muscles, increased warmth of the affected side, and tenderness between the heads of the gastrocnemius muscle. Such signs are present in around one-third of pulmonary embolism patients.

....

Pneumothorax

Pneumothorax refers to air in the pleural space. A pneumothorax occurs when damage to the lung causes air to leak from the lung, through the visceral pleura into the pleural space. Such damage may occur either spontaneously or less commonly following trauma (see Table 5.17).

Effects

The presence of air in the pleural space abolishes the negative pressure within the space, which provides the suction force that maintains the inflation of the lungs.

Symptoms

The air within the pleural space may cause pleuritic pain while the lung collapse causes breathlessness.

Table 5.17 Causes of pneumothorax

Spontaneous
Any lung disease, especially emphysema
Subpleural bleb, usually in young adults (mostly men) with otherwise normal lungs

Trauma
Iatrogenic, following pleural aspiration or central line insertion
Chest wall injury

Signs

- Expansion is reduced.
- Percussion is hyper-resonant.
- VR and TVF are reduced.
- Breath sounds are vesicular but reduced.

Tension pneumothorax

In this condition, air in the pleural space accumulates creating sufficient pressure to force the mediastinum and its contents away from the side of the pneumothorax. This is a dangerous development.

Causes

In most cases of pneumothorax, the leak closes off as the lung deflates. In the case of a tension pneumothorax, the opening from the lung into the pleural space not only persists but acts as a valve so that air enters the pleural space in inspiration but cannot exit on expiration. Tension pneumothorax usually follows trauma and only rarely occurs spontaneously.

Effects

This is an emergency situation. As the pressure in the pleural space builds up, not only does the lung collapse, but the mediastinum is pushed further towards the opposite side until venous return to the heart is reduced with a consequent reduction in cardiac output.

Symptoms

- Pleuritic pain.
- Severe breathlessness.

Signs

- Expansion is minimal.
- Percussion is hyper-resonant.
- VR and TVF are absent.
- Breath sounds are absent.
- Often accompanied by hypotension, cyanosis, and tachypnoea. There may be signs of mediastinal displacement with the trachea and apex beat shifted away from the affected side.

Spirometry

The spirometer is a machine that measures the volume of air blown into it.

There are two key measurements:

- **forced vital capacity (FVC)**—the volume of air expelled by a maximal expiration, from an initial position of full inspiration
- **forced expiratory volume over 1 second (FEV_1)**—the volume of air expelled in the first second, again from an initial position of full inspiration.

The ratio of FEV_1/FVC is usually calculated. This is normally around 70% (somewhat higher in young people). In small airways obstruction, both the FEV_1 and FVC are reduced but the FEV_1 disproportionately so—so that the FEV_1/FVC ratio is reduced. In pulmonary fibrosis, again both FEV_1 and FVC are reduced but the FVC disproportionately more so—so that the FEV_1/FVC ratio is increased.

Peak expiratory flow rate

The PEFR is the maximal rate of flow of expired air. The measurement is obtained using a peak expiratory flow meter (Fig. 5.19). As in spirometry, the patient should start after taking a full inspiration. However, rather than a prolonged expiration, the aim is to blow as hard as possible into the meter. The meter measures this maximal flow rate. The PEFR is reduced in small airways obstruction and as such is commonly used to monitor asthma control.

Bronchoscopy

This is where a fibreoptic instrument (similar but smaller to that used in gastroscopy, see Chapter 7) is passed into the bronchial tree to inspect it for pathology. Only proximal lesions close to the bronchial tree are usually suitable in day-to-day practice, students will more often be tested on patients with pleural effusions and consolidation (see Tables 5.18 and 5.19). The latter is particularly uncommon in examinations, as pneumonia is an unpredictable illness the signs of which usually resolve in a matter of weeks with treatment.

Key diagnostic clues

In day-to-day medicine, the key signs are those pointing to severity of asthma or COPD such as pulse and respiratory rate and any added auscultatory sounds. However, as regards Finals, the key signs are clubbing, expansion (as measured by both inspection and palpation), and percussion or auscultation especially at the bases of the lungs posteriorly.

Key signs for Finals

- **Pulmonary fibrosis.** Clubbing, fine crackles at bases of lungs bilaterally posteriorly.
- **Bronchiectasis.** Clubbing, coarse crackles at bases of lungs bilaterally posteriorly.
- **Pleural effusion.** On affected side—expansion reduced, very (stony) dull to percussion, reduced breath sound intensity, reduced TVF and VR, trachea may be deviated away from affected side.
- **Consolidation.** On affected side—expansion reduced, dull to percussion, bronchial breathing, increased TVF and VR.

Some advice relating to examination problems now follows.

Some advice relating to examination problems

General

Do not waste time looking for the respiratory system examination routine that will completely satisfy all examiners. It does not exist! Use the one given in this chapter.

The instruction

The examiner will usually ask you to 'examine the respiratory system'. Occasionally, they will say 'examine the chest'. These both mean the same thing. However, if the examiner is more specific, such as 'auscultate at the bases', you must

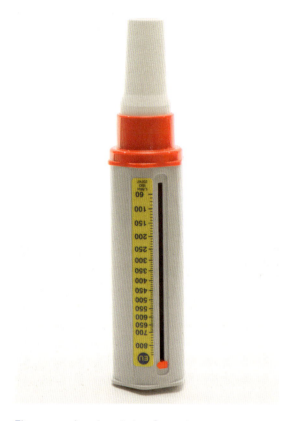

Figure 5.19 A peak expiratory flow meter.

for this procedure (peripheral lesions are best investigated using CT scanning with or without fine needle biopsy). As well as observing lesions there is also the facility to biopsy specimens for histological analysis, aspirate fluid for culture and cytology, and sometimes remove mucus plugs or other thickened secretions that can cause respiratory embarrassment.

Finals section

In this section, some specific issues dealing with Finals will be discussed. This is not a summary section. For revision, I suggest you read the key points throughout the chapter and the examination summary and do the questions at the end of the chapter.

In exams, the examiners need patients with consistent signs. Thus, patients with pulmonary fibrosis and bronchiectasis are common Finals diagnoses whereas

Table 5.18 Common Finals cases

Pulmonary fibrosis

Bronchiectasis

Pleural effusion

Table 5.19 Common day-to-day cases

Asthma or COPD

Pleural effusion

Consolidation

Pulmonary fibrosis

Bronchiectasis

do just as they request. With such requests, the possibility of confusion here is in how to fit in the 'general look'. This should be done, as always, while preparing the patient for examination. In the OSCEs written instructions are given; see the following examples.

Moving infirm patients

Always proceed with the aim of carrying out the full examination requested, asking the patient's permission as you go. If the examiner feels that moving such a patient is inappropriate, they will stop you.

Positioning

Even if the patient is already sitting in bed at an angle of around 45°, you should alter their position, albeit minimally, to make it clear to the examiner that you know the patient should be at that angle.

Hands

Clubbing is the key sign. You need to make a clear decision on its absence or presence. Clubbing is much more common in examination patients so if you think it is present, you are probably correct. Try not to spend longer than 30 seconds.

Face

With respect to Horner's, it can be very easy to overdiagnose anhidrosis and ptosis. The clearest sign in Horner's

is the miosis; if this is not present it would be unwise to diagnose Horner's. SVC obstruction is very easy to overlook; just make sure you consider it as a possibility before moving on.

Neck

While the JVP can be an important sign in the respiratory system, it is nowhere near as fundamental as it is in the cardiovascular system. If you cannot see it, do not spend ages analysing why. Simply consider it not elevated.

Inspect front of chest from end of bed

This is the best way of identifying unilateral disease. Pleural effusion, pneumothorax, and consolidation all cause a reduction in expansion on the affected side—so concentrate. Three breaths in and out is enough: more than this is unlikely to enlighten you further but may cause the patient to become light-headed.

Palpate apex beat

As for the JVP, the apex beat is a sign that can be difficult to assess while not adding much information to the respiratory examination. It is often impalpable as in COPD and even if you do suspect that it is not in the normal position, there are lots of cardiac reasons to explain this. So, if you cannot feel the apex beat, move on quickly. If you think the apex beat is in an abnormal position it would be unusual to find a respiratory cause to explain this.

Percussion, tactile vocal fremitus, breath sounds, and vocal resonance

It is clearly important to examine over the whole of the chest. However, you will need to combine brevity with thoroughness.

Percussion

Practise percussion as much as possible (perhaps more than other signs) because your technique will be seen as an indicator of how much time you have spent with patients. Even if you get the case wrong, the examiner cannot fail to be impressed if your percussion technique is slick.

Tactile vocal fremitus and vocal resonance

Stick to 'ninety-nine'. You do not want to stand out (other than for your expertise).

Examination of the front of the chest as a whole

In the examination setting, common cases such as pulmonary fibrosis, bronchiectasis, and pleural effusion may produce little in the way of signs on the front of the chest. So if you have not found any abnormality by the time you begin examination of the back of the chest, do not worry. It is the bases posteriorly that usually hold the answer.

Axillae

The axillae should be examined while examining the front of the chest. Sometimes, you will realize that in the heat of the moment, you have forgotten to do this. If this is the case, it is quite reasonable to examine the axillae from behind.

Putting the signs together

The signs should make sense. If you find an area of dullness, the breath sounds should also be altered (reduced in pleural effusion or bronchial in consolidation) as should the TVF and VR (reduced in pleural effusion and increased in consolidation). It is reasonable to perhaps expect that one or two of the five key features (expansion, percussion, TVF, breath sounds, and VR) do not quite add up, but to find one isolated abnormality is very unlikely. Clubbing combined with crackles has three key causes (Table 5.20).

Wash your hands

Do not forget this important procedure, which also provides a pause for thought.

Presentation

VR at the back is the last part of the examination of the chest itself. While doing this, formulate your thoughts as to what you have found overall.

Good luck!

OSCE examples

History-taking station

You are an FY1 in the medical admissions unit. An 83-year-old man presents with increasing shortness of

Table 5.20 Causes of clubbing and bilateral basal crackles

Idiopathic pulmonary fibrosis
Bronchiectasis
Asbestosis

breath and a cough. Take a focused history of the patient. Form a list of differential diagnoses and come up with a range of initial investigations. You do not need to examine this patient. You have 8 minutes in total. The examiner will stop you after 6 minutes and ask you to present the history and formulate a management plan.

Remember:

- Introduce yourself to the patient.
- Take a focused respiratory history covering cough, sputum production, exercise tolerance, haemoptysis, shortness of breath (SOB), chest pain.
- Ascertain the patient's usual level of functioning.
- PMH including COPD, asthma, cardiac symptoms.
- Social history, including smoking.
- Drug history, including inhalers, nebulizers, oxygen, and allergies.
- Thank your patient.
- The main differentials would be pneumonia and exacerbation of COPD although congestive cardiac failure is a possibility.
- Check observations (e.g. HR, BP, RR, temperature, oxygen saturation).The main investigations would include bloods (full blood count (FBC) to check WCC, U&E for kidney function, CRP for signs of infection. Chest radiograph to differentiate between pneumonia, exacerbation of COPD, and to rule out heart failure. Arterial blood gases (ABG) if patient is sufficiently ill to determine if hypoxic ± respiratory failure.

Examination station

You are a junior doctor working in the emergency department. A 79-year-old who is a smoker presents with a 3-week history of haemoptysis. You should examine this patient's respiratory system. On completion of the examination, give a list of basic investigations. The examiner will then show you a radiograph which you should interpret (see Fig. 5.20). There is no need to take a history. You have 15 minutes in total.

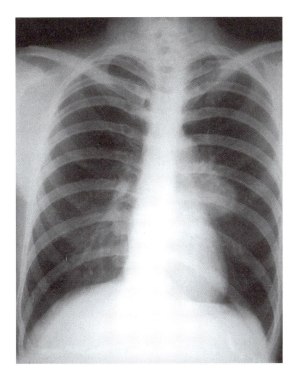

Figure 5.20 Radiograph showing unilateral hilar enlargement.

You will be expected to:

- Introduce yourself to the patient and gain consent for the examination.
- Wash your hands/use alcohol gel provided.
- Get your general look in: does the patient look cachexic; check from the end of the bed/couch to see if both sides of the chest are expanding equally.
- Conduct a full respiratory examination including general inspection, hands, face, neck, palpation, percussion, auscultation front and back.
- Don't forget to check for lymphadenopathy.
- Thank your patient and wash your hands/use alcohol gel provided.
- Ask for supplementary tests if not already available—sputum sample, chest radiograph, peak flow.

Radiograph shows unilateral hilar enlargement and in conjunction with the history makes the diagnosis of bronchial carcinoma highly likely. Further investigation would include CT of the thorax and abdomen, and bronchoscopy.

Questions

1 Give three causes of chronic cough not due to chest disease.
2 What are the three commonest causes of clubbing?
3 Give two features that suggest that an acute asthma attack is severe.
4 Give four causes of haemoptysis.
5 What circumstances would require urgent action in a case of haemoptysis?
6 Give four physical signs of SVC obstruction.
7 Compare percussion note, breath sounds, and TVF in lung consolidation, lung collapse, and pleural effusion.
8 What examination features would you expect with a left-sided pneumothorax?
9 Describe the characteristics of bronchial breathing. In which conditions might you encounter it?
10 What is whispering pectoriloquy and when might you encounter it?

References and further reading

British Thoracic Society/Scottish Intercollegiate Guidelines Network; British guidelines on the Management of Asthma (revised) Jan 2012; Lim WS, Baudouin SV, George RC, et al. BTS guidelines for the management of community acquired pneumonia in adults: update 2009; *Thorax* 2009; **64**:iii1–iii55.

Buller AJ, Dornhorst AC. The physics of some pulmonary signs. *Lancet* 1956; ii:649–51.

Coury C. Hippocratic fingers and hypertrophic osteoarthropathy. A study of 350 cases. *British Journal of Diseases of the Chest* 1960; **54**:202–9.

Cretikos MA, Bellomo R, Hillman K, et al. Respiratory rate: the neglected vital sign; *Medical Journal of Australia* 2008; **188(11)**: 657–9.

Currie GP, Gray RD, McKay J. Chronic cough. *BMJ* 2003; **326**:261.

Goldhill DR, McNarry AF, Mandersloot G, et al. A physiologically-based early warning score for ward patients: the association between score and outcome. *Anaesthesia* 2005; **60**:547–53.

Hirschberg B, Biran I, Glazer M, Kramer MR. Hemoptysis: etiology, evaluation and outcome in a tertiary referral hospital. *Chest* 1997; **112**:440–4.

Hooker EA, O'Brien DJ, Danzi DF, Barefoot JAC, Brown JE. Respiratory rates in emergency department patients. *Journal of Emergency Medicine* 1989; **7**:129–32.

Irwin RS, Curley FJ, French CL. Chronic cough. The spectrum and frequency of causes, key components of the diagnostic evaluation, and outcome of specific therapy. *American Review of Respiratory Disease* 1990; **141**:640–7.

Lee BR, Yu JY, Ban HJ, et al. Analysis of patients with hemoptysis in a tertiary referral hospital. *Tuberculosis and Respiratory Diseases (Seoul)* 2012; **73(2)**:107–14.

Lim WS, van der Eerden MM, et al. Defining community acquired pneumonia severity on presentation to hospital: an international derivation and validation study. *Thorax* 2003; **58**:377–82.

Mackowiak PA, Wasserman SS, Levine MM. A critical appraisal of 96.8° F, the upper limit of the normal body temperature, and other legacies of Carl Reinhold August Wunderlich. *JAMA* 1992; **268**:1578–80.

Martin JF, Kristensen SD. Finger clubbing. *Lancet* 1991; **338**:947.

Murphy RLH, Holford SK, Knowler WC. Visual lung-sound characterisation by time-expanded wave-form analysis. *New England Journal of Medicine* 1977; **296**:968–71.

Smith GB. Measuring pulse and breathing rates—simple, yet complex. *Resuscitation* 2011; **82**:1367–8.

Thirumaran M, Sundar R, Sutcliffe IM, et al. Is investigation of patients with haemoptysis and normal chest radiograph justified? *Thorax* 2009; **64**:854–6.

6 Neurological system

CHAPTER CONTENTS

Introduction

The neurological examination is one that often fills medical students (and some doctors) with a sense of dread. In fact it is one of the easiest examinations to perform and has the added benefit that all the signs elicited are very obvious; for example, the presence of a tremor or a brisk reflex. This is in contrast to those elusive diastolic murmurs in the cardiovascular system or that palpable splenic tip in the abdominal system. However, be warned that if you try to learn everything in one go, you will be overstretched. Your approach should be to learn small digestible chunks until you can put it together. This chapter has a helpful structure to guide you. Start off with the symptoms and then when you get to the examination, learn the cranial nerves, then the motor system, followed by the sensory system, etc.; or in any order you wish. The aim will be to zip it all together once you are proficient into one seamless neurological examination. To help you make sense of your examination there is a section devoted to analysing your findings, to help you to pinpoint where a lesion is, as well as making a diagnosis. There is also a section on important presentations following this, together with a 'Neurological diseases and investigations' section for you to dip in and out of so you can put your clinical findings into context. However, before you can do this it is important to have some basic knowledge of neuroanatomy as this will aid you in your understanding of how neurological problems occur and ultimately how to diagnose them.

Basic neuroanatomy

The two important subdivisions of the peripheral nervous supply to the limbs are the motor and sensory systems. In the motor system, impulses originate in the cerebral cortex and terminate at a muscle in the periphery to initiate movement, whereas the sensory system operates in the opposite direction, carrying information from receptors in the skin for example, up to the brain.

Motor pathways

Impulses from the motor cortex in the cerebral hemispheres travel along upper motor neurons (UMNs) in the corticospinal tracts to the internal capsule. This is an area of the brain where nerve fibres become tightly packed. From here, they travel through the midbrain, pons (*ponz*), and medulla (*med-duller*) (collectively known as the brainstem). The majority of fibres cross the midline of the medulla in a process called decussation (*de-cuss-ay-shun*). More precisely, this occurs in an area called the pyramids of the medulla and hence the corticospinal tracts are also known as the pyramidal (*pi-ram-id-al*) tracts.

Having crossed over, the corticospinal tracts descend to different levels within the spinal cord. Some end in the cervical cord to supply the arms while others continue to the lumbar levels to supply the legs. They terminate in the 'anterior horns', which are projections of the grey matter within the spinal cord as seen on transverse section. Here they synapse with anterior horn cells, the axons of which are known as lower motor neurons (LMNs). These transmit impulses along the limbs to the target muscle. This pathway is important for control of movement by the cerebral cortex. Other descending tracts are also involved but the corticospinal pathway is the only one you need to know in detail. See Fig. 6.1.

Differentiating upper and lower motor neuron lesions

As illustrated previously, the two main components of the motor pathway are the UMN, originating in the cerebral cortex and the LMN, originating in the anterior horns of the spinal cord; UMN and LMN lesions produce very different clinical pictures, although weakness is common to both. See Table 6.1 for a comparison of UMN and LMN lesions.

Upper motor neuron lesions

The UMN, under cortical control, acts to modify the activity of the LMN. It can stimulate the LMN to achieve voluntary movement, but has predominantly inhibitory effects at rest. If the UMN is damaged, then loss of this descending inhibition from the cortex leads to increased reflexes and tone. This is mediated by the spinal reflex. Wasting is mild and occurs late in UMN lesions since the muscle is still innervated by the LMN. UMN or 'pyramidal' weakness has a characteristic distribution, being more pronounced in weaker muscle groups. Hence in the arms, the relatively weak action of triceps is overcome by the biceps, leading to a flexor posture of the limb. By contrast, pyramidal weakness in the legs results in an extensor posture of the limb because the extensor power of the quadriceps is greater than the flexor action of the hamstrings. Two further neurological signs, which are found in UMN but not LMN disease, are the plantar response (one of the superficial reflexes) and clonus (*clone-us*).

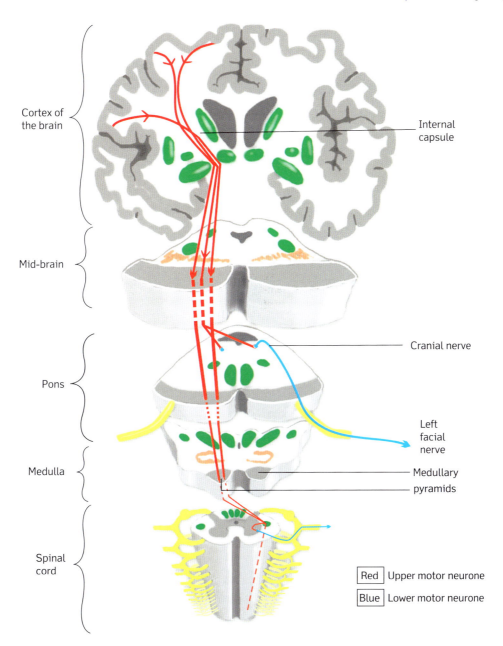

Cortex of
the brain

Internal
capsule

Mid-brain

Pons

Cranial nerve

Left
facial
nerve

Medulla

Medullary
pyramids

Spinal
cord

| Red | Upper motor neurone |
| Blue | Lower motor neurone |

Figure 6.1 The pyramidal system.

Lower motor neuron lesions

The LMN forms the final common pathway to the muscle. If it is damaged, no impulses reach the target muscle, which becomes wasted and flaccid. Reflexes are diminished or absent because the muscle cannot contract.

Visible contractions of muscle fibres known as fasciculations (*fa-sick-you-lay-shuns*) may be present. These are a characteristic feature of motor neuron disease. In contrast to UMN lesions, LMN pathology causes weakness that tends to predominantly affect the distal musculature.

Table 6.1 Comparison of upper and lower motor neuron lesions

	Upper motor neuron lesion	Lower motor neuron lesion
Inspection	Wasting, often mild	Wasting more marked
	No fasciculations	Fasciculations may be present
Tone	Increased	Reduced/normal
Distribution of weakness	Extensors > flexors (arms), flexors > extensors (legs)	Distal > proximal
Reflexes	Increased	Reduced
Plantar response	Extensor	Flexor/absent

Spinal reflex

See Fig. 6.2. Although the pathway from the motor cortex to the target muscle seems long, it takes less than a second from initiation of a thought to contraction of a muscle. Occasionally even more rapid responses are required, so there are shorter pathways that do not travel up to the cortex. These form a local reflex arc between the muscle and the spinal cord, enabling the body to perform swift protective movements without requiring conscious thought.

Mechanism

Voluntary muscle contains 'spindle fibres'—adapted muscle fibres that act as sensory organs. When the tendon is tapped, stretching of the spindle fibres occurs, stimulating sensory impulses. These impulses pass along sensory afferent tracts to the spinal cord ('afferent' indicates that the tracts are entering the spinal cord). These directly synapse with the efferent fibres (that is, fibres leaving the spinal cord), which are LMNs, resulting in muscle contraction. This type of reflex is known as a stretch reflex, because reflex contraction of the muscle is triggered by stretching of the spindle fibres. This is in contrast to superficial reflexes, which are triggered by sensory receptors in the skin, for example the plantar reflexes.

Control of movement

When voluntary movements are initiated by the cerebral cortex, other areas of the central nervous system are activated to ensure that muscle contraction is smooth and coordinated. The two most important of these are described here.

Cerebellum

The cerebellum (*serry-bell-um*) is located posterior and inferior to the cerebral hemispheres. It also consists of two hemispheres, each involved with control of movement

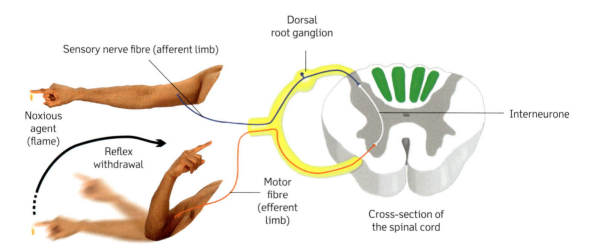

Figure 6.2 The spinal reflex.

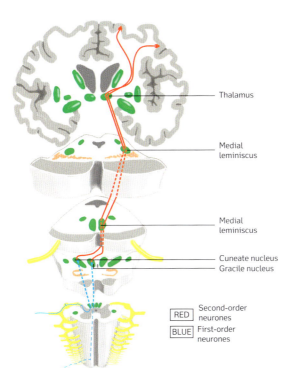

Thalamus

Medial leminiscus

Medial leminiscus

Cuneate nucleus
Gracile nucleus

RED Second-order neurones
BLUE First-order neurones

Figure 6.3 The dorsal columns.

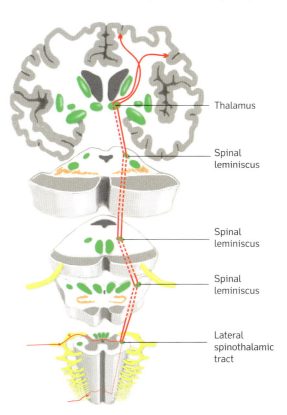

Thalamus

Spinal leminiscus

Spinal leminiscus

Spinal leminiscus

Lateral spinothalamic tract

Figure 6.4 The spinothalamic tracts.

of the **same** side of the body. They are linked by a midline structure called the vermis (*ver-miss*). The latter is concerned with the function of the trunk muscles and is involved in the maintenance of posture.

Basal ganglia

The basal ganglia are a group of structures situated within the cerebral hemispheres, deep to the cortex (subcortical). They consist of the corpus striatum (*core-puss-try-ate-um*), the substantia nigra (*sub-stan-sha-nigh-gra*), and the subthalamic nucleus. The function of the basal ganglia is less well understood than the cerebellum, but they are also involved in normal muscle function. Diseases affecting these structures will be described later.

Sensory pathways

There are two main sensory pathways. One is the dorsal column system, which, as its name suggests, transmits impulses in the dorsal part of the cord relating to vibration, joint position sense, and pressure (see Fig. 6.3). The other is the spinothalamic (*spy-no-tha-lam-ick*) pathway, which carries pain and temperature information (see Fig. 6.4). Light touch is carried by both pathways, but principally in the dorsal columns. In the dorsal columns, impulses from receptors pass along the peripheral nerve to the spinal cord and ascend on the ipsilateral side (meaning the same side) of the cord before crossing at the medulla. In contrast, the spinothalamic tracts decussate much earlier, either at the same level as their entry into the cord or a few segments above. They then ascend in the contralateral (opposite) half of the cord. Impulses from both tracts pass to the sensory cortex of the cerebral hemispheres, via the thalamus (*tha-la-muss*). Damage at any point in these pathways may lead to abnormalities in the appreciation of sensation.

Tip

Students often forget which tract travels on which side of the cord. The mnemonic **disc** will help: **d**orsal tracts are **i**psilateral; **s**pinothalamic tracts are **c**ontralateral.

Dermatomes

The skin can be divided up into areas known as dermatomes (*der-mat-omes*), each supplied by a specific spinal cord segment. For example, the skin over the tip of the shoulder lies within the C5 dermatome, because impulses from here will enter the cord at the fifth cervical segment (see Fig. 6.5). Unfortunately for students, it is important to have some idea about the distribution of dermatomes. This is because if there is a sensory disturbance that conforms to a dermatomal distribution it gives a clue as to where the lesion is.

Symptoms

Blackouts and syncope

What are they?

A blackout is a colloquial term for a loss of consciousness. Patients sometimes use the word 'collapse'. This word is less specific and embraces patients who fall to the floor with or without loss of consciousness. Neither terms are medical in origin but are in widespread use by the general public.

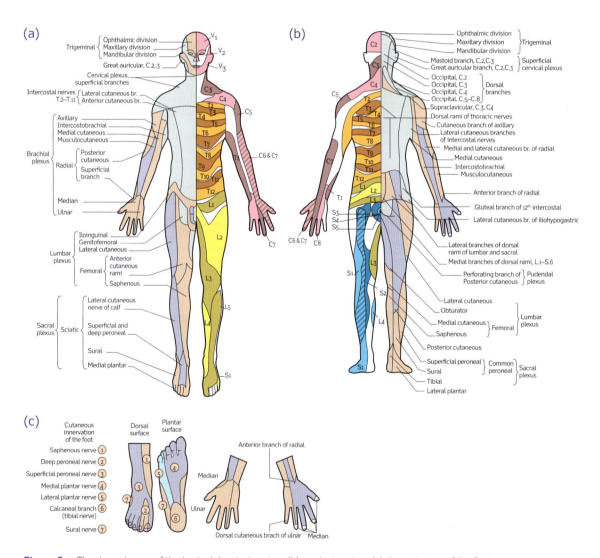

Figure 6.5 The dermatomes of the body: (a) anterior view, (b) posterior view, (c) dermatomes of the foot.
Adapted by permission of Oxford University Press from Fig. 1(a) and (b) (pp. 21.110 and 21.112), *Oxford Textbook of Medicine* (2nd edn, Vol. 2), edited by Weatherall, D. J. et al. (1987), reproduced by permission of Oxford University Press from *Brain's Clinical Neurology* by R. Bannister.

Syncope (*sin-cup-ee*) is a medical term and refers to a sudden transient loss of consciousness and postural tone with spontaneous recovery. The underlying problem is usually within the cardiovascular system.

What to ask

A blackout can be a challenging symptom for the history-taker. The story may be vague, there may be no eyewitness account (a vital component in the investigation of blackouts) and the causes can be wide ranging. When asking questions about blackouts, it is worth dividing your enquiry into

- questions about the blackout itself
- questions about events leading up to the blackout
- questions about events following the blackout.

Instead of rushing to a diagnosis, try and reach it in stages. The answers you receive should allow you to determine which 'system' may be at fault. In a previously fit person the systems that are principally affected are the cardiovascular system, where there is a temporary decrease in the flow of blood to the brain (e.g. due to cardiac arrhythmia) and the neurological system, where consciousness is disturbed usually because of epilepsy. The first thing to establish is what your patient means by their terminology. Ask, 'What do you mean by blackout or collapse?' Many patients use these terms interchangeably and they can be used to not only describe loss of consciousness, but dizziness, vertigo, a fall, or even the loss of memory. If the description remains vague you may have to ask a leading question, 'Did you pass out?' Always be on your guard for the uncertain response, 'I don't think so' or 'I might have done'. Take these answers with a pinch of salt. Also, try not to get frustrated with your patient. Remember that events can happen extremely quickly. This point highlights the value of an eyewitness account.

Questions about the blackout itself

- **'How long were you unconscious for?'** At first sight this seems a stupid question but sometimes a helpful bystander may inform them how long they passed out for. Or they may use detective work to deduce how long they were unconscious, for example, 'I had just put on a CD and when I came round it was still Adele playing, so it must have been two minutes at the most.' Usually syncope lasts less than a minute. Neurological causes can last several minutes and occasionally hours.

- **'Have you had blackouts before?'** If they have, try and get an accurate account of how many and how recent.

Clearly, five blackouts in the space of a week is worrying and needs urgent investigation. One previous attack, 20 years ago, occurring in explicable circumstances—for example, after prolonged standing on the spot (vasovagal [*vay-z-owe-vay-gal*] syncope, also known as fainting), is less worrying. Establish if they ever had faints at school or in childhood as they may still retain the propensity for syncopal events.

- **'Are you able to prevent an attack?'** Sometimes patients with syncope recognize the light-headed, pre-syncopal feeling as a warning that they may pass out. If they are able to sit down or lie down quickly they may abort an attack. Patients with epilepsy can never prevent an attack once it begins.

Questions about events leading up to the blackout

- **'How was your health on the morning of the blackout?'** This establishes a baseline for their health. An older person who is unwell may be at the limit of their ability to compensate so that any additional stress—e.g. standing too long or antihypertensive treatment—may be sufficient to cause syncope.

- **'What were you doing just before the blackout?'** Loss of consciousness while sitting or lying down is unlikely to be due to syncope. Blacking out following exertion could be due to aortic stenosis. A common scenario is the patient who has been standing for long periods, particularly in a warm environment. These are essential prerequisites for vasovagal syncope.

- **'Did you have any chest pain or palpitations before the blackout?'** This question probes the possibility of a cardiovascular cause for the blackout, for example, myocardial infarction or arrhythmias. If the answer is yes then further questions need to be asked to refine the diagnosis (see Chapter 4).

- **'Did you have pain anywhere else?'** This question is a check for other possible causes: for example, headache—subarachnoid haemorrhage? stroke? hypoglycaemia?

- **'Did you have any unusual feelings or symptoms before blacking out?'** This question is important. A light-headed feeling, a hot or cold feeling rising up the body (or down) accompanied by nausea, sweating, and occasionally ringing in the ears could be the result of syncope. More unusual symptoms such as a strange feeling, taste, smell, or nausea (often difficult to describe) prior to the blackout may be the aura preceding an epileptic fit. Patients with known epilepsy learn to recognize their aura as a warning of an impending fit.

• **'What was the last thing you remember before blacking out?'** This gives your patient another opportunity to recall any of the above.

Questions about events following the blackout

• **'What is the first thing you remember when you came round?'** This is another important question. If they remember being on the floor and were instantly aware of their surroundings, this would suggest a cardiovascular cause leading to a syncopal attack. However, if the first thing they remember is coming round in the ambulance or hospital (despite eyewitness accounts of the patient being conscious), this would strongly favour epilepsy as a possible cause. Following a seizure, epileptics are frequently confused and often have no recollection of events for minutes, hours, and occasionally days afterwards. This is described as the post-ictal (*ick-tal*) state.

• **'Did you injure yourself?'** People who have epileptic seizures lose control of their limbs and can fall to the floor unprotected and sustain injuries. Also ask, 'Did you bite your tongue?' This injury may suggest the possibility of epilepsy (although it can occur with other forms of loss of consciousness if the tongue is caught accidently in the teeth).

• **'Did you wet yourself?'** This is an embarrassing question, but if your patient has lost bladder control this is strongly suggestive of epilepsy. However, be wary of older patients or patients with existing continence problems as they may lose bladder control regardless of the reason for losing consciousness.

Do not forget other aspects of your history, which may give supporting evidence.

Past medical history

Ask the patient if they have epilepsy. It is surprising how some patients do not volunteer this up front. Also check if they have diabetes. A prolonged episode of hypoglycaemia can lead to unconsciousness (therefore a blood sugar level should always be checked on any unconsious patient). Also check if they have had any previous neurosurgery, as seizures may be a complication of this surgery.

Drug history

Check if the patient is on anticonvulsant medication and if it has been taken regularly. Are they on antihypertensive, antianginal, or anti-Parkinson's medication as they can lead to postural hypotension. Tricyclic anti-depressant drugs can lower the seizure threshold in susceptible people, leading to fits.

Family history

Ask if there is a family history of epilepsy or heart disease.

Social history

Check especially for alcohol consumption. Alcoholics may drink until they are stuperose and may still deny that they have a problem (often leading to protracted and fruitless investigations). They may also develop seizures if they drink excessively in a session, or paradoxically if they abstain from drinking. Also check if the patient drives. If they do drive they must be told **not** to drive until the cause of their blackout has been determined. Those diagnosed with epilepsy must be seizure free for 1 year before they can resume driving. If you are lucky enough to interview an eyewitness, it is useful to ask many of the questions you asked the patient. This allows you to gauge which aspects of the history are reliable. An eyewitness account is even more important if your patient is confused. A description of the blackout and events just before and after are the most valuable aspect of their account. Ask the following questions.

• **'Did they become pale before losing consciousness?'** Pallor suggests a cardiovascular cause.

• **'Did they shout or cry out?'** In epilepsy there is often an involuntary shout or groan during the tonic phase (see 'Neurological diseases and investigations' section), before the patient falls to the floor. Care must be used when interpreting this observation because sometimes a person may cry out when they stumble or trip. Therefore make sure that the witness is sure that an accidental fall did not occur before ascribing the shout to epilepsy.

• **'Did they fall without protecting themselves?'** When someone trips they automatically attempt to break their fall with their arms. With epilepsy, because all voluntary muscle control is absent, patients fail to protect themselves when they fall to the ground (often leading to injury).

• **'Did they lower themselves to the floor?'** Patients with syncope can recognize they are about to pass out and try to get on to the floor before they fall to the floor. Patients with abnormal illness behaviour or malingerers also get themselves on to the floor (often exhibiting strange movements when on the floor to mimic a fit). Have an index of suspicion for this type of patient if they give a story of multiple blackouts without injury.

• **'Did they go rigid and then start jerking their limbs?'** This is the classical description of a seizure and is highly suggestive of epilepsy. However, even with this description the diagnosis may still not be clear cut.

Some people who hit their head or who become temporarily anoxic (lack of oxygen) can also develop seizures, which are not due to epilepsy.

- **'How long were they unconscious?'** See above.
- **'Were they confused when they came round, and if so how long did this last?'** The greater the duration of confusion the greater the chances are that you are dealing with epilepsy.

Do not be alarmed if the diagnosis is not clear following your history (and examination). This is common. Try to determine whether the cause is cardiovascular or neurological (usually epilepsy) in nature. This is important, as it will guide your subsequent investigations. Table 6.2 will help you to make the distinction. If this was not difficult enough, many of the criteria that help to differentiate a cardiovascular cause from a neurological one are blurred when dealing with older people and these are also highlighted in Table 6.2. Be flexible and be prepared to change your working diagnosis as more information is gathered

on many occasions. Above all, remember that even the experts get it wrong. People have been wrongly labelled as epileptic or have had the diagnosis overlooked by neurologists. This highlights the difficulty of this particular symptom and why a detailed assessment is vital. Therefore be meticulous and patient and be prepared to see these patients on many occasions before the vital clue is unearthed.

Dizziness

What is it?

Dizziness is a common description that people use to describe a variety of symptoms. These include light-headedness, wooziness, vertigo, feeling unsteady, confusion, and anxiety. Dizziness is rarely life threatening, especially if it is infrequent and short lived, for example, lasting a few seconds only. The true significance of dizziness lies in its underlying cause. A patient who is ill, for example, with an infection, may report

Table 6.2 Contrasting symptoms of cardiovascular and neurological causes of blackout with modifications for the older patient

Feature	Usual distinction		Modification in older patients
	Faints	**Fits**	
Posture	Usually occur in the upright position	Not position dependent	Faints in older people are not position dependent because they are often due to position-independent pathology
Onset	Gradual	Sudden	Loss of consciousness may be quite abrupt in syncope in an older person; partial complex seizures may have a gradual onset
Injury	Rare	More common	A syncopal attack may be associated with significant soft tissue or bony injury in an older person
Incontinence	Rare	Common	An individual prone to incontinence may be wet during a faint; partial seizures will not usually be associated with incontinence
Recovery	Rapid	Slow	A fit may take the form of a brief ('temporal lobe') absence; a faint associated with a serious arrhythmia may be prolonged
Post-event confusion	Little	Marked	A prolonged hypoxic episode due to a faint may be associated with prolonged post-event confusion
Frequency	Usually infrequent and usually with a clear precipitating cause	May be frequent, without a precipitating cause	Faints associated with cardiac arrhythmias, low cardiac output, postural hypotension, or carotid sinus sensitivity may be very frequent

Adapted from Table 3 (p.21), *Epilepsy in elderly people* by Raymond Tallis (1995), with permission from Martin Dunitz.

Key points

- Always determine what your patient means by a blackout
- Always try and get an eyewitness account of the blackout
- Determine what the patient's health was like leading up to the blackout
- Ask if there were any symptoms such as chest pain or palpitations before the event
- If the patient bit their tongue and was incontinent and confused after the blackout, this is strongly suggestive of epilepsy
- If the blackouts happen while the patient is standing and some events are prevented by sitting or lying, this is strongly suggestive of syncope

dizziness when they exert themselves. This will be more noticeable if they have been bed bound for long periods. Dizziness in this context does not require investigation unless it becomes prolonged. Your history should identify patients who are at risk of blackouts. When dizziness is the prelude to a blackout, it is called presyncope (*pre-sin-cup-ee*).

Causes

See Table 6.3.

What to ask

First ask, 'What do you mean by dizziness?' The answer to this is crucial, as it will determine your next sequence of questions. Be prepared to ask supplementary questions to refine your patient's answer, for example, 'Is it a light-headed feeling?' (syncope? hypoglycaemia?), 'Did the room spin round?' (vertigo?), or 'Do you feel your balance is poor?' (ataxia?). Then ask, 'Did you feel that you were going to pass out?' If the answer to this is yes, this increases the chance of the patient's event being presyncopal (beware that this is subjective, and someone who is very anxious may swear blindly that they were even going to die). Also ask, 'Were you able to stop yourself passing out?' Many people will attempt to sit or lie down during a dizzy episode and this may abort an attack if it is due to reduced blood flow to the brain. Now ask, 'What was your health like just before the attack?' (this establishes a baseline for their health), 'What were you doing just before the dizzy episode?' 'Did you have any chest pains or palpitations?' 'Did you have any pains

Table 6.3 Causes of dizziness

Physiological
Warm environment[a]
Overexertion[a]
Anxiety
Hyperventilation
Cardiovascular
Low cardiac output[a]
Congestive heart failure[a]
Myocardial infarction[a]
Cardiac arrhythmia[a]
Vasovagal syncope[a]
Postural hypotension[a]
Neurological
Transient ischaemic attack[b]
Vertigo
Acute labyrinthitis
Ménière's syndrome
Benign positional vertigo
Epilepsy[a]
Endocrine
Hypoglycaemia[a]
Addison's disease[a]
Myxoedema
Thyrotoxicosis
Anaemia
(All causes)
Hypoxia
Respiratory disease
Cardiovascular disease

[a] Also causes blackouts.
[b] Only causes blackouts if posterior circulation transient ischaemic attack.

Key points

- Always determine what your patient means by dizziness
- Discover what their health was like before the attack
- Ask if there were any other symptoms associated with the attack, for example, chest pain or palpitations
- Ask if they have ever lost consciousness or felt that they were about to lose consciousness
- Check what medications they take
- Worrying features that warrant further investigations include blackouts, focal neurological signs, and chest pain or palpitations

elsewhere?' and 'Did you have any other symptoms?' The relevance of these questions is explained in the blackout section.

Other worrying symptoms that suggest the need for further investigation include

- blackouts
- diplopia or blurred vision
- hearing loss
- dysphasia (a disorder of language)
- limb weakness
- sensory abnormalities
- chest pain or palpitations.

Vertigo

What is it?

Vertigo is the false perception (hallucination) of movement. The patient feels the environment is spinning or swaying, when this is clearly not the case. Any person can experience vertigo by spinning round rapidly on the spot. This sets up a rotational current in the fluid of the semicircular canals (SCCs), which in turn stimulates the hair cells within the current. This informs the brain that the body is spinning. However, when you stop, the fluid within the canals still has momentum and will continue to stimulate the hair cells, fooling the brain into thinking the environment is still rotating. Disease of the vestibular system can also fool the brain into thinking that the environment is spinning. The resultant vertigo can be so severe that the

patient can fall to the floor. They may also suffer with nausea and may vomit.

Causes

See Table 6.4

A description of the causes of vertigo listed in Table 6.4 can be found in the 'Neurological diseases and investigations' section.

What to ask

Most people will complain of dizziness rather than vertigo. Therefore you will only establish that true vertigo exists by probing what they mean by dizziness. If the answer is vague then you may have to ask the leading question, 'Does the room and its contents spin around?' Also ask the following supplementary questions.

- 'Did you feel sickly?'
- 'Have you vomited?'
- 'Were you able to walk around during an attack?'
- 'Has your hearing been affected?' (Ménière's syndrome?)
- 'Have you ever heard a ringing or buzzing sound in the ears?' (Ménière's syndrome?)
- 'Does it occur when you change your position, e.g. turning to one side in bed?' (BPPV?)

Table 6.4 Causes of vertigo

Acute labyrinthitis
Benign paroxysmal positional vertigo (BPPV)
Ménière's (*many-airs*) syndrome (*Prosper Ménière (1799–1862), French ENT surgeon*)
Acoustic neuroma (*new-roma*)

Key points

- Vertigo is the hallucination of movement
- With true vertigo the patient will be unable to walk and will fall to the ground
- Vertigo is usually accompanied by nausea and sometimes vomiting
- Always ask about hearing impairment and tinnitus when faced with vertigo

Headache

A headache is a common symptom and most people have experienced this at some time in their life. It is important to deduce whether the headache has an innocent or a sinister cause. To do this you need to be familiar with the common causes and how they present (see Table 6.5). You will also need to know the rarer causes and their presentations so you do not miss a potentially treatable condition before it becomes too advanced for treatment. The approach to headache is similar to that of pain elsewhere in the body.

What to ask

This can be broken into two sections: (1) questions about the headache itself and (2) questions about the potential causes of headache.

Table 6.5 Causes of headache

Primary
Migraine
Tension headache
Cluster headache
Secondary
Trauma
Referred from eyes, face, sinuses, teeth, and neck
Meningitis or encephalitis
Subarachnoid haemorrhage
Space-occupying lesion[a]
Drugs
Temporal arteritis
Other medical conditions, for example, hypoglycaemia and infections

[a] A 'space-occupying lesion' (SOL) is a non-specific term to describe any lesion in the brain that occupies space. This could be a tumour, abscess, or haematoma (other rarer causes exist). Because the cranium is a closed container any additional swelling will lead to a rise in intracranial pressure and to the symptoms described below. As a general rule a SOL in the posterior fossa will lead to rapid rises in intracranial pressure as there is very little space for the brain to expand into, whereas tumours in the anterior fossa can grow to relatively large sizes before any rise in pressure causes symptoms. Additional symptoms may be experienced depending on the area of brain affected. A primary cause of headache is where there is no obvious underlying cause for the headache. A secondary cause is where the headache is due to an obvious underlying medical cause.

Questions about the headache itself

Begin with an open question, 'Tell me about your headache'. This gives your patient an opportunity to give their version of events. However, there are key facts you need to establish (if they are not forthcoming in their account).

- **'Where is the headache?'** The site of pain can sometimes point you towards a specific condition. Tension headache can be experienced 'like a band' around the head. Migraine tends to be unilateral and temporal arteritis causes tenderness over the temporal arteries in the temple region.

- **'Was the onset sudden or gradual?'** Headache of sudden onset is of great concern. If the pain literally comes on in seconds, and is severe, 'like being hit by a baseball bat', this could represent a subarachnoid haemorrhage. These patients require urgent investigation. Some variants of migraine can also have a rapid onset. Otherwise most other causes of headaches usually have a gradual onset.

- **'Have you experienced headache like this before?'** Recurrent headaches experienced over many years are unlikely to be due to a sinister cause. Causes of recurrent headache include tension headache, migraine, and sinusitis. If headache is recurrent try to get an idea of the frequency of headache. Is it every fortnight or is it daily? Do the headaches occur in a cluster (cluster headaches?—see 'Neurological diseases and investigations' section) or are they related to menstruation (migraine can be triggered by the hormonal changes associated with the menstrual cycle). Also determine whether the frequency of headache has changed. This could represent the development of a SOL and therefore requires further investigation. It is now appreciated that migraine and sometimes tension headache can change their character and frequency following regular dosing with medication and become a chronic daily headache. This is called a transformed migraine. The cure for this situation is weaning off the analgesia. This can be difficult to achieve because the patient may experience rebound headache on stopping or reducing their analgesia and will be reluctant to discontinue their medication. They may be convinced that something sinister is going on and that the return of the headache is proof that they need even stronger medication. This process needs to be managed skilfully with firm guidance and counselling.

- **'How long does the headache last?'** Most benign causes of headache are short lived, lasting from a few hours to a couple of days. Other headaches are persistent so long as the underlying cause remains active, for example, temporal arteritis or meningitis. Other active disease may not produce a continuous headache but one that is intermittent or that can be aggravated by certain manoeuvres, for example, cerebral tumour worsening with straining, coughing, or sneezing.

- **'How severe is the headache?'** This feature can be misleading but still needs to be documented because of the impact on the patient's life. Some benign causes, for example, migraine, can cause excruciating pain and prevent the patient from working. Conversely intracerebral tumours may only produce a dull, nagging headache, which can be shrugged off easily.

- **'Can you describe the headache?'** The character of the pain is always difficult to describe so you may have to give options. Is the pain burning in nature, sharp, or throbbing? A feeling of diffuse pressure over the top of the head or a band-like constriction may suggest a tension headache. Throbbing pain may suggest a tension headache or migraine. A sharp, shooting (lancinating) pain suggests nerve root irritation or neuralgia. A burning pain may also suggest a neuralgia.

- **'Does the pain come on at a particular time of the day?'** A headache that is present on waking or wakes a person from sleep should raise the suspicion of a SOL in the brain. This feature is not specific to SOLs because other headaches such as migraines can also mimic this. A headache that gets worse at the end of the day may be due to a tension headache.

- **'Does anything bring on the pain (precipitating factors)?'** Sometimes the cause of the headache is clear cut, for example, following trauma or drug ingestion. Sometimes the precipitant is less obvious, for example, the original stressor in chronic tension headache may have been forgotten over the months. Migraines may be precipitated by stress, fatigue, changes in sleeping habits, menstruation, and alcohol.

- **'Does anything make the pain worse (aggravating factors)?'** The headache due to a SOL can worsen if the patient bends forwards or if they strain in the toilet. The headache of sinusitus may also worsen if the patient bends forwards. With temporal arteritis, there is tenderness over the temporal arteries at the temples and sometimes over the occiput when the patient combs their hair.

- **'Does anything make the pain better (relieving factors)?'** This question is less helpful. Patients with migraine and tension headache find they may get temporary relief if they can get off to sleep. Some people may find a measure of relief with analgesia but run the risk of developing a transformed migraine or rebound headache if they rely heavily on medication.

- **'Do you have any other symptoms (associated factors)?'** With migraine, patients may suffer an aura. This tends to be visual, in the form of flashing lights (photopsia) or zigzag lines (fortification spectra or teichopsia *[tie-cop-sia]*). They may develop blind spots (scotomas) (*sco-toe-maz*) or visual field defects. Most migraine sufferers develop photophobia (aversion to light) and nausea with occasionally vomiting. Patients with meningitis may have associated photophobia and nausea. For symptoms of other conditions see the next section on the potential causes of headache.

Questions about the potential causes of headache

Causes of headache that you should know and their associated features are described in the following list. Please note that a fuller account of these can be found in the 'Neurological diseases and investigations' section.

- **Migraine**. Unilateral headache (occasionally bilateral), pulsatile in nature, aggravated by exercise or bending, may experience visual aura, for example, zigzag lines; motor aura, for example, hemiplegia; or sensory aura, for example, hemianaesthesia. The aura usually lasts less than 1 hour and is usually (but not always) followed by headache. Also associated with nausea, vomiting, photophobia, phonophobia (aversion to sound), and osmophobia (aversion to smells).

- **Tension headache**. Usually bilateral headache, 'tight' like a band or a diffuse pressing sensation. Occasionally photophobia or phonophobia (never both together as in migraine).

- **Cluster headache**. Severe unilateral headache, sometimes burning quality, also ipsilateral (same side) conjunctival injection (red eye), lacrimation, nasal congestion and rhinorrhea *[rhino-rear]* (runny nose), miosis (*my-owe-sis*) (small pupil), and ptosis (*toe-sis*) (drooping eyelid). May have a cluster of attacks with remissions.

- **Trauma**. Severity of pain usually lessens with time from incident. Can occur weeks to months after event. It can be difficult in late-onset headache or those of prolonged duration to know whether they are truly due to trauma or are a function of an anxiety or depressed state (or seeking compensation). Also associated with dizziness, decreased concentration, anxiety, and depression. Headache may also be as a result of intracranial bleeding. In this situation, clinical features may be due to raised intracranial pressure, that is, nausea, vomiting, focal neurological signs, seizures, and altered conscious level.

- **Meningitis**. Severe headache, nausea, photophobia, neck stiffness. Other symptoms depend on infecting organism: viral—sore throat, arthralgia, and muscle pain; bacterial—late complications (focal neurological signs and fits, petechial rash). If you suspect meningitis and are faced with a petechial rash (a purply-blue pinpoint rash) that does not blanch when a glass tumbler is placed over it (see Fig. 14.6) or more confluent bruising, this is probably the onset of septicaemia as a result of meningococcal infection. This is a medical emergency and the patient should be given antibiotics immediately (preferably penicillin or cephalosporin).

- **Encephalitis**. Decreased conscious level, focal or generalized fits, focal neurological signs, neck stiffness.

- **Subarachnoid haemorrhage**. Severe headache of sudden onset, nausea, photophobia, neck stiffness.

- **SOL**. Dull headache worse in the morning and with straining, nausea, vomiting, may be focal neurological signs, seizures, personality changes (see 'Neurological diseases and investigations' section).

- **Drugs**. A variety of drugs may cause headache. The principal group are the vasodilators, for example, nitrates or calcium channel blockers. Other drugs include caffeine, alcohol, and the contraceptive pill. Associated features will depend on the individual drugs involved but common features are nausea and dizziness. Illicit drugs including cocaine, amphetamine, and cannabis also cause headache. Withdrawal of chronically administered drugs including analgesics, alcohol, and illicit drugs may also cause headache. Associated features in this situation include sweating, tremor, dizziness, and irritability. A rarer mechanism for drug-induced headache is an aseptic meningitis (an inflammation of the meninges not due to an infection). Drugs implicated include non-steroidal anti-inflammatory drugs and intrathecal (*in-tra-thee-cal*) (into the spinal fluid) chemotherapy, for example, vincristine or intravenous immunoglobulin.

- **Referred pain**. Headache can be referred from eyes, ears, face, sinuses, teeth, and neck. Acute-angle closure glaucoma is worthy of mention because its recognition will not only reduce misery but will potentially save vision in the affected eye. Pain is around and above the affected eye and can be severe. Associated features include a red eye, an oval poorly reactive pupil, coloured haloes seen around light sources (due to corneal clouding), nausea, and vomiting.

- **Temporal arteritis**. Headache localized to temples or occiput, malaise, pain on chewing (jaw claudication),

Key points

- Sudden onset of headache (within seconds) suggests a subarachnoid haemorrhage and is a medical emergency
- The severity of headache is not proportional to the severity of the underlying cause
- A headache that is present on waking, which worsens with straining, is a SOL until proven otherwise.
- A headache with fever, photophobia, and neck stiffness is meningitis until proven otherwise (if a purpuric rash is also present, give antibiotics straightaway as this is an absolute emergency)

Raynaud's (*ray-nose*) phenomenon of the tongue, visual loss, associated with polymyalgia rheumatica (therefore proximal muscle pain and stiffness).

- **Other medical conditions**. Associated features depend on the underlying condition. Hypoglycaemia is worth summarizing—sweating, nausea, dizziness, confusion, aggression, and coma.

Special senses

Visual loss

Visual loss is a frightening symptom and a careful history needs to be taken to avoid missing potentially treatable lesions that may lead to permanent blindness. Sudden visual loss is also an opththalmological emergency.

Important questions to ask

'Was the loss of vision sudden or gradual?'

Sudden onset suggests causes such as vitreous haemorrhage or retinal detachment and vascular causes such as stroke. Transient visual loss can be caused by emboli from arteriosclerotic plaques. Patients will describe a curtain coming down in front of one eye. This usually lasts 20–30 minutes before the 'curtain' lifts again. This is called amaurosis fugax (*am-more-roe-sis-few-gax*) and is an important symptom as it may signal the possibility of an impending stroke. Visual loss of gradual onset may be caused by cataracts, age-related macular degeneration (ARMD), or primary open-angle glaucoma (*glaw-coma*). With gradual onset, the loss of vision may be insidious and not recognized until late on in the disease process. This is particularly important in the case of primary open-angle glaucoma because if it is detected early enough, that is, by screening, it can be treated.

'What is the nature of the visual loss?'

It is important to know what your patient means by loss of vision. For some people this means a loss or blurring of detail (visual acuity). For others this will mean some form of visual field defect, for example, homonymous hemianopia (*hu-mon-ee-muss-hemi-an-owe-pia*). Others will complain of a loss of central vision (because of diseases affecting the macula of the eye) and others may complain of poor vision at night (nyctolopia (*nick-ta-low-pia*).

'Are there any associated features?'

- **Floaters**. These are shapeless blobs of varying sizes, which float around in the patient's field of vision. They are usually caused by changes in the **vitreous gel** (this sits behind the lens of the eye and in front of the retina and forms the majority of the volume of the eye). Some people have experienced small faint floaters all their life and these are particularly noticeable when looking against a well-lit background, for example the sky. If there are new floaters this may represent the vitreous gel separating from the retina (posterior vitreous detachment) and can cause a tear in the retina leading to vitreous haemorrhage or a retinal detachment. This is usually associated with flashing lights. In all cases of new floaters urgent ophthalmological review is required.

- **Flashing lights**. These suggest traction on the retina. Vitreous or retinal detachment may be the cause. Flashing lights (called photopsia) (*foe-top-sia*) may occur transiently in the build-up to a migraine.

- **Photophobia**. An aversion to light may be experienced with anterior uveitis. Photophobia may also be experienced in meningitis, encephalitis (*en-keffer-light-iss*), migraine, and with corneal problems.

- **Diplopia**. This is double vision and will be explained fully in the context of eye movements.

- **Headache and vomiting**. These are non-specific features and may be found in a number of conditions. It may be part of the syndrome of migraine or may develop with SOLs such as brain tumours or cranial infections like meningitis or encephalitis. It could also be due to acute-angle closure glaucoma. If the cause for headache and vomiting is not obvious, ask if the patient has seen coloured haloes around light sources. This is due to corneal clouding and is highly suggestive of this form of glaucoma.

- **Nyctalopia**. This is the disturbance of night vision, which is uncommon. It can be due to vitamin A deficiency or may be an early sign of retinitis pigmentosa (*ret-ee-night-iss-pig-ment-toes-ah*)—a genetic condition that initially affects peripheral vision and later leads to blindness (see 'Neurological diseases and investigations' section).

Past medical history

Drug history

A drug history is always important. Drugs that affect the eye include:

- **chloroquine** (*clo-roe-quin*) (occasionally used for rheumatoid arthritis)—bull's-eye retina (this is one of the forms of retinopathy produced by chloroquine leading to pigmentation at the centre of the macula surrounded by an area of hypopigmentation; this gives the appearance of a bull's-eye)

- **steroids**—cataracts

- **ethambutol** (treatment for TB)—optic neuritis.

Family history

Some conditions can be inherited, for example, optic atrophy, some forms of cataracts, and diabetes mellitus.

> **Key points**
> - Sudden visual loss is an ophthalmological emergency
> - Ask for associated features such as headache, photophobia, and floaters, which could be pointers to the underlying diagnosis
> - Always check a drug history (including illicit drugs)

Hearing loss

Hearing loss is a debilitating symptom, which can lead to social isolation and depression. Its effects are more pronounced if both ears are affected and the loss is severe. The effects of hearing loss are also determined by the person's stage of life. Severe, bilateral hearing loss in a baby, will prevent them acquiring normal speech. In an adult hearing loss will interfere with work and social activities.

Important questions to ask

'Was the loss of hearing sudden or gradual?'

Sudden hearing loss can occur with trauma, for example, a blow over the external auditory meatus (*me-ate-us*) or rapid changes in pressure within the ear canal (called barotrauma) (*barrow-traw-ma*) following an explosion, rapid descent in an aircraft, and so on. Sudden hearing loss is an ear, nose, and throat (ENT) emergency and the patient requires urgent assessment to make sure the cause is treatable. Gradual hearing loss can occur with ageing (sometimes called presbyacusis) (*press-by-a-cue-sis*) or following repeated exposure to loud noise.

'Is one ear affected or both?'

Most people can cope with hearing loss of any severity in one ear. In fact, if the hearing loss is gradual the patient may not realize they have a hearing problem. Sometimes it is the spouse or friends who notice that they have to repeat themselves or that the volume of the television is unusually loud.

'Is there pain along with the hearing loss?'

Pain in the absence of trauma is usually due to an inflammatory cause. Infections by microorganisms can inflame the pinna and external auditory meatus (called an otitis *[owe-tight-iss]* externa) or the middle ear (called an otitis media). There are conditions that can cause referred pain to the ear, for example, tonsillitis, but in these conditions hearing is usually unimpaired.

'Is there a discharge from the ear?'

Otitis externa and otitis media can also produce a discharge. Pain usually precedes the discharge, particularly with otitis media because it requires the perforation of the eardrum before the inflammatory contents can escape. Both otitis externa and otitis media can become chronic. Permanent hearing loss is not a problem with otitis externa. By contrast this is a danger with chronic otitis media and this condition should always be referred to a specialist if suspected. In both cases aural discharge can be recurrent or continuous.

'Have you had any head injury or a blow over the ear?'

In causes of sudden deafness ask about the possibility of trauma, no matter how trivial. A simple slap over the external auditory meatus is capable of generating sufficient pressure to perforate the eardrum.

'Do you hear any ringing, whistling, or buzzing in the ears?'

Tinnitus is the perception of abnormal noises by the ear. Tinnitus can be as devastating as hearing loss to the sufferer. Ask, 'When are the noises most troublesome?' This is usually at night or in quiet surroundings, particularly when the patient is not distracted by other tasks. Tinnitus is sometimes due to an awareness of the patient's own physiological function, for example, the rushing noise due to blood flow within the ear. Often tinnitus is a marker for hearing loss. Therefore patients with tinnitus should be referred for a hearing assessment.

'Tell me about your occupation or hobbies'

A patient's occupation (past and present) or their hobbies may be important in the genesis of hearing loss. Any environment that subjects a person to excessive noise over a sustained period of time may cause hearing loss, particularly for the higher frequencies (at-risk occupations include those in the aviation industry, road drilling, shipbuilding, motor sports, and musicians (rock/pop and classical) and at-risk hobbies include shooting, listening to loud music, nightclubbing). Certain at-risk jobs should provide ear protection. You should check that these have been provided and that your patient has worn them.

'What medications are you on (or have you taken?)'

Certain drugs can cause hearing loss. Usually a person has to be exposed to very high doses intravenously to achieve a toxic level for the cochlear nerve. These drugs are described as ototoxic (*owe-toe-toxic*) and include furosemide, salicylates, and aminoglycoside antibiotics, for example, gentamycin.

'How does your hearing loss affect you?'

Always try to find out what impact hearing loss has on your patient. A small loss to a telephonist may be more

Key points
- Deafness is a cause of social isolation and depression
- Sudden deafness is an ENT emergency
- Always ask about tinnitus
- Always ask about regular exposure to noise with occupation, hobbies, or other lifestyle activities
- Always take a drug history

devastating than a greater loss to a retired labourer. Knowing the problems your patients face can guide your strategies in dealing with them: for example, the provision of hearing aids and other assistive devices such as flashing doorbells and lip-reading programmes.

Disturbance of smell

Loss of smell

The medical term for the loss of smell is anosmia (*an-oz-me-a*). Hyposmia is a decrease in the ability to appreciate smell. Anosmia is an unpleasant symptom as it decreases our appreciation of food flavours. It also robs the sufferer of a vital warning system, for example the detection of leaking gas or food going rotten. It is rare for a patient to complain solely of the loss of smell. It is a common accompaniment of upper respiratory ailments such as 'colds' or influenza and is usually recognized as a temporary complication by the sufferer. The most common cause of permanent anosmia is head injury. This is because bundles of primary sensory neurons perforate the cribriform (*cribri-form*) plate of the ethmoid (*eeth-moid*) bone before synapsing with the olfactory bulb. If the brain is subject to an accelerating force (either forwards or backwards), these fibres can be sheared at this point. The questions you need to ask can be deduced by knowing the causes shown in Table 6.6.

Table 6.6 Causes of anosmia

Temporary
Upper respiratory tract infection
Allergic rhinitis (*rhine-eye-tiss*), e.g. hay fever
Nasal polyps
Permanent
Head injury
Cranial surgery
Tumours of the anterior fossa (at the front of the brain), e.g. olfactory groove meningioma
Drugs or chemicals
Long-term application of nasal spray
Ammonia

Key points

- The sense of smell combines with taste to produce a wide range of flavours
- A temporary loss or reduction in the sense of smell and food flavours may occur with upper respiratory tract infections
- Head injury is the most common cause of anosmia
- Do not forget drugs as a cause of smell or taste disturbance

Parosmia

This is sometimes called dysosmia and is the distortion or perversion of the sense of smell. If any environmental reasons for bad smells are ruled out this may be a manifestation of temporal lobe epilepsy (and is a hallucinatory symptom). Uncommonly it can be the aura of a patient with migraine. With a child the possibility of a foreign body up a nostril should always be borne in mind. Patients may also experience parosmia during regeneration of a damaged olfactory nerve.

Disturbance of taste

Loss of taste

The medical term for the loss of taste is ageusia (*ay-goo-sia*) (a term not used very often). Hypogeusia is the decrease in the ability to appreciate taste. Many people notice a 'loss of taste' when they have a cold or other upper respiratory tract infection. This highlights the large contribution smell provides for the taste experience. In fact the sense of taste is based on five taste receptors: the classic salt, sweet, sour, bitter, and the more recently discovered umami (*oo-mar-me*). Umami is mediated by glutamate (an amino acid) and gives a savoury chicken-like taste. It does not enhance the classic four taste sensations and cannot be synthesized by any combination of sweet, sour, salt, or bitter. The experience of taste is a product of these receptors and smell to produce a flavour, hence it is flavour that is lost when smell is affected. Practically, your patient will not make this semantic distinction, therefore always ask, 'Has there been a change in your sense of smell also?' Again the questions you need to ask can be deduced by knowing the causes of decreased taste sensation or loss of taste (given in Table 6.7).

Table 6.7 Causes of a loss of taste

Facial nerve palsy (in the facial canal proximal to the chorda tympani branch)
Dry mouth, e.g. Sjögren's (*show-grens*) syndrome, heavy smoking
Drugs (antibiotics, anti-cancer chemotherapy, digoxin, angiotensin-converting enzyme inhibitor, and amiodarone)

Motor symptoms

Muscle weakness

Muscle weakness is an important and distressing symptom. The first thing to decide is whether there is true muscular weakness. Some people use the term to describe fatigue. Other patients will claim they have weakness in their arms or legs but in fact it is pain that limits their movement. If there is true muscle weakness, find out if it is the proximal or distal muscle groups that are affected. If it is an asymmetrical weakness, is there a specific muscle group or muscle that is affected? One characteristic form of weakness occurs with myasthenia gravis (*my-ass-theen-ia-grah-vis*). The patient may start the day with full strength but become easily fatigued as their levels of neurotransmitter become depleted. Ascertain the following.

- How long has the weakness been noticed?
- Does it affect all limbs or just the arms or legs?
- Does it affect one or both arms (or one or both legs)? (nerve or root lesion?)
- Does the weakness affect the proximal muscles or the distal muscles? Does the patient have difficulty combing their hair or have difficulty rising from a chair (proximal myopathy)? Do they have difficulty gripping objects or unscrewing jam jars? (peripheral neuropathy? or peripheral nerve lesion?)
- Can the patient stand?
- Can the patient stand on one leg?
- Is the patient able to walk without difficulty?
- Does the patient drag their leg when walking?
- Does the patient feel as if they are drunk when they walk? (This suggests a balance problem, although some patients may feel that this is weakness.)
- Does the weakness vary substantially throughout the day? If yes, follow this up and determine whether it is

a dramatic weakness following activity (myasthenia gravis) or merely just a normal response to exhausting everyday tasks.

- What other activities do they have difficulty with?
- Is there a history of trauma?

> **Key points**
> - Determine if there is true muscular weakness
> - Ask how the weakness affects their activities and abilities
> - Is there a pattern of weakness, for example, proximal > distal, asymmetry
> - If a patient experiences dramatic fatiguability in muscular function consider myasthenia gravis

Involuntary movements

These are important conditions that can cause a patient distress because of their lack of control over these movements and the subsequent embarrassment this can cause in public. As they are dynamic, a one-dimensional description cannot do them justice but they will make sense once you see examples during your training. The main categories of involuntary movements are summarized in Table 6.8. Of these, tremors are the category that you will see most commonly and is therefore discussed in more detail.

Tremor

What is it?

A tremor is an involuntary movement that usually affects the limbs. The hands are most commonly affected, but the feet, head, lips, tongue, and eyelids can be involved. It is a repetitive rhythmic movement and can be coarse or fine.

Table 6.8 Types of involuntary movements

Tremor
Chorea
Athetosis (*ather-toe-sis*)
Hemiballismus (*hemi-ba-liss-muss*)
Dystonia (*dis-tone-ia*)
Myoclonus (*my-owe-clone-us*)
Tics

They can be divided into four main types: postural, pill-rolling, intention or flapping tremor.

Postural tremor

These are sometimes called physiological tremors because they are exaggerations of the normal physiological tremor that everybody possesses. (The hands shake imperceptibly at 5–8 Hz). This can become exaggerated for various reasons when it is known as a postural tremor. They are very common; you may have had experience of tremors related to anxiety or fear (observe the hands of your fellow students at exam times). These tremors can be seen at rest but they become more apparent if you ask your patients to hold out their hands in front of them.

Causes

See Table 6.9.

Benign essential tremor is inherited as an autosomal dominant trait. This tremor is often improved by alcohol and can be treated with β-blockers. It differs from other postural tremor in that it can be quite coarse in nature and has often been mistaken for Parkinson's disease.

'Pill-rolling' tremor

This is a slow (4–6 Hz), fine, resting tremor. The name derives from the repetitive movement of finger and thumb, as if a pill were being rolled between them. A pill-rolling tremor is typical of parkinsonism. Parkinsonism is a syndrome comprised of the triad of a resting tremor, rigidity (increased tone or stiffness), and bradykinesia (slow movements). Parkinsonism can be idiopathic, when it is known as Parkinson's disease. It can also be caused by drugs (dopamine antagonists, for example, metoclopramide and haloperidol) and viral encephalitis.

Intention tremor

The hallmark of an intention tremor is that it is absent when the limb is at rest but becomes evident on movement.

Table 6.9 Causes of a postural tremor

Fear or anxiety
Fatigue
Caffeine-containing drinks (e.g. coffee)
Drugs; for example, ventolin, lithium, theophylline (*thee-offi-lin*)
Withdrawal of alcohol
Thyrotoxicosis (see Chapter 11)

It behaves differently from other tremors in that its amplitude does not remain constant. As a movement begins the limb may demonstrate small horizontal oscillations, which can quickly progress to much larger ones. (In some cases the limb can swing back and forth very wildly indeed.) It is often associated with past-pointing (dysmetria). In the less dramatic cases the tremor may diminish or vanish altogether as the movement progresses and may re-emerge as the arm nears its target. A true intention tremor signifies a cerebellar disorder. Other associated signs are ataxia, dysarthria (slurred speech), and nystagmus. (Common causes of cerebellar signs in an examination are cerebrovascular disease or MS.)

Flapping tremor

Also called asterixis (*ass-stir-ix-iss*), this is an important sign in hepatic encephalitis, renal failure, and type II respiratory failure. Type II respiratory failure is when the patient hypoventilates (breathes insufficiently) causing the carbon dioxide level in the blood to increase. The recognition of this tremor is dealt with in Chapters 5 and 7.

What to ask about a tremor

- **'When did the tremor start?'** Was it a gradual or sudden onset? A gradual onset may be due to a progressive disease like Parkinson's disease. An acute onset could be caused by a stroke or starting a new drug.

- **'Is it worse at any particular time of day?'** An early morning tremor may be due to alcohol withdrawal. A benign essential tremor can be exaggerated by tiredness and therefore be more pronounced in the evening.

- **'Is there anything that makes it better?'** Alcohol may improve benign essential tremor. Holding an object in the hand can improve a pill-rolling tremor.

- **'Is there anything that makes it worse?'** Many tremors can get worse with anxiety, especially if the patient is conscious of being closely observed.

- **'How does it affect you?'** Does it prevent the patient from doing certain tasks?

- **'Do you have any other symptoms?'** Dysarthria, poor balance, and intention tremor are associated with cerebellar disease. Stiffness, difficulty standing up, turning over in bed, and increased incidence of falls are associated with parkinsonism.

- **'Is there anyone in your family who has (or had tremors)?'** Benign essential tremor can be inherited as an autosomal dominant trait, so one of the parents should have the disease. There are genetic conditions that can affect the cerebellum, for example, Freidrich's ataxia, which have a variable inheritance.

Chorea

What is it?

These are irregular, jerky movements that can affect most muscle groups in a random sequence. In old textbooks the movements are often described as 'quasi-purposeful' which means the movements **almost** seem intentional. Many sufferers will go to great lengths to disguise these movements by making them seem **totally** intentional. Therefore if they are seated and their leg jumps, they will 'hijack' this movement and cross their leg and make it look like a planned manoeuvre. Similarly, if their arm jerks upwards, they may use the movement to scratch their nose. This behaviour may be so successful that people do not suspect the patient has chorea. The first thing you might notice is that your patient may seem a little fidgety or restless. You might even feel that their behaviour is a little eccentric. This should alert your mind to the possibility of chorea. Their face may exhibit grimacing and frequent changes of expression. If you were to ask the patient to put out their tongue they would be unable to maintain it in a constant position. Instead it would move in and out repeatedly and is sometimes called a trombone tremor of the tongue. If you shook hands with your patient when you first met, you may have noticed their grip fluctuating. This waxing and waning of the grip has been likened to a milkmaid's grip. (Those of us who are not cows can only guess what a milkmaid's grip must be like.) Finally, when you are engaged in history-taking you may observe your patient grunting on occasion. This is due to the involuntary contraction of the diaphragm, which forces air out through the larynx.

Causes

See Table 6.10.

Table 6.10 Causes of chorea

Huntington's chorea
Sydenham's chorea (associated with rheumatic fever) (*Thomas Sydenham (1624–1689), English physician*)
Thyrotoxicosis
Polycythaemia (*polly-sigh-theme-ia*) rubra vera
Pregnancy
Systemic lupus erythmatosus (SLE)

Athetosis

What is it?

This is a slow 'snake-like' writhing movement that tends to affect the peripheries, including the hands, feet, and face. Sometimes chorea and athetosis coexist and the resulting condition is known as choreoathetosis.

Hemiballismus

What is it?

This abnormal movement is so violent that it causes the flailing of one or both limbs on one side of the body. The cause is a lesion of the contralateral subthalamic nucleus (a component of the basal ganglia) usually as a result of a stroke. Thankfully this condition does not occur very often in clinical practice.

Dystonia

What is it?

Part of the body assumes an abnormal posture due to a sustained contraction of a particular muscle group. It may be focal, affecting one or a few muscle groups only, or generalized.

Focal dystonias

These may be familiar through their colloquial names, for example, writer's cramp and wry neck (spasmodic torticollis *[taut-i-coll-iss]*). With writer's cramp the muscles of the hand and forearm contract as the person attempts to write. They may manage to write a few lines (or even less) before the task has to be abandoned. Until recently this used to be thought of as a psychiatric disorder. Spasmodic torticollis is the (sometimes) painful contraction of the sternomastoid muscle, which twists the neck to one side (torticollis) (see Fig. 6.6). Sometimes other neck muscles can be involved leading to forward flexion (antecollis) or backward extension (retrocollis).

Generalized dystonias

These tend to be seen more commonly in children as a result of birth trauma, metabolic, or neurodegenerative disorders. An idiopathic form exists, idiopathic torsion dystonia (old name, dystonia musculorum deformans [*dis-tone-ia-mus-cue-lore-um-de-four-mans*]), which may have a genetic basis. Again, this is seen more commonly in childhood. Sufferers may exhibit a torticollis, the back may twist or arch backwards and the arms typically rotate

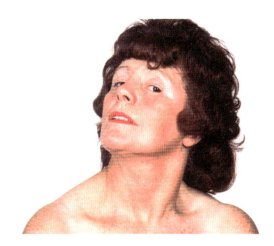

Figure 6.6 Spasmodic torticollis. Note the dystonic contraction of the left sternomastoid leading to the abnormal posture of the head.
Reprinted from Fig. 6.52 (p. 6.18), *Atlas of Clinical Neurology* (2nd edn), by G. David Perkin, Fred Hochberg, and Douglas C. Miller (1993), Mosby Publications, with permission from Elsevier.

inwards and extend, with the wrists flexed. They may walk with their feet plantarflexed and inverted, forcing them to walk stiffly on tiptoes. These extreme postures can be held for hours and in advanced cases only disappear during sleep.

Myoclonus

What is it?

This is a process where a person experiences brief, shock-like jerks that may be restricted to a muscle group (focal) or be more generalized, the latter usually as a component of juvenile epilepsy. They are distinct from chorea in that they are usually rhythmical and do not flit from one muscle group to another. Myoclonus can occur in normal people, for example, on falling asleep. The small number of beats that affect the legs can be sufficient to cause the affected person to wake.

Extensor spasm

This is a non-specific feature of UMN disease and is a sudden jerky movement (usually of the hip). It can be uncomfortable and even painful for the patient. It is thought to be due to the release of inhibitory impulses of the dorsal reticulospinal fibres on the LMNs.

Associated reactions

This can also occur in longstanding, UMN pathology (usually stroke). When a patient changes the posture of a limb or performs an involuntary act, for example, a yawn, there may be an accompanying movement of a normally paralysed limb; for example, a hemiplegic leg may flex in response to the yawn. Its importance lies in the false promise it conveys. A patient may feel that movement is returning in the limb and be filled with optimism, only to find their hopes dashed later on.

Tics

What are they?

These are irregular jerky movements that are repeated continually. They differ from other forms of involuntary movements in that they can be voluntarily suppressed. These movements tend to affect the face and upper body and common movements include exaggerated blinking, grimacing, sniffing, shoulder shrugging, and so on. One disorder that exhibits complex tics is Gille de la Tourette (*jeel-de-la-tour-ett*) syndrome (*George Albert Édouard Brutus Gille de la Tourette (1857–1904), French neurologist*). More recently the name has been shortened to Tourette syndrome and has captured the medical imagination because of the outrageous behaviour that can be seen with this syndrome. Some tics can be repetition of obscene gestures. Sufferers also exhibit vocal tics, which include grunting, barking, and in some cases swearing.

Sensory system

Pain

The subject of pain, especially of neurological origin (neurogenic [*new-roe-jen-ick*] pain) is a complicated one and there are whole textbooks devoted to the problem. The following represents a simplified means of dealing with pain in the spine and limbs.

Local pain

Local pain arises from the pain-sensitive structures involved in the spine, pelvis, and legs. These include soft tissue such as ligaments, muscles, and joints as well as the bones themselves. There is usually a clear relationship with trauma, which is often volunteered by the patient. The pain can be superficial, where it has a sharp 'light' quality and is easily localized by the patient. It does not interfere with muscle function. Deep pain tends to be dull and not so readily localized. In addition there may be decreased muscle activity around any inflammation or even frank spasm to protect the area. Further neurological problems can occur if nearby nerves are involved in an injury; for example, a fracture at the head of the fibula may damage the common peroneal (*peh-roe-knee-al*) nerve. This can lead to a foot drop and loss of sensation of the anterior and lateral aspect of the leg and the dorsum of the foot.

Referred pain

This is even more difficult to localize as the area where the pain is experienced is remote from its site of origin. Pain can be referred from the spine, the pelvis, and even the abdominal or pelvic viscera. The pain can assume almost any character depending on the structure involved. The importance of referred pain is the potential for misdiagnosis.

Neuropathic pain

This is pain caused as a result of nerve damage in the central nervous system. Sometimes the term 'neurogenic pain' is used and means practically the same thing. Neuralgia (*new-ral-ja*) also means nerve pain although in latter years it has been tagged on to the end of specific nerves to represent a particular condition, for example, trigeminal (*try-jemmy-nal*) neuralgia. Neuropathic pain tends to be burning in nature, diffuse, and poorly localized. It can also be symmetrical in the case of a peripheral neuropathy. It can be difficult to treat but some patients respond to the anti-depressant amitriptyline (*am-ee-trip-ta-lean*) or the anticonvulsant carbamazipine (*car-ba-maz-ee-peen* or *car-ba-maze-ee-peen*).

Radicular pain

This is a form of neuropathic pain with characteristic qualities. It is an episodic, shooting pain, which is conducted along a narrow path. When this form of pain is particularly severe it is described as lancinating. The best example of this form of pain is sciatica. Protrusion of an intervertebral disc (prolapse) can irritate adjacent nerve roots. As well as some localized pain at the site of the prolapse there is also transient shooting pain usually felt down the back of the leg. Manoeuvres like coughing, straining, stretching, or sneezing can irritate the nerve roots and provoke the pain.

There are other aspects of neuropathic pain that you may encounter occasionally in your reading.

- **Allodynia** (*allo-din-nia*). This is an abnormal and unpleasant sensation produced by normal stimuli. This is sometimes called dysaesthesia (*dis-as-theez-ya*).
- **Hyperalgesia**. This is where the pain threshold is lowered, so that the slightest stimulation can cause pain, for example, blowing on the skin can evoke pain.
- **Hyperpathia**. This is where the pain threshold is elevated, so that a painful stimulus is not felt until it becomes very forceful. When it is experienced the full magnitude of the noxious stimulus is felt.

What to ask

With regards to neurogenic pain it is best to concentrate on questions regarding the pain itself. Begin with an open question, for example, 'Tell me about your pain.' But be prepared to ask some supplementary questions.

- 'Where is the pain?'
- 'How long did it last?'
- 'Did it come on suddenly or gradually?'
- 'Is the pain constant or intermittent?'
- 'Can you describe the pain?' Give some examples to help—for example, sharp, burning, shooting, or aching.
- 'Does the pain radiate anywhere?' For example, down the back of the leg or the front of the leg.
- 'Did anything bring the pain on?' For example, trauma, or movement of a limb.
- 'Does anything aggravate the pain?' For example, coughing, sneezing, or bending.
- 'Does anything relieve the pain?'

The responses to these questions may suggest neurogenic pain. If so, ask about associated neurological

Key points

- Neuropathic pain tends to be diffuse and burning in nature
- Trauma may cause neurological dysfunction through damage to nearby nerves
- Always bear in mind the possibility of referred pain so as to avoid the dangers of misdiagnosis
- Radicular pain is a transient shooting pain that is conducted in a narrow band

symptoms. As with many symptoms you also have to decide whether your patient is exaggerating the degree of pain or underplaying it. This is a skill you will learn to develop through your training.

Paraesthesia

This is the feeling of pins and needles or a continual prickly feeling. It is usually caused by damage to larger myelinated fibres. Most people have experienced this at some point, for example, if they have slept on their arm overnight. This example also demonstrates that a non-neurological cause of paraesthesia exists, that is, disruption of arterial blood supply. Be aware that some patients have difficulty describing the sensation of paraesthesia and may call it pain instead. This phenomenon is not necessarily accompanied by objective sensory impairment and it is therefore difficult to localize the source of the lesion (an exception to this is the radicular distribution of paraesthesia in shingles).

Numbness

This is a decrease or absence of sensation and is usually accompanied by a loss of proprioception (*pro-pree-owe-sep-shun*). Always ask the patient what they mean when they say 'numb'. Several expressions are often used by patients to explain numbness, for example, heaviness, dead feeling, cold, no sensation, 'it does not feel the same as the other leg', and so on. It is useful to ask further questions to define the problem further. Ascertain the following:

- Can they feel their pyjamas, gloves, socks, or tights when they wear them?
- Can they tell the difference between hot and cold materials?
- Can they tell the difference between different surfaces on the floor—carpets, tiles, or wooden floor?

Sometimes patients will volunteer that it feels as if they are walking on cotton wool or eggshells. Any loss of pain sensation in the long term can lead to burns, scars, or trophic ulcers. If pain sensation is profound this can lead to deranged joints (Charcot's (*shark-owes*) joints) (*Jean Martin Charcot (1825–1893), French neurologist*). The patient will be unaware of any of these injuries at the time they occur but may notice the changes later on or if relatives or friends draw their attention to it.

A sudden loss of sensation indicates an acute lesion and the possible causes include vascular events affecting the sensory cortex, subcortical structures, or even the spinal cord. Demyelination (*de-mile-lin-ay-shun*), such as with a transverse myelitis (*mile-eye-tiss*) or multiple sclerosis, may also be possible (this is true of any neurological abnormality). A more gradual onset of numbness that ascends up the arms or legs over a period of time may suggest a peripheral neuropathy especially if it occurs in a 'glove and stocking' distribution. It is well known for patients with spinal cord compression to have a band of numbness, paraesthesia, or hyperaesthesia at the proximal limit of sensory loss. If you suspect spinal cord compression then you must make sure you ask about bowel and bladder function as these are red flag symptoms. If the patient has developed urinary retention and constipation then it is a medical emergency and the spinal cord compression must be relieved to prevent permanent damage.

Key points

- Always ask what a patient means by numbness
- The patient may complain that they are walking on cotton wool, eggshells, and so on
- Chronic loss of sensation can predispose to burns, scars, trophic ulcers, and even deranged joints (Charcot's joints)

Tip

If you find a sensory level and suspect spinal cord compression then you must enquire about bladder and bowel function. Urinary retention and constipation with suspected spinal cord compression is a medical emergency.

Completing the neurological history

Past medical history

- Has the patient had any recent viral illnesses? This may suggest causes such as transverse myelitis or Guillain–Barré (*ghee-on-ba-ray*) (*George Charles Guillain (1876–1961), French neurologist, Jean Alexandre Barré (1880–1967), French neurologist*) syndrome.
- Have they had previous operations that may have damaged nearby nerves or a laminectomy involving the spine, which may suggest previous back problems such as a prolapsed intervertebral disc?

- Do they have important current illnesses, for example, diabetes mellitus or rheumatoid arthritis, which may predispose to nerve injury such as peripheral neuropathy or mononeuritis (*mono-new-right-iss*) multiplex?

Drug history

Some drugs are notorious for causing injury:

- **isoniazid** (ice-so-nigh-a-zid)—treatment for tuberculosis—peripheral neuropathy
- **rifampicin** (riff-amp-i-sin)—treatment for tuberculosis—peripheral neuropathy
- **vincristine** (vin-christine)—chemotherapy.

Family history

A family history is important for some conditions, for example, Huntington's chorea (*cu-rear*) (*George Sumner Huntington (1851–1916), American physician*)—autosomal dominant and Duchenne muscular dystrophy (*do-shen-muscular-dis-truffy*) (*Guillaume Benjamin Amand Duchenne (1807–1875), French neurologist*)—X-linked recessive.

Review of systems

Always perform a review of systems looking for possible clues, for example, multisystem disorders or malignancy that may have effects in other systems as well as the neurological system.

The review of systems also gives you another chance to check on bowel and bladder function if you have forgotten to ask about them in your initial questions, particularly if there is the possibility of spinal cord compression. There are other conditions that may predispose to constipation and urine retention, for example, Parkinsons's disease (*James Parkinson (1755–1824), English physician*), stroke, and so on, either primarily through the disease process or through its treatments. However these do not present the emergency that spinal cord compression does.

Importance of examining the neurological system

There is no substitute for the hands-on clinical evaluation of the nervous system. Although we have ready access to powerful diagnostic tools such as MRI and CT scans, they are of little value if poor clinical evaluation leads to the deployment of the wrong test in the wrong place. Although diagnosis is your ultimate aim, one of your early

objectives will be to work out **where** in the complex neurological system a lesion is. That is why there is a great emphasis on distinguishing an UMN lesion from a LMN lesion. This will help to differentiate lesions that are in the brain and spinal cord from those of nerve roots, plexuses, and peripheral nerves. There are also other patterns of presentations that you should be familiar with and these are described in the following section, particularly in the analysis section near the end. Although we present a format for learning the various aspects of the neurological system, as your confidence and experience grows you can start to play around with the order of your assessments as the clinical situation demands. You will assess speech as you meet the patient for the first time and as you take the history. Experienced neurologists will examine the gait as the patient enters their consulting rooms rather than at the end because there is a rich seam of neurological data that can be exploited simply from watching the patient walk. The final message is that the key to eliciting the various signs is practice. With a good technique the signs can be easy to elicit but with a sloppy technique they can just as easily become confusing. Learn to use the tendon hammer in particular, as this is to the neurologist what the stethoscope is to the cardiologist. It can feel very alien when you first use one but with time and practice you will soon get those reflexes twitching with confidence.

Neurological system examination summary

Preparation

1 Get your equipment ready.
2 Introduce yourself to the patient and ask for permission to examine.
3 Get the patient in position.
4 Wash your hands.
5 While doing 2–3, have a 'general look'. Pain/discomfort? Mood? Are they unsteady? Is there generalized wasting? Is there a walking aid nearby?
6 Assess their speech.

Examine the cranial nerves

7 Ask if there is any change in their sense of smell (I tested) or taste (I and VII tested) (DF 2/10).
8 Check visual acuity (II tested) (DF 6/10), assess the visual fields (II tested) (DF 7/10), test the pupillary

light and accommodation reflexes (II and parasympathetic III tested) (DF 5/10), and perform fundoscopy (II tested) (DF 9/10).

9 Inspect for ptosis and a squint (DF 3/10) and check eye movements: look for nystagmus and ask about diplopia (III, IV, and VI tested) (DF 8/10).

10 Test facial sensation (V tested) (DF 6/10), assess the muscles of mastication (V tested) (DF 4/10), test corneal reflex (V tested) (DF 3/10), and assess the jaw jerk reflex (V tested) (DF 6/10).

11 Assess the muscles of facial movement (VII tested) (DF 6/10).

12 Assess hearing (VIII tested) and perform Weber's and Rinné's tests (VIII tested) (DF 8/10).

13 Assess movement of the soft palate (IX and X tested) and assess sensation of the soft palate (IX and X tested) (DF 5/10).

14 Assess the trapezius and sternomastoid muscles (XI tested) (DF 4/10).

15 Assess the tongue and tongue movements (XII tested) (DF 4/10).

Examine the motor system

16 Inspection: look for wasting (DF 4/10), fasciculations (DF 6/10), and involuntary movements (DF 7/10).

17 Assess muscle tone at the: wrist, elbow, shoulder, hip, and knee (DF 6/10).

18 Test for clonus if relevant (DF 4/10).

19 Test power, proximally to distally (DF 5/10) in arms and legs.

20 Test reflexes: biceps (DF 5/10), supinator (DF 7/10), triceps (DF 6/10), knee (DF 4/10) and ankle (DF 9/10).

21 Elicit the plantar reflex (DF 8/10).

22 Other reflexes.

23 Test coordination: finger–nose test (DF 6/10); check alternating hand movements (DF 4/10) and heel-shin test (DF 3/10).

Examine the sensory system

24 Assess sensation: light touch (DF 6/10), pain (DF 6/10), proprioception (DF 6/10), and vibration sense (DF 5/10).

25 Get your patient to stand and perform Romberg's test (DF 5/10).

26 Assess gait (DF 7/10).

27 Other signs.

28 Make sure your patient is comfortable and thank them for their time.

29 Wash your hands.

30 Analyse your findings.

31 Present your findings.

Examination of the neurological system in detail

Preparation

1 Getting prepared (get your equipment ready)

You will need to collect your equipment to take to the bedside. For a complete examination of the neurological system you will need the following:

- cotton wool
- ophthalmoscope
- tuning fork (256 or 516 Hz to perform the Rinné and Weber tests)
- tuning fork (128 Hz to test vibration sense)
- red hatpin
- tongue depressor
- bedside Snellen chart (*Herman Snellen (1834–1908), Dutch ophthalmologist*)
- tendon hammer
- neurology pins ('neuropins')

2 Introduce yourself to the patient

Put out your hand to shake the patient's hand. Say something like, 'Hello I'm James Parkinson, a first-year student. Do you mind if I examine the nerves of your face, arms, and legs?'

3 Get the patient in position

The cranial nerve examination is best performed out of bed, with you and your patient sitting on a chair at equal heights and with the patient's face almost at arm's length from you. This is ideal in a clinic, or primary care setting. If you are on a ward then your patient can sit on the edge of the bed with you seated opposite on a chair. Make sure that the bed is raised or lowered so that you are both roughly face to face. If your patient is too frail it is best to leave them in bed but it will mean that you will have to lean over the bed to be approximately face to face with your patient—but be warned, this will be tiring for you.

4   Wash your hands

Germs are no respecter, so please don't be a hospital vector!

5   While doing steps 2–3, be having a 'general look'

While introducing yourself and getting your patient into position, perform your general look. This has to be brief but packed with as many clues as you can digest. Does your patient look in pain or discomfort? Pay particular attention to their mood. This is important for any system but particularly for a neurological examination. Depression may be the end result of a chronic problem or may conversely be the cause of multiple non-specific symptoms. It is also worth remembering that someone who looks apathetic and depressed may be exhibiting decreased facial expression (hypomimia [*high-poe-mim-ia*]) which may be a sign of Parkinson's disease. A euphoric patient may have a frank psychiatric disorder but may occasionally have conditions in which emotional lability is a recognized feature, such as multiple sclerosis or stroke. These points highlight the great deal of overlap between neurology and psychiatry. Observe the patient's face, is there any facial asymmetry (VIIth nerve palsy?), or eyelid or pupil abnormality? Does the mouth droop or the voice sound unusual when they respond to your introduction? Any abnormality will give you a point of focus for your examination. Look for kyphoscoliosis, as there is an association with certain neurodegenerative conditions, for example, Friedreich's ataxia. Also watch the patient as they get on to the bed/chair. Are they unsteady? This could suggest weakness in the legs or a cerebellar lesion. A patient with proximal weakness will try and support their thighs with their hands and lift their legs on to the bed. Also look for clues around the bedside, for example, a hearing aid or a pair of glasses, a diabetic sticker (peripheral neuropathy, mononeuritis multiplex, or diabetic amyotrophy (*ay-my-ot-roe-fee*), a walking aid such as a walking stick, or even a wheelchair.

6   Assess speech

An assessment of speech is extremely important and is another feature that can be assessed during the history-taking. As you listen you should be alert to any abnormalities of speech and voice production. As speech is also a window into the cognitive function of your patient, any abnormality in language production may also give you

vital clues to potential disorders of the brain. There may also be impairment of memory leading to a history that is vague and lacking in detail or where your patient may repeat themselves without insight.

Speech and voice production

There are two main aspects of speech production to be aware of and that is the volume or power of the sound produced and the articulation of the vocal apparatus that give shape to the sound and encodes it with meaning. Any abnormality in either of these two properties can cause dysphonia (*dis-fone-ia*) or dysarthria (*dis-are-three-a*).

Dysphonia: what is it?

This is an abnormality in the production of sound volume and quality (aphonia means no sound produced at all).

How to recognize

Your patient's voice will sound very quiet, hoarse or breathy in quality.

Causes

See Table 6.11

Table 6.11 Some causes of dysphonia

Vocal cords	
Voice abuse	Shouting, crying, singing
Infection	Laryngitis (viral, bacterial, fungal)
Tumour	Benign (cysts, nodules); malignant (squamous cell carcinoma)
Acid reflux	GORD, LPR
Trauma	Intubation, penetrating injury of larynx
Damage to nerve supply	Surgery (thyroidectomy, heart/lung surgery), lung cancer
Drugs	Steroid inhalers
Endocrine	Hypothyroidism
Neurological	Parkinsons disease, bulbar palsy, pseudobulbar palsy, myasthenia gravis
Psychogenic	

GORD, gastro-oesophageal reflux disease; LPR, laryngopharyngeal reflux

Tip

As the majority of causes of dysphonia are due to vocal cord lesions they will usually need investigation by an ear, nose, and throat (ENT) surgeon.

Dysarthria: what is it?

This is an abnormality in the articulation of word formation (anarthria means no articulation produced at all).

How to recognize

Your patient's speech will sound slurred or will have a disordered rhythm or unusual intonations rendering the speech difficult to understand. Some people advocate that patients repeat phrases such as 'British constitution' to demonstrate dysarthria but this is not necessary as it will be obvious during normal speech.

Causes

See Table 6.12.

Tip

If you have a patient with dysarthria that cannot be explained by simple causes such as local factors, tiredness, or drugs then they must have a neurological assessment and not be ignored.

Language disorders

When we speak, the ideas we want to communicate are usually thought through before we select the appropriate words and construct a meaningful sentence around the grammatical rules of our country and peer group. Different areas of the brain work seamlessly to provide a meaningful output that often appears instant and fluid. Damage to any of these key centres can lead to recognizable defects in communication. Any disorder of language is called dysphasia (*dis-faze-ia*) and traditionally aphasia (*a-faze-ia*) was reserved for patients without any language function. However currently many countries and interested groups are using the term aphasia in preference to dysphasia because they believe that it helps to distinguish it from other similar and confusing terms such as dysphagia and dysphonia. Although there are a number of language disorders, only three are considered here: (1) expressive dysphasia, (2) receptive dysphasia, and (3) global dysphasia.

Expressive dysphasia: what is it?

This is caused by a lesion in Broca's area in the frontal lobe. It leads to difficulty in patients finding the right word or idea to express themselves.

How to recognize

The speech is hesitant with a stop–start rhythm, as the patient gropes and searches for the right word(s) to express themself. Hence this has also been called non-fluent dysphasia, motor dysphasia as well as Broca's dysphasia. The patient's understanding is usually intact and can be tested by a number of tasks such as, 'Show me something that you drink out of.' The complexity of the tasks can be increased to determine a more subtle problem with comprehension and is part of the service offered by a speech therapist. Note that there may be other neurological dysfunction such as a hemiparesis, so a patient will ultimately need a full neurological examination.

Receptive dysphasia: what is it?

This is caused by a lesion in Wernicke's area of the temporal lobe. This leads to difficulty in comprehending speech.

Table 6.12 Some causes of dysarthria

Local	
Infections of mouth/throat	Candida, ulcers, tonsillitis
Ill-fitting dentures	
Excessive tiredness	
Drugs	Alcohol, sedatives, opiates
Neurological	Stroke, head injury, cerebral palsy, cerebellar disease, bulbar palsy, pseudobulbar palsy

How to recognize

The output of an affected patient will appear bizarre and may not bear any relationship to any question you may have asked. They may speak total nonsense fluently and seem oblivious to it. Hence this has also been called fluent dysphasia, sensory dysphasia, as well as Wernicke's dysphasia. The speech may contain made-up words called neologisms (*knee-owe-low-jiz-ums*), or words may be used as substitutes for other words, e.g. ball for spoon, termed paraphasia. Occasionally the speech is so corrupted by neologisms and paraphasias that it becomes meaningless and is called jargon dysphasia.

Global dysphasia: what is it?

This is caused by damage to both Broca's and Wernicke's areas leading to a mixed picture of comprehensive and expressive dysfunction. When severe there may be little language production at all.

....
Tip

All forms of dysphasias should have an early referral to a speech and language therapist.
....
Tip

If you are not succeeding with your efforts to communicate:

- Ensure that the patient does not require a hearing aid.
- Try speaking a little slower or with shorter sentences.
- Try asking closed questions where you get yes or no answers only.
- Have a pen and paper handy to write or draw to aid communication.

Speech therapists have cards with symbols to represent common everyday themes that can also help in instances where writing is not recognized.
....

Examination of the cranial nerves

There are 12 cranial nerves each arising from the brainstem. They provide important motor and sensory function to the head and neck including the eyes, ears, and some internal organs (Table 6.13). Damage to any one of them will cause motor or sensory loss to the areas supplied. In addition the special senses such as sight, hearing, smell, and taste can also be affected. Knowledge of the function of each nerve is therefore vital to

enable you to deduce any abnormality you may encounter. Although there are 12 separate nerves, their functions overlap. When examining the nerves at least for the first few attempts it is easier to think of them as individual nerves and perform the relevant examination. This will ensure none are missed out. It is actually a bit more complicated than this because each nerve may have more than one test and not all parts of each nerve can or will be tested. With more experience it will become smoother and you and the patient will move around less. Finally, try to think ahead all the time, while doing one test you should be thinking about the next thing you are going to say or do to the patient. Eventually examining the cranial nerves will become second nature and your thoughts will be focused on picking up the abnormality!

Olfactory nerve (cranial nerve I)

7 Ask if there is any change in their sense of smell (I tested) or taste (I and VII tested) (DF 2/10)

The olfactory nerve is responsible for the sense of smell. In the clinical setting, the sense of smell is rarely tested objectively (there are bottles with standard smells that exist for this purpose but the author has yet to see them used). Practically this nerve is assessed by a crude screening question, 'Do you have any problems with your sense of smell?' If your patient says no, then it is unlikely they have anything wrong with this particular nerve (the exception would be a unilateral loss of smell which could be compensated by the other nostril). 'If they say yes, make sure you ask this supplementary question. 'Do you have a cold or blocked nose at the moment?' If they say yes this simple question will stop you going off on an unfruitful tangent. If they do not have a cold you will have to question them further to find the cause of their lack of smell. You can go on to confirm their lack of smell by testing it with some strong recognizable smells, for example, orange or coffee. Get your patient to close their eyes and make them occlude one nostril by pressing it firmly from the outside with a finger (a finger up the nostril looks uncouth and may unearth untold horrors!). Now get them to take a sniff and to try and identify the aroma. Then occlude the other nostril and repeat the test. If any abnormality is found the nostrils should be inspected for foreign bodies or polyps. Ideally experts (i.e. ENT specialists) should do this.

When you ask your screening question for smell, it is timely to ask about taste also (nerve VII). As taste is

Table 6.13 The functions of the cranial nerves

I	Olfactory nerve	Sense of smell
II	Optic nerve	Visual acuity, visual fields, colour vision, and pupillary light and accommodation reflex (sensory part)
III	Oculomotor nerve	Eye movements and pupillary light and accommodation reflex (motor part)
IV	Trochlear (*trock-leer*) nerve	Eye movements
V	Trigeminal (*try-jemmy-nal*) nerve	Facial sensation, muscles of mastication, and corneal reflex (sensory part)
VI	Abducens nerve	Eye movements
VII	Facial nerve	Facial muscles, taste to the anterior two-thirds of the tongue, stapedius muscle, and corneal reflex (motor part)
VIII	Vestibulocochlear (*vest-tib-you-low-cock-leer*) nerve	Hearing and balance
IX	Glossopharyngeal (*gloss-owe-fa-ren-jeel*) nerve	Sensation of palate and pharynx and the gag reflex (sensory part)
X	Vagus (*vague-us*) nerve	Palatal and pharyngeal muscles, sensation of the respiratory system, and the gag reflex (motor part)
XI	Accessory nerve	Sternomastoid and trapezius muscles
XII	Hypoglossal nerve	Motor supply of the tongue

intimately related to smell, if smell is affected it is likely that taste will be as well (as anyone who has had a blocked nose can testify). If, however, the sense of smell is unaffected but taste is, then you will need to enquire further to see if you can determine a possible cause for the loss of taste.

Optic nerve (cranial nerve II)

8 Check visual acuity (II tested) (DF 6/10), assess the visual fields (II tested) (DF 7/10), test the pupillary light and accommodation reflexes (II and parasympathetic III tested) (DF 5/10), and perform fundoscopy (II tested) (DF 9/10)

The optic nerve is responsible for vision. Begin by asking if the patient has any problems with their eyesight: 'Do you wear glasses or contact lenses?' and 'Are you short or long sighted?' This may provide some initial clues and enables you to make allowances for longstanding problems. If your patient is wearing spectacles ask them politely, 'Could you please take off your glasses?' Inspect the eyebrows, eyelids, sclera, and pupils. Is there any difference between the eyes? Look specifically for drooping eyelids (ptosis), any deviation of the eyes (strabismus or squint, see later), unequal pupils, or a prosthetic eye. Learning how to spot a prosthetic eye is not usually taught but it is worth knowing so you do not end up with egg on your face. Sometimes the colour of the prosthetic eye is a brilliant white compared with the normal sclera. It sometimes has a shinier appearance and fails to move in any direction (some modern prostheses can exhibit limited movement but this still looks unrealistic). It is simplest to examine the optic nerve in five stages: visual acuity, visual fields, colour vision, pupil light and accommodation reflexes, and fundoscopy.

Visual acuity

What is it?

This is the ability of the eye to discriminate fine detail.

How to examine

Most people have had their eyesight checked and so should be familiar with the technique. Ideally a Snellen chart is used at 6 m. This is cumbersome in the bedside setting so a 3 m 'end-of-the-bed' version is available. Make sure the patient is wearing their distance glasses (it is so embarrassing to diagnose a severe defect only for the patient to pipe up 'Of course, if I was wearing my glasses I could have read it, no problem!'). The Snellen chart is made up of letters of decreasing size as you read down the chart. Each line is of a standard size so that the vision of your patient can be compared to that of a population of people with healthy sight. You must test one eye at a time. Simply asking the patient to close one eye is inadequate. Some patients find this difficult and even if they succeed it can alter the vision of the eye under test. Ideally an occluder should be used but most people ask the patient to cover their eye with a hand and check they are not cheating,

Tip

Double check that those patients who do wear glasses have fully covered their eye.

Say to your patient, 'Please cover your right eye with your right hand and read the top letter for me. Carry on reading down the chart.' Even when the patient wants to give up, encourage them to continue. The aim is to get your patient to read down the chart until they are unable to read the letters on a particular line. This is the limit of their visual acuity and you should note which line this is. The lines are numbered, usually 60 at the top down to 5 or 6 at the smallest letters at the bottom. You should find this limit for the other eye too. The visual acuity for each eye is represented by a fraction. The top figure represents how far your patient should be away from the Snellen chart when reading it. It is measured in metres and is usually 6. The bottom figure represents the lowest line the patient can read. Most charts label the lines, from top to bottom, 60, 36, 24, 18, 12, 8, 6, and 5. These figures are chosen because most people should be able to read the top line at 60 m, the next line at 36 m, and so on. Therefore people with normal vision can read at least the 6 line (often when their vision is corrected with glasses) and therefore have 6/6 vision. You may have heard the term 20/20 vision—this is the equivalent when the distance is measured in feet rather than metres. If your patient can only read the top

line their vision is represented as 6/60. This means they can read at 6 m what a healthy person can read at 60 m. If the patient is unable to read the top letter (which is very poor sight) move the chart to 3 m (if they can read it here their vision is 3/60) or even 1 m. If the patient still has difficulty reading the first line, see if they can count fingers at 1 m, recognize hand movements, or finally, perceive light.

Tip

If you do not possess a standardized visual chart, you can assess vision crudely by getting the patient to read any material close by, for example, a newspaper or your name badge. This will identify any gross visual disturbance or disparity between the eyes. Again check to see if they normally wear reading glasses. If they cannot see any reasonably sized print, see if they can count fingers held up in front of them.

Visual fields

What are they?

When you look at an object, you not only see your point of interest with good-quality colour vision (by virtue of the macula, an area of the retina rich in cones, which are the colour-sensitive photoreceptors) but you are also aware of surrounding items. For example, as you read this text you may be aware of the immediate environment, such as the desk the book may be resting on. The rest of the retina supplies this 'peripheral' vision by virtue of mainly rods, which are the non-colour-sensitive photoreceptors and which give a poorer image quality. Visual fields examination represents a mapping out of the patient's peripheral vision and the aim is to discover any areas of visual loss within them.

How to examine

The bedside method of testing visual fields is called the confrontation test. Basically compare your visual fields (which are hopefully normal) with your patient's. To do this the examination position is critical (see Fig. 6.7). The patient may already have their left eye covered with their left hand following their visual acuity assessment. If so, you should cover your right eye with your right hand. To make a direct comparison between your and your patient's visual fields it is essential that your face is on the same level and about 1 m apart (like looking in a mirror).

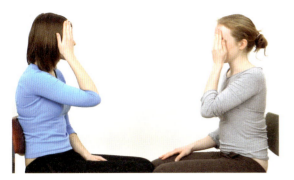

Figure 6.7 Position for testing visual fields.

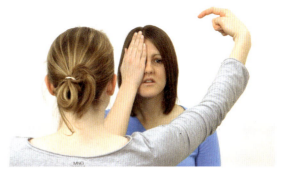

Figure 6.8 Testing the visual fields by confrontation. Bring the target in from the periphery.

Say, 'I want you to look directly into my left eye and I want you to keep your head and eyes still at all times.' You want your patient to look straight ahead while you bring in your visual source from the periphery. Wiggling your index finger makes a crude but acceptable target. To be more accurate you could use a light source, counting fingers, or a white or better still red neurological hatpin to assess the visual fields. Make sure your target is equidistant between you and the patient. The length of your arms will limit the extent of the visual fields that you can test. Say to your patient, 'Tell me when you can see my finger moving.' When the patient says, 'now', you can confirm your findings by stopping and starting your finger movements, 'Are my fingers still moving?' It is traditional to examine the visual fields in four quadrants: upper temporal, upper nasal, lower temporal, and lower nasal (Fig. 6.8). You should bring your finger in from the extremity of each quadrant as a bare minimum. Your aim is to map out as much of the visual fields as is possible.

Once you have checked out the field of the patient's right eye, say to your patient, 'Uncover your left eye please, and now cover your right eye with your right hand.' This time you will cover your left eye with your left hand and ask the patient to look at your right eye. Now map out the field for the other eye.

Tip
You may find it difficult to test the nasal fields without swapping the hand that covers your own eye, that is, if your right hand is covering your right eye, you will be using your left hand as the target. This will feel natural until you reach your nasal fields where your inclination will be to force your left arm across your body. Rather than get into this clumsy position, simply cover your right eye with your left hand and use your right hand as the target.

Remember your fingers are crude targets and may miss a subtle defect or not define a defect very well, so after using fingers as a target use your red neurological pin. The retina is very sensitive to the colour red and lesions of the optic nerve or chiasma may manifest with red objects appearing washed out, or even white. This process is called 'red desaturation' and may be the first indication of a problem before an area of blindness develops. Also use the neurological pin to map out the blind spot. The blind spot is a physiological scotoma (see later) and corresponds to the optic disc (where there are no photoreceptors as this is the exit point for the optic nerve). Using your neurological pin, move it slowly in from the temporal side of the eye being tested level with the eye. Your patient should continue to look at your eye as before. They should be aware of the red tip of the pin as it moves slowly inwards until a point is reached where the tip vanishes. If you move the pin further inwards, the tip should reappear again. This 'vanishing' point is only momentary and can be easily missed. Try this on yourself to see how small this point is. Just focus on a point in the distance and bring in a target from the temporal side of the eye you are testing. Make sure that your other eye is closed because the fields of both eyes overlap. This will give you a feeling for what is 'normal'. If however you can move the pin around in a larger area around the blind spot with the tip remaining invisible then this may be an enlarged blind spot and is a feature of papilloedema (*pap-ill-ee-deema*).

Tip
Practise these manoeuvres on yourself first until you feel confident to perform them on a patient.

Tip

Inevitably during many visual field assessments you will find patients turning their heads or gazing directly at your fingers. If this happens don't become exasperated, just keep reinforcing the command, 'No—please keep your head still and just look straight into my eyes.'

Abnormal findings

There is a range of deficits you may pick up from total blindness in one eye to small areas of visual loss (called scotomas). Sometimes the pattern of visual loss can give you a clue to the location of a lesion (see Fig. 6.9). It is useful to know the following definitions.

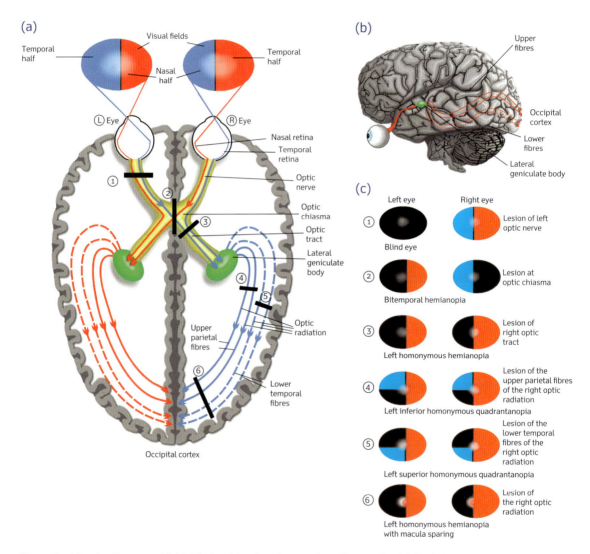

Figure 6.9 Visual pathways and field defects arising from lesions along these paths. (a) Axial slice through the brain at the level of the eyes. (b) Lateral view of the brain. (c) Visual defects associated with lesions indicated. Nerve impulses travel down the optic nerves (the nasal fibres crossing at the chiasma) before travelling along the optic tracts to relay in the lateral geniculate bodies. The impulses then travel along the optic radiation to terminate in the occipital cortex. Ultimately the right occipital cortex is responsible for the left half of the visual fields and the left occipital cortex is responsible for the right. The brain is able to synthesize the visual stimuli and correct the inversion of the images to produce meaningful vision.

- **Hemianopia**. This is the loss of one half of a field of vision.

- **Homonymous hemianopia**. This is the loss of the same half of the visual field in each eye, for example, the left half of the left and right eyes (see Fig. 6.9).

- **Quadrantanopia** (*quad-ran-tan-owe-pia*). This is the loss of one-quarter of a field of vision.

When interpreting schematic representations of visual fields you need to remember that the image is inverted on the retina. Light rays from the top of an object will be the bottom-most point of the image on the retina. Also light from the temporal half of a field will strike the nasal portion of the retina and light from the nasal half of a field will strike the temporal portion of the retina. The other feature to remember is that nerve fibres from the left and right temporal retinae do not cross the midline at the optic chiasma and therefore terminate in the ipsilateral occipital cortex. The fibres from the nasal retinae do cross the midline at the optic chiasma and therefore end in the contralateral occipital cortex (see Fig. 6.9).

Colour vision

This is not normally tested in a routine clinical setting but can be assessed using Ishiara charts to look for colour blindness.

Pupillary light and accommodation reflexes

Pupillary light reflex: what is it?

This is the constriction of the pupil when a light is shone in the eye and helps to limit the amount of light entering the eyes in bright conditions. In normal circumstances both pupils will constrict when light is shone in one eye. Therefore the reflex is described as direct in the eye being illuminated and consensual in the other eye. On shining a light into someone's eyes, the nerve impulse travels up the optic nerve (cranial nerve II), relaying in the brainstem before passing down the parasympathetic branch of the oculomotor nerve (cranial nerve III). This causes the pupil of that eye to constrict through the sphincter pupillae muscle (direct reflex). Impulses also pass to the oculomotor nerve of the other eye, leading to constriction of that pupil also (consensual reflex). See Fig. 6.10.

Pupillary light reflex: how to examine

First inspect each pupil and make sure that they are equal in size and that they are round and regular. Any asymmetry in pupil size or shape needs to be explained. A small difference in pupil size of about a millimetre is acceptable and may be physiological, especially if this relationship is maintained both in bright and poor illumination and is variable between eyes. Pupils that are constricted are called miotic (the process of constriction is called miosis)

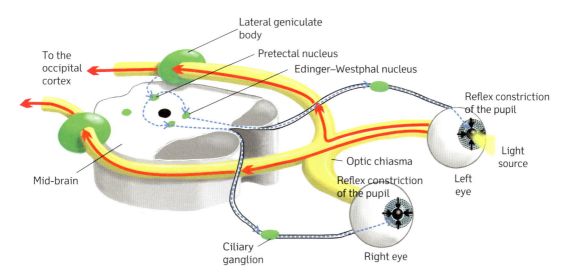

Figure 6.10 Pathways associated with the pupillary light reflex. A light shone into the left eye leads to nerve impulses conducted in the normal way along the optic chiasma to the lateral geniculate body (some impulses continue to the occipital cortex). The brightness of the light triggers impulses along another (reflex) pathway leading to the pretectal nucleus and then to both Edinger–Westphal nuclei (the parasympathetic nucleus of nerve III). Further impulses travel via the ciliary ganglion to the sphincter pupillae muscle of both eyes which contract in response to limit the light entering the eyes.

and pupils that are dilated are called mydriatic (*mid-dree-attic*) (the process of dilatation is called mydriasis (*mid-dree-ay-sis*)). Healthy pupils will be constricted in bright sunshine and dilated in poor light. Despite this range in size they should still display the direct and consensual reflex (although it is much harder to spot the change in size when the pupils are small to begin with).

Warn your patient, 'I am going to shine a light into your eyes . . . it will be a little bright.' Your pen torch should be brought in from the side of the face and shone in the same eye on two successive occasions (shine the light for no more than a split second). The first time, look at the same pupil for the direct reflex and the second time look into the other pupil for a consensual response. It is sometimes taught to put a hand vertically from the nose to the forehead (to stop some light shining in both eyes), but this technique looks clumsy and is unnecessary. Now do the same to the other eye. You should have used your torch on four separate occasions.

....

Tip

It can be difficult to spot the constriction if the pupils are small to begin with. If this is the case try to reduce background light as much as possible, for example, closing blinds or switching off the bedside lamp. Or take your patient to somewhere dimly lit and try again.

....

Pupillary accommodation reflex: what is it?

When you look into the distance and then switch your focus to an object close to your eyes, the adjustment process is called accommodation. During this process your eyes turn inward marginally (converge) and the pupils constrict to limit the light received to the approximate area of interest. As before the impulse travels up the optic nerve and relays in the brainstem, before returning down the oculomotor nerve to constrict the pupil.

Pupillary accommodation reflex: how to examine

Choose a distant point that is at least 6 m away (ideally the further away the better). It is better to give the patient an object to focus on rather than just telling them to gawp into the distance. Say something like, 'Look at the number one on the clock on the far wall.' Observe the size of the pupils and wait until you are certain they are focusing on the distant object. Have your near target, preferably a very small picture, a small letter, or your index finger close to your patient's face (at a distance of about 15 cm) and then quickly ask them to look at your target. Observe the pupils and see if they constrict as they focus on the object. Be careful to get a good look at both pupils because in some conditions the pupils will remain constricted for some time and so you will not be able to repeat the test. The reaction is often very minimal so it can be easily missed! This test was important in the days when syphilis was rife, when patients sometimes exhibited Argyll-Robertson (*are-guile-robert-son*) pupils (*Douglas Moray Cooper Lamb Argyll-Robertson (1837–1909), Scottish ophthalmologist*). In this condition the pupils are small and irregular and the key feature is that they do not react to light but constrict with accommodation. Nowadays this is rarely seen, although it can occur in some people with diabetes.

....

Tip

Choose somewhere slightly elevated for the distant point and keep your finger slightly above the level of the patient's eyes when you ask them to focus on it. This prevents the upper eyelid from obscuring your view of the pupils (see Fig. 6.11).

....

(a)
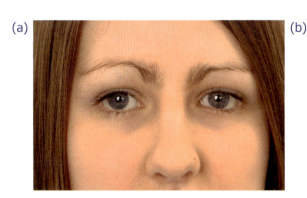

(b)
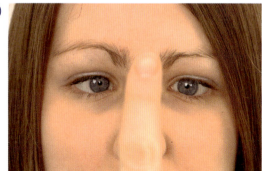

Figure 6.11 Testing the accommodation reflex: (a) looking into the distance, (b) focusing on finger: note the convergence of the eyes and constriction of the pupils.

Abnormal findings

- **Pinpoint pupils**. Caused by bilateral instillation of miotic eye drops, for example, pilocarpine (*pile-owe-carp-een*), opiate overdose, brainstem stroke (pontine), bilateral Horner's syndrome (*Johann Friedrich Horner (1831–1886), Swiss ophthalmologist*), and old age.

- **Dilated pupils**. Caused by bilateral instillation of mydriatic eye drops, for example, tropicamide (*trow-pick-amide*), fear or anger, drug overdose, for example, anticholinergic drugs, and brainstem stroke (midbrain).

- **Unilateral miosis**. Caused by miotic eye drops in the affected eye, Horner's syndrome (see Fig. 13.14), and Holmes–Adie (*homes-ay-dee*) pupil (*Sir Gordon Holmes (1876–1965), English neurologist; William John Adie (1886–1935), Australian-born British physician*).

- **Fixed oval pupil (not reactive to light or accommodation)**. Caused by acute untreated glaucoma.

- **Grossly irregular pupil (not reactive to light or accommodation)**. Caused by previous trauma and adhesions of the iris to the lens, which occurs in iritis (called posterior synechiae (*sign-ee-key-eye*)).

- **Unilateral mydriasis**. Caused by mydriatic eye drops in the affected eye and nerve III palsy.

- **Argyll-Robertson pupils**. Small irregular pupils (not reactive to light but react to accommodation). Caused by syphilis and diabetes mellitus.

- **Marcus Gunn pupil (relative afferent pupillary defect (RAPD))** (*R. Marcus Gunn (1850–1909), Scottish ophthalmologist*). This is due to either damage of the optic nerve, for example, due to retrobulbar neuritis secondary to multiple sclerosis or massive retinal damage, for example, a retinal detachment. A RAPD can be demonstrated by the swinging light test. First shine a very bright light in one eye from the side for 3 seconds. If this eye is normal, both pupils will constrict briskly. Quickly swing the light over to the other eye. If the second eye is affected the pupil is seen to dilate rather than constrict. This is because the nerve impulse is conducted poorly along the damaged optic nerve so that what you see is the pupil relaxing from its original consensual response when you shone your torch in the first eye. After 3 seconds quickly swing the light back to the first eye and now note both pupils will constrict again. You can keep swinging between the eyes to check your findings. To make yourself look slick, perform this test just after testing the direct and consensual pupil reactions.

....
Tip
When faced with pupillary abnormalities also check for drooping eyelids (ptosis). The presence of ptosis will exclude many causes but not a nerve III palsy or Horner's syndrome.
....

Fundoscopy

What is it?

The fundus (*fun-duss*) in this context is synonymous with the retina. Fundoscopy is the examination of the retina and the structures that enter and leave it using an instrument called an ophthalmoscope (sometimes the technique is called ophthalomoscopy but this is rather a mouthful). In reality, when you become skilled at performing fundoscopy you can inspect other structures of the eye including the lens and abnormalities in the vitreous humour.

How to examine

Everyone who has tried fundoscopy knows how difficult it is. There are four stages that you have to master before you can become proficient at this procedure:

1 being familiar with the ophthalmoscope (see Fig. 6.12)

2 being familiar with using the ophthalmoscope on a patient

3 being familiar with the normal fundus

4 learning what different abnormalities can affect the fundus.

First, familiarize yourself with the controls of the ophthalmoscope. There is usually a dial, which can be turned by the index finger of either hand depending on which eye you are examining. The dial alters the lenses within the instrument. These range from positive lenses (these may have red numbers and are used to focus your view in long-sighted (hypermetropic) patients) to negative lenses (these may have black numbers and are used to focus your view in short-sighted (myopic) patients). Some models of ophthalmoscopes use red numbers for negative lenses and black for positive lenses, so be wary. There is also a switch to activate the light. On most models you will press in a switch and rotate a collar or the base of the ophthalmoscope to turn the light on. There may also be controls to alter the size, strength, and colour of the beam. A small beam is used when looking

CASE 6.1

Problem. You are performing fundoscopy and are struggling to see any landmarks in the fundus. Why is this?

Discussion. Initially your technique may be to blame as you become familiar with using the ophthalmoscope. Many people have difficulty using their non-dominant eye while holding the instrument with their non-dominant hand. Only practice will solve this. However, the biggest stumbling block to visualizing the fundus is constricted pupils. Most people attempt to view the fundus in broad daylight and are destined to fail. The pupils need to be dilated with short-acting eye drops like tropicamide. The next best thing is a room that can be made dark enough to allow the pupil to dilate sufficiently.

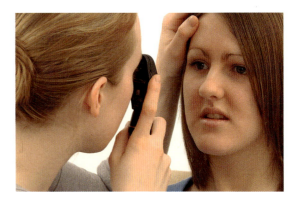

Figure 6.13 Using the ophthalmoscope.

through a small pupil in order to minimize reflections, but the larger the beam the better in a dilated patient. The green light or 'red free' is used to increase contrast when looking at red things on the retina. Small haemorrhages are therefore easier to see.

Now it is time to try and use the instrument on a patient. See Fig. 6.13. To optimize the view of the fundus, your patient's pupils should be adequately dilated. The best method for achieving this is with short-acting eye drops. Unfortunately unless you are in a specialist eye clinic, it is more likely that your patient will not have this done. The next best thing is to find a room that can be darkened sufficiently to allow your patient's pupils to dilate—the pupils will constrict when you shine your light in though! If your patient wears glasses, these must be removed. If you wear glasses, however, it is perfectly acceptable for you to leave them on (as it reduces the need to correct for both your own vision and the patient's with the opthalmoscope). See Case 6.1 for common difficulties in seeing the fundus.

....

Tip
It can be difficult to tell if the light has been activated, so point the ophthalmoscope towards your palm and look for a small circle of light. When you have finished using the ophthalmoscope it is even more important to check that it has been switched off completely. So point it at your palm again and make sure the light has gone. This is because it is very easy to leave it on and drain the batteries, leaving the ward without a functioning opthalmoscope (it is amazing how some wards do not even have a stock of spare batteries).
....

Tip
Practise getting the feel of the ophthalmoscope and use it with both hands. Get used to turning the dials with the index finger of either hand, before trying it on a patient.
....

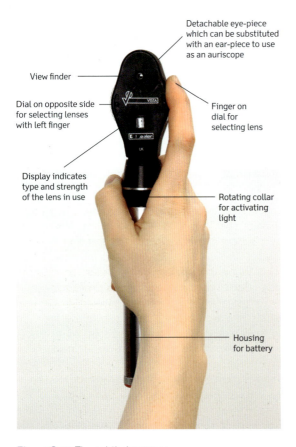

Detachable eye-piece which can be substituted with an ear-piece to use as an auriscope

View finder

Dial on opposite side for selecting lenses with left finger

Finger on dial for selecting lens

Display indicates type and strength of the lens in use

Rotating collar for activating light

Housing for battery

Figure 6.12 The ophthalmoscope.

To look in the patient's right eye, hold the ophthalmoscope in your right hand and use your right eye. You will have to examine from the right hand side of the patient. Similarly, for the patient's left eye, use your left eye and left hand and examine from the left-hand side of the patient. You have to get very close to your patient, so make sure you have had a shower and not eaten garlic the previous night! Now hold your ophthalmoscope steady and peer through its aperture. Some people emphasize that your redundant eye should remain open. As you improve you will be able to do this but in the early stages it is easier to keep the eye shut.

Get your patient to look slightly upwards for two reasons: first, so their eyelids do not obscure the pupils (you may have to use the thumb of your other hand to gently pull the upper eyelid out of the way) and second, so that when you move in from the side you 'hit' the optic disc almost immediately (the optic disc is an important reference point). Say to your patient, 'Look straight ahead please, where the ceiling joins the wall, try and concentrate on that spot even if I get in the way.' While you have the patient at arm's length elicit the red reflex in both eyes. You should see a red reflection just like the red eyes on an amateur photograph. An absent or reduced reflex implies an opacity somewhere in the path of the retina. The most common cause is a cataract. Move in slowly until you see the retina. Focus the ophthalmoscope by using the negative lenses if the patient is short sighted and the positive lenses if the patient is long sighted.

Now identify the optic disc. The optic disc represents the exit point of the nerve fibres from the retina to become the optic nerve. Once in focus, comment upon its three Cs: the colour, the contour, and the cup. The colour of the optic disc is usually a light pinky-orange. If there is optic atrophy (see later) the disc becomes a pale yellow colour. Papilloedema produces a reddy-pink disc. The contour of the disc is usually well defined. With papilloedema the margin of the whole disc becomes indistinct and blurred (see Figs. 6.17 and 6.18). The optic cup is the small oval aperture within the optic disc, which transmits the blood vessels to the retina. The diameter of the cup is normally small compared to that of the optic disc (see Fig. 6.14). If there is ischaemia of the optic nerve or if there is glaucoma (a condition with raised intraocular pressure (IOP) and a damaged optic nerve causing visual field defects) there is loss of the nerve fibres and this leads to an increase in the cup diameter relative to the optic disc, a process called 'cupping'. Determining what constitutes 'glaucomatous cupping' is subjective and has led to disagreement. For the non-ophthalmologist, if there is any doubt send your patient to an expert for further evaluation.

There are four 'arcades' of arteries and veins radiating from the optic disc, each extending into the superior and inferior temporal and the superior and inferior nasal quadrants. Follow each in turn, noting the appearance of the vessels and the surrounding retina. Now get the patient to look up, down, left, and right to see the peripheries of the retina. Some signs such as pigmentation in retinitis pigmentosa may only be seen when looked for in the peripheries. This will give you a good systematic method of reviewing the fundus. Now say to your patient, 'Look directly into the light for me . . . I know it is difficult.' This will enable you to assess the macula. You may have to refocus the ophthalmoscope. Finally, 'rack back' through the positive lenses and review the more anterior structures of the eye. These include the vitreous for floaters and even the iris.

The only way to appreciate what a normal fundus looks like is to see as many as you can. It is worth looking at ophthalmology atlases, which will show you the variety of normal funi that exist. See Fig.6.14.

Similarly, the best way to learn about pathology is to study the appearances in an ophthalmology atlas and take any opportunity you can to see these in real patients if you hear about them. Ophthalmology clinics and diabetic eye clinics are the best places to see common abnormalities. Figures 6.15–6.18 show the appearances of important abnormalities you should be conversant with.

Papilloedema

What is it?

Papilloedema refers to the appearance of the fundus in response to raised intracranial pressure. As a consequence of this pressure the eye goes through a sequence of changes.

1 Initially there is a loss of venous pulsation and the veins may become more dilated and tortuous. Not many clinicians have the expertise to spot these early changes.

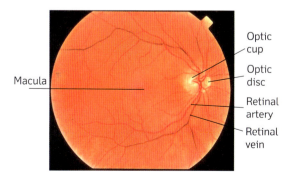

Figure 6.14 Normal fundus.

(a)

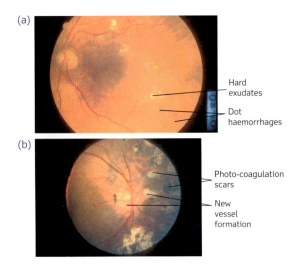

Hard exudates

Dot haemorrhages

(b)

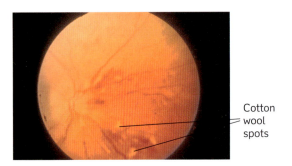

Photo-coagulation scars

New vessel formation

Figure 6.15 Diabetic retinopathy: (a) background retinopathy, (b) proliferative retinopathy.

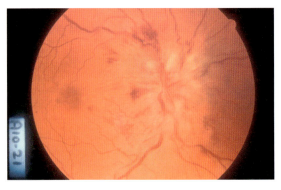

Figure 6.17 Papilloedema secondary to malignant hypertension.Note the veins seem to disappear on approaching the optic disc or loop over the swollen margin. Also note the flame-shaped haemorrhages.

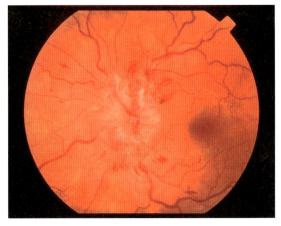

Cotton wool spots

Figure 6.16 Hypertensive retinopathy showing cotton wool spots.

2 Then the optic cup becomes pinker and indistinct.

3 The contour of the optic disc becomes blurred and vessels seem to disappear at the margins of the disc, rather than running straight into the optic cup.

4 The whole of the optic disc becomes pink and swollen.

5 Other changes may be seen depending on the underlying cause, for example, malignant hypertension—flame-shaped haemorrhages radiating from the optic disc.

Causes of papilloedema

- raised intracranial pressure
- SOL (e.g. cerebral tumour, intracranial haematoma, or cerebral abscess)
- malignant hypertension (see Fig. 6.17)
- benign intracranial hypertension (BIH)

Figure 6.18 Papilloedema secondary to central retinal vein occlusion. Note similar appearance of the optic disc; however, haemorrhages are scattered more widely than in malignant hypertension.

- severe hypercapnia (*high-per-cap-knee-a*)
- complication of meningitis
- central retinal vein thrombosis (see Fig. 6.18).

The presence of papilloedema indicates the need for further investigation. It is also a cautionary sign when considering a lumbar puncture. If a lumbar puncture is performed in the presence of raised intracranial pressure there is the risk of 'coning', where the brainstem is forced down through the foramen magnum with lethal consequences. A CT scan **must** be performed before consideration of a lumbar puncture in the presence of papilloedema. However, the absence of papilloedema does not rule out the possibility of raised intracranial pressure (because the eye changes may lag behind the onset of raised pressure).

Key points

- With any visual disturbance, always check visual acuity with a standardized assessment chart, for example, Snellen chart
- With any visual disturbance, always check the visual fields
- If the pupils are not equal in size this must be explained
- Always observe the response of the pupils to light and accommodation
- Fundoscopy is a vital technique and must be mastered
- Only perform fundoscopy with the pupils properly dilated either with short-acting dilating eye drops or a sufficiently darkened room, otherwise you are doomed to fail
- Make sure that you are familiar with the range of normal fundi that can be found
- Make sure that you are familiar with the appearances of common diseases you are likely to see in everyday practice
- A swollen optic disc is an indicator of raised intracranial pressure
- Do not do a lumbar puncture in the presence of papilloedema without a normal CT scan to check it is safe to do so
- Do not do a lumbar puncture without a CT scan if the history suggests raised intracranial pressure even if the optic discs are normal

Therefore do not do a lumbar puncture if the history suggests the possibility of raised intracranial pressure, even if the discs are normal.

Oculomotor (III), trochlear (IV), and abducens (VI) nerves

9 Inspect for ptosis and a squint (DF 3/10) and check eye movements: look for nystagmus and ask about diplopia (III, IV, and VI tested) (DF 8/10)

Inspect for ptosis

What is it?

Ptosis is the medical term for a drooping eyelid. Normally with ptosis, the lower margin of the eyelid passes just below the upper border of the pupil when a person

Table 6.14 Causes of ptosis

Myogenic	Horner's syndrome, IIIrd nerve palsy,
Neurogenic	Myasthenia gravis, myotonia dystrophica
Tendon	Involutional (= old age)
Others	Trauma, infection, inflammation, tumours, and congenital

is awake. The lid can droop sufficiently to encroach on the visual axis. At this point the lid will interfere with the patient's upper field of vision.

Significance

The levator palpebrae (le-vay-tor-pal-pe-bray) is the main muscle that elevates the eyelid and is supplied by the cranial nerve III. Muller's muscle also helps lift the eyelid to a small degree and is supplied by the sympathetic system. This is why the eyes appear more open when the body is in a frightened state and why a complete lesion of cranial nerve III produces a complete ptosis whereas a lesion of the sympathetic system (Horner's syndrome) produces a partial ptosis.

Causes

Causes of ptosis are given in Table 6.14. They are easy to remember if you think of the different anatomical structures required to lift the eyelid, that is, the nerves, muscles, tendon, and of course the 'other' group as well. It is important to remember some causes of pseudoptosis, that is, cases that look like ptosis but are not really. These include the fellow eyelid being retracted, for example, in thyroid eye disease or the globe being sunken in enophthalmos, for example, after a blow-out fracture of the orbit.

What to look for

A complete ptosis is obvious. Mild degrees of ptosis can be easily missed. Make sure that your patient is looking directly ahead and focus on the eyelids (if they are looking up or down the appearance of the eyelids will be misleading). Does one seem to droop more than the other? If it does, quickly check there is no obvious infection or swelling there. Also quickly check pupil size. A tiny pupil (miotic) may suggest a Horner's syndrome and a large pupil (mydriatic) that does not react to light suggests a nerve III lesion. Bilateral ptosis, which is mild, is very hard to spot. However if you notice both eyelids encroaching on the visual axis, this is abnormal. See Figs 6.19–6.21.

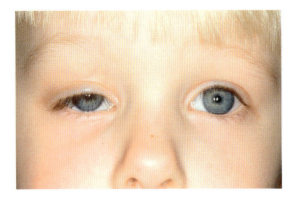

Figure 6.19 Congenital ptosis. Note the right pupil is of comparable size to the left.

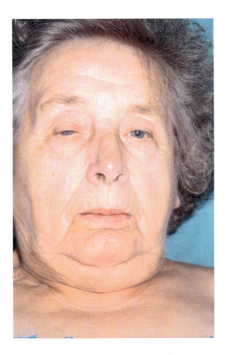

Figure 6.20 Bilateral ptosis due to myasthenia gravis. Ptosis improved with injection of cholinesterase inhibitor.

Tip
With most forms of ptosis the patient compensates by contracting their frontalis (*front-ay-lis*) muscle (the muscle that makes the forehead wrinkle) to produce a modest elevation of the eyelids. The exceptions to this rule are the myopathic causes of ptosis where this muscle may also be affected.

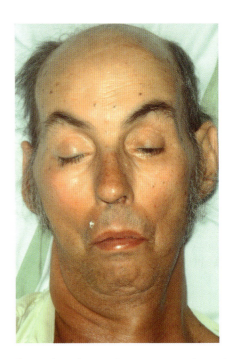

Figure 6.21 Bilateral ptosis due to myotonia dystrophica. This patient has the typical facies of the condition. There is 'hollowing out' of the temples because of wasting of the temporalis muscles. There is also wasting of the masseters of the cheeks and of the sternomastoids. As this is a myopathic cause the patient is unable to wrinkle his forehead to improve his ptosis.

Tip
If the ptosis is sufficient to compromise the upper field of vision, the patient may tilt their head backwards to improve their field of vision.

Inspect for a squint

What is it?

The eyes are normally aligned in parallel and move together as a unit. A squint (medical term strabismus [*stra-biz-muss*]) is where one of the eyes deviates from the parallel. If the affected eye turns inward this is called a convergent squint. If the affected eye turns outwards this is called a divergent squint. Squints can be further classified as concomitant or paralytic.

A concomitant squint is where the deviation remains constant whichever direction the person looks. It is termed incomitant if this is not the case. A paralytic squint is where the affected eye has a weakened extraocular muscle. The angle of deviation is maximal when looking in the direction of action of the paralysed muscle.

Significance

Concomitant squints are usually found from childhood onwards and may be congenital or due to refractive errors (see Chapter 14). The developing brain suppresses the image from the affected eye, preventing diplopia. If this suppression occurs during a child's critical development period, which is up to about the age of 8 years, the eye may never develop to be as strong as the other, that is, it will produce amblyopia (*am-blee-owe-pia*) (otherwise known as a 'lazy eye'). Refractive errors need to be corrected with spectacles. Amblyopia is usually treated by covering the good eye, in a bid to force the use of the lazy eye. This form of squint therefore must be rectified before the image from the affected eye is irreversibly suppressed. Paralytic squints are usually due to lesions of the cranial nerves III, IV or VI (the squint due to nerve IV is subtle). Patients with paralytic squints need further evaluation to find an underlying cause.

Check eye movements: look for nystagmus and ask about diplopia

All three cranial nerves supply the extraocular muscles and are responsible for the smooth and coordinated movement of the eyes (this is conjugate eye movement). Problems with any of these nerves will impair eye movements and lead to double vision.

Nystagmus: what is it?

This is the involuntary, repetitive oscillation of one or both eyes. Each oscillation can be of equal rate where the nystagmus (*nis-stag-muss*) is called pendular, or there can be a fast and a slow phase when it is termed jerky. With jerky nystagmus the direction of nystagmus is determined by the direction of the fast phase, for example, if the eye flicks out quickly to the right and slowly returns to the left, the direction of nystagmus is to the right. Nystagmus is usually in the horizontal plane but occasionally can occur in the vertical plane (where you should be suspicious of a brainstem lesion). It can also be rotatory usually due to vestibular lesions). If nystagmus is severe it can be observed at rest. Otherwise it has to be provoked by eye movements (the basis of clinical testing).

Nystagmus: significance

Nystagmus is a problem maintaining the posture of the eye or conjugate eye movements. The problem can be

Table 6.15 Causes of nystagmus

Physiological (optokinetic nystagmus, endpoint nystagmus, and vestibular stimulation)
Congenital
Visual impairment
Vestibular disease (BPPV)
Central lesions
Cerebellar disease

BPPV, benign paroxysmal positional vertigo

anywhere along a pathway that includes the eye itself, the vestibular system, the cerebellum, the brainstem, and their complex interconnections. Paradoxically it is not the fast phase of nystagmus that is abnormal. Rather it is the slow phase, which represents the aberrant drift of the eye away from the visual source and the fast phase is the compensatory flick back to the target.

Nystagmus: causes

See Table 6.15

- **Physiological**. These are normal responses of the eye to various stimuli. Optokinetic nystagmus is the jerky nystagmus that can sometimes occur when tracking a fast-moving target, for example, watching scenery going by in a car. Endpoint nystagmus is the jerky nystagmus that can occur at the extremes of gaze. Vestibular stimulation will occur if a person spins repeatedly. They become dizzy and may exhibit jerky or rotational nystagmus. Vestibular stimulation can also occur by introducing cold water into the ear canal. This is called caloric testing and is a recognized test of labyrinthine function.

- **Congenital**. This is present at or soon after birth. The nystagmus is usually seen in all directions of gaze and is pendular in nature. It is often familial and has no other serious consequences.

- **Visual impairment**. People with severe visual impairment have difficulty fixing on a target; the eye roves around and the associated nystagmus is pendular in nature.

- **Vestibular disease**. The vestibular system is concerned with maintaining balance. Lesions affecting its peripheral apparatus, for example, semicircular canals, can cause a jerky or rotational nystagmus. The direction of nystagmus is away from the affected side.

CASE 6.2

Problem. A 43-year-old woman presents to an acute admissions unit with a sudden onset of vertigo. The room spins around a vertical axis and is associated with nausea. She has no deafness or tinnitus. You check her eye movements and you notice nystagmus to the left in all directions of gaze. What is the diagnosis?

Discussion. This story sounds typical of an attack of acute labyrinthitis. There is a sudden onset of true vertigo without tinnitus or deafness, which distinguishes it from Ménière's syndrome. With vestibular disease the direction of nystagmus is away from the affected side, in this case the affected organ is the right labyrinth.

Associated diseases that affect this apparatus include viral labyrinthitis and Ménière's syndrome. Associated symptoms may include vertigo, tinnitus, and deafness. These forms of nystagmus tend to be self-limiting. See Case 6.2.

- **Central lesions**. A central lesion in this context means a problem in the central nervous system (or brain essentially). The areas that are affected are usually the posterior fossa (an area of the brain that houses the cerebellum) or the brainstem. A tumour, demyelinating diseases such as multiple sclerosis, or a stroke affecting these areas can cause vertigo and nystagmus (which may behave like benign positional vertigo). The difference with central lesions is that there is no delay before the onset of nystagmus, it is not fatiguable, and head movements in any direction can provoke it (see 'Hallpike–Dix manoeuvre' section).

- **Cerebellar disease**. The cerebellum is also concerned with balance and the coordination of movement. Lesions of the cerebellum lead to ataxia (unsteadiness) and a jerky nystagmus with the direction towards the affected side. A wide range of diseases can affect the cerebellum including tumours (see Case 6.3), multiple sclerosis, stroke, alcohol, inherited disease, and degenerative disorders. As the eyes move look for any abnormal oscillation of the eyes. Also nystagmus may be more complex than has been described. Some conditions can affect more than one organ or neural pathway producing a hybrid nystagmus, for example, an acoustic neuroma can affect the vestibular nerve causing nystagmus and as it grows it can also compress the brainstem and affect central vestibular or cerebellar pathways.

CASE 6.3

Problem. A 59-year-old man presents with a 4-week history of headache, which is worse in the morning and associated with nausea. He is also unsteady on his feet and finds himself lurching to the right. He had fallen on the morning of presentation and felt he needed to be checked over. You examine him and notice he is thin and anxious with tar staining of the fingers of his right hand. He has papilloedema on fundoscopy and has nystagmus on looking to the right. You perform a full neurological examination and discover that he has an intention tremor of his right hand and exhibits past-pointing with it. He has a wide-based gait and tends to stagger to the right especially when he turns around. What is the diagnosis?

Discussion. His story is worrying. The neurological signs you have unearthed suggest two problems. The headache, which is worse in the morning and the papilloedema point towards raised intracranial pressure. The nystagmus to the right, the intention tremor, the past-pointing of the right hand, and his staggering to the right, suggest a lesion in the right cerebellar hemisphere. There is a strong possibility that the gradual progression of symptoms is produced by a tumour. Primary tumours are rare in adults and it is more likely that this represents secondary spread. A further clue in the history is that he has tar staining of his fingers. It is likely that he is (or was) a heavy smoker and this could represent a bronchial carcinoma with metastases to the right cerebellar hemisphere (or a paraneoplastic syndrome). This man needs a CT/MRI scan of the brain as well as a chest radiograph.

Diplopia: what is it?

This is the resultant double vision caused (usually) by extraocular muscle dysfunction.

Diplopia: significance

Commonly this is because of damage to the nerve supply to the extraocular muscles, that is, nerves III, IV, and VI. Other mechanisms are discussed later. Normally, eye movements are controlled by six extraocular muscles working together in pairs (see Fig. 6.22). Remembering their function is relatively easy as their name reflects their actions (with notable exceptions), for example,

- superior rectus—elevates the eye superiorly
- inferior rectus—depresses the eye inferiorly

- lateral rectus—pulls the eye laterally (called abduction)

- medial rectus—pulls the eye medially (called adduction).

The exceptions are the 'obliques,' which have complex paths prior to their insertion on to the globe of the eye, such that their actions are opposite to that suggested by their name:

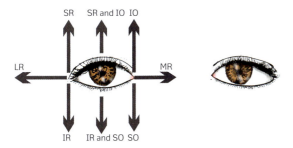

Figure 6.22 The direction of action of the eye muscles. MR, medial rectus; LR, lateral rectus; SR, superior rectus; IR, inferior rectus; IO, inferior oblique; SO, superior oblique.

- inferior oblique—elevates the eye;

- superior oblique—depresses the eye.

As Fig. 6.22 demonstrates, eye elevation and depression are more complicated. The superior and inferior recti muscles have their greatest effect when the eye is abducted. The superior and inferior oblique muscles have their greatest effect when the eye is adducted. When the eye is midway between abduction and adduction, the superior rectus and inferior oblique combine to elevate the eye and the inferior rectus and the superior oblique combine to depress the eye. Note that some of the extraocular muscles also have rotational effects but you do not need to know these (a technique for identifying a nerve IV palsy in the presence of a nerve III lesion uses this principle).

Neural centres in the brainstem and cerebral cortex coordinate eye movements so that light from an object will fall on corresponding points of the retina of each eye (usually the macula). This binocular input allows the brain to build up a three-dimensional picture of the environment. If, however, one of the extraocular muscles is weak, the corresponding light rays from an object will strike a different and more peripheral portion of the retina of the affected eye leading to a fainter double image (see Fig. 6.23).

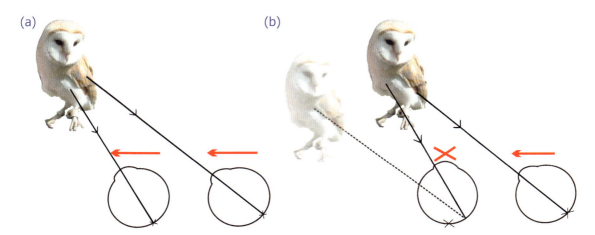

Figure 6.23 The mechanism of diplopia due to the paralysis of the left lateral rectus muscle. The eyes work as a functional pair. (a) Both eyes look to the left to view an object. Each eye moves together to allow focusing of the image on each macula allowing the object to be seen with the greatest clarity. Note the slightly different (but overlapping) aspects of the object seen with each eye leading to a 3D view (the depth perception associated with stereoscopic vision). (b) With a left nerve VI palsy the left eye is unable to look to the left (abduct). Light from the object is only able to strike the periphery of the retina where there are fewer photoreceptors. As the brain is used to the eyes working in tandem, it will extrapolate where it believes the light rays would originate from if the eye was moving normally. Hence a second *false* outer image. As the density of photoreceptors is less than at the macula this false image is also fainter. Finally there is a loss of depth perception because of overlap of the visual fields.

There are three important things to remember about diplopia, as they will help in locating the affected eye.

- The greatest separation of images occurs when the eye is trying to look in the direction of action of the weakened muscle, for example, if the lateral rectus is weak, the greatest separation of the image occurs when the eye tries to abduct.
- The outer image is always the false image.
- The affected eye always produces the false image.

Nystagmus and diplopia: how to examine

The aim of examination is to stress the extraocular muscles and to observe for any abnormal oscillation of the eyes or any failure of eye movement in any direction. To examine, hold your finger about 1 m away from the patient. Ensure your patient does not turn their head as they follow your finger. Say, 'I would like you to keep your head still and to follow my finger by moving your eyes only.' Also add, 'Please tell me if you see double at any time'. Now slowly move your finger through a 'H' configuration. It does not matter which part of the 'H' you start on, so long as you trace along its entirety (see Fig. 6.24). You will have to judge how far you move your finger but it should only be to a point where your patient's eyes can comfortably view it without straining or moving their head. If eye movements are normal both eyes should track your finger smoothly to the extremes of your 'H' configuration (without evidence of nystagmus).

Even if it is not volunteered, double check and ask, 'Did you have double vision at any point?' Occasionally a weakness of the ocular muscle is subtle enough to go unnoticed during testing. If diplopia is present the cover test can identify which eye is at fault.

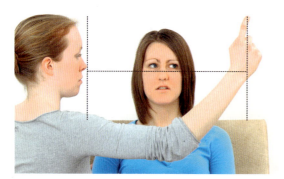

Figure 6.24 Testing eye movements for diplopia and nystagmus.

If nystagmus is present determine whether it is jerky, pendular, or rotational and if it is jerky, work out its direction. You will not be able to deduce the cause of the nystagmus solely on the basis of eye movements. You will need a history and full neurological examination to enable you to do so.

....

Tip

As you become proficient you will be able to look for nystagmus and a failure of eye movement at the same time.

....

Tip

If you see any deviation in eye movement and the patient does **not** experience diplopia, this usually means that the patient is blind in one eye.

....

Nerve III palsy

See Fig. 6.25.

Functions of cranial nerve III

Elevates the eyelids (via the levator palpebrae), constricts the pupil (via the sphincter pupillae muscle of the iris), and innervates the superior rectus, inferior rectus, and medial rectus muscles.

Features of a nerve III palsy

A combination of inspection and examination is needed to diagnose a nerve III palsy.

- Ptosis of the affected eye (paralysis of levator palpebrae)
- If you elevate the eyelid you may notice two features:
  - dilated pupil (paralysis of sphincter pupillae)
  - the position of the eye is depressed and abducted (down and out) because of the unopposed actions of the superior oblique and the lateral rectus muscles, that is, a divergent squint.
- Very little eye movement occurs and diplopia is evident in nearly all directions of gaze.

When all the above criteria are present this is known as a complete nerve III palsy. Sometimes you may only get a partial ptosis and an unaffected pupil. This used to be called an incomplete or partial nerve III palsy; now it is called a nerve III palsy with pupillary sparing.

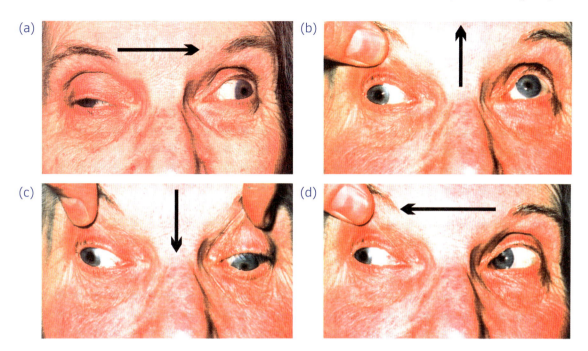

Figure 6.25 Nerve III palsy: (a) divergent squint more pronounced when attempting to look to the left; (b) failure of the right eye to elevate; (c) failure of down-gaze in the right eye; (d) successful abduction of the right eye indicating functioning lateral rectus (and nerve VI).

Reprinted from Fig. 14.38(a)–(d) (p. 14.13), *Atlas of Clinical Neurology* (2nd edn), by G. David Perkin, Fred Hochberg, and Douglas C. Miller (1993), Mosby Publications, with permission from Elsevier.

Tip

The pupillary fibres run on the outside of nerve III where they are vulnerable to compression. Therefore if the pupil is involved in a nerve III palsy, consider a compressive lesion such as a posterior communicating artery aneurysm. If the pupil is spared consider a vasculitic cause or diabetes mellitis.

Tip

To check if nerve IV is intact in the presence of a nerve III palsy, observe the eye as you move your finger down. The affected eye will already be in a depressed position. If the nerve IV is intact the eye will rotate inwards in response.

Causes

Posterior communicating artery aneurysm, multiple sclerosis, brainstem infarct, brainstem neoplasm, raised intracranial pressure, diabetes mellitus, and hypertension.

Nerve IV palsy

Function of cranial nerve IV

The only function of the nerve IV is to supply the superior oblique muscle (which depresses the eye in the adducted position).

Features of a nerve IV palsy

A nerve IV palsy is unusual.

- The patient may have a slight tilt of their head away from the affected eye as a compensatory manoeuvre to minimize the diplopia. (The weak superior oblique enables the unopposed superior rectus to slightly elevate the eye. There is also a slight outward rotation of the eye. The subtle tilt of the head helps to realign the images from both eyes.)

- Diplopia is noted when the eye is made to look down and away from the affected eye and the images will be one above the other. The patient will have difficulty reading and walking downstairs because these activities rely on the superior oblique muscle.

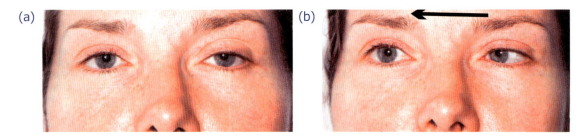

Figure 6.26 Nerve VI palsy: (a) mild convergent squint; (b) failure of the right eye to abduct.
Reprinted from Fig. 14.38(a) and (b) (p. 11.4), *Atlas of Clinical Neurology* (2nd edn), by G. David Perkin, Fred Hochberg, and Douglas C. Miller (1993), Mosby Publications, with permission from Elsevier.

Causes

Trauma, multiple sclerosis, infarct, and neoplasm of the brainstem.

Nerve VI palsy

See Fig. 6.26.

Function of cranial nerve VI

The only function of the nerve VI is to supply the lateral rectus muscle (which abducts the eye).

Features

- The affected eye will be pulled inward because of the unopposed action of the medial rectus muscle (this appearance is called a convergent squint).
- There may be voluntary ptosis as the patient attempts to suppress the diplopia (to check for this pseudoptosis, gently close the eyelid of the unaffected eye and the patient should open the lid of the affected eye to see).
- Diplopia will occur in nearly all directions of gaze (except adduction of the eye). It will be maximal when there is attempted abduction of the eye and the images will be side by side.

Causes

Multiple sclerosis, brainstem infarct, brainstem neoplasm, mononeuritis multiplex, and raised intracranial pressure.

Other causes of ocular palsies

Occasionally you may be faced with ophthalmoplegia that does not follow the normal rules, that is, it does not have the characteristics you would expect in a nerve III, IV, or VI palsy. For example, you discover a superior rectus and a lateral rectus palsy in the same patient. A nerve III palsy

Table 6.16 Other causes of ocular palsies

Disease of the orbit, e.g. a blow-out fracture
Proptosis
Extraocular muscle infiltration, e.g. thyroid eye disease
Extraocular muscle weakness, e.g. myasthenia gravis
Lesion of higher pathways, e.g. internuclear ophthalmoplegia (INO).

never selectively affects one muscle group. All the muscles it supplies (superior, medial, and inferior recti) will show signs of weakness. This together with a nerve VI palsy makes for an unlikely combination. Other causes of ocular palsies that need to be considered are in Table 6.16.

A blow-out fracture of the floor of the orbit will allow the eye to recede into the socket. There may be entrapment of the inferior rectus or inferior oblique impairing their function. Proptosis can put the extraocular muscles at a mechanical disadvantage. Thyroid eye disease can cause ophthalmoplegia either because of exophthalmos or by infiltration of the muscles. The superior rectus and lateral rectus muscles are the most commonly affected and the infiltration will gradually lead to progressive weakness. In chronic cases fibrosis can tether the muscle altogether. Myasthenia gravis is a disorder of the neuromuscular junction (see Fig. 6.20) and leads to the depletion of the neurotransmitter acetylcholine preventing the transmission of the nerve impulse in skeletal muscle. There is a variable ptosis and ophthalmoplegia. Muscular weakness is worse with repeated activity and becomes more noticeable towards the end of the day. (Internuclear ophthalmoplegia is described in the 'Neurological diseases and investigations' section.)

Key points

- With jerky nystagmus the direction of the fast phase of nystagmus represents the direction of nystagmus
- With diplopia there are three important facts to remember:
  - the greatest separation of images occurs when the eye tries to look in the direction of the paralysed muscle
  - the outer image is always the false image
  - the affected eye always produces the false image
- A nerve III palsy causes ptosis, an eye that looks down and out (a divergent squint), sometimes a dilated pupil, and eye movements that are very restricted
- A nerve IV palsy causes diplopia when the patient reads or walks downstairs
- A nerve VI palsy causes a convergent squint and a failure of abduction of the eye

Monocular diplopia

The final point about diplopia is that it can occur as a result of disease in one eye which is called monocular diplopia. It used to be taught that if diplopia persisted when one eye was covered, then it was likely that the patient was hysterical or malingering. Although these diagnoses must be borne in mind, it is now appreciated that monocular diplopia can be due to cataracts, scarring of the cornea, pathology of the iris, or vitreous or aqueous humour. These conditions can refract and split the light rays from an object to form a double image.

Trigeminal nerve (cranial nerve V)

10   Test facial sensation (V tested) (DF 6/10), assess the muscles of mastication (V tested) (DF 4/10), test corneal reflex (V tested) (DF 3/10), and assess the jaw jerk reflex (V tested) (DF 6/10)

The trigeminal nerve is the largest cranial nerve and has three large branches: the ophthalmic branch, the maxillary branch, and the mandibular branch. Through these branches it provides sensation to the face and front half of the head, sensation to the mucous membranes and sinuses, and the motor supply to the muscles of mastication.

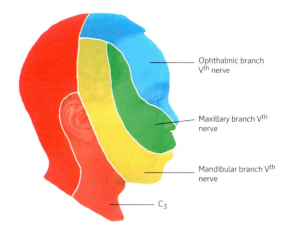

Figure 6.27 The sensory divisions of the head and neck.

Test facial sensation

All three branches of the trigeminal nerve carry sensory fibres from the face and head. The areas they serve are represented in Fig. 6.27. Sensory abnormalities are more common than motor abnormalities in lesions of the trigeminal nerve.

Take a piece of cotton wool and roll part of it in your fingers to form a wisp. Say to your patient, 'Close your eyes please and say yes if you can feel me touching you. Does it feel like you would expect cotton wool to?' This qualification is important with all modalities of sensory testing because the stimulus may be felt but may have a completely different quality; for example, it could feel like pins and needles or be experienced as pain with some neurological problems. Only dab once, so that you test light touch sensation. Compare each side, maxillary branch to maxillary branch, mandibular branch to mandibular branch, and so on. If you find an abnormal area you must test the area in detail and try and work out its limits. Now check pain sensation by repeating your testing but this time with your neuropins. Say to your patient, 'Close your eyes and tell me if this feels sharp or blunt.' You can also check temperature sensation very crudely by using the cold tines of a tuning fork. This is a useful exercise if you are not sure whether pain sensation is impaired (some patients' responses can be inconsistent). If it is impaired the cold tuning fork is often perceived as warm.

Assess the muscles of mastication

For the uninitiated, these are the muscles that are responsible for chewing. The main muscles are the masseters (*mass-itters*) (cheeks) and the temporalis (*temp-or-ale-iss*) muscles (temples), both responsible for clenching the teeth together, and the pterygoids (*terry-goids*), which move the jaw from side to side.

A quick inspection of the face is useful, looking for wasting of the temporalis muscle. If this muscle is wasted it leads to a 'hollowing out' of the temples. Otherwise the rest of the examination relies on you palpating the muscles. Say to your patient, 'Clench your teeth for me'. Feel for the masseter by pressing on the cheeks either side of the mouth. While the teeth are still clenched, also feel for the temporalis by placing your fingertips on either temple. Get the patient to relax and feel the tension disappear from the temples.

Also get the patient to open their jaw against resistance. Use your thumb applied to the undersurface of the jaw to apply the resistive force. Practise on yourself and other patients to learn how much force the jaw can overcome.

In patients with a motor weakness it takes little force to keep the mouth from opening and sometimes the jaw can slew to one side (if there is a weakness of the pterygoids on that side). Finally, place an index finger on one side of the jaw and ask your patient to push their jaw against it. This tests the pterygoid muscles directly. Now do the same on the other side. Using this technique you may pick up a subtle weakness on one side that might not be obvious on direct observation.

Test corneal reflex

What is it?

The corneal reflex is a useful protective mechanism for the eyes. When either cornea is touched, it results in the reflex blinking of both eyes. The sensory impulse is conducted by the trigeminal nerve (afferent limb) and the motor response occurs via the facial nerve (efferent limb). This is an important reflex to test (although it is often overlooked) because it can be the earliest sign of a nerve V palsy, for example, due to an acoustic neuroma.

How to examine

Say to your patient, 'I am going to dab this piece of cotton wool on to your eye; it may feel a little uncomfortable. Look straight ahead for me and keep your eyes wide open.' With the patient looking forwards bring the wisp of cotton wool in from the side of the face and gently dab the cornea (see Fig. 6.28).

Aim for the transparent area at the front of the eye and not the white sclera. You **must** approach from the side, or your patient will blink because of the visual threat. If you touch the eyelids the patient will also blink and your examination will be invalid again. The best method is a

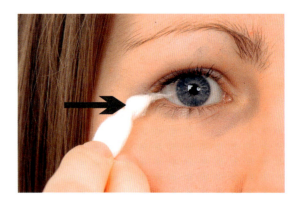

Figure 6.28 Eliciting the corneal reflex.

bold and swift movement in from the side with the cotton wool (avoiding the eyelids). As you near the cornea, slow your movement so that you apply the slightest touch on the cornea. Then remove the cotton wool rapidly before the patient has a chance to blink. Check that both eyelids blink appropriately before testing the other eye. If the corneal sensation is impaired, when you touch the cornea, there will be no blinking (blinking may also be impaired if there is a LMN nerve VII palsy, but this will be more obvious). The final thing to note is that most people have an automatic rate of blinking. So you have to time your dab in between this regular rate so that your movement and the patient's blinking do not coincide.

Assess the jaw jerk reflex

What is it?

The jaw jerk is like any other reflex elicited in the body, except the muscle involved is the masseter muscle. The stretch stimulus provided by the tendon hammer is detected by the proprioceptive end-organs in the muscle and is conducted via the sensory fibres of the trigeminal nerve. After negotiating the reflex arc, the impulse is conducted down the motor fibres of the same nerve back to the masseter muscle.

Significance

It has some minor clinical value in locating a lesion within the central nervous system. If an abnormal reflex is obtained it indicates that the lesion is above the pons of the brainstem. An exaggerated reflex can only be demonstrated in the presence of bilateral UMN lesions, for example, bilateral cortical infarcts. Its value is in excluding spinal cord compression as a cause of bilateral UMN signs in the arms and legs. The utility of this test has been diminished because of the availability of CT and MRI scans that can readily image the brain and upper cervical cord.

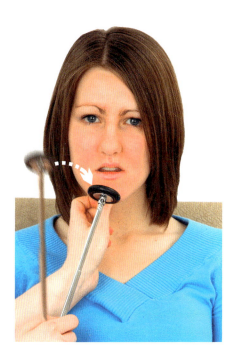

Figure 6.29 Demonstrating the jaw jerk.

How to examine

See Fig. 6.29. This test can look quite brutal and may frighten your patient. You need to reassure them beforehand. Say to them, 'Relax now, open your mouth, and let your jaw hang loose. Don't open it wide, just let it sag open. Now I'm going to tap very gently with this tendon hammer on to my finger . . . it won't hurt.'

The normal response is for the jaw to flick down a short distance. If there is a bilateral UMN lesion the reflex will be brisk. When you see it for the first time a brisk jaw jerk will be unmistakable. The jaw bounces down as if it was on a piece of elastic and the jaw may close altogether. Sometimes you can see a wave of contraction at the sides of the

Key points

- The corneal reflex may be the earliest sign of a nerve V palsy
- Always approach from the side when testing the corneal reflex and make sure you touch the cornea and not the sclera
- Sensory dysfunction of cranial nerve V is more common than motor dysfunction
- The jaw jerk is of limited value and is only abnormally brisk in the presence of bilateral UMN lesions

jaw. Although the reflex is described as brisk, its duration of action is slightly longer than a normal one. The term 'exaggerated reflex' is probably a more accurate one.

Facial nerve (cranial nerve VII)

11 Assess the muscles of facial movement (VII tested) (DF 6/10)

The facial nerve supplies the muscles of facial expression. It also has other specialist functions, which are useful to know as they may help pinpoint where an abnormality is (in a LMN lesion only). Nerve VII is one of the most common cranial nerves to be affected by disease (deafness and blindness are usually due to disease of the sensory organs rather than the cranial nerves themselves). It is worth knowing the neuroanatomy of this particular nerve to understand the variety of features associated with its dysfunction (see Fig. 6.30). The LMN of the facial nerve arises in the pons (part of the brainstem). The axon winds around the nerve VI nucleus before leaving the lateral aspect of the brainstem. At this point it joins the nervus intermedius (*nervous-inter-me-de-us*), the specialized part of the facial nerve that carries taste fibres, as well as fibres that stimulate lacrymation (tearing of the eye) and salivation. The facial nerve crosses the cerebellopontine angle with the vestibulocochlear nerve (nerve VIII) and both enter the internal auditory canal (where nerve VIII supplies the ear and balance organs). The facial nerve travels in the facial canal and relays in the geniculate ganglion (*jen-nick-you-let*) before giving off three branches:

- **Greater superficial petrosal (*pet-rose-al*) nerve**. This supplies the lacrymal gland and salivary glands to produce tears and saliva.
- **Nerve to stapedius (*sta-pee-dee-us*)**. This supplies the tiny stapedius muscle, which contracts in the presence of loud noises to dampen the movement of the stapes at the cochlea.
- **Chorda tympani nerve**. This supplies taste sensation to the anterior two-thirds of the tongue.

The facial nerve then exits the skull through the stylomastoid foramen and runs in the substance of the parotid gland, dividing into a number of branches that supply the muscles of the face.

How to examine

Inspection will often lead you towards the diagnosis. Discovering a unilateral nerve VII palsy is the easy part. There

(a)

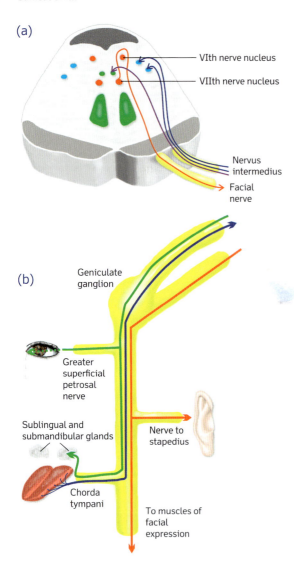

VIth nerve nucleus

VIIth nerve nucleus

Nervus
intermedius

Facial
nerve

(b)

Geniculate
ganglion

Greater
superficial
petrosal
nerve

Sublingual and
submandibular glands

Nerve to
stapedius

Chorda
tympani

To muscles of
facial
expression

Figure 6.30 Neuroanatomy of cranial nerve VII in the brainstem and its subsequent branches: (a) brainstem at the level of the pons showing the facial nerve nucleus and surrounding structures; (b) branches of the facial nerve.

will be obvious asymmetry of the face with drooping of the corner of the mouth on the affected side and flattening of the nasolabial (*nay-zo-lay-be-al*) groove (the skin crease linking nose and the corner of the mouth on either side, which accentuates when you smile). You will be expected to work out if it is a UMN lesion, that is, the nerves from the cortex supplying the facial nerve, or a LMN lesion, that is, the facial nerve itself. The upper half of the face (the

frontalis and orbicularis oculi *[orb-ick-you-lar-iss-ock-you-lie]* muscles) has dual innervation from both the left and the right side of the cerebral cortex. However, the lower half of the face is innervated from the contralateral cortex only.

UMN VII lesion

If there is an abnormality of the right cerebral cortex, for example, due to a stroke, the upper half of the left side of the face will still receive impulses from the left cerebral cortex via the left facial nerve and will appear normal. However, the lower half of the face does not have this dual innervation and weakness at this level will be evident.

LMN VII lesion

In contrast to this, if the right facial nerve is affected by, for example, a Bell's palsy (*Sir Charles Bell (1774–1842), Scottish surgeon*), both the upper and lower half of the face will be affected because the final common pathway, which delivers the motor impulses to the facial muscles, is disrupted. See Fig. 6.31.

It is easiest to work down the face testing the muscle groups as you go (see Fig. 6.32). Say to your patient, 'Raise your eyebrows' (frontalis muscle); you may have to demonstrate this yourself so they know what you want. Some patients find this difficult to do and if this is the case ask them to follow your finger upwards with their eyes while keeping their head still. As they strain to follow your finger above their natural horizontal gaze, the forehead will automatically wrinkle (unless there is a LMN lesion on one side of the face). Now say, 'Close your eyes tight and stop me opening them' (orbicularis oculi muscle). A normal person will be able to bury their eyelashes tightly under the lower lid. Now place both your thumbs on each eyelid and gently attempt to open them. If the muscles are strong this can be quite difficult to do. However, a mild lower motor weakness on one side will allow you to peel back the eyelid easily with your thumb. In a severe LMN palsy, the eyelid may fail to close altogether and you may see the eyeball turning upwards to display the white sclera (this is called Bell's phenomenon). The eyeball turning upwards is a normal process but it is usually hidden behind a closed eyelid. If the eyelid does not close then the eye is in danger. The eyelid provides protection from dirt and grit and if this barrier is missing the cornea can become ulcerated and infected. If the risk is high, doctors may sew part of the upper and lower eyelids together to protect the eye (this operation is called a tarsorrhaphy *[tar-sorra-fee]*). Now say to your patient, 'Blow your cheeks out' (buccinator *[buck-sin-ate-ter]* muscle). Press both cheeks with your fingers and make sure the tension feels roughly the same on either side. A difference will suggest a lesion on the weaker side. Say, 'Show me your

(a)

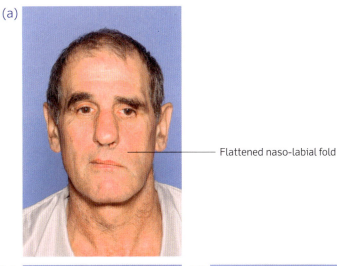

———— Flattened naso-labial fold

(b)   (c)   (d)

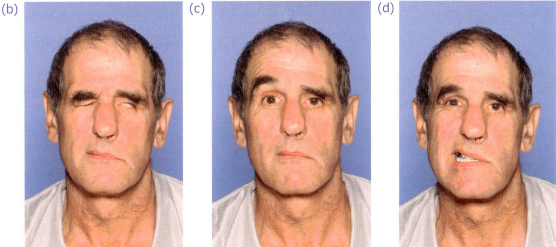

Figure 6.31 A left LMN facial nerve lesion. (a) The patient at rest. Note the drooping of the lips on the left and flattening of the nasolabial fold. (b) Screwing the eyes up tight: note Bell's phenomenon on the left. (c) Raising the eyebrows: the patient is unable to raise the eyebrow on the left side with lack of wrinkling of the frontalis muscle on that side. This confirms that this is a LMN lesion rather than a UMN lesion. (d) Showing the teeth: there is lack of movement of the mouth on the left.

teeth' (orbicularis oris muscle). You may have seen droop-ing of the corner of the mouth on initial inspection and this manoeuvre should exaggerate any weakness. Normally you should get a complete view of their teeth but a weakness on one side will lead to those teeth being obscured by the paralysed lips. Be on the look out for those older patients with a sense of humour who when you say, 'Show me your teeth' will point to their dentures in a denture pot.

Tip

Do not get your patient to smile as a test of facial expression. This is because the descending pathways used to express emotions are different from the UMNs that are under voluntary control. As a result the patient may be able to smile spontaneously and give the false impression that there is no weakness.

(a)   (b)   (c)

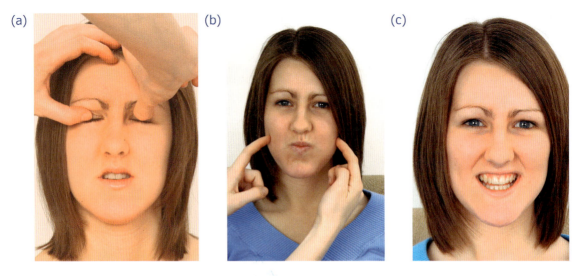

Figure 6.32 Testing the facial nerve: (a) screwing the eyes up tight, (b) blowing the cheeks out, and (c) showing the teeth.

Tip

Occasionally you may get caught out by a patient with bilateral facial nerve palsies as there will be no asymmetry of the face. The key to spotting this condition is to observe that there is very little movement of the facial muscles when you get the patient to run through the above regime.

Abnormal findings

It is worth considering the sites in the nervous system where the facial nerve is vulnerable to injury. The following sequences illustrate these; see also Fig. 6.30.

UMN lesion

- contralateral facial nerve palsy
- only lower face affected because of dual innervation of the upper face
- also possible contralateral hemiplegia.

Causes

- stroke
- tumour
- multiple sclerosis.

LMN lesion

The pattern of other cranial nerve involvement plus other clinical features may give further clue to the location of the lesion.

The pons

- ipsilateral facial nerve palsy
- ipsilateral nerve VI palsy (nerve VI and nerve VII are at the same level in the pons)
- contralateral hemiplegia (the corticospinal tracts do not cross the midline until lower down in the medulla).

Causes

- stroke
- tumour
- multiple sclerosis.

Cerebellopontine angle

- ipsilateral facial nerve palsy
- ipsilateral nerve VIII palsy
- ipsilateral nerve V palsy
- ipsilateral cerebellar signs (possibly IX, X, and XI palsy also)

- in addition, the facial nerve palsy at this level will lead to dysfunction of the three major branches:
  - greater superficial petrosal nerve—leads to a loss of lacrimation and salivation
  - nerve to stapedius—leads to hyperacusis (*high-per-a-cue-sis*) (this is the unpleasant exaggeration of normal sound due to the lack of damping that is normally produced by the contraction of the stapedius muscle)
  - chorda tympani nerve—leads to loss of taste over the anterior two-thirds of the tongue.

Causes

- acoustic neuroma (see 'Neurological diseases and investigations' section)
- meningioma.

Facial canal

- no other cranial nerves involved at this level
- the location of the lesion within the facial canal will dictate the clinical symptoms. The three branches described above come off the facial nerve in the order written. Therefore a lesion after the greater superficial petrosal nerve but before the nerve to stapedius will spare lacrimation and salivation but will still lead to hyperacusis.

Causes

- Bell's palsy (see 'Neurological diseases and investigations' section)
- Ramsay-Hunt syndrome (*J. Ramsay-Hunt (1874–1937), American neurologist*) (see 'Neurological diseases and investigations' section)
- fracture of the skull base
- spread from otitis media.

Distal to stylomastoid foramen

At this point the facial nerve has exited the skull and is travelling through the substance of the parotid gland, dividing into its final branches to supply the facial muscles. Some of the facial muscles may be spared depending on which branches have been affected.

Causes

- cancer of the parotid gland
- surgery to the parotid gland
- sarcoidosis.

Bilateral facial nerve palsies

- bilateral strokes (cause of UMN lesions)
- multiple sclerosis (cause of UMN lesions)
- myasthenia gravis
- muscular dystrophy (some forms, for example, facio-scapulo-humeral dystrophy)
- Guillain–Barré syndrome
- sarcoidosis
- bilateral Bell's palsy.

Vestibulocochlear nerve (cranial nerve VIII)

12 Assess hearing (VIII tested) and perform Weber's and Rinné's tests (VIII tested) (DF 8/10)

The vestibulocochlear nerve is responsible for hearing and balance although it is only the auditory aspect of the nerve that is routinely tested.

Assess hearing

It is only possible to make a crude assessment of hearing during the cranial nerve examination. There may be clues before you start your assessment. Your patient may have a hearing aid or you may notice that you have to repeat your questions or instructions many times. Some doctors advocate occluding one ear and asking the patient to identify a ticking clock or fingers being rubbed together. Another more sensitive approach involves whispering numbers into either ear. This has the advantage that you can vary the volume you use to state the numbers. Say to your patient, 'I am going to rub your earlobe and I want you to repeat the numbers I whisper to you.' It is important that you rub the earlobe of the ear that is **not** being tested. This creates a noise that 'masks' this ear and prevents it from assisting the ear under test. If the patient does have a hearing impairment and the other ear is not masked, this ear may pick up the sounds and lead to the false impression that hearing in the tested ear is unaffected. Most people will be able to repeat your numbers back. If the patient cannot hear you, then raise the volume of your voice. This suggests some hearing impairment. If you have to shout into the ear, you will draw the correct conclusion. If you suspect hearing loss you should go on to perform Weber's (*webbers*) and Rinné's (*rin-ayz*) tests to differentiate between conductive and sensorineural deafness.

Key points

- You must determine whether a facial nerve lesion is UMN or LMN in origin
- The forehead has bilateral cortical representation and is only paralysed if there is a LMN lesion or bilateral UMN lesions
- A facial nerve palsy of LMN type may render the ipsilateral eye unprotected
- Smiling is a misleading test of the facial nerve
- Beware of missing bilateral facial nerve palsies

Conductive deafness

What is it?

This is the inability of the outer and middle ear to conduct sound to the inner ear. This can be due to disease anywhere from the external auditory meatus to the stapes (also called the stirrup, one of the tiny 'ossicle' bones of the ear that articulates with the oval window of the cochlea, see Fig. 6.33).

Causes

See Table 6.17

Sensorineural deafness

What is it?

This is due to damage to the cochlear (the sense organ, which is a shell-like apparatus that converts acoustic vibration into neural impulses) or to the cochlear nerve, which together with the vestibular nerve conducts sensory input to the brain as the vestibulocochlear nerve.

Causes

See Table 6.18

Perform Weber's and Rinné's tests

Weber's test

Weber's test (*F. E. Weber-Liel (1832–1891), German otologist*) is sometimes described as a lateralizing test, that is, it is used to determine which ear is affected (in practice it is not as clear cut as this as you need information from Rinné's test to help with this). You need a 512 Hz tuning fork, which is smaller than the ones normally lying about the wards (256 Hz will do). Vibrate the tuning fork and place it in the middle of the patient's forehead. Ask, 'Can you hear the noise? Does it sound the same in both ears or can you hear it louder in one than the other?' If your patient has healthy hearing, they should hear the noise

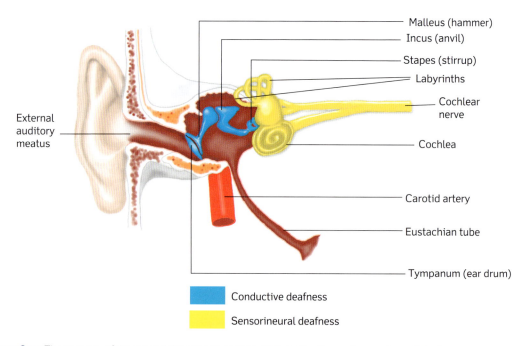

Figure 6.33 The anatomy of the ear and the apparatus involved in conductive and sensorineural deafness.

Table 6.17 Some causes of conductive deafness

Otitis externa
Otitis media
Paget's disease (affecting the ossicles)
Perforated eardrum

Table 6.18 Some causes of sensorineural deafness

Presbycusis (due to ageing)
Noise-induced deafness
Ototoxicity due to drugs, for example, high-dose frusemide or gentamycin.

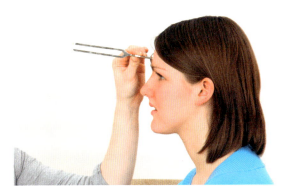

Figure 6.34 Weber's test.

equally in both ears. If they hear the noise louder in one ear, this either means there is a conductive deafness in the ear perceiving the louder sound or there is a sensori-neural deafness in the other ear (see Figs. 6.34 and 6.35). To help distinguish between the two possibilities you need to perform Rinné's test. One further point to note is that the tuning fork can be heard equally by both ears in the presence of hearing impairment. In this case, hearing loss will be approximately equal for each ear.

Rinné's test

See Fig. 6.36. Rinné's test (*Friedrich Heinrich Adolf Rinné (1819–1868), German ENT surgeon*) relies on the princi-ple that in the healthy individual, air conduction is better than bone conduction. If this is the case it is described as a positive Rinné's test. Find the mastoid process. This is the bony prominence just behind the ear. Set the tuning fork vibrating and place the base on this spot. Say to your patient, 'Tell me when you can no longer hear the tuning fork.' When your patient indicates that they can no longer hear the tuning fork, move the tuning fork so that the end of the prongs are just by the entrance to the ear. Ask them, 'Can you hear it now?' The healthy patient should hear it. If the patient does not hear the tuning fork this implies

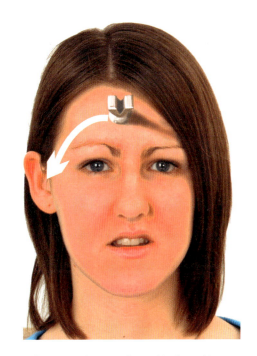

Figure 6.35 Lateralization of sound to the right ear.

(a)   (b)

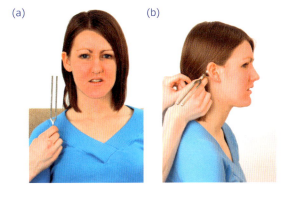

Figure 6.36 Rinné's test: (a) air conduction; (b) bone conduction.

CASE 6.4

Problem. You examine a middle-aged man who has been complaining of pain in the left ear for a fortnight. He has noticed the hearing has deteriorated in that ear and you confirm this clinically by whispering various numbers into each ear. You perform Weber's and Rinné's tests. With Weber's test the sound from the tuning fork is heard loudest in the left ear and the Rinné's test is negative in that ear. Can you explain this?

Discussion. This case is straightforward. The patient has already indicated that the problem is with his left ear and you have confirmed that the hearing is impaired. Weber's test indicates that either there is a conductive hearing loss in the left ear or a sensorineural hearing loss in the right ear. A negative Rinné's test is where bone conduction is better than air conduction. Therefore a negative Rinné's test in the left ear confirms a conductive hearing loss in the left ear. This man needs his ear examined with an otoscope for signs of an otitis media.

CASE 6.5

Problem. You examine an elderly woman who has been described as 'hard of hearing' by her son. She says she is not bad when speaking 'one on one' in a quiet room but struggles with conversation if there is a lot of background noise. Her eardrums are normal on otoscopic examination and you perform Rinné's and Weber's tests. She hears the tuning fork directly in front of her and both ears are Rinné positive. Explain the results.

Discussion. This case is tricky. The history suggests the patient has some hearing impairment but superficially she performs normally with the tuning fork tests. However, you must remember that a positive Rinné's test can either indicate normal hearing or sensorineural hearing loss. It is therefore possible that this woman has bilateral sensorineural hearing loss, which is roughly equal in both ears, leading to a Weber's test that is heard equally in both ears. An audiogram is needed to assess the hearing more accurately before any strategies such as hearing aids can be employed.

---

a conduction defect in that ear. This is described as a negative Rinné's test. If the patient has a sensorineural deficit in the tested ear you will elicit a positive Rinné's test (so long as the hearing loss is not so bad that they cannot hear the tuning fork). Any hearing deficit that you find needs to be assessed more fully by an audiological department.

Cases 6.4 and 6.5 explore some of the challenges you might face when interpreting the results of these examinations.

··

Tip

Another way of performing this test is to set the tuning fork vibrating and put the tines in front of the ear. Then, using the same force, set the tuning fork vibrating again and this time place it on the mastoid process; ask the patient which was louder. The interpretation remains the same as above.

··

Tip

Never diagnose hearing impairment until you have checked the ear for wax. Most opthalmoscopes are multipurpose and can be used as an otoscope (*owe-ta-scope*) (sometimes called an auriscope). The head screws off and you can put on the otoscopic attachment. This

allows you to clip on earpieces of different sizes. Switch the light on in the normal ear and carefully introduce the earpiece into the auditory canal of the ear. With your free hand you need to pull the ear firmly upwards and backwards (much the same position that teachers used to pull the ear of a naughty child, before it was outlawed). This straightens out the auditory canal and allows you to get a good view of the eardrum. If this view is obstructed by a lot of brown gunky stuff, your patient has a lot of earwax. This needs to be removed before the ears can be tested formally.

··

Key points
- Determine whether hearing loss is conductive or sensorineural
- Conductive deafness may be reversible whereas sensorineural deafness is usually irreversible
- Make sure that wax has been removed from the ear before referring for a formal hearing assessment
- Rinné's test helps to determine whether hearing loss is conductive or sensorineural in nature
- Weber's test helps to determine which is the affected ear

Glossopharyngeal (IX) and vagus (X) nerves

13 Assess movement of the soft palate (IX and X tested) and assess sensation of the soft palate (IX and X tested) (DF 5/10)

As lesions of cranial nerves IX and X rarely occur in isolation they will be considered together. I will only discuss those functions that are routinely tested. The glossopharyngeal nerve (IX) is a mixed nerve with motor, sensory, and some parasympathetic activity. It carries sensory input from the palate and the pharynx and taste from the posterior third of the tongue. It provides the afferent limb of the gag reflex. The vagus nerve (X) is also a mixed nerve with motor, sensory, and parasympathetic activity. It provides the motor supply to the pharynx, soft palate, and larynx and provides the efferent limb of the gag reflex.

Assess movement of the soft palate

Say to your patient, 'Can you open your mouth, please.' Now shine a torch into the back of the mouth and look at the soft palate. Be familiar with what a normal soft palate looks like. It should be symmetrical and divided roughly into two by the fleshy uvula that dangles down (see Fig. 6.37). The patient's tongue may obscure your view. If this happens you will need to use a tongue depressor. Say, 'I'm just going to press down on your tongue with this stick. It might be a little uncomfortable.' For this reason it is best not to dilly-dally once it is in the mouth. Check for asymmetry. Now ask your patient to say 'aaah!' The soft palate should elevate and the uvula should stay central. If there is unilateral weakness of the soft palate the uvula is pulled away from the weakened side.

Assess sensation of the soft palate

With the mouth still open say to your patient, 'I am just going to touch the back of your mouth gently with this stick—let me know if you can feel it.' Using your orange stick gently touch the back of the palate, withdraw your stick, and wait for your patient's response. Now touch the opposite side and ask your patient to compare the two sides. It is very easy to trigger the gag reflex doing this. If you do, apologize to your patient.

Gag reflex

What is it?

If the posterior wall of the pharynx is stimulated, there follows a choking or gagging response as the pharynx constricts and elevates as a protective measure.

How to examine

This is an unpleasant reflex to elicit for the patient. Say something like, 'And now I'm just going to touch the back

(a)

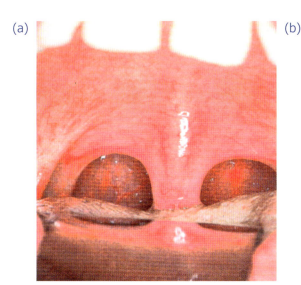

(b)

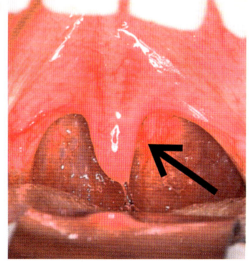

Figure 6.37 Nerve X palsy: (a) uvula in the midline; (b) on elevation the uvula moves away from the weaker side.
Reprinted from Fig. 14.63(a) and (b) (p. 14.22), *Atlas of Clinical Neurology* (2nd edn), by G. David Perkin, Fred Hochberg, and Douglas C. Miller (1993), Mosby Publications, with permission from Elsevier.

Key points

- Lesions of the lower cranial nerves rarely occur in isolation
- The soft palate elevates **away** from the weakened side
- The glossopharyngeal nerve supplies the afferent limb of the gag reflex and the vagus nerve supplies the efferent limb
- An absent gag reflex can be a normal variant
- A gag reflex that is absent unilaterally or is absent bilaterally with symptoms such as dysphagia, dysphonia, or aspiration is abnormal

of your throat very briefly. I am afraid it might cause a choking sensation, but it needs to be done and will be over quickly . . . well done.' Use your tongue depressor and gently touch the back of the throat on one side. In the normal circumstance the patient will gag. Both sides of the throat need to be tested although it can be very difficult to cajole your patient into having it done a second time. A brief apology afterwards might convince them you are not a sadist. If a gag reflex is not elicited you need to ask the patient if they felt the tongue depressor touch the back of the throat. If they did not, it suggests that the afferent limb of the reflex (nerve IX) is affected (or possibly nerves IX and X together). If they felt the stimulus it suggests that only the efferent limb is affected (nerve X).

It is important to note that an absent gag reflex can be found in normal people. It is only if the reflex is absent unilaterally or if the patient presents with symptoms, for example, dysphagia, aspiration of fluids into the lung, and so on that this finding will be significant.

Tip

As the gag reflex is an unpleasant test, eliciting the gag reflex should not be part of the normal examination routine. Only perform it if your patient has relevant symptoms such as dysphagia, nasal regurgitation of fluids, or dysphonia.

Accessory nerve (XI)

14 Assess the trapezius and sternomastoid muscles (XI tested) (DF 4/10)

This nerve innervates trapezius and sternomastoid (full name—sternocleidomastoid) muscles together with a contribution from the spinal cord.

Trapezius

Say to your patient, 'Shrug your shoulders.' Show the patient how to do it and then watch for asymmetry. Get them to repeat the movement but this time say, 'Stop me pressing your shoulders down.' Place both your hands on their shoulder and press down. Feel if there is any gross difference in muscle power on each side.

Sternomastoid

Say to your patient, 'Turn your head to the right.' Again demonstrate how to do this so that the head is looking over the shoulder. Then say 'Keep your head in that position and stop me pushing it back to the middle.' Gently push your hand against the patient's jaw and increase the pressure gently (see Fig. 6.38). Also palpate the belly of the left sternomastoid muscle as it contracts. Then say, 'If you could turn your head to the left side now,' and now test the other side remembering to palpate the right sternomastoid muscle.

Hypoglossal nerve (XII)

15 Assess the tongue and tongue movements (XII tested) (DF 4/10)

Cranial nerve XII is the motor nerve supplying the intrinsic muscles of the tongue. Like the facial nerve, each

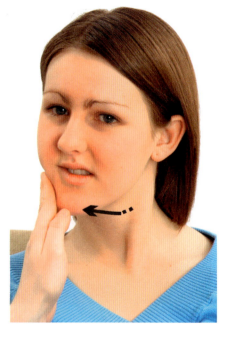

Figure 6.38 Testing the left sternomastoid muscle: note the contraction.

hypoglossal nerve has bilateral cortical representation. Therefore a unilateral supranuclear lesion will not have any discernible effect on tongue function. Bilateral cortical infarcts will produce a 'spastic tongue', which has limited movement and cannot be protruded from the mouth. This is part of the syndrome of pseudobulbar palsy (see later). A unilateral lesion of nerve XII (LMN) will produce wasting of the tongue, with possible fasciculations on the side of the lesion.

Say to your patient, 'Open your mouth please.' Look at the patient's tongue. Is it wasted and fasiculating? (see 'Bulbar palsy'). Now assess the tongue movements. Ask, 'Can you put your tongue out for me . . . and move it from side to side.' If there is a unilateral weakness of the tongue it will deviate to the weaker side with protrusion (see Fig. 6.39). If any doubt remains, also say to your patient, 'Push out your cheek with the tip of your tongue.' Using this method you can use your index finger to press the cheek to gauge the amount of force the patient can generate with the tongue and compare both sides.

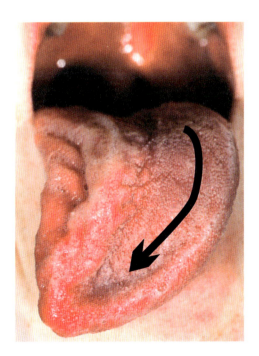

Figure 6.39 Nerve XII palsy. Note the wasting of the right side of the tongue with deviation towards this weakened side.
Reprinted from Fig. 14.67 (p. 14.23), *Atlas of Clinical Neurology* (2nd edn), by G. David Perkin, Fred Hochberg, and Douglas C. Miller (1993), Mosby Publications, with permission from Elsevier.

> **Tip**
> When you get slick at examining the cranial nerves you will assess the tongue while you are assessing the soft palate with the patient's mouth open.

Jugular foramen syndrome

Isolated lesions of the lower cranial nerves rarely occur. Instead a group may be affected, often in recognizable combinations, for example, the jugular foramen syndrome. This is the unilateral combination of cranial nerve IX, X, and XI lesions. A right-sided lesion will cause the soft palate to elevate and pull the uvula across to the left. There will be loss of taste and sensation to the posterior third of the tongue and pharynx and a decreased gag reflex on the right. The right shoulder may droop lower than its opposite counterpart and there will be difficulty shrugging it. Also there will be an inability to turn the head to the left.

Cause

Tumour of the skull base, for example, meningioma.

Bulbar palsy

The pons and medulla of the brainstem are sometimes referred to as the bulb because of their anatomical appearance. A bulbar palsy is the term reserved for bilateral dysfunction of the lower cranial nerves IX, X, and XII. The tongue is wasted, flaccid, fasciculates, and lacks movement. The patient will suffer with dysphagia, which is worse with liquids, which regurgitate up the nose. They will also have dysphonia. Because of difficulty swallowing liquid, saliva pools in the mouth and periodically the patient will pause to swallow it.

Causes

The causes of bulbar palsy include

- motor neuron disease
- Guillain–Barré syndrome
- polio.

Pseudobulbar palsy

This is due to bilateral UMN lesions. The tongue is spastic and cannot be moved rapidly from side to side. There is dysphagia with nasal regurgitation of liquids. Saliva cannot be swallowed and may drool from the mouth. The speech is high pitched and monotonous

Key points

- The tongue will deviate **towards** the weakened side
- A bulbar palsy occurs with a bilateral LMN lesion
- A bulbar palsy causes a wasted fasciculating tongue with dysphagia (nasal regurgitation of liquids) and an indistinct, low-volume speech
- A pseudobulbar palsy causes a 'spastic' poorly moving tongue with dysphagia (nasal regurgitation of liquids), a high-pitched monotonous speech, drooling, and a brisk jaw jerk

(has been likened to Donald Duck speech). There will usually be evidence of bilateral hemiparesis with bilateral extensor plantars and the jaw jerk will be brisk. The patient may exhibit emotionalism and may cry or laugh inappropriately.

Causes

- bilateral strokes
- multiple sclerosis.

Examine the motor system

16 Inspection: look for wasting (DF 4/10), fasciculations (DF 6/10), and involuntary movements (DF 7/10)

Wasting

With your patient relaxed on the couch or bed (see Fig. 6.40), look specifically for wasting.

If you detect any wasting, you need to know if it is generalized or confined to a specific muscle group. Generalized wasting could simply be the result of any debilitating illness including cancer. In a neurological context wasting may suggest motor neuron disease or any other pathology affecting the LMNs. Check for asymmetry, which could suggest a root or a specific nerve lesion? Gross wasting and shortening of a limb of long standing may suggest previous poliomyelitis (the patient may wear a built-up shoe to compensate for the unequal leg lengths). Wasting of the thighs preferentially may suggest a proximal myopathy (any associated tenderness of the muscles should make you consider poly/dermatomyositis). One characteristic pattern of wasting can be seen with Charcot–Marie–Tooth disease (*Jean Martin Charcot (1825–1893), French neurologist; Pierre Marie*

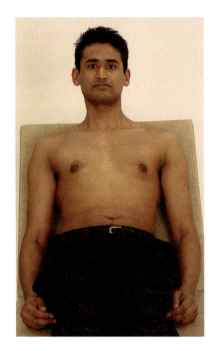

Figure 6.40 Examination position.

(1853–1940), French neurologist; Howard Henry Tooth (1856–1925), English physician) (also known as hereditary sensory motor neuropathy (HSMN); see Fig. 6.41). The wasting begins distally and spreads up the leg sometimes stopping mid-calf. The appearance produced is often likened to an inverted champagne bottle. It is also associated with pes cavus (an abnormally pronounced plantar arch), as is Friedrich's ataxia. UMN lesions seldom cause muscle wasting but if it is present it is often due to chronic disuse and is less marked. Wasting can be isolated and subtle; for example, localized wasting of the thenar eminence supplying the thumb in carpal tunnel syndrome (see 'Neurological diseases and investigations' section). Do not be afraid to palpate the muscle bulk to confirm wasting. Wasted hypotonic muscle tends to be flabby, soft, and insubstantial (compare this with your own muscles unless you happen to be flabby, soft and insubstantial).

Fasciculations

These occur in LMN lesions and represent spontaneous discharges from motor units. They are visible as small contractions that look like the transient writhing of a worm under the skin. You may have to observe the arms for several minutes before you see one.

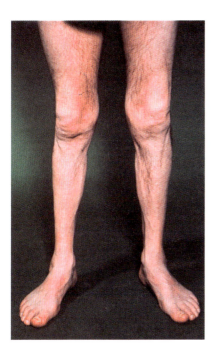

Figure 6.41 Hereditary sensory motor neuropathy (Charcot–Marie–Tooth disorder).
Reprinted from Fig. 2.2 (p. 2.2), *Atlas of Clinical Neurology* (2nd edn), by G. David Perkin, Fred Hochberg, and Douglas C. Miller (1993), Mosby Publications, with permission from Elsevier.

Tip

If you have not spotted any fasciculation within 30 seconds I would suggest you continue with the rest of your examination but keep a wary eye out for them periodically and even at the end of your examination.

Involuntary movements

Look carefully at the hands and see if there is an obvious resting tremor. You can ask your patient to put their hands out to accentuate a postural tremor. Focus on the thumb and

Key points

- Wasting (in the absence of malnutrition, cachexia, or disuse) is a manifestation of an LMN lesion
- Fasciculations are also LMN phenomena
- Always check for involuntary movements, which may give useful clues

see if there is a pill-rolling quality that could point to Parkinson's disease. Do you only notice a tremor on movement but not at rest? (This could represent an intention tremor and should be tested formally; see 'Intention tremor'.)

The other forms of involuntary movements have been described in the 'Symptoms' section. If you are unsure what an unusual movement pattern is, try to describe it as best you can. Even better, get the patient's written consent and video the movement sequence on your mobile phone for an expert to identify.

17 Assess muscle tone at the wrist, elbow, and shoulder, hip, and knee (DF 6/10)

Tone

What is it?

Tone is the resistance felt when moving a joint through its range of movement.

Significance

In a normal, relaxed individual there is very little resistance as any joint is moved through its range of movement. In pathological circumstances there can be an increase in the resistance (hypertonia) as the joint is moved or a decrease (hypotonia).

Hypertonia

Hypertonia may have characteristics that point to the underlying nature of a lesion. UMN lesions cause what is known as 'clasp-knife' rigidity (also called spasticity). The increased tone is felt throughout the majority of the range before the tone 'gives way' in much the same way that a clasp knife does when it is opened. In Parkinson's disease, two types of increased tone are seen, the typical one being 'cogwheel' rigidity, which is similar to the intermittent resistance felt when turning a cogwheel. The other is 'lead pipe' rigidity, named because the resistance felt is said to be similar to that when bending a lead pipe (!), that is, sustained resistance throughout the range of movement (at last medical terms that are self-evident!).

Hypotonia

Hypotonia is subtle and is due to a LMN lesion. There is practically no resistance to movement (sometimes described as flaccidity).

How to examine

See Fig. 6.42. Before you start testing you need to make your patient as relaxed as possible. Check that they

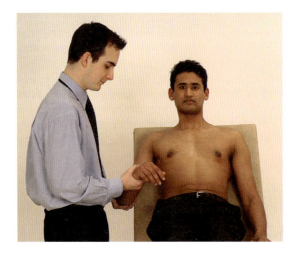

Figure 6.42 Assessment of tone in the arms. The starting position before moving the joints through their range of movement.

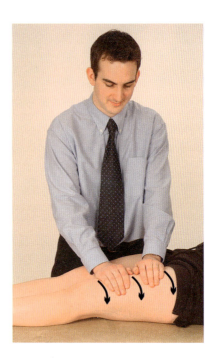

Figure 6.43 Examination of tone in the legs.

do not have pain in any of their joints. Say something like, 'I am going to move your arm about and I need you to be as relaxed as you can. Don't try to help me, just stay as loose as you can.' Muscle tone is tested at the wrist by holding the fingers of the arm being tested and gently flexing and extending the wrist. Now assess tone at the elbow. Maintain your grip on the fingers and pronate (palm downwards) and supinate (palm upwards) the forearm, followed by flexing and extending at the elbow. Finish off by abducting and adducting the (flexed) arm at the shoulder. Although each joint is described individually the aim is to create a continuous movement of the arm that will allow each joint to be assessed sequentially (experienced neurologists are so adept at this that it sometimes looks as if they have created a Mexican wave on one side of the body). As you gain in confidence you will find that you can switch your attention rapidly from one joint to the next.

Tip

Try to make your movements of varying amplitudes and unpredictable when assessing any joint, so that your patient does not get into a 'rhythm' and try to second-guess you. This often ends in them trying to help you by moving the limb which invalidates your assessment of tone.

Now switch to the legs (see Fig. 6.43). Again check to make sure that there is no pain in any joints. Say to your patient, 'Let your leg go nice and floppy, just relax and let me do the moving.' Then place the flat of both your hands on your target leg and gently rotate it inwards and outwards (as if you were using a rolling pin to flatten dough). Now place both hands under the knee and quickly lift them about 15 cm (6 inches) and then let go (this movement should flex the knee partially). A normal leg should be rolled very easily; there should be little resistance when the knee is displaced upwards and it should flop back readily on to the bed (repeated practice on patients with normal tone should help you generate a 'feel' for this). With a spastic leg there is much more resistance and the knee is difficult to flex. A hypotonic leg is floppy like a rag doll; it will be flexed quite easily and will readily flop back on to the bed.

Key points

- Make sure your patient is relaxed (and remains relaxed) when testing tone
- Hypertonia indicates a UMN lesion
- Hypotonia indicates an LMN lesion
- Hypertonia is easier to detect than hypotonia

CASE 6.6

Problem. You are assessing the tone of your patient's upper limbs and you are unsure if it is increased.

Discussion. The most common cause of a slight increase in tone is an unrelaxed patient, which can fool the unwary. Some patients will contract their muscles in a bid to help you move the arm. The resistance you feel is the opposing force of the muscle when you reverse the movement of the arm. Stress to the patient that they need to relax. You also need to monitor the arm carefully. Feel the weight of the arm: does it flop into your arm when you take it? Watch the arm carefully and make sure no muscles contract during your assessment. If they do, your assessment of tone is invalid. If the patient still cannot relax, try distracting them. Ask them to move the opposite arm or leg up and down, while you quickly assess tone in the arm. Usually if the tone is pathologically increased, there will be other signs to support this, for example, mild weakness and hyper-reflexia.

Cases 6.6 and 6.7 give further tips on assessing tone.

Tip
When assessing tone at the knee, pay particular attention to the leg just after you have flexed it upwards and have removed your displacing force. If the patient is relaxed the leg should flop back naturally on to the bed. However, if they are not relaxed, the leg remains in the flexed position and does not flop back on to the bed. You should also see the tell-tale contraction of the quadriceps muscle and if this is the case your assessment of tone is void and needs to be repeated.

18 Test for clonus if relevant (DF 4/10)

Clonus

What is it?

Clonus is a rhythmical jerking movement, which can be produced by applying a rapid stretch (and sustaining that stretch) to a muscle. The jerking represents an initial reflex

CASE 6.7

Problem. You have assessed the tone of a patient and are unsure if there is hypotonia.

Discussion. This one is difficult. The difference between a normal patient and one with hypotonia is very subtle. Here it is speculated that if you asked a sample of physicians to diagnose pathological hypotonia with blindfolds on, the number of correct responses would be close to what you would expect by chance. The author would only diagnose it in the context of other LMN signs, for example, weakness, wasting, fasciculation, and decreased or absent reflexes.

contraction to protect the muscle, followed by relaxation. If you maintain a stretch on the muscle it will contract and relax again and may enter an iterative cycle of contraction and relaxation, which can be sustained for numerous beats (>5 beats usually indicates pathology).

Significance

The presence of sustained clonus implies the presence of an UMN lesion affecting the limb under test.

How to examine

Clonus is traditionally demonstrated at the ankle or knee. To elicit ankle clonus, simply grasp the forefoot and dorsiflex it sharply (but not violently) and maintain some upward pressure at the end of the range of movement (this maintains a stretch on the tendon). If clonus is present you will feel the foot start to jerk up and down. Keep pressing up on the foot as this will provide the stretch that will maintain the phenomenon. See Fig. 6.44. To elicit knee clonus, grip the lateral borders of the patella (kneecap) between your thumb and other fingers. Now pull it down sharply as far as it will go and then maintain some downward pressure. If clonus is present the patella will jerk up and down rhythmically.

Tip
A more elegant way of demonstrating knee clonus is to place your index finger at the top of the patella and strike it gently downwards with a tendon hammer. Remember to maintain some downward pressure with your index finger at the end of the manoeuvre.

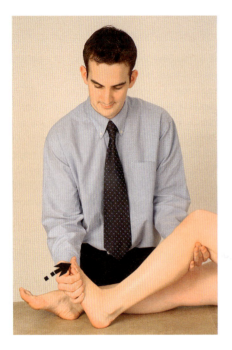

Figure 6.44 Eliciting ankle clonus.

19 Test power, proximally to distally in the arms and legs (DF 5/10)

It is important to remember that your assessment of power has to take into account what you would normally expect for that individual. So a healthy little old lady would score just as well as Arnold Schwarznegger. The most common standardized scale used to grade power is the MRC scale. There are five grades of power: 0 = nil; 1 = flicker of movement; 2 = movement if gravity is eliminated; 3 = movement against gravity but not against resistance; 4 = movement against resistance but abnormally weak; and 5 = normal.

There are several ways to test power, but the best technique is to demonstrate exactly what you want the patient to do and get them to copy you. First, ask them to hold their arms outstretched (palm upwards) in front of them. This is a good screening test for any mild weakness. An UMN lesion of one arm will cause it to drift downwards and pronate. Now test each muscle group in turn, starting at the shoulders. Always compare the two sides.

Shoulder abduction and adduction

Demonstrate by holding your arms out to the side in a horizontal position, with the elbows flexed: 'Put your arms up like this; now, don't let me push them down' (abduction, using nerve roots C5 and C6; see Fig. 6.45). During this

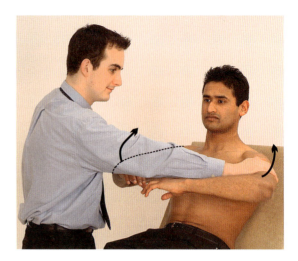

Figure 6.45 Testing the power of shoulder abduction. Note the arrows represent the direction of force generated by the patient.

movement, you need to provide resistance by pressing on the mid-shaft of the upper arms. If your patient has full strength it will be difficult to budge the arm (grade 5/5). If you can move the patient's arm with a little difficulty the patient has grade 4/5 power. If the patient can just about abduct their arm but are unable to resist your opposing force their power is grade 3/5. If the patient cannot abduct their arm against gravity you need to alter the position of your patient. Ask them to lie flat and then to abduct their arm. This eliminates the effect of gravity because the movement required is now parallel to the floor. If they are now able to perform this movement they have a power grading of 2/5. If they cannot and only a flicker of movement occurs, the grade is 1/5. If no flicker of movement occurs the grade is 0/5. Repeat your assessment for adduction (adduction, C6, C7, C8; see Fig. 6.46). Ask your patient to adopt the same position as for abduction but this time, put your arms under your patient's and say, 'Now try to press your elbows in to your sides.' Grade the power as before but note that adduction will occur with the help of gravity in this position. Therefore for grades 2/5–3/5, you have to make an educated guess as to the grade of power (rather than suspend your patient upside down to test adduction against gravity). As you assess more patients, this guess will become more precise within the subjective limits of the scale.

Elbow flexion and extension

Ask your patient to put their fists up like a boxer: 'Bend your elbows in front of you like this; now pull me towards you' (elbow flexion, C5, C6; see Fig. 6.47). 'Now push me

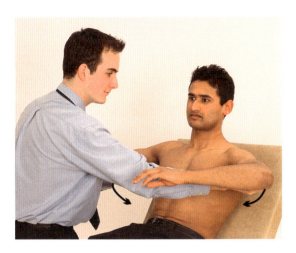

Figure 6.46 Testing the power of shoulder adduction.

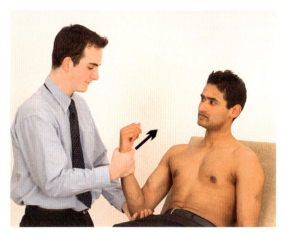

Figure 6.47 Testing the power of elbow flexion.

away' (elbow extension, C7, C8; see Fig. 6.48). Grade the power as before. If your patient has grade 2/5 power, that is, they cannot flex the arm against gravity, you will have to hold their upper arm and abduct it to 90°. With the arm horizontal, flexion will take place without gravity and you can grade the power according to the response. As with shoulder adduction, extension of the elbow will occur with the aid of gravity. Therefore you will have to make a reasonable guess for grades 2/5–3/5. It is also important that when you assess extension you make sure the patient's palms are facing their face, otherwise you will not just be testing triceps (C7) but getting extra help from brachioradialis (*bray-kio-ray-di-ay-liss*) (C5, C6) as well.

Wrist extension (dorsiflexion) and wrist flexion (palmar flexion)

Check each wrist in turn, holding the forearm steady with your left hand and providing resistance with your right hand. Say to your patient 'Make a fist. Now cock your wrists up like this; don't let me bend them down' (wrist extension, C5, C6, C7; see Fig. 6.49). As your patient extends their wrist, apply downward pressure with your right hand. If your patient is unable to do this, turn the wrist into a semi-pronated position to eliminate gravity, then repeat. When you have assessed extension keep their wrist cocked, and place your right hand underneath it. Say 'Push down against my hand' (wrist flexion, C6, C7, C8; see Fig. 6.50). Use your left hand to hold their forearm so that they are only using the wrist flexors to push against you rather than their entire arm. As with shoulder adduction and elbow extension, wrist flexion is also aided by gravity. The strength in the two hands should be similar, although the dominant limb may be slightly stronger.

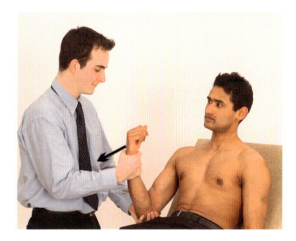

Figure 6.48 Testing the power of elbow extension.

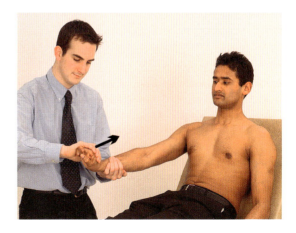

Figure 6.49 Testing the power of wrist extension.

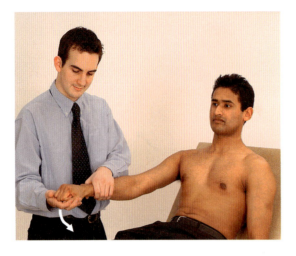

Figure 6.50 Testing the power of wrist flexion.

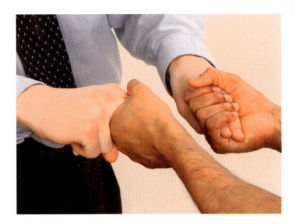

Figure 6.51 Testing grip strength.

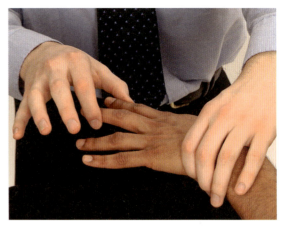

Figure 6.52 Testing finger abduction.

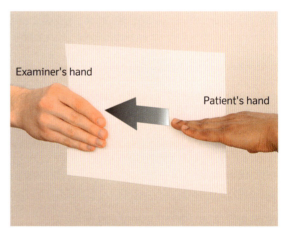

Figure 6.53 Testing finger adduction.

If appropriate, test the power of the fingers

If your history or observation suggests that there may be neurological problems with the hands then power can be tested as follows:

- **'Grasp my fingers as tight as possible.'** Offer the patient two of your fingers to hold (see Fig. 6.51). This assesses the strength of finger flexion. The muscles being tested are flexor digitorum profundus (*flex-or-digit-or-um–pro-fund-us*) and flexor digitorum superficialis (*soup-er-fishy-ale-iss*). They are supplied by branches from the median and ulnar nerves (their innervation is principally from spinal root C8) (opposition of the thumb is supplied by T1).

- **'Hold your hand out straight, don't let me bend your fingers.'** This assesses finger extension. The muscle is

extensor digitorum, supplied by the radial nerve fibres and is innervated chiefly from the root C7.

- **'Spread your fingers out wide, don't let me push your fingers together.'** This assesses finger abduction. This tests the dorsal interossei (*inter-ross-ee-eye*) muscles. Supplied by the ulnar nerve fibres, from spinal root T1 (see Fig. 6.52).

- **'Grasp this piece of paper between your fingers as tightly as possible. Stop me from pulling it out.'** Here you are assessing finger adduction. The muscles being used are the palmar interossei. Also supplied by the ulnar nerve, arising from spinal root T1 (see Fig. 6.53).

- **'Point your thumb towards the ceiling. Don't let me push it down.'** This is assessing abduction of the

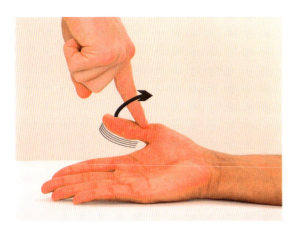

Figure 6.54 Testing abduction of the thumb. The arrow represents the direction of force generated by the patient.

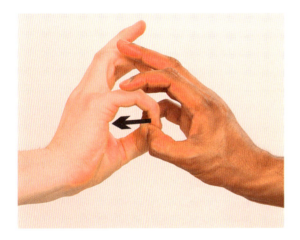

Figure 6.55 Testing opposition of the thumb.

thumb. The muscle being tested is abductor pollicis brevis (*ab-duck-tor-polly-sis-brev-iss*), supplied by fibres from the median nerve arising from T1 (see Fig. 6.54).

- **'Place your thumb and little finger together to form a ring. Don't let me pull them apart.'** This is assessing opposition between the thumb and little finger. The major muscle used is opponens pollicis (*op-poe-nens-polly-sis*), which is supplied by a branch of the median nerve (see Fig. 6.55) (root T1). Movement of the little finger is via a branch of the ulnar nerve (C8).

Froment's sign

See Fig. 6.56. Froment's (*fro-ments*) sign (*Jules Froment (1878–1946), French physician*) is a test that demonstrates

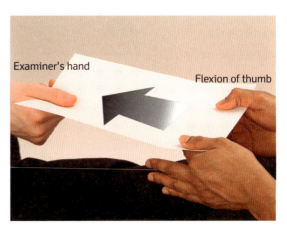

Figure 6.56 Froment's sign. Note flexion of the patient's right thumb. This 'trick movement' is adopted because there is a paralysis of adductor pollicis brevis (supplied by the ulnar nerve).

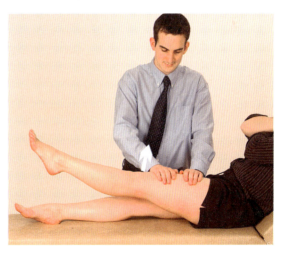

Figure 6.57 Assessing the power of hip flexion. Arrows represent the direction of force generated by the patient.

the inability of the thumb to adduct in an ulnar nerve lesion (see the 'Peripheral nerve lesions' section). Ask your patient to grip a piece of paper between their thumb and index finger (this requires adduction of the thumb). In the presence of an ulnar nerve palsy the grip is achieved by flexing the thumb.

Hip flexion and extension

See Figs. 6.57 and 6.58. Say to your patient, 'Lift up your leg, don't let me push it down' (hip flexion L1, L2, L3). As they raise their leg, place your hand on the top of the thigh and push down. If the patient is unable to raise

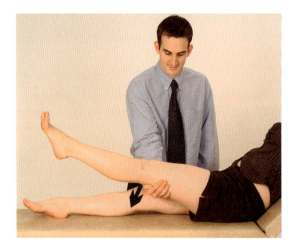

Figure 6.58 Assessing the power of hip extension.

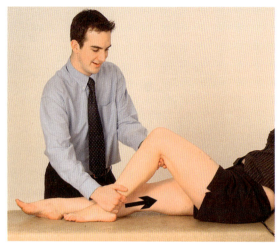

Figure 6.59 Assessing the power of knee flexion.

their leg against gravity (by MRC definition less than grade 3/5), get them to lie on their side to eliminate gravity from the movement (the side opposite to the leg being tested). Now get them to flex their hip again. If they can, this is grade 2/5. If they cannot and there is only a flicker of contraction, this is grade 1/5. No contraction is grade 0/5.

Do the same for the other leg. Now put your hand under the thigh and say to your patient, 'Push down with your leg' or 'Pull your leg into the bed' (hip extension L5, S1). Remember that this movement is aided by gravity and therefore you also have to make an empirical judgement for grade 2/5–3/5.

The purists may suggest that you lie your patient face down on the bed and raise their leg so that gravity is a factor again but this is not necessary and leads to your patient having to change position numerous times.

Hip abduction and adduction

Place your hands on the lateral aspect of each thigh and say, 'Spread your legs apart and push against my hand' (abduction L4, L5, S1). Now place your hands on the inner aspect of each thigh and say, 'Pull your legs together' (adduction L2, L3, L4). Compare both hip movements together and grade them. Gravity is not a major influence on these movements and therefore grades 2/5–3/5 will have to be estimated.

Knee flexion and extension

See Figs 6.59 and 6.60. Now get your patient to bend their knees up in the air. As they do this place your hand

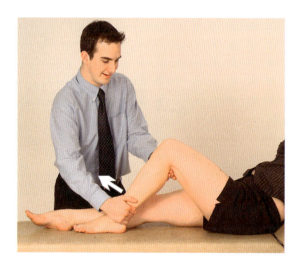

Figure 6.60 Assessing the power of knee extension.

on the back of the calf and say, 'Pull me towards you as hard as you can' or 'Pull your heel in towards your bottom' (flexion L5, S1) and resist the subsequent movement. Now test the other leg. Then move your hand to the front of the shin and say, 'Push me away now as hard as you can' (extension L3, L4) and resist it. Grade the power for both legs as before.

Dorsiflexion and plantarflexion of feet

See Figs. 6.61 and 6.62. Say, 'Cock your feet up.' When the patient has complied, place your hands on the dorsum of the foot and say, 'Don't let me push them down'

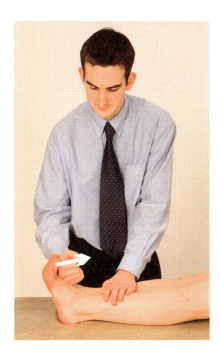

Figure 6.61 Assessing the power of dorsiflexion.

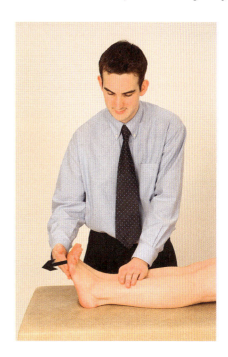

Figure 6.62 Assessing the power of plantarflexion.

(dorsiflexion L4, L5). Resist the movement. It is possible to assess both feet at the same time by placing the legs alongside each other and then providing resistance with the back of your hand and forearm on the dorsum of the feet. Now place your hands on the soles and say, 'Push me away now' and resist the movement (plantarflexion S1). Grade all movements as before.

Tip

If a patient has a foot drop do not assume that they cannot plantarflex their foot. You will have to physically dorsiflex the foot before asking them to push their foot down. You may be surprised to find that this movement may be unaffected.

Inversion and eversion of the foot

These movements are not often tested but are useful if motor deficits have been found in your previous assessments. Ensure that the patient's leg is fully relaxed on the bed. Now place your fingers on the medial border of their sole and say, 'Turn your foot in towards my

fingers . . . don't let me move it' (inversion L4). Remove your fingers and place them on the lateral border of the foot and say, 'Turn your foot out towards my fingers . . . don't let me move it' (eversion S1). Make sure that the only part of the leg that moves is the foot. Check both feet and grade accordingly and remember that both these movements are relatively weak compared to the larger muscle groups.

Toe extension and flexion

Place your thumb or index finger on the nail of the big toe and say, 'Cock up your big toe' and resist the action (extension L5). Now place your digit on the sole of the big toe and say, 'Push your toe away' and resist again (flexion S1).

Tip

While you are assessing power, every now and then glance at your patient's face and make sure that they are not grimacing with pain. If the power is limited it is worth asking whether it was pain or lack of power that restricted their performance because some patients will suffer in silence.

Key points

- Assessing power is subjective and you need to judge what is normal for an individual (for example, older person compared with Arnold Schwarznegger in his prime)
- Try to recall the root values of the muscles being tested as this may help in localizing the neurological lesion
- Make sure your patient gives their maximum effort (but without resorting to a trial of strength)
- Make sure it is a lack of power and not pain which is reducing performance

Table 6.19 Grading of reflexes

–	Absent
–/+	Present with reinforcement
+	Normal
++	Brisk but normal
+++	Abnormally brisk (hyper-reflexia)

20 Test reflexes: biceps (DF 5/10), supinator (DF 7/10), triceps (DF 6/10), knee (DF 4/10), and ankle (DF 9/10)

When assessing the reflexes, you need to look for a contraction in the muscle concerned as well as movement of the arm itself, because the latter may not be obvious if the contraction is weak. The left-sided reflexes are more difficult to elicit and require more practice. In all cases the patient must be relaxed. The best position is with both arms folded loosely across the upper abdomen and the legs relaxed on the bed. You may have to stress to the patient to relax a number of times when attempting the reflexes. When you elicit a response you should grade it according to the scale in Table 6.19.

Biceps

(Root value: C5, C6) See Figs. 6.63 and 6.64. Hold the tendon hammer loosely at the end with your right hand (if you are right handed) and place your left thumb just below and parallel to the skin crease in the antecubital (*anti-cube-it-al*) fossa. The right biceps tendon will be palpable here as a thick cord. Extend your right wrist, then flick it gently into flexion and let the heavy end of the hammer swing down with gravity to hit your left thumb. You do not need to apply any force. If the reflex is elicited then there is no need to give the patient repeated wallops to make sure. Repeat on the left biceps tendon to compare directly (see Case 6.8).

Supinator

(C5, C6) See Figs. 6.65 and 6.66. Place your left index and middle fingers at the site of the tendon, which is three-quarters of the distance along the forearm from the

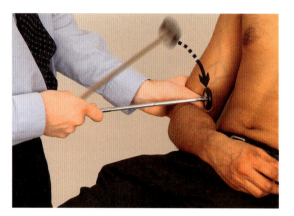

Figure 6.63 Eliciting the right biceps reflex. Make sure your patient is adequately relaxed.

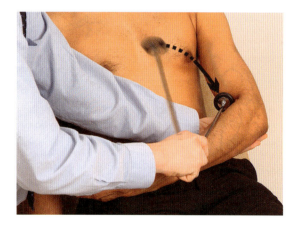

Figure 6.64 Eliciting the left biceps reflex.

antecubital fossa, on the radial aspect. The tendon itself can be difficult to feel but do not panic, the reflex is likely to be elicited despite this. The hammer is used in exactly the same way as for the eliciting the biceps reflex. Now check the opposite side.

CASE 6.8

Problem. When you elicit the biceps reflex the right one seems brisker than the left. Is this significant?

Discussion. It may be, but before you can say it is, you need to satisfy certain criteria. Was the patient relaxed when you tested each reflex? If they were relaxed for the right biceps but tense for the left this could lead to the discrepancy you observed. Therefore make sure your patient is relaxed throughout your assessment. The other factor to consider is your technique. You need to make sure the tendon hammer strikes each tendon with equal force. If you actively tap the tendon (rather than let it swing down with gravity) it is possible that you may have hit the right biceps tendon harder than the left. Practise letting gravity take over the downswing and in time you will be assured that you are eliciting each reflex with an equivalent stimulus. With experience you will control these factors and make a valid comparison of the reflexes.

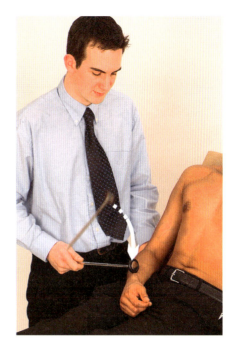

Figure 6.65 Eliciting the right supinator reflex.

Triceps

(C6, C7) See Figs. 6.67 and 6.68. This is a flat tendon that can be palpated running vertically upwards from the posterior aspect of the elbow tip just above the bony prominence (the olecranon [oh-leck-ran-on]). This time, the tendon is tapped directly rather than with your fingers interposed. The left side is particularly tricky and the arm needs to be pulled across the chest towards you to enable you to elicit the reflex. As you cannot directly see the tendon you will have to aim in the general direction just above the elbow. If you can carry off the procedure without slapping the patient in the face, you are doing well. Case 6.9 showcases further difficulties in obtaining reflexes which are also applicable for the legs.

Knee jerk

(L3, L4.) See Fig. 6.69. Say to the patient, 'Just relax your legs and let them rest in my hands'. Gently insert your hand underneath the knee and gently lift the knee off the bed. Check to make sure the full weight of the leg is resting on your arm. If it is not and you can see them contracting their quadriceps muscle, reinforce your request to relax. Strike the patellar tendon, which lies between the patella and its insertion at the tibial tuberosity (about 4–6 cm below). Watch for the leg jerking forwards or if this is not obvious, the contraction of the quadriceps muscle above. Observe the response you get and then do the other knee and compare.

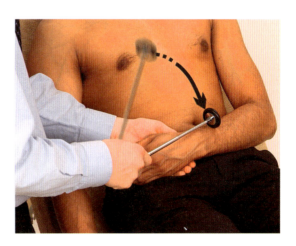

Figure 6.66 Eliciting the left supinator reflex.

Ankle reflex

(L5, S1.) See Figs. 6.70 and 6.71. The ankle jerks can be particularly awkward to demonstrate. First warn your patient, 'I am going to move your leg and I need you to stay completely relaxed'. Now flex the knee and laterally rotate the leg letting the leg flop naturally to the side (some people place the ankle on the opposite leg before rotating the leg under test). Dorsiflex the ankle

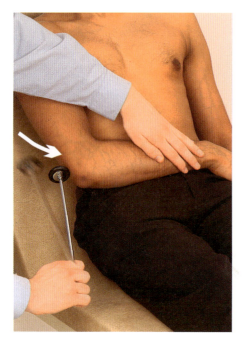

Figure 6.67 Eliciting the right triceps reflex.

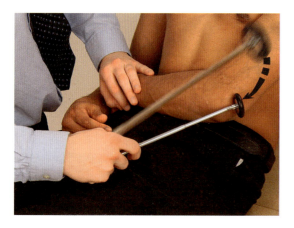

Figure 6.68 Eliciting the left triceps reflex.

with your non-dominant hand to put the Achilles tendon on stretch and strike the tendon, just above its attachment to the heel. Observe for plantar flexion and also for contraction of the calf muscle. The left ankle jerk is even more fiddly as your non-dominant arm is forced up in an awkward arch as you dorsiflex the left foot and you have to swing your tendon hammer within this arch at an unusual angle to strike the tendon. The potential for tying yourself in an embarrassing knot has never been so

CASE 6.9

Problem. You are trying to elicit the reflexes in the arms but cannot get them—why?

Discussion. This could be due to a number of factors. Your technique may be faulty; for example, you might not be striking the tendons precisely (the supinator can be easy to miss at first), so double check that you are controlling the tendon hammer and aiming correctly. A common cause of absent reflexes is a tense patient. So make sure the patient is relaxed and keep monitoring for signs of muscle activity (as for assessing tone). You may have to persevere for several minutes before complete relaxation is achieved. Only when you are satisfied that the reflexes are unobtainable with your patient fully relaxed should you attempt to elicit them with reinforcement. If they are absent with reinforcement, then this suggests LMN pathology such as a peripheral neuropathy.

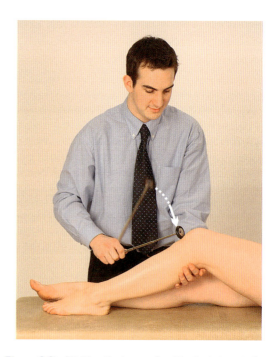

Figure 6.69 Eliciting the knee reflex. The technique is the same for both knees.

high; practice is the key. Grade the reflexes as before and attempt reinforcement if you cannot elicit a response. The authors advocate walking around the bed or couch and performing the left ankle jerk as they do the right. It

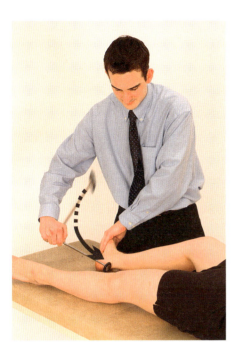

Figure 6.70 Eliciting the right ankle jerk.

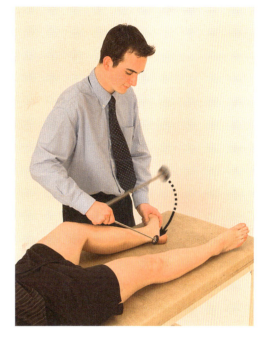

Figure 6.71 Eliciting the left ankle jerk.

is simple to perform and at the end of the day it is the result that is crucial (providing the ankle jerk is elicited with an equivalent stimulus to the right to enable a valid comparison).

Tip

Another less elaborate way of eliciting the ankle jerks is to keep the legs relaxed and lying on the bed. You need to be standing on the right side of the bed facing towards the feet. In this position, you simply dorsiflex the foot with your non-dominant hand and then strike this hand with the tendon hammer. This procedure is not recommended for an examination situation (currently).

Reinforcement of reflexes

If you are unable to elicit a reflex then it is acceptable to try once more. If you still cannot demonstrate it, you need to attempt reinforcement (see Fig. 6.72). Explain to the patient that they need to relax and when you say 'Now!' they need to clench their teeth (providing they have got their teeth in, of course). Timing is essential here. You need to time the swing of the hammer so that

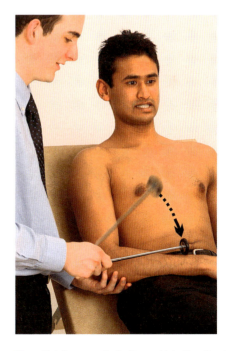

Figure 6.72 Reinforcement of reflexes. Note the clenched teeth just at the point of contact of the hammer with the tendon.

you strike the tendon as the patient clenches their teeth (or gums). This manoeuvre is important because you cannot say a reflex is absent until you have been unable to elicit it with reinforcement. This part of the examination is often forgotten. If hyper-reflexia is elicited there are various other reflexes which you can go on to test, including Hoffman's, the pectoral, the deltoid, and the finger reflexes.

If any of the lower limb reflexes are absent despite adequate relaxation, reinforcement can be attempted as follows. Get your patient to interlock the fingers of both hands together (palms facing each other and the fingers of the topmost hand hooking into the curled up fingers of the hand below). Ask the patient to pull them apart when you give the word. Say, 'Now!' on the upswing of your tendon hammer. If your timing is right you should strike the tendon at the same time as your patient starts performing the manoeuvre. This is sometimes known as Jendrassik's (*jen-drass-icks*) manoeuvre (*Erno Jendrassik (1858–1921), Hungarian physician*) (see Fig. 6.73). Grade your response as before.

21 Elicit the plantar reflex (DF 8/10)

See Fig. 6.74. This is the most important of the superficial reflexes. It is a reflex contraction that occurs as the result of a scratch-like stimulus to the skin. This reflex is tested using a firm stimulus on the sole of the foot. Warn the patient beforehand: 'I'm just going to scratch the bottom of your foot'.

Using the blunt tip of a key or an orange stick, apply a firm stroke starting at the heel, moving upwards along the lateral border and across the metatarsophalageal joints of the toes taking care not to touch the ball of the big toe. This can cause flexion of the big toe, sometimes called a withdrawal response. Observe the first movement of the big toe carefully. A normal response is a downgoing (flexor) response of the big toe. If the response is an upward extension of the big toe, this is abnormal and it is termed an extensor plantar or a positive Babinski response (*Joseph Jules François Felix Babinski (1807–1875), French neurologist of Polish descent*). A positive Babinski response is indicative of an UMN lesion (note that there is no equivalent 'negative Babinski response' for a normal flexor response). Some people advocate looking for a fanning movement of the other toes to help in deciding whether a plantar is upgoing but this can be misleading, so stick to observing the big toe only. See Cases 6.10 and 6.11. An absent response is encountered in severe peripheral neuropathy due to severe sensory impairment, total paralysis, or even when the patient is tense.

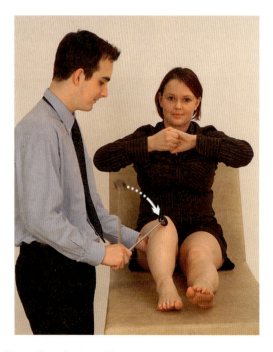

Figure 6.73 Jendrassik's manoeuvre.

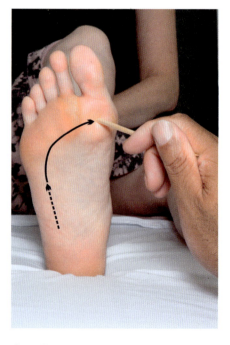

Figure 6.74 Eliciting the plantar reflex.

CASE 6.10

Problem. You are concluding your neurological examination and have found no abnormalities, but when you elicit the plantar reflex the toe goes upwards. Is this a positive Babinski response?

Discussion. The likely answer is no. You would only expect a positive Babinski response in the presence of an UMN lesion, in which case you would elicit other related signs such as spasticity, clonus, or hyper-reflexia. You may also see a positive Babinski response in an unconscious patient or in someone with an encephalopathy, which is not the case here. The likeliest scenario is the withdrawal response. This is usually elicited in someone who is anxious or ticklish. A full-blown response includes an upgoing big toe accompanied by a rapid flexion at the knee as the leg is lifted away from the noxious stimulus. The key to the true plantar response is the very first movement of the big toe. This requires close observation of the big toe (pray that your patient has washed their feet). The very first movement is fleeting but is downgoing before the withdrawal response. Often this first movement is so difficult that many members of a medical team disagree. If you are faced with uncertainty, remember to weigh up the consequences of a positive sign in the context of other clinical features. In this case there were no other neurological features to make a positive Babinski response tenable.

CASE 6.11

Problem. You have been told to examine a patient who has just been admitted acutely with a left hemiplegia (*hemi-plea-jah*). You find that he has no movement of the left arm (grade 0/5) or leg, the tone is not increased, and you are unable to elicit any reflexes in the arm or leg. You are confused because you know a stroke is the cause of a UMN lesion but your findings are completely the opposite of what you would expect.

Discussion. If you see a patient in the very early stages of a stroke, they often have a flaccid paralysis, that is, decreased tone, absent reflexes, and lack of plantar response. Over the next few hours or days you will see the classic signs of a UMN lesion emerge, that is, increased tone, hyper-reflexia, and an upgoing plantar. The same phenomenon can be seen shortly after an acute injury to the spinal cord.

Key points

- Make sure you use a blunt instrument such as a key or orange stick to elicit the plantar reflex
- An upgoing plantar is consistent with an UMN lesion
- The first direction of movement of the big toe is the crucial one
- An upgoing plantar is termed an extensor plantar response or a positive Babinski sign

22 Other reflexes

Just about any muscle with a tendon that is accessible can be shown to have a reflex. There are also a small number of superficial reflexes. Their value is that in certain cases they may help in the localization of a lesion.

Pectoral reflex

(C5, C6) With the pectoral reflex, tapping on the lateral insertion of pectoralis major (by placing your fingers on the lateral chest wall and pressing them up to the shoulder just above the armpit) causes a slight muscle contraction, which jerks the shoulder forward. This movement is exaggerated in hyper-reflexia.

Deltoid reflex

(C5). The deltoid reflex is elicited by tapping the insertion of the deltoid muscle (by placing your fingers on the lateral aspect of the shoulder where the bulk of the muscle starts to converge on the upper humerus). If successful you may see a slight movement of the arm away from the body. Again the reflex becomes more exaggerated in hyper-reflexia.

Finger jerks

(C8) See Fig. 6.75. Place two fingers across the palmar aspect of the patient's proximal phalanges and take their weight with them. The patient's hand should be facing palm downwards and relaxed. Swing the tendon hammer up to tap your own fingers. The impact should cause slight flexion of the patient's fingers. This reflex is not easily seen normally but becomes more prominent in hyper-reflexia.

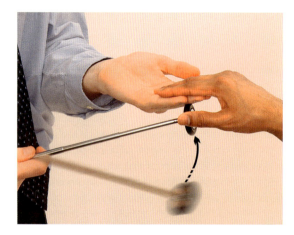

Figure 6.75 Finger jerks.

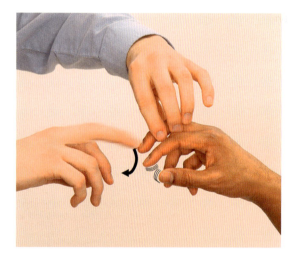

Figure 6.76 Hoffman's reflex. Flicking the distal phalanx of the middle finger leads to the flexion of the index finger and thumb.

Hoffman's reflex

See Fig. 6.76. Hoffman's reflex (*Johann Hoffman (1857–1919), German neurologist*) is elicited by holding the middle phalanx of the patient's middle finger between your left index finger and thumb, with their palm facing downwards. Their hand must be relaxed. Flick the distal phalanx downwards with your right thumb. If hyper-reflexia is present the patient's thumb will be seen to flex with the stimulus.

Abdominal reflex

See Fig. 6.77. The abdominal reflex is another superficial reflex and is tested with a scratch provided by the tip of a patella hammer or key. First apply a scratch in the

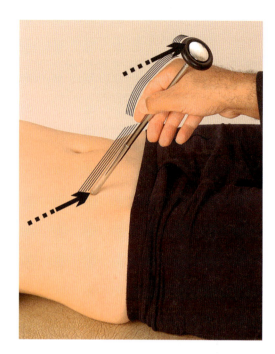

Figure 6.77 Eliciting the abdominal reflex.

subcostal region parallel to the costal margin from the flanks towards the midline (D6–D8). Repeat again at the level of the umbilicus (D10), followed by a stroke parallel to the iliac crest in the iliac fossa (D11, D12). Also check the opposite side. A normal response is a brisk contraction of the muscles of the anterior abdominal wall directly below the stimulus. If this is absent it may suggest an UMN lesion above the root supply of the area stimulated. However, this can be absent in anxious or obese patients and is therefore not a reliable sign. It has a minor role in supporting other UMN signs that you may have demonstrated.

Cremastric reflex

(L1.) In the male, stroking the inner thigh, gently, with the tip of a patella hammer tests for the cremastric (*cream-ass-ter-rick*) reflex. Observe for the contraction of the scrotum on the same side. This is due to the contraction of the cremastric muscle.

Anal reflex

(S4, S5.) If the skin around the anus is scratched lightly, the external sphincter contracts in response.

Bulbocavernosus reflex

(S2, S3, S4.) If the glans penis (the 'helmet' part of the penis) is gently squeezed, the bulbocavernosus (*bulb-owe-cavern-owe-suss*) muscle contracts in response.

Key points

- Make sure your patient is relaxed throughout the examination
- Try to recall the root values of the reflexes as this will aid in the localization of the lesion, for example, knee jerk (L3, L4)
- Hyper-reflexia indicates an upper motor lesion above the level of the reflex arc
- An absence of reflexes indicates a lower motor lesion at the level of the reflex arc
- Make sure you are particularly proficient in eliciting the left ankle jerk
- Always attempt reinforcement before saying a reflex is absent

This is best appreciated by palpating the underside of the penis lightly with a finger to feel its contraction. This reflex is rarely tested and it goes without saying that if you are going to do it, you will need to explain it very carefully! (You do wonder about the motivations of those pioneering physicians who closely observed the first cremasteric, anal, and bulbocavernosus reflexes!)

Primitive reflexes

Primitive reflexes are a collection of reflexes that are present during babyhood but are eventually suppressed by the increasing activity of the frontal lobes. Damage to the frontal lobes may lead to the re-emergence of these reflexes.

- **Snout/pout reflex**. This can be elicited by tapping the lips very gently with a tendon hammer. The test is positive if the lips pout in response.

- **Rooting reflex**. If the upper lip is stroked on either lateral extremity, the patient will move their mouth towards the finger (like a baby searching for a nipple).
- **Palmomental** (*palm-owe-mental*) **reflex**. Stroke the palm of one hand while looking at the lower lip and jaw on the same side of the face. An abnormal response is a contraction of the ipsilateral mentalis (*men-tail-iss*) muscle of the lower lip.

The utility of these reflexes is limited. They remain impressive signs to delight your colleagues with.

23 Test coordination: finger–nose test (DF 6/10) check alternating hand movements (DF 4/10), heel-shin test (DF 3/10)

It is worth noting that these tests are difficult to interpret if the patient has marked limb weakness, so do not waste time attempting them if the power is grade 3 or less.

Finger–nose testing

See Fig. 6.78. Hold your index finger at arm's length from the patient. Ask them to touch it with their right index finger then to touch their nose. It is worth doing a dry run by grasping the patient's finger and guiding them to each target so they get the idea. Tell them to repeat the sequence several times, as quickly and accurately as possible. Note that if your index finger is held too close to the patient, you may miss subtle incoordination. Your instructions must be clear, otherwise you run the risk of the patient lurching towards you to touch your nose! If the patient has a cerebellar lesion the finger–nose test may bring out an

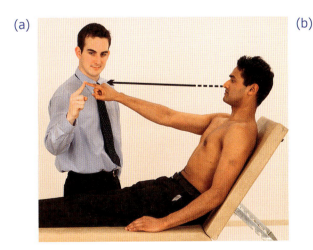
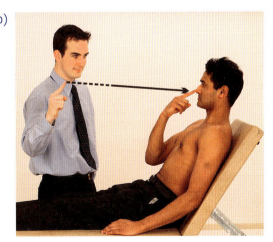

Figure 6.78 The finger–nose test.

(a)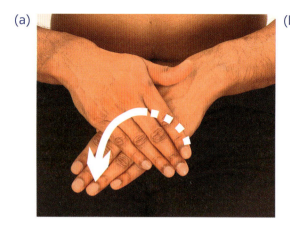

(b)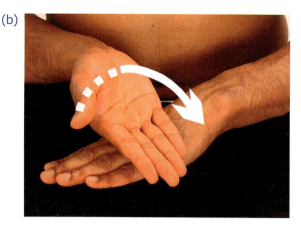

Figure 6.79 Examining for dysdiadochokinesia.

intention tremor. In other words the tremor occurs when the patient attempts to carry out skilled actions such as aiming for a target at arm's length. This is in contrast to a parkinsonian tremor, which occurs at rest. The patient may also exhibit 'past-pointing' (dysmetria (*dis-met-ria*)) in which they miss the target altogether.

Alternating hand movements

Demonstrate what you want your patient to do, that is, tap your right hand on to your left, first with the palm then with the dorsal aspect. Continue to alternate quickly. In cerebellar lesions, this test will be carried out slowly and clumsily and is called dysdiadochokine-sia (*dis-die-owe-dough-co-kin-easier*) (see Fig. 6.79). A simpler form of this is to ask the patient to tap the back of one hand repeatedly as fast as they can using the fingers of the other hand. Similar results will be obtained.

....

Tip
Ask if the patient is right or left handed, because the non-dominant hand is often slightly more clumsy than the dominant one.

....

In another technique you might see occasionally, the examiner will ask the patient to hold their arms out in front of them with their eyes closed and maintain that position even when the arms are pushed down. The examiner then gently pushes down on one of the forearms. A normal person will resist this movement and quickly restore the arm to roughly its former position. A patient with cerebellar

dysfunction may bounce their arm up and down, making it oscillate wildly from its original position in a bid to restore its posture.

Heel–shin

See Fig. 6.80. Make sure the patient is lying flat in the bed with both legs straight. Ask them to lift the leg and place the heel on to the opposite knee. Then get them to slide the heel along the shin until it reaches the ankle. Now ask them to lift the heel back up to the knee and repeat this cycle a few times (about three times is sufficient). It is useful to do a rehearsal by getting hold of the patient's leg and guiding it through the sequence of events. Once the patient has started it is also helpful to remind them of their objectives, for example, 'Slide down the shin . . . to the ankle', 'Now lift it up', 'Go back to the knee', and 'Slide down again'. A normal person can do this quickly and efficiently. A person with incoordination will find that their foot might shake on the shin and veer away from the ankle (you may see the heel drop off the shin before reaching the ankle). Sometimes people may make it to the ankle but the clue to some degree of incoordination is that the movement is slow, hesitant, and very deliberate. If you are suspicious of incoordination go on to check the patient's gait as well as looking for evidence of this in the upper limbs (and nystagmus). You can increase the sensitivity of this test by holding your finger about a metre above the patient's foot and asking them to touch it with their big toe after they have reached the ankle. If they are unable to locate your finger with their toe, this is further evidence that could support a cerebellar lesion. From this point they can begin the cycle again by putting their heel back on the knee. Go on to check the other leg.

(a)
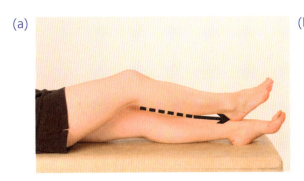

(b)
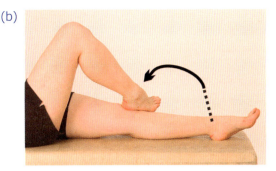

Figure 6.80 Performing the heel–shin test.

A further supplementary test you could perform if you sus-pect incoordination in the legs is the foot tapping test.

Foot tapping

This is the lower limb's equivalent of tapping the back of your hand. Simply place the palm of your hand near the forefoot of the leg being tested. It should be close enough for the foot to make contact when it is plantarflexed. Say to your patient, 'Tap your foot as fast as you can'. Although the foot is naturally clumsier than the hand a normal person can still tap fairly rap-idly, that is, between three and five taps per second. Anything slower than this suggests incoordination. The problem with this test is that it is not very specific for cerebellar disorder. The incoordination you demonstrate here could simply be natural clumsiness. However if other features of incoordination are present elsewhere this does provide further evidence.

24 Assess sensation: light touch (DF 6/10), pain (DF 6/10), proprioception (DF 6/10), and vibration sense (DF 5/10)

By convention, each part of the sensory examination begins distally, moving proximally up the arms. In practice it does not matter where you start assessing sensation so long as you are systematic and thorough. Remember that any sensory loss should fit into one of four main patterns.

- **Global sensory loss**. The entire limb is affected, for example, in stroke.
- **Peripheral neuropathy**. 'Glove and stocking' distri-bution.
- **Dermatomal sensory loss**. Often two or more adja-cent dermatomes are involved, in which case the cause is a peripheral nerve lesion, for example, a median nerve. Occasionally just one dermatome is affected, usually due to compression of a single nerve root as it exits the spinal cord.
- **Dissociated sensory loss**. There is loss of certain modalities of sensation but preservation of others, for example, loss of pain and temperature sensation but intact appreciation of light touch and proprioception, as in syringomyelia (*si-ring-owe-mile-ia*) (see 'Neur-ology and investigation' section).

Light touch

Impulses for light touch travel principally up the dorsal columns in the spinal cord as described earlier. Damage to any component of the sensory pathway from the sense organs in the skin, along the course of the nerves in the limbs and the pathways in the spinal cord, up to the cere-bral cortex can lead to disorder of light touch appreciation.

How to examine

Examination is performed using a piece of cotton wool. First, make one end into a wisp and then gently dab the skin (once only) over the top of the sternum. Ask the patient to confirm that they can feel it and that it feels soft, as they would expect cotton wool to feel (some patients may have altered perception while still being able to feel

> **Key points**
> - Do not test coordination in the presence of limb weakness (grade 3/5 or less) or in the presence of involuntary movements
> - An intention tremor, past-pointing, and dysdiadochokinesis indicate a cerebellar lesion
> - The non-dominant hand is usually clumsier than the dominant hand

CASE 6.12

Problem. A 45-year-old woman was admitted via the emergency dpartment with difficulty walking. She had a 2-week history of progressive leg weakness and stiffness. In addition, she noticed some numbness in both legs. There were no bowel or bladder symptoms. When asked about previous symptoms she recalled a time in her twenties, where she experienced blurring of the vision in her right eye, which resolved after a few days. On examination, she was apyrexial and had evidence of incoordination, dysdiadochokinesia, and an intention tremor, with past-pointing in the left arm. She had increased tone in both legs, plus clonus in the right leg. Power was reduced to 3/5 in the right leg and 4/5 in the left leg. There was generalized hyper-reflexia. There was also sensory loss extending up the legs to the umbilicus (*um-be-like-us*). Her cranial nerve examination was normal except for nystagmus to the left. What is the diagnosis?

Discussion. At first sight this case seems a nightmare, overflowing with all sorts of neurological signs. You need to try and digest the information, breaking it up into smaller pieces and see if you can recognize any patterns. Start with the motor system. The collection of signs in the left arm (together with the nystagmus to the left in the cranial nerves) should make you think of a cerebellar lesion in its left hemisphere. The signs in the legs are different. They point to bilateral UMN lesions affecting the legs (this pattern is called a spastic paraparesis). However there are no UMN signs in the arms, which means that the lesion has to be below the nerve supply to the arms, which points to its location being at the thoracic level or lower in the spine. There are a number of causes of a spastic paraparesis but the presence of a sensory level is worrying. It suggests spinal cord compression and the level demonstrated on examination (up to the umbilicus) further localizes the lesion within a few spinal segments around the T10 level. This is a neurological emergency and urgent MRI (or a CT myelogram) needs to be done.

However, spinal cord compression does not explain the left-sided cerebellar signs. To do this you would have to think of a second condition unrelated to the cord compression (for example, stroke) to explain everything. Although this is possible the patient would be unlucky to have two different pathologies at the same time. A much better explanation for her condition is multiple sclerosis (MS). Plaques of demyelination can be found scattered throughout the central nervous system, which can lead to unusual patterns of neurological signs that are not easy to explain at first sight. Another characteristic of MS is its relapsing and remitting nature. This means that your patient may suffer a neurological deficit before it improves or disappears altogether. The episode in her twenties sounds suspiciously like optic neuritis (see 'Neurological diseases and investigation' section) and is a common symptom of MS. Despite the high probability of MS in this case it is prudent to exclude spinal cord compression as mentioned earlier because mistakes have been made in similar circumstances; for example, patients assumed to have MS have later been found to have spinal cord tumours.

the stimulus). Next dab the skin of one of the fingers of the right hand. Instruct the patient: 'Say yes if you can feel this and does it feel the same as on the chest.' If an affirmative response is given continue in the same manner moving up the arm and alternating from the lateral to the medial aspects of the arm so that you can compare the stimulus across different dermatomes (see Fig. 6.5). Repeat the process in the left arm. An alternative method is to dab the same dermatome on each arm to directly compare, then move up the arms as before. There is no fixed number of times you need to dab, but an average number would be about eight for each arm. If an area of sensory loss is identified, dab once more to confirm your findings then attempt to map out its boundaries. This will help you to identify which of the four patterns of sensory loss the deficit corresponds to. A similar process is used for the legs. See 6.12 for the contribution sensory loss makes to a complex case.

Tip

If you find sensory loss in the lower limbs you must always check the sensation around the anus (S4) and check the anal tone with a finger (a lax patulous anus may indicate an S5 lesion). You will also need to pay particular attention to the function of the bowels and bladder. Find out if the patient has become constipated or has had difficulty passing urine recently (and check for a palpable bladder). The latter two problems are associated with spinal cord compression.

Tip

A crude but rapid screen for the possibility of spinal cord compression involves searching for a sensory level with your finger. Quickly touch the sternum as your reference point and confirm that the patient can feel your finger. Then start at one toe and if the sensation is abnormal, run your finger slowly up the leg on to the abdomen. You should ask the patient to let you know when the sensation feels normal. This technique can alert you to other neurological deficits but you must always follow this up with a more conventional and thorough assessment as described above.

. . . .

Pain

Pain, along with temperature sensation, travels principally along the spinothalamic tracts in the spinal cord to the brain.

How to examine

A pin-prick is used as a surrogate for pain. The assessment is performed using special 'neurotips', which are available on the wards. Never use venepuncture needles as these are more painful and may draw blood. Again, begin at the sternum. Warn the patient that you are now using something sharp and gently tap the skin with the tip. Ask them to confirm that it feels sharp. Then move on to the arms as before, but ask them to say 'sharp' each time they feel the pricking sensation; or 'dull' if this is the case. If a sharp sensation is perceived as dull then this either indicates that the appreciation of pain is abnormal or that you have been too timid with your stimulus, so be bold and try to achieve a similar 'tap' with each test. If the patient is unable to detect the stimulus at all, the area is said to be anaesthetic. Feel free to directly compare any area with the sternum again to verify your findings, particularly if they are subtle.

Proprioception

Proprioception is the ability of a person to sense the position of any of their joints in space without the aid of their eyes. Hence this is also called 'joint position sense'. Stretch receptors in joints send information about joint position via the dorsal columns to the brain.

How to examine

Ask your patient to watch what you are doing. Hold both sides of the proximal phalanx of your patient's thumb between your left index finger and thumb. Using your right hand hold the distal phalanx in the same way and flex the

CASE 6.13

Problem. You are assessing proprioception in the right thumb. Sometimes your patient gets the position right and sometimes they get it wrong. Are they messing around?

Discussion. Very rarely will this be the case (although you do have to be aware of the potential malingerer). Patients with an intact dorsal column system are able to give the correct answer even with small increments in movement, so an inconsistent response suggests that your patient is guessing the answer. This is because patients often feel obliged to give a response even when they are unsure. Often in this situation you will be able to detect uncertainty in their expression and voice. If you suspect they are guessing do not be afraid to ask them if this is the case. The danger with a patient guessing is they may get it right by chance, throwing you off the scent. Also check if there is any difficulty with vibration sense and light touch if you have not done so already, as these modalities are mainly transmitted along the same tracts.

interphalangeal (*inter-falan-jeel*) joint. Tell them that this is 'down'. Next extend the joint and tell them that this is 'up'. Ask the patient to close their eyes. Wiggle the distal phalanx up and down a few times then stop in either position and ask the patient to say which position they think it is in. Repeat this a few more times using different positions. If they get them all correct, proprioception is normal and there is no need to test the arm further. If they answer incorrectly repeat the test to confirm your findings then go on to examine the next proximal joint, that is, the wrist, to assess how widespread the problem is (see Case 6.13). Exactly the same technique can be employed on the big toe for proprioception in the foot. Another crude method exists for screening for a proprioceptive loss in the hands. Ask your patient to put their hands out in front of them and close their eyes. Then instruct them to place each index finger in turn on their nose. A normal person will be able to locate their nose without any difficulty even with their eyes shut.

Vibration sense

Vibration sense is the ability to appreciate a vibrating stimulus. The physiological advantage of this is unclear but it is an observation that the medical profession has made use of. It is likely that the stimulus predominantly travels along the dorsal columns. It is one of the first modalities to be affected in certain conditions, for

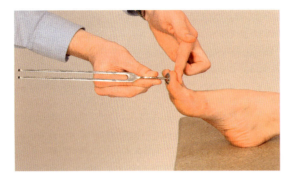

Figure 6.81 Testing vibration sense.

example, peripheral neuropathy. It is often absent distally in healthy, elderly people.

How to examine

See Fig. 6.81. Remember to use a 128-Hz tuning fork (the smaller 512-Hz fork is used for testing hearing). You should find the frequency value inscribed on the tuning fork. Try to avoid making the fork vibrate by hitting a hard surface such as the bedside locker. Sufficient stimulus can be achieved simply by springing the two prongs together with your thumb and index finger. Make the fork vibrate, then place the end on the sternum and ask the patient to confirm that they can feel it vibrating (or 'buzzing'). Make it vibrate again then touch the distal interphalangeal joint of their right thumb and ask, 'Can you feel the buzzing/vibration now?' If they can, then vibration sense is normal and you can proceed on to the left arm. If it is abnormal you need to move to the wrist (and then the elbow if necessary) and repeat the test. Note that testing is performed over bony areas because these are better for transmitting a vibrating impulse. A similar procedure is used for the legs starting initially with the big toe. If it is felt at the big toe then vibration sense is normal. If the vibration is not detected then work up to the medial or lateral malleoli, then the shin, the patella, or even the iliac crest until it is perceived. Document the level at which vibration is first detected.

Tip

Always make sure you ask, 'Can you feel it buzzing?' because if you simply ask if they can feel the tuning fork, some patients will say 'yes' when they feel the pressure/coldness on the skin rather than the actual vibration which is the focus of your assessment.

Other modalities of sensation

Temperature and two-point discrimination are not routinely tested.

Temperature sensation

Temperature sensation (DF 3/10) can be tested with test tubes of cold (approximately 7 °C) and warm (approximately 40 °C) water. Be quick while doing this test, as the temperature should be maintained relatively constant throughout the test. If the temperature is too hot or cold then you run the risk of stimulating pain fibres in addition, which will be unpleasant for your patient and confuse your results. In clinical practice the crude test of using the cold tines of a tuning fork is more commonly used.

Tip

Check briefly before placing the tuning fork on the patient's skin to make sure it feels cold because after a few exposures to the skin the fork will warm up, giving misleading results.

Two-point discrimination

Two-point discrimination (DF 7/10) can be tested using a paper clip opened out so that the two ends are 5 mm apart and can be used to touch the skin simultaneously. A normal result is where the patient can feel the two stimuli as

Key points

- For any sensory modality (except proprioception) always compare the sensation elicited to that on the sternum
- Also compare sensation in equivalent dermatomes of each arm and proximal to distal to discern patterns of sensory loss
- Remember the root values of the dermatomes as this will help in localizing a lesion
- Never use a venepuncture needle to assess pain
- Always use a 128-Hz tuning fork for vibration sense
- Make sure the patient appreciates the buzzing sensation in vibration testing rather than cold or pressure sensation
- If you suspect spinal cord compression, look for a sensory level
- Anal sensation and anal tone are a valuable adjunct to sensory testing and should never be forgotten

because vision is a very potent aid to balance and this test uses this fact to detect its presence.

CASE 6.14

Problem. You are preparing to perform Romberg's test on a patient. As they stand you notice that they seem unsteady and sway continually around their centre of gravity. When you ask them to close their eyes, they over-balance. You conclude that they have a positive Romberg's test but when you demonstrate this to the consultant on a teaching round the next day, they say you are wrong. Why?

Discussion. The key to a true positive Romberg's test is that the patient should be steady before they close their eyes. If they are unsteady before they close their eyes this suggests a different pathology. Cerebellar ataxia can lead to unsteadiness and this will be exaggerated when the eyes are closed (look for other cerebellar features, for example, nystagmus, dysdiadochokinesia, incoordination, intention tremor, and past-pointing).

two separate points on sensitive areas of the body such as the fingers. If the two ends are any closer they are usually perceived as a single stimulus. In disease states such as a peripheral neuropathy the distance at which two points can be perceived separately increases, in some cases to several centimetres.

25 Get your patient to stand: perform Romberg's test (DF 5/10)

Watch carefully as your patient attempts to stand and notice the ease or difficulty with which they assume an upright posture.

Romberg's test; what is it?

Romberg's test (*Moritz Heinrich Romberg (1795–1873), German neurologist*) is a test looking for sensory ataxia. This condition is the result of abnormal joint position sense in the feet and simply means that the patient has a tendency to be unsteady because of a lack of proprioception. This unsteadiness may not be initially apparent

Key points

- Romberg's test checks for sensory ataxia
- Make sure your patient is steady before getting them to close their eyes
- If the patient becomes unsteady when the eyes are closed the test is positive and indicates sensory ataxia (due to loss of joint position sense)

How to examine

When the patient stands, ask them to put their feet fairly close together and to 'get their balance.' Stand close to the patient and extend your arms to the front and the back of the patient. Once they are steady, ask them to close their eyes. A normal person will be able to maintain their balance without problem. Someone with sensory ataxia will begin to sway and may even fall over, hence the need to have your arms ready to catch them should this look likely. See Case 6.14 for a false positive test.

26 Assess gait (DF 7/10)

Gait: What is it?

This simply means the way in which a person walks (and not the mobile barrier in your garden fence).

Significance

No neurological examination of the legs is complete without watching a patient's gait. Walking is a complex activity dependent on many factors including muscles, joints, intact nerves, and higher brain centres. A problem in any one of these areas can lead to a change in the normal walking pattern. A doctor should be able to recognize the main patterns of abnormal gait as these can give useful insights into the possible underlying mechanisms. Once you are confident in spotting the major patterns you will find you will be able to predict the signs you should find in a neurological examination (a knack that will save time in the busy clinics and surgeries that you will inherit in the future.)

How to examine

If you have not had the opportunity to see the patient walk (or if you are in an examination situation) it is useful to ask the patient, 'Do you have difficulty walking?' If they say no, observe them safely from a distance. If they say yes, then you have to supervise them closely. Get close enough so that you can catch them if they look as if they are going to fall over. Get your patient to turn round and to walk back. Turning is an even more complex manoeuvre and may unmask problems in people who may only be mildly affected by a disorder.

Tip

If the patient is prone to stumbling, it is worth getting someone else to be on hand to catch your patient (preferably out of your line of sight) so that you can be free to analyse the gait unhindered by safety concerns.

Most students can recognize a normal gait pattern as they have seen thousands (subconsciously) by the time they reach medical school. The key things to look for are as follows.

- **Stability**. Is your patient stable or unstable?
- **Stride length**. Are the steps taken regular or does the stride length vary? Are the steps taken short and shuffling?
- **Gait pattern**. This is the manner in which the patient walks, which will now be described.

Antalgic gait

Antalgic (*ant-al-jick*) gait is the pattern of walking readily recognizable as a 'limp'. Any cause of pain, in any part of the leg, which is severe enough, will force the sufferer to keep as much weight off the affected limb as possible.

Ataxic gait

This implies an unbalanced or unsteady gait. The usual cause is a cerebellar lesion, although vestibular (*vest-tib-you-lar*) or labyrinthine (*lab-i-rin-thine*) lesions are also possible. Look at the patient's stance before they start walking. They usually stand with their feet wide apart to maximize their stability (hence sometimes called a broad-based gait). Despite this, some patients remain unsteady and may sway or lurch to the affected side (that is, an ipsilateral cerebellar hemisphere lesion) and can be mistaken for drunks. In milder forms, when you get the patient to turn they may stagger (or even fall, so beware). If you still suspect a cerebellar disorder but the patient has performed normally, put more stress on them by getting them to walk as if on a tightrope by putting the heel of one foot in front of the toe of the other foot. Normal people will be able to do this reasonably well but ataxic people will reel all over the place.

Hemiplegic gait

This is associated with a stroke and depends on its severity. The patient's posture will give some clues. Their stroke leg may be adducted and extended, with a plantarflexed foot. The arm on the same side may also be adducted, internally rotated, and with both the wrist and elbow flexed. As the hemiplegic leg is usually weak and stiff, the patient tends to swing it round in a circular movement (called circumduction) rather than lift it off the ground.

Spastic gait

This is basically a bilateral version of the hemiplegic gait (although the arms do not adopt the above posture

in a spinal cord lesion). As both legs are adducted and plantarflexed, this gives the patient the appearance of a pair of scissors (the gait is sometimes called a scissors gait). Each leg has to sweep stiffly around the other adducted knee in turn. Sometimes the patient looks as if they are wading through mud or quicksand. With milder disease the patient may just walk more stiffly than normal.

Steppage gait

This occurs with lesions causing foot drop, for example, lateral popliteal nerve palsy, L5, S1, root involvement, or peripheral neuropathy. The patient is unable to dorsiflex the foot to get it clear of the ground. Instead they have to raise their whole leg to achieve this before the foot is 'slapped' back onto the floor. This slapping gives a further audible clue to the trained observer. If the lesion is bilateral, the gait resembles a dressage horse performing an exaggerated canter.

Stamping gait

This resembles the high stepping gait but is due to sensory loss in the feet rather than a motor disturbance. The feet rather than slapping down passively are actively 'stamped' down by the patient. The patient has impaired joint position sense and is therefore unsure of where their feet are in space. Stamping provides a much greater stimulus, which increases the chance of proprioceptive feedback. In severe cases the patient has to look down at their feet to be sure of what their feet are actually doing.

Parkinsonian gait

The patient's posture is flexed and when they walk it is with short shuffling steps, with very little arm swing. Sometimes the patient has difficulty starting off and seems stuck in a pose. This is called freezing and can happen during the walk. Because of their flexed posture when they lean forwards to start moving, their centre of gravity falls outside their base of support (that is, their legs), which makes them unstable. They then have to hurry to 'chase their centre of gravity' or they will topple over (this is called a festinant (*fest-in-ent*) gait). A useful analogy for this is the sprint start (try it yourself), where the athlete is in the set position. Their centre of gravity is well outside the support from their legs (but is inside that provided by the arms and legs). If you were to remove the arms the athlete would fall to the ground, but they overcome this instability at the start of the race by driving hard and fast with their legs until their centre of gravity is once again acting through the support provided by their legs.

Myopathic gait

This is due to proximal muscle weakness, which affects the hip girdle muscles. These muscles keep the pelvis horizontal as the other leg is swung through. However, when they are weak the pelvis dips down on the side which is off the ground. Then when this leg is planted on the floor the pelvis is elevated on that side but dips down on the other side. This process repeats itself, leading to an oscillation of the pelvis that resembles the waddling of a duck (hence sometimes called a waddling gait).

Apraxic gait

This is a form of 'higher level' gait disorder which means that the centres in the brain responsible for automatic movements, for example walking, are dysfunctional. This is despite adequate power and coordination to fulfil the task. There is often difficulty in initiating the walk and the gait is wide based with the feet seemingly stuck to the ground. This gives the walk a shuffling quality that has been likened to skating on ice. The patient also tends to lean backwards and can fall in this direction also. With the initial freezing and shuffling, this gait can sometimes be mistaken for a parkinsonian gait. Other variations of this gait include taking small steps (given a French term 'marche à petit-pas' (*marsh-a-pet-tea-pah*)) or having a variable step length, that is, taking some small and then some longer steps. The smooth pattern of walking is disrupted and the patient may even stop walking before setting off on the same leg they had just landed on. Also watch them turn. A normal person will execute this effortlessly but your patient will take several small steps to complete the turn. An analysis of the footprints made by such a person shows that they make up the points of a star and again this is given a French term ('marche à l'étoile' (*marsh-a-lay-twarl*)).

Hysterical gait

This can take many forms but the key feature is inconsistency (both in history and examination). The gait

may change when repeated and often the underlying neurology is normal or does not fit the predicted gait pattern (an old-fashioned term for this is astasia abasia, which is a hysterical term for a hysterical gait).

26 Other signs

Agnosia

What is it?

Agnosia (*ag-nose-ia*) is an inability of the cerebral cortex to recognize or interpret stimuli delivered from intact sense organs and pathways. The area responsible for this interpretation is mainly the parietal cortex of the non-dominant hemisphere. In over 90% of right-handed people and about 70% of left-handed people the right hemisphere is non-dominant. Clinically the two important forms of agnosia are visual and tactile. It is appropriate to test for agnosia if you suspect your patient has a disorder causing cortical dysfunction, such as a stroke. Tactile agnosia (sometimes called astereognosia (*ay-stereo-ag-nose-ia*)) is the inability to recognize familiar objects by touch.

How to examine

You must first demonstrate that sensation is intact in the hand being assessed. When you are satisfied in this regard you can begin testing by asking the patient to close their eyes and then putting a pen or key, for example, into the affected (usually left) hand. They will be unable to recognize it until you put it into the right hand or let them open their eyes to see it.

Neglect

What is it?

In this condition the patient disregards, and in extreme cases denies, the existence of the affected side. It can also be caused by a lesion in the non-dominant parietal cortex (occipital lobe lesions may be associated with visual neglect).

How to examine

Again ensure that sensation is intact and ask the patient to close their eyes. Now touch the normal arm (again, usually the right arm) and ask them to tell you with which arm they felt the touch. They should be able to give the correct response. Repeat on the left arm and they may say that they feel the touch but are unable to localize it in the body. An extension of this test is to touch both arms simultaneously. Ask the patient to say on which side the touch was

Key points

- No neurological examination is complete without watching the patient walk
- Familiarity with the different gait patterns can give major clues to the underlying problem
- Always check if they have a problem walking beforehand (or if they need walking aids)
- When you watch a patient walk **make sure** you or someone else is on hand in case the patient stumbles

felt. A normal response would of course be 'both'. However a patient with neglect will only detect stimulus on the unaffected arm and will indicate that arm only. This inability to detect a stimulus in the presence of a competing stimulus presented at the same time is called 'sensory extinction' or 'sensory inattention'. A further way of demonstrating neglect is to ask your patient to draw a clock face and fill in the numbers representing the hours. With neglect they will only fill in one half of the clock (being totally unaware of the other half).

Apraxia

What is it?

Apraxia (*ay-pracks-ia*) is the inability to perform previously learned activities despite having intact (or only mildly impaired) motor function. It is again a feature of damage to the non-dominant parietal cortex.

How to examine

Having demonstrated that your patient has reasonable power (at least 4/5), ask them to perform an everyday task such as dressing or reading a book. They will be unable to do so and will appear lost, stopping frequently to ponder their next move; they may do bizarre things, for example, trying to put their trousers over their heads.

Tip

It is important to be aware of the presence of parietal syndromes, such as agnosia, apraxia, and neglect when you qualify because they all have one other thing in common. The rehabilitation team may recognize that the patient has good motor or sensory function but are dismayed by the patient's lack of progress. They may wrongly stigmatize a patient and brand them as lazy and poorly motivated. This in turn can decrease the patient's morale, leading to further impairment of their rehabilitation, which rapidly becomes a vicious cycle. In fact these are the patients who often require more support and rehabilitation.

Examining for neck stiffness (nuchal rigidity)

This manoeuvre is only performed if you suspect that the patient has meningism *(men-in-jism)*. The likeliest reason for looking for this sign is if you believe the patient has meningitis (see 'Neurological diseases and investigations' section). It can also be found in subarachnoid haemorrhage.

How to examine

Both hands are placed behind the head in a cradling fashion. The neck is then gently flexed forwards. If the patient has meningism, they will find this painful and will actively resist the movement. The diagnosis of meningitis demands clinical judgement and experience certainly helps. This judgement will be based on the history and examination. An experienced clinician may still perform a lumbar puncture even in the absence of Kernig's sign, Brudzinski's sign, or neck stiffness if they believe the clinical situation demands it.

Kernig's sign

Kernig's sign (*Vladimir Kernig (1840–1917), Russian physician*) is one of the classical tests for meningism (see Fig. 6.82). Along with Brudzinski's sign it is suggested that these signs are produced because the motor nerve roots are irritated as they are put on stretch as they pass

(a)

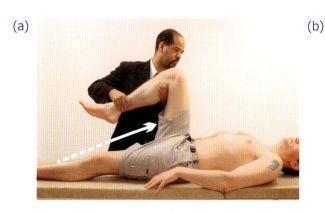

(b)

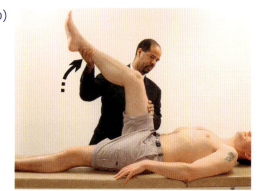

Figure 6.82 Eliciting Kernig's sign.

through the inflamed meninges. Although both signs are regarded as classical, their sensitivity is very poor. They will be negative in many cases that will go on to be proven meningitis.

How to examine

With the patient lying on their back, flex their hip to 90° as well as their knee. Then slowly extend the knee as far as you can. With meningism, you will be unable to extend the knee beyond 135° without eliciting pain and resistance. Some patients who are not very limber may also experience difficulty extending their knee fully. However, you should be able to coax them beyond 135° and there is no pain associated.

Brudzinski's sign

Brudzinski's (*brew-zin-skiz*) sign (*Jósef Brudzinski (1874–1917), Polish physician*) is another test for meningism. Again with the patient lying supine, place one hand behind the patient's head and the other on their chest. Then lift the patient's head while pressing down firmly on the chest to prevent the patient from rising off the bed. If the patient has meningism they will flex their hips and knees.

Hallpike–Dix manoeuvre

The Hallpike–Dix manoeuvre (*Margaret R. Dix (1922–1981) and Charles Hallpike (1900–1979), British neurologists*) is used in the investigation of vertigo (see Fig. 6.83). It is principally used to diagnose benign paroxysmal positional vertigo (BPPV) (see 'Neurological diseases and investigations' section) but it may unearth other disease as well. Before testing, first check that your patient does not have neck problems. Now sit your patient on a couch. Your aim is to get the patient to lie down on the couch so that their head and neck will dangle over the top of the couch. Either

sit them on the couch and estimate where they need to be to enable you to do this, or go through a 'dry run' by getting them into the required position and then getting them to sit up from there (be aware that you may stimulate vertigo while doing this). Now grasp the head and turn it 45° to one side. Warn your patient that you are going to lower them over the edge of the couch and it may set off their vertigo. If the vertigo occurs, tell them to keep their eyes open if at all possible and not to try to sit up (all natural reactions to the vertigo). Then briskly push the patient backwards until they are lying flat and continue to lower their head until it is about 30° below the level of the couch. Observe their eyes and be prepared to wait up to 10 seconds before anything happens.

If they have BPPV, after a latent period nystagmus may develop along with vertigo. The nystagmus is usually rotary, with the top part of the cornea rotating downward towards the affected ear. This is usually short lived, lasting no more than 20 seconds. If the patient sits up, they may experience milder vertigo and nystagmus can be seen but in the opposite direction to what was previously seen. If you repeat the test, vertigo and nystagmus may return but the duration will be less. After two or three repetitions this reaction will no longer be elicited and the nystagmus is termed fatiguable. If you do not elicit any reaction the first time, turn the patient's head 45° to the other side and repeat the manoeuvre. Sometimes with brainstem lesions, nystagmus may also be provoked with this test. In these cases there is usually no latent period before the onset of nystagmus and it does not fatigue with testing.

28 Make sure your patient is comfortable and thank them for their time

This is only polite.

29 Wash your hands

While you do this, you should continue to make sense of your findings.

30 Analysing your findings

You should attempt to interpret your results as you go along. Try to work out the significance of the signs you have elicited and gradually build up a picture of possible diseases (much like a jigsaw or identikit picture). Refine your thoughts with the information gained from your history-taking and do not be afraid to let your thoughts

(a)   (b)

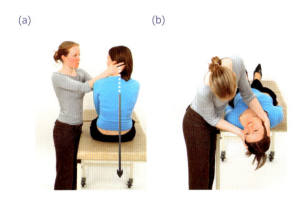

Figure 6.83 The Hallpike–Dix manoeuvre.

range beyond the neurological system. The neurology you unearth could be the result of disease in another system, for example, lung cancer with brain metastases or a paraneoplastic syndrome. As you learn more about neurological diseases you will automatically build on this framework and learn to spot emerging patterns that will guide you towards the location of a lesion if not the diagnosis itself. Although some diagnoses can be made from your neurological examination it is best to try and work out **where** the lesion is rather than what it is initially. Begin by asking the following.

1 Is the **motor** system affected or the **sensory** system affected? If both are affected begin by analysing the motor system first as this is the quickest to do and is less subjective.

2 If the motor system is affected, which of the following is it?

- a UMN lesion?
- a LMN lesion?
- a cerebellar lesion?
- an extrapyramidal lesion?

For cerebellar and extrapyramidal lesions the location is reasonably obvious but with UMN and LMN lesions there is still some work to be done.

3 If it is a **UMN** lesion is it **unilateral** or **bilateral**? (UMN = hypertonia, clonus, hyper-reflexia, extensor plantar.)

4 If it is a lesion causing **unilateral UMN** signs, where in the central nervous system is it? In both unilateral and bilateral UMN lesions you need to try and home in on the cause. The lesion can be anywhere from the spinal cord up through the brainstem to the cerebral cortex. The author finds the best way of 'pinning down' a unilateral UMN lesion is by analysing the pattern of weakness (in conjunction with other useful features) on either side of the midline.

Cortical lesions

	R	L
Face	weak	normal
Arm	weak	normal
Leg	weak	normal
Plantars	↑	↓

In this example the right side of the body is weak and as this is controlled by the contralateral cortex, the lesion is likely to be in the **left cerebral cortex**. Other features pointing to a cortical origin include disturbance of higher functions, including language, that is, dysphasias, neglect, hemianopias (*hemi-an-owe-pee-a*), decreased conscious level, and so on. The vascular territory affected will further influence the pattern of deficits.

Internal capsule

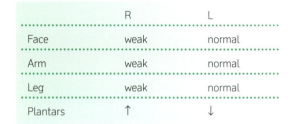

	R	L
Face	weak	normal
Arm	weak	normal
Leg	weak	normal
Plantars	↑	↓

Another possible cause of this configuration is a lesion in the internal capsule. Here all the motor and sensory fibres converge into a narrow area and hence a small lesion can lead to a major deficit. As this area is 'subcortical' there is no hemianopia, dysphasia, and so on.

Brainstem

	R	L
Face	normal	weak
Arm	weak	normal
Leg	weak	normal
Plantars	↑	↓

The key feature of a brainstem lesion is an ipsilateral deficit of a cranial nerve combined with a contralateral hemiplegia. In this example there is a lesion of the VIIth nerve on the **left side**, which will be an LMN lesion as it is at the level of the VIIth cranial nerve nucleus. However at this level the corticospinal tracts have not reached their crossing point further down in the medulla and therefore the arm and leg on the right side will be affected. Other cranial nerves can be affected, for example, an ipsilateral nerve III palsy with a contralateral hemiplegia (Weber's syndrome).

Spinal cord

	R	L
Face	normal	normal
Arm	normal	normal
Leg	weak	normal
Plantars	↑	↓

Any motor lesion below the brainstem (where the cortico-spinal tracts have crossed) will affect the limbs on the ipsilateral side. This example suggests a spinal cord lesion on the right side. As the arms are normal, this indicates that the lesion is below the level of its nerve supply. The likeliest position for the lesion is the thoracic cord (or possibly a high lumbar lesion). Additional sensory information will help in pin-pointing the lesion. If there is total involvement of one half of the spinal cord the resulting neurological pattern is called the Brown-Sequard (*seck-card*) syndrome (see Case 6.15).

5 If it is a lesion causing **bilateral UMN** signs, where in the central nervous system (CNS) is it? The method recommended for homing in on a lesion causing bilateral UMN signs is to look at the pattern of reflexes.

Cortical

Jaw jerk	brisk	
	R	L
Arm	brisk	brisk
Leg	brisk	brisk
Plantars	↑	↑

For a cortical lesion to cause bilateral UMN lesions, it has to span the midline (called a parasagittal (para-saj-it-tal) lesion). The resulting bilateral UMN weakness is called a spastic paraparesis. The brisk jaw jerk is the key to the cortical origin here. It implies a bilateral UMN lesion that must be above the brainstem. However a normal jaw jerk does not exclude a cortical origin. Therefore a CT or MRI scan of the brain is recommended. Causes include bilateral CVAs, MS, and a parasagittal tumour.

High cervical cord

Jaw jerk	normal	
	R	L
Arm	brisk	brisk
Leg	brisk	brisk
Plantars	↑	↑

This configuration suggests a lesion in the cervical cord. The brisk reflexes in the arms suggest the lesion is higher than its nerve supply. The normal jaw jerk suggests that the lesion is below the brainstem. However a normal jaw jerk does not exclude the possibility of a cortical lesion and so a CT or MRI scan of the head is important before focusing on imaging the cervical cord. A high cervical lesion such as transection of the cord following trauma can be fatal above C3 because this is the nerve supply to the diaphragm and would lead to respiratory failure. The paralysis of all four limbs is described as a quadriparesis or tetraparesis.

Cervical cord

Jaw jerk	normal	
	R	L
Arm	brisk/↓/absent	brisk/↓/absent
Leg	brisk	brisk
Plantars	↑	↑

This example suggests very strongly that the lesion is in the lower cervical cord. The mixture of brisk reflexes and diminished or absent reflexes (UMN and LMN signs) can lead to accurate localization. The diminished or absent reflexes (LMN) indicate the level of the lesion. The interrupted pyramidal tracts below this lesion will cause brisk reflexes in the area of supply, for example, an intervertebral disc pressing on the cord at the level of C5/C6 will cause LMN signs at C5/C6 (absent reflexes at C5/C6 = absent biceps/absent deltoid) and UMN signs at C7 and below (brisk reflexes at C7 = brisk triceps/brisk finger jerks).

CASE 6.15

Problem. A 57-year-old man was having difficulty walking and felt his right leg seemed stiff on occasion. He also noticed that his left leg felt funny but he could not elaborate further. You suspect a neurological cause and perform a full neurological examination. There are no cranial nerve abnormalities and the jaw jerk was normal. There were no neurological findings in the arms either. In the right leg you find increased tone and seven beats of clonus. There is grade 4/5 power in the leg, with hyper-reflexia and an extensor plantar. You also demonstrate loss of light touch, vibration sense, and proprioception in the right leg. In the left leg, the tone, power, and reflexes are normal except that you cannot elicit a plantar response. There is the loss of pain and temperature sensation in the left leg up to the umbilicus. What is going on?

Discussion. Using the knowledge you have gained from the preceding chapters and the simple stepwise approach just described, you can begin to break down what seems to be a complex case.

1 There are both motor and sensory components to the case, so concentrate on the motor side.

2 In the right leg the increased tone, clonus, hyper-reflexia, and extensor plantar point to a UMN lesion (the left leg seems normal from a motor perspective).

3 As it is a unilateral UMN problem you need to observe the pattern of weakness on either side of the midline. This looks like a monoparesis of the right leg as the cranial nerves and the arms are not affected. This suggests that the lesion is below the nerve supply of the arms, which puts it at the level of the thoracic spinal cord or below (but not below the L3, L4 as the knee jerks are brisk). As the corticospinal tracts have already crossed in the brainstem,

the lesion must be on the same side as the UMN signs, that is, the right half of the thoracic spinal cord (anteriorly).

4 Already you have a good idea where the lesion is likely to be but you still have to explain the sensory features (which appear bizarre at first glance).

5 Start with the right leg. There is the loss of light touch, vibration sense, and proprioception. This indicates damage to the dorsal columns. Pain and temperature sensation is normal on this side indicating a dissociated sensory loss, which supports a spinal cord lesion. As the dorsal column fibres do not decussate until high up in the cord, the loss of these modalities will be on the same side as the lesion, that is, the right half of the thoracic cord (posteriorly).

6 The left leg exhibits the loss of pain and temperature sense. Unlike the dorsal columns, the spinothalamic tracts cross within two segments of the spinal cord. Therefore the lesion will be on the right half of the thoracic spinal cord (laterally) also. There is further information here. The sensory loss extends to the umbilicus, which approximates to the T10 level. As the fibres cross within two spinal segments, the true level of the lesion should be around T8 in the spinal cord.

You can see the supporting role the sensory analysis played in this example (the sensory level did help in pin-pointing the lesion further). This case is known as the Brown-Sequard syndrome (*Charles Édouard Brown-Sequard (1817–1894), French neurologist/ physiologist*). It is seen rarely (particularly with the full-blown features) because it represents damage to an entire half of the spinal cord, which is not easy to produce naturally. It is useful however as an excellent teaching exercise in matching clinical signs with spinal cord anatomy.

Thoracic cord

Jaw jerk	normal	
	R	L
Arm	normal	normal
Leg	brisk	brisk
Plantars	↑	↑

This configuration suggests the lesion is below the level of the nerve supply to the arms, that is, below T1 of the thoracic cord. The brisk reflexes in both knees suggest that the lesion must be above L3/L4. This puts the lesion in the thoracic cord (more accurately between T1 and L3). Weakness that just affects the legs is called a paraparesis.

6 If it is a lesion causing **LMN** signs is it **unilateral** or **bilateral**? (LMN = wasting, fasciculations, hypotonia, diminished or absent reflexes, flexor plantars.)

7 If it is a lesion causing **unilateral LMN signs**, where in the peripheral nervous system is it? Again you need to try and home in on the cause. This is a little easier than for a UMN lesion. A lesion can be anywhere from the anterior horn cell in the spinal cord to the muscle end plates. It is easier to consider either a root lesion or a peripheral nerve lesion.

Root lesion

Spotting the difference between a root lesion and a peripheral nerve injury can be difficult as their presentations can be similar. The author tends to try and match the root values of the affected muscles with the root values of affected tendon reflexes and dermatomes. For example, **root lesion C5**—wasted and weak deltoid, supraspinatus (*soup-ra-spin-ate-us*), and infraspinatus:

- **movement affected**—shoulder abduction through the full range of movement (180°)
- **tendon reflexes affected**—deltoid (C5) absent and biceps (C5, C6) diminished or absent
- **dermatome affected**—C5 affected over the whole of the shoulder (pain may also be experienced in this area).

Compare this with an **axillary nerve lesion**—wasted and weak deltoid (teres (*terry's*) minor is not accessible to testing):

- **movement affected**—shoulder abduction **but** only after the first 90° of abduction
- **tendon reflexes affected**—none
- **sensory loss**—some sensory loss (or pain) over a small area of the shoulder tip.

Although many features are similar the distinguishing features are as follows.

	Root lesion	Axillary nerve palsy
Shoulder abduction	full 180° weak	second 90° weak
Tendon reflexes	absent deltoid	normal
	↓ biceps	normal

Peripheral nerve lesion

The previous example highlights the need to know the consequences of lesions to important nerve supplies to the limbs. This is the only way you can detect the patterns they produce (and sadly there are no shortcuts). Some important nerves are discussed in the following paragraphs.

8 If it is a lesion causing **bilateral LMN** signs, what is it? The emphasis here is different. Instead of trying to localize the lesion, the emphasis is on recognizing the pattern and hence the type of lesion.

- Bilateral proximal weakness affecting the arms and legs suggests a proximal myopathy (reflexes are unaffected and there are no sensory features).
- Bilateral distal weakness affecting the arms and legs suggests a motor peripheral neuropathy (reflexes ↓ or absent).
- It is a mixed motor/sensory peripheral neuropathy if there is an associated sensory loss in a glove and stocking distribution (do not forget that only the arms or the legs need be affected).

9 Is it a **sensory** lesion (or mixed)?

10 Analysing sensory impairment can be done for an isolated sensory lesion or a mixed motor/sensory lesion. In both cases the approach is the same. In mixed lesions it is recommended that the motor component is analysed first for the following reasons.

- In the author's neurological routine the motor system precedes the sensory system.
- The sensory examination is more subjective and can vary because of your technique (unequal stimuli) or the patient's personality (stoical versus obsessive).
- In some areas the overlap of adjacent sensory nerves can reduce the sensory deficit you would expect (this is particularly true in the arms).
- Sometimes an area of sensory impairment (or pain) can extend beyond the boundaries you would expect for a particular nerve supply.

The author simply separates sensory deficits into four main categories:

- affecting the whole limb (cortical/subcortical lesion?);
- affecting dermatomes (root lesion? peripheral nerve lesion?);
- distal limbs affected (peripheral neuropathy?);
- dissociated sensory loss (spinal cord lesion?).

See Fig. 6.84 for a flowchart summarizing the previous analyses.

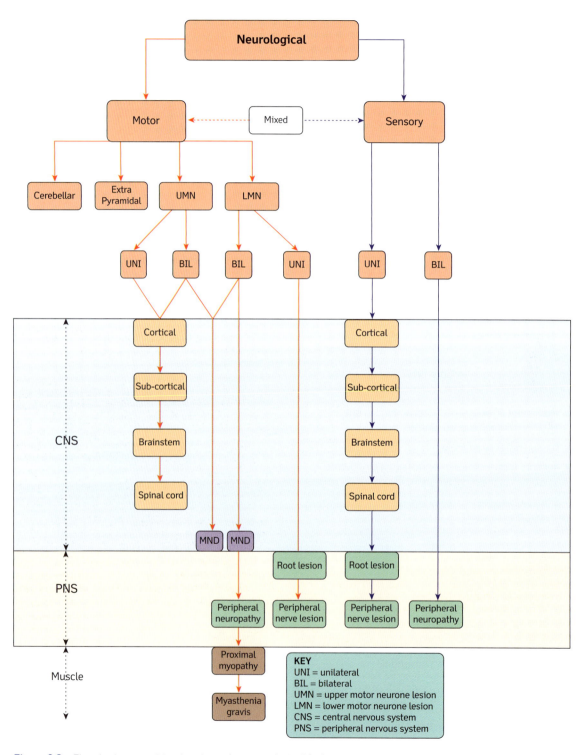

Figure 6.84 Flowchart summarizing how to analyse neurological findings.

Some important clinical presentations

Peripheral nerve lesions

Arms

Ulnar nerve palsy

A palsy is an old-fashioned term for paralysis. The ulna nerve arises from the medial cord of the brachial plexus (a network of nerve fibres, in turn arising from the nerve roots C5, C6, C7, C8, and T1, which eventually supplies the upper limb). It provides the motor and sensory supply to the medial aspect of the forearm and hand. Its root value is **C8, T1**. It can be damaged (1) at the elbow, following a fracture or stab wound or (2) at the wrist, by a stab wound as the nerve runs superficial to the flexor retinaculum (*ret-in-ack-you-lum*) (a fibrous band of connective tissue that forms a roof over the carpal tunnel).

Injury at the elbow

This causes wasting of the small muscles of the hand (except the thenar eminence (the mound of muscle at the base of the thumb) supplied by the median nerve).

- **Motor:** paralysis of abduction and adduction of the fingers (the patient will be unable to keep a piece of paper between their fingers, see earlier) and paralysis of adduction of the thumb (adductor pollicis brevis is the only muscle of the thenar eminence supplied by the ulnar nerve). There will be a positive Froment's sign. The combination of weakness and wasting together with the unopposed action of non-paralysed muscle leads to the production of a clawed hand (see Fig. 6.85).

(a)   (b)

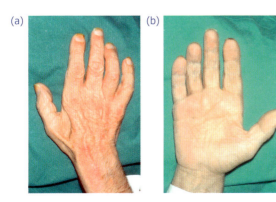

Figure 6.85 Ulnar claw hand.

- **Sensory:** loss of sensation over the medial half of the hand and medial one and a half digits on both palmar and dorsal surfaces.

Injury at the wrist

As for the elbow except there is (1) no involvement of the medial forearm muscles and (2) sparing of the sensation over the medial half of the dorsum of the hand.

Function

Despite these deficits the hand is still useful because the thumb and index finger remain functional both in motor and sensory terms and the vital pincer grip can be maintained.

Radial nerve palsy

The radial nerve arises from the posterior cord of the brachial plexus, (C5, C6, C7, C8, T1). It mainly supplies the triceps muscle (producing extension at the elbow), the long extensors of the forearm (extending the wrist and fingers), and sensation over the posterior aspect of the arm, forearm, lateral half of the hand, and lateral three and a half digits.

It can be damaged (1) in the axilla, due to upward pressure from a crutch or a drunk falling asleep with their arm dangling over the back of a chair, or due to downward traction on the nerve following a fracture dislocation of the neck of the humerus or (2) in the spiral groove of the humerus. This is a groove in the posterior aspect of the shaft of the humerus. The radial nerve can be injured due to a fracture of the shaft of the humerus or due to pressure from callus formation following a fracture or to a tightly fitting plaster cast. It can also occur in an unconscious patient if the back of the arm rests against a hard surface for a long time.

Injury in the axilla

- **Motor:** paralysis of the triceps muscle leading to loss of extension at the elbow and paralysis of the long extensors of the forearm leading to a wrist drop (see Fig. 6.86).
- **Sensory:** small area of anaesthesia over the posterior surface of the lower arm and forearm and a small variable area of loss over the lateral half of the dorsum of the hand and over the base of the thumb. Note that the area of loss is much less than expected due to overlapping innervation from neighbouring cutaneous nerves.

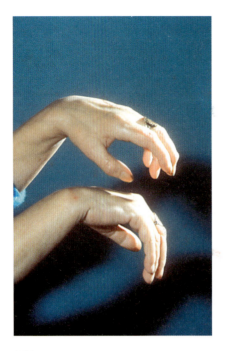

Figure 6.86 Bilateral wrist drop due to radial nerve palsy.

Injury in the spiral groove of the humerus

As above, except no paralysis of the triceps if the nerve is damaged in the distal part of the spiral groove and only a variable area of sensory loss around the root of the thumb.

Function

Motor function is affected adversely because of the wrist drop. In this position the long flexors of the forearm cannot flex the fingers and therefore grip is impaired. This can be overcome by passively extending the wrist, which allows the flexors to function and restore finger grip.

Median nerve palsy

The median nerve arises from the medial and lateral cords of the brachial plexus (C5, C6, C7, C8, T1). It mainly supplies the long flexor muscles of the forearm (except the medial component, which is supplied by the ulnar nerve), the muscles of the thenar eminence (except adductor pollucis brevis, which is supplied by the ulnar nerve), and sensation over the lateral half of the palm and lateral three and a half digits (palmar surface only). It can be damaged (1) at the elbow following a supracondylar (*soup-ra-con-dill-are*) fracture of the humerus, (2) at the wrist following a stab wound proximal to the flexor retinaculum, or (3) at the wrist due to compression in the carpal tunnel.

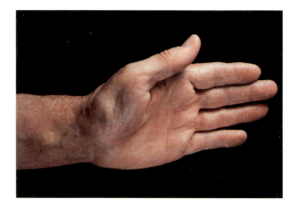

Figure 6.87 Carpal tunnel syndrome.
Reprinted from Fig 2.39 (p.217), *Atlas of Clinical Neurology* (2nd edn), by G. David Perkin, Fred Hochberg and Douglas C. Miller (1993), Mosby Publications, with permission from Elsevier.

Injury at the elbow

It causes wasting of the thenar eminence leading to a 'flattened' hand.

- **Motor:** wrist flexion is weak with deviation to the medial side due to the unopposed action of the flexor muscles under ulnar nerve control. There will be no finger flexion of the index and middle finger but there will be weak flexion of the ring and little finger because there is some innervation from the ulna nerve. The thumb is practically useless as flexion, abduction, and opposition is lost.
- **Sensory:** loss of sensation over the lateral half of the palm and the lateral three and a half digits (palmar surface).

Injury at the wrist following a stab wound proximal to the flexor retinaculum

As above, except the long flexors of the forearm are not affected.

Function

This is the most disabling nerve injury of the hand. The hand is rendered useless because of the loss of sensation over the thumb and index finger and the loss of the pincer grip.

Injury at the wrist due to compression in the carpal tunnel (carpal tunnel syndrome)

This is compression of the median nerve at the wrist as it travels under the flexor retinaculum. It causes wasting of the thenar eminence (see Fig. 6.87) and pain and tingling

Table 6.20 Causes of carpal tunnel syndrome

Idiopathic
Pregnancy, menopause, oral contraceptive pill
Rheumatoid arthritis
Myxoedema
Acromegaly
Amyloidosis
Gout

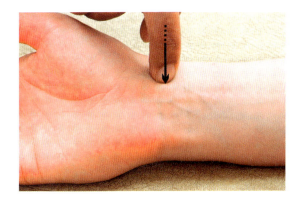

Figure 6.88 Tinel's test.

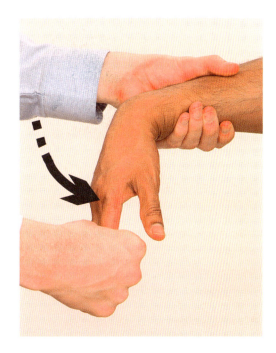

Figure 6.89 Phalen's test.

in the arm, hand, and lateral three and a half digits. This tends to be worse at night and is relieved by shaking the hands on waking. If Tinel's sign or Phalen's sign are positive this may add further weight to the diagnosis. Causes of carpal tunnel syndrome are given in Table 6.20.

Tinel's sign

See Fig. 6.88. This is an additional test if you suspect a carpal tunnel syndrome. To elicit Tinel's (*tin-elz*) sign (*Jules Tinel (1879–1952), French neurologist*) you percuss over the median nerve as it runs through the carpal tunnel at the wrist. To locate the nerve get your patient to flex their wrist slightly. This accentuates the tendon of palmaris longus (*pal-ma-riss-long-us*). Roll your index finger laterally over the tendon and tap about an inch from the wrist crease (in those patients who lack this tendon, locate the radial artery and aim slightly medial to this position about an inch from the wrist crease). The test is positive if the patient feels tingling or pain over the first three and a half digits of the hand, that is, paraesthesia in the distribution of the median nerve.

Phalen's sign

See Fig. 6.89. Phalen's (*fail-enz*) sign (*George Phalen (1911–1998), American orthopaedic surgeon*) is a further test you can perform if you suspect carpal tunnel syndrome. Ask the patient to flex the wrist of the affected hand for a minute. Patients with carpal tunnel syndrome develop paraesthesia in the distribution of the median nerve. The symptoms resolve quickly when the wrist is relaxed.

Legs

Sciatic nerve injury

This is the largest nerve in the body and is the continuation of a plexus of nerves from L4 and L5 along with S1, S2 and S3. It exits the pelvis between the greater trochanter and the ischial tuberosity into the buttock before descending in the posterior aspect of the thigh. It then divides into two main branches at the popliteal fossa, the tibial nerve (L3, L4, L5, S1, S2, S3) and the common peroneal nerve (L4, L5, S1, S2). It can be damaged by trauma such as fractures of the pelvis or posterior dislocation of the femur particularly in road traffic accidents. It can occasionally be injured by intramuscular injections in the buttock if the proper procedure is not carried out (IM injections should be targeted at the upper outer quadrant of the buttock to avoid this).

- **Motor:** This leads to foot drop as there is weakness of all the muscles below the knee particularly the dorsiflexors of the foot. Knee flexion will be weak.
- **Sensory:** There is loss of sensation over the posterior aspect of the whole leg and over the ankle and foot.

Common peroneal nerve palsy

Also known as lateral popliteal nerve palsy (L4, L5, S1, S2), this is commonly seen in patients who are bed bound for a long time or in patients with a plaster cast for a fracture of the leg. This is due to the injury of the lateral popliteal nerve around the neck of fibula.

- **Motor:** When the whole nerve is involved, foot drop ensues due to the weakness of dorsiflexors of the ankle and toes.
- **Sensory:** There is loss of sensation over the whole of the dorsum of the foot. Partial lesions will have less extensive sensory impairment.

Spinal cord compression

Extrinsic compression

Due to extradural or intradural, extramedullary lesions (see 'Neurological diseases and investigations' section).

Clinical features

- The patient may complain of localized back pain near the site of the lesion.
- In addition, if there is nerve root irritation there could be radicular pain experienced in the distribution of the nerve which can be precipitated by movement or sneezing.
- The patient may have mild spastic paraparesis with UMN signs below the level of the lesion. So the legs will have increased tone and feel stiff to the patient. They may also feel that they are dragging their legs when they become tired. Other signs in the leg may include clonus, hyper-reflexia, and bilateral upgoing plantars.
- They may have sensory involvement which may begin in the feet and ascend up the legs and trunk producing a sensory level. Below this level sensation in all modalities will usually be reduced or absent. This sensory level will typically be 2–3 spinal segments below the level of the lesion.

- Autonomic features may occur including bladder and bowel dysfunction. Initially there may be difficulty with initiating micturition, or urinary frequency but later urinary retention will occur which is a danger sign in spinal cord compression. The coexistent development of constipation is another red flag sign. A less well known feature is the development of a sweat level. There may be absent sweating below the level of the lesion due to sympathetic nerve involvement.

It must be pointed out that this is the expected feature for bilateral spinal cord involvement. However if roughly one half of the spinal cord is involved this will produce signs consistent with the Brown-Sequard syndrome (see Case 6.15).

....

Tip

A sweat level can be demonstrated by running your finger or a tuning fork slowly up the legs and trunk. In the absence of sweating your finger/tuning fork will glide effortlessly up the body but will 'catch' where there is an abrupt change in the skin as it becomes tackier where sweating resumes.

....

Intrinsic compression

Due to intradural, intramedullary lesions.

Clinical features

- Lesions within the cord usually occur centrally and disrupt the decussating fibres crossing to the lateral spinothalamic tract.
- Initially the patient may complain of pain in distribution of the nerves affected by the lesion.
- Later there may be subtle sensory loss to pain and temperature in the same area supplied by the affected nerves.
- The anterior horn cells at the affected level can be damaged and there may be LMN signs at that particular spinal level with loss of reflexes. As the tumour increases in size, the area of spinothalamic loss expands in a cape-like distribution over the shoulders, back, and upper arms. As the sacral fibres are the most peripheral, there is usually 'sacral sparing' of sensation bilaterally even with very large tumours. Corticospinal tracts are affected late and then UMN signs will be displayed in the legs.

- If the lesion occurs in the cervical cord then the sympathetic nerves can be affected and produce a unilateral or bilateral Horner's syndrome.

- Dorsal column involvement is very rare.

Cauda equina syndrome

This is the collection of signs caused by damage to the bundle of lumbar and sacral nerve roots emerging from the termination of the spinal cord.

Clinical features

- Low back pain.

- There may be pain in the leg depending on which nerve roots are irritated. Later there may be motor weakness and/or sensory loss in the distribution of the nerve roots.

- A typical pattern of sensory loss is saddle anaesthesia around the buttocks, upper thigh posteriorly, perineum and anus. If a rectal examination is performed the anal tone will be diminished leading to a lax sphincter.

- Sciatica, either unilateral or bilateral.

- Bladder disturbance, leading to difficulty in micturition and then urinary retention.

- Bowel disturbance leading to constipation.

- Sexual dysfunction.

31 Present your findings

If you are sure of the diagnosis, mention it at the beginning, for example:

This young man has amyotrophic lateral sclerosis, motor neuron disease. He has a spastic paraparesis, as evidenced by the posture of both legs, increased tone bilaterally and ankle clonus. He has grade 3/5 power bilaterally, exaggerated knee and ankle jerks with bilateral extensor plantar response, gross bilateral wasting of distal and proximal muscles with fasciculations. He has preserved sensation and coordination and no bladder involvement.

If the diagnosis is not obvious, do not panic. Students mistakenly believe that reaching a correct diagnosis is the single most important part of the examination. Your examiners are far more concerned with how competent your method of examination is and whether or not you have a courteous attitude to the patient. If you are unsure of the diagnosis then present your findings together with a reasonable differential diagnosis and possibly suggest further investigations, which may help resolve the situation.

For example,

There is increased tone in the arms bilaterally, with decreased power grade 4/5 in both arms. There is generalized hyper-reflexia in both arms with positive Hoffman's sign and finger jerks. This patient has evidence of upper motor neuron lesions in both arms and the possibilities include multiple sclerosis, motor neuron disease (although I did not see any wasting or fasiculations), a lesion in the cervical cord, or bilateral strokes. To try and determine the cause, I would normally take a full history and examine other aspects of the neurological system including legs and cranial nerves so as to guide my investigations. These might include MRI or a CT scan of the brain and cervical cord.

This final point is so important because it would be a waste of time and resources organizing a CT scan of the brain if you elicit signs that point to LMN pathology.

Neurological diseases and investigations

In earlier parts of this chapter, various medical conditions have been mentioned. In this section these will now be described. In general these descriptions are brief, though some important topics are described in more detail.

The brain

Meninges

The brain and spinal cord are covered by three membranes called the meninges. It is useful to understand the relationship of the meninges to the brain and spinal cord as it is helpful in understanding the various lesions that can afflict the CNS. The three layers are the dura mater (*d-your-a-may-tah*), the arachnoid (*a-rack-noy-d may-tah*) mater, and the pia mater (*pee-a-may-tah*).

Dura mater

The dura mater (Latin for 'hard mother') is the outer layer which is tough and fibrous and encases the brain. It also extends through the foramen magnum to cover the spinal cord throughout its extent as far as the S2 level.

As the cranial and spinal nerves exit the brain and spinal cord respectively the dura forms protective sheaths around them and becomes continuous with the connective tissue surrounding the nerve.

Arachnoid mater

Underneath the dura mater is a more delicate membrane called the arachnoid mater. It gets its name because its fibres resemble that of a spider's web. It is separated from the dura mater by a potential space called the subdural space. In the brain the arachnoid mater bridges the sulci (rather than following their contours) and in certain areas the membrane projects into venous sinuses to form arachnoid villi. At this point cerebrospinal fluid (CSF) can diffuse into the bloodstream. The arachnoid mater also continues through the foramen magnum to envelop the spinal cord under the dura mater.

Pia mater

The pia mater (Latin for 'soft mother') is a thin membrane which is highly vascular and is the innermost of the three membranes. It is closely applied to the brain surface and therefore follows all the gyri and sulci. It also fuses with specialized cells in the ventricles (called ependymal cells) to form the choroid plexuses. These participate in the formation of CSF. This CSF is essential for nourishing the cells of the brain and spinal cord as well as removing cellular waste. It also acts as a shock absorber to protect the CNS along with the meninges. The CSF circulates around the brain in a predetermined pattern around the ventricles and into the space between the pia mater and the arachnoid mater, called the subarachnoid space. The CSF eventually diffuses into the bloodstream via the arachnoid villi in the superior sagittal sinus.

Meningitis

A variety of infective (and non-infective) agents can inflame the meninges. Infective causes include viral, bacterial, protozoal, or fungal agents and non-infective causes include drugs and malignant cell infiltrates.

Viral meningitis

Any virus can cause meningitis. It is difficult to get an accurate picture of which organisms are the most common because many people with viral meningitis may not present themselves for medical help. The majority of those who present to hospital will not have viruses isolated (if they are looked for at all). With these reservations, the most common viruses are the enteroviruses such as echovirus and cocksackie (cock-sacky) virus. Clinically the

patient may have a prodrome of an influenza-type illness, for example, lassitude, muscle and joint pains, and fever. In addition they may develop severe headache and neck stiffness (a sign of meningeal irritation, called meningism). This form of presentation should lead to further investigation including lumbar puncture.

Bacterial meningitis

Bacteria may infect the meninges through blood-borne (haematogenous (he-mat-todger-nuss)) spread or there may be more direct spread following complications of head trauma, otitis media, or sinusitis.

The most common organisms are Neisseria meningitidis (nice-eerier-men-in-jitty-dis) (also called meningococcus) (men-in-go-cock-us), Streptococcus pneumoniae (strep-toe-cock-us-new-moan-i-ee) (also called pneumococcus) (new-mow-cock-us), and Haemophilus influenzae (heem-off-ee-lus-in-flu-en-zee). Clinically the patient will present with headache, neck stiffness, photophobia, vomiting, and drowsiness. Later complications such as fits, cranial nerve palsies, or hemiplegias may supervene. There may also be obstruction to the flow of CSF called hydrocephalus leading to a rise in intracranial pressure. Meningococcal meningitis is the form that everybody fears as rapid deterioration can occur with septicaemia and the patient can become comatose within hours. There is a high mortality rate associated with it.

One of the signs of septicaemia is the development of a purpuric rash that does not blanch. Lay sources of medical information tell the public to put a glass tumbler over the rash and apply gentle downward pressure. If the rash remains visible then the likelihood is high that this represents a serious development of meningitis (see Fig. 14.6). If in doubt the patient should get an immediate injection of penicillin without waiting for confirmatory tests. The investigation of choice is a lumbar puncture. However, if focal neurological signs, fits, or depressed conscious level are evident, then a CT scan should be performed first.

Other causes of meningitis

It is worth considering other infective and non-infective causes of meningitis in patients who are immunocompromised, for example, patients with AIDS or leukaemia or transplant patients on immunosuppressive drugs. In these cases unusual organisms such as fungi, amoebae, or tubercle bacilli may be responsible. Suspect these if your patient does not respond to first-line antibiotics (as recommended by your local hospital formulary). Occasionally malignant cells can invade the meninges, for example, leukaemic cells, and produce an inflammatory reaction. There should, however, be clues to the malignant process else-where in the body or blood film, as well as clues in the CSF.

Encephalitis

There are a variety of viral agents that can infect the brain directly. In the UK, herpes simplex is the most common cause of encephalitis, although with the increasing number of HIV infections this will assume greater notoriety in the future. Some organisms seem to have a predilection for certain areas of the brain, for example, herpes simplex—the temporal lobes and the virus in encephalitis lethargica—the basal ganglia. In other countries more 'exotic' viruses may cause spectacular disease and may be transmitted by a range of vectors including mosquitoes and ticks.

Clinically there is an acute onset of headache usually associated with a fever. There is usually a fluctuating conscious level and there may be evidence of focal signs such as cranial nerve palsies or hemiparesis. There may be meningism and seizures may occur. Investigations usually include a CT scan to rule out other pathology such as brain tumour, a lumbar puncture, and sometimes electroencephalography, because the diagnosis may still not be clear following these procedures. The treatment includes supportive measures such as intravenous fluids, anti-convulsive therapy, and intravenous aciclovir (*ay-sigh-clo-veer*) or other similar anti-viral treatment, if herpes simplex encephalitis is suspected.

Space-occupying lesion in the cranium

Because the cranium is a closed box any mass lesion will increase the pressure within the confined space as there is nowhere for the pressure to be dissipated. Lesions include tumours, haemorrhage, and abscesses.

Regardless of the nature of the cause symptoms include:

- Headache which is worse in the morning on waking, when lying down, when bending forwards, or coughing and sneezing.
- Nausea and vomiting.
- Seizures both focal and generalized.
- Occasionally a nerve VI palsy. During its long intracranial course the sixth nerve can become compressed against the tip of the petrous bone as the brainstem is pushed downwards. An isolated nerve VI palsy should raise the possibility of raised intracranial pressure. In this circumstance this is known as a false localizing sign (because the lesion is not located in the brainstem as you might predict).

- Other features will be dictated by the site of the lesion e.g. hemiparesis, personality change, confusion, etc.

Eventually the pressure becomes so great that the brainstem can be forced downwards through the foramen magnum; this phenomenon is called **coning** and is a fatal complication.

Central nervous system tumours

These can be primary or secondary.

- **Primary brain tumours** arise from the variety of nerve cells (and other cell lines) within the brain and spinal cord. Table 6.21 is not comprehensive but reflects the tumours you are more likely to hear about or are mentioned previously in this chapter.
- **Secondary tumours** are the commonest form of tumour to affect the brain or spinal cord. They usually spread from lung, breast, bowel and kidney primaries.

Astrocytoma

Astrocytes are one of the glial cells that support the neurons in their function. An astrocytoma is the commonest benign tumour and can be found in the brain and rarely in the spinal cord (intramedullary). Histologically different grades exist from the well-differentiated tumour to the most malignant, poorly differentiated tumour which is locally invasive.

Table 6.21 Primary brain tumours

Neuroepithelial	
	Astrocytoma
	Oligodendroglioma
	Ependymoma
	Glioblastoma multiforme
Meningeal	
	Meningioma
Tumours of cranial and spinal nerves	
	Neurofibroma
	Neuroma
Haemopoietic tumours	
	Lymphoma
Pituitary tumours	

Oligodendroglioma

Oligodendrocytes are another of the supportive glial cells, some of which help to produce and maintain the myelin sheath of neurons. Oligodendrogliomas tend to be slow growing. They can occasionally be found in the spinal cord (intramedullary).

Ependymoma

Ependymal cells are glial cells which line the cerebral ventricles and tend to be in contact with the CSF. An ependymoma can rarely cause spinal cord compression (intradural tumour; either intramedullary or extramedullary) or cauda equina syndrome.

Meningiomas

These are benign slow-growing tumours that arise from the dura mater. They cause symptoms depending on where they are situated. They can grow in the spinal cord where they produce intradural extramedullary tumours.

Neurofibroma

This is a hybrid tumour consisting of Schwann cells and fibroblasts. They tend to affect spinal nerves but can involve cranial nerves. In the spine they produce intradural extramedullary tumours which are slow growing. As they grow through the intervertebral foramina, this narrow opening gives the tumour a 'waist' and eventually a dumbbell appearance. There is also an association with the syndrome of neurofibromatosis. There are two main types of neurofibromatosis which both have an autosomal dominant inheritance but with a variable penetrance meaning that many of the possible features of the syndrome will manifest in one individual but only a handful in others. Type 1 neurofibromatosis is more common and is also called Von Recklinghausen's (*wreck-ling-house-enz*) disease (*Friedrich Daniel Von Recklinghausen (1833–1910), German pathologist*). It is associated with cutaneous lesions such as café-au-lait spots (usually more than five of these brownish pigmented lesions), subcutaneous neurofibroma, and skin fibromata. In a rare form of neurofibromatosis there can be an exuberant overgrowth of neurofibromas leading to gross deformities. It was initially thought that the 'Elephant Man' was a product of this rare variant. This is now disputed and another even rarer syndrome (Proteus syndrome) has been suggested as the cause. About 1% of patients with neurofibromatosis will have phaechromocytoma (*fay-chrome-owe-site-owe-ma*) (a tumour of the adrenal medulla).

Neuromas

These are sometimes called schwannomas or neurilemmomas. They are slow growing and behave similarly to neurofibromas. They are also found on spinal nerves or on cranial nerves. In the spine they are a cause of intradural extramedullary tumours. If the vestibular portion of cranial nerve VIII is affected it is called an acoustic neuroma.

Acoustic neuromas

Ninety-five per cent are unilateral and 5% are bilateral. There is an association with neurofibromatosis (type 2) especially with bilateral tumours. Sensorineural hearing loss is the initial symptom and it may be gradual enough to be dismissed by the patient as part of the ageing process. Occasionally hearing loss can be sudden (any sudden hearing loss warrants investigation by an ENT surgeon). Other symptoms include tinnitus and vertigo.

The tumour is slow growing and may enlarge over many years. As it enlarges it may compress surrounding cranial nerves and neural structures. There may be a LMN facial nerve palsy. The trigeminal nerve may be affected, leading to a depressed corneal reflex and facial numbness. Very large tumours can occasionally cause dysphagia by affecting the lower cranial nerves IX and X. They may also compress the brainstem and cerebellum causing raised intracranial pressure and ataxia. The investigation of choice is an MRI scan, although high-resolution CT scanners can detect tumours as small as 1 cm. The treatment is surgical excision.

Glioblastoma multiforme

These are highly malignant tumours which are poorly differentiated on histological examination. They are very invasive and the prognosis is usually poor. It can rarely produce an intramedullary tumour of the spinal cord.

CNS lymphoma

Lymphomas are malignant tumours of the lymphatic cells which are an integral part of the immune system. As the immune system permeates every part of the body a lymphoma can manifest in the brain and spinal cord as well as other parts of the body. If they arise in the brain or spinal cord they are termed a primary CNS lymphoma. If they metastasize to the brain from other primary tumours elsewhere in the body then they are secondary tumours. This distinction is important because the treatment approach to primary and secondary CNS lymphoma is different. Primary CNS lymphomas are more common in immunosuppressed patients and usually have a poor prognosis. The commonest type of lymphoma seen is the non-Hodgkin's B-cell lymphoma.

Pituitary tumours

The pituitary is a small gland responsible for a large array of hormones that regulate the body's growth, development and metabolism. Like the conductor in an orchestra the pituitary exerts effects on other glands in the body such as the adrenals, thyroid, sex organs, etc. Unlike the other tumours it does not grow to a size where it causes raised intracranial pressure. Instead it causes complications because of local expansion such as compression of the optic chiasma or optic nerve superiorly. If the tumour is a functioning adenoma it may produce systemic effects by the overproduction of a particular hormone. Thus excess production of prolactin leads to galactorrhoea, excess growth hormone causes giantism in prepubertal individuals and acromegaly in adults, excess thyroid stimulating hormone causes thyrotoxicosis, etc.

Intracranial haemorrhage

This is bleeding within the skull or brain. It is usually classified according to which structures within the cranial cavity the blood accumulates. Therefore bleeding can be extradural, subdural, subarachnoid, intraventricular or intracerebral. Sometimes you may see the terms intra-axial or extra-axial haemorrhage. Extra-axial means outside the CNS, and intra-axial means within. In the context of intracranial haemorrhage this means outside and inside the brain respectively. The relationship between these terms is demonstrated in Table 6.22.

Extradural haemorrhage

This usually occurs acutely because of a head injury leading to a skull fracture. The fracture can lead to the rupture of blood vessels (usually the middle meningeal vessels) which bleed into the potential space between the skull and the dura. If the middle meningeal artery is involved there may be a rapid rise in intracranial pressure.

Table 6.22 Extra- and intra-axial haemorrhage

Extra-axial haemorrhage
Extradural (or epidural) haemorrhage
Subdural haemorrhage
Subarachnoid haemorrhage
Intra-axial haemorrhage
Intraventricular haemorrhage
Intracerebral haemorrhage

Symptoms depend on the severity of the trauma. In serious cases the patient may die or remain comatose. In less severe cases the patient may not lose consciousness or may lose it for a short period only. If these patients are seen in the emergency department, they must be given written head injury instructions so a guardian or carer can respond to any developing complications. This is because a proportion of patients with extradural haematoma have what is called a lucid period before they deteriorate.

Clinical features

The patient may develop headache, vomiting, dizziness or blurred vision. There may be increasing confusion. The development of a unilateral dilated pupil is an ominous sign. This is because as the intracranial pressure rises and begins to distort the brainstem, the third nerve can become compressed. As the parasympathetic pupillary fibres are peripherally placed, these are damaged preferentially leading eventually to a fixed dilated pupil (compare with nerve III palsy). This is why pupillary size and reactivity are one of the features assessed in the Glasgow Coma Scale (GCS). As the brainstem is pushed further across, the opposite nerve III also becomes compressed and ultimately both pupils become fixed and dilated. There may be other neurological signs such as the development of hemiparesis or even seizures. If any of these signs develop then this is a medical emergency. Diagnosis can be made by CT scanning or MRI and the treatment is usually surgical intervention to remove the clot.

Subdural haemorrhage

This can be acute or chronic.

Acute

The acute form may occur after a high-impact injury which subjects the brain to large acceleration and deceleration forces. These forces may be sufficient to rupture the veins that bridge the subdural space leading to the accumulation of blood in that space. This can lead to a rapid increase in intracranial pressure. Again this is a medical emergency and surgical evacuation is required to relieve the pressure. The mortality rate is high for acute subdural bleeds.

Chronic

The chronic form occurs more commonly in older people, alcoholics, and children. In some older people and alcoholics there is cerebral atrophy which leads to shrinkage of the brain and a corresponding enlargement of the subdural space. The bridging veins become stretched and tend to be more friable. As a result they are more prone to rupture even with minimal trauma. In up to 50% of cases a history of trauma cannot be accurately determined. Shortly after a bleed occurs a membrane forms around the haematoma. Sometimes the haematoma slowly resolves but in other cases it continues to grow. Why this happens is unclear and there have been two main theories that attempt to explain this. The osmotic theory suggests that the breakdown of protein within the clot increases the osmotic pressure in the haematoma hence drawing fluid through the enclosing membrane. However, this has largely been discredited because it has been demonstrated that the osmotic pressure is equal in the haematoma and surrounding fluid. The current view is that recurrent bleeding into the haematoma is the more likely cause.

It can take weeks or months for the symptoms to become manifest. The elderly patient may present with increasing confusion and/or fluctuating drowsiness. They may suffer vague headaches and focal neurological deficits may be found. They may also develop seizures. Subdural haematomas can mimic many different neurological conditions and the key to the diagnosis is considering its possibility in the first place. It can be diagnosed by CT scan or MRI scan and treatment can be conservative either if the lesion is small and not causing raised intracranial pressure or if the patient has multiple comorbidities where the risk of surgery is too great. Treatment is surgical evacuation usually through burr holes.

Subarachnoid haemorrhage

This is a bleed into the subarachnoid space, usually as a result of the rupture of an intracranial aneurysm or arteriovenous malformation. Clinically this haemorrhage leads to the sudden onset of severe headache 'like being hit with a baseball bat'. If the haemorrhage is severe the patient may collapse and die. Otherwise they may become comatose within hours. They may also develop fits and focal neurological signs (an expanding aneurysm may produce signs prior to a haemorrhage, for example, posterior communicating artery aneurysm leading to a complete nerve III palsy).

Those with milder degrees of haemorrhage may have headache with neck stiffness (neck stiffness may be absent in 30% of cases). The initial investigation is by CT or MRI scan.

If no blood is seen this does not rule out a subarachnoid haemorrhage and a lumbar puncture should be performed to look for xanthochromia (zan-throw-chrome-ia) (a breakdown product of blood) in the CSF. This is usually seen 5–12 hours after a haemorrhage and can be present in the CSF for up to 40 days. Patients with a proven subarachnoid haemorrhage need cerebral angiography and any aneurysm demonstrated needs clipping to prevent a further bleed.

Intraventricular haemorrhage

This is commoner in infants and particularly premature babies. Why it occurs in children is not clear but it is assumed that the blood vessels in premature babies in particular are very fragile. Small bleeds may not cause any long-term sequelae but larger bleeds can lead to hydrocephalus and also raised intracranial pressure. In adults this is usually due to severe trauma and the prognosis is poor. There is no specific treatment for this condition and a number of experimental treatments using diuretics, repeated lumbar punctures, streptokinase and ethamsylate in children have proven disappointing.

Intracerebral haemorrhage

See 'Stroke'.

Stroke

This is one of the most common neurological cases. A stroke is defined as a sudden onset of focal neurological deficit due to a vascular event. Eighty per cent are due to thrombosis or thromboembolism (from a carotid artery plaque or the heart). Other causes you should be aware of include intracranial haemorrhage for example, rupture of an intracerebral artery, subarachnoid (sub-arack-noid), subdural (sub-due-ral), or extradural haemorrhage (see Table 6.22) or spontaneous haemorrhage in a patient taking aspirin or warfarin and vasculitic disorders (including SLE, infective endocarditis, and temporal arteritis).

Risk factors

The risk factors are hypertension, hypercholesterolaemia (high-per-coal-est-er-ol-eem-ia), diabetes mellitus, smoking, increasing age, positive family history, and hyperviscosity states (e.g. polycythaemia, oral contraceptive). In thromboembolic stroke important additional factors include atrial fibrillation and recent myocardial infarction. The primary risk factors for intracerebral haemorrhage include hypertension, anti-platelet and anti-coagulant drugs, and bleeding disorders.

Symptoms

The symptoms depend on the area of brain affected and are described individually in the following sections. As mentioned earlier in the chapter, strokes tend to cause an absence of symptoms, so beware of diagnosing a patient with stroke disease if they present with 'positive' symptoms such as paraesthesia. Another common misconception is that strokes cause blackouts; this is rarely the case.

Classification of stroke disease

One method used is based on the duration of symptoms: transient ischaemic attack if duration is less than 24 hours; stroke if duration is greater. A more recent method has attempted to correlate the clinical features with the blood supply to the brain, which will be outlined next. This classification is more useful because it gives a rough guide to the prognosis of a stroke patient and is simple enough to be used in research protocols.

Blood supply to the brain

The blood supply is categorized into anterior and posterior subdivisions. The anterior circulation is derived from the carotid arteries. These give rise to the anterior and middle cerebral arteries, which take part in a circle of anastomosing vessels on the base of the brain known as the circle of Willis. From this circle further vessels arise, which supply the substance of the brain. The posterior circulation is derived from the two vertebral arteries that ascend in the neck and join to form the basilar artery. Branches from this, for example, the posterior cerebral artery, form the posterior part of the circle of Willis.

Classification of stroke

- **Total anterior circulation syndrome (TACS)**. This is the result of infarction of the entire area supplied by the carotid circulation on one side. Clinically there is a triad of
  - contralateral motor or sensory loss
  - hemianopia
  - disorder of language—dysphasia (if the left hemisphere is involved) or neglect/agnosia (if the right hemisphere is involved).

  Prognosis is poor and risk of recurrence is low.
- **Partial anterior circulation syndrome (PACS)**. This is the term used when only two of the above three clinical features are present. Prognosis is more favourable than for TACS. Risk of recurrence is high, hence the importance of identifying and treating risk factors for stroke.
- **Lacunar syndrome (LACS)**. Unlike TACS or PACS, which are usually caused by large vessel thrombosis, a lacunar (*la-koon-ar*) infarct is caused by disease of a small vessel within the substance of the brain. A typical presentation would be an isolated motor or sensory loss or ataxia of a limb. However, a significant deficit

may nevertheless result, for example, a lacunar infarct of the internal capsule may cause a dense hemiparesis, via involvement of the pyramidal tracts. Prognosis is good and risk of recurrence is high.
- **Posterior circulation syndrome (POCS)**. This refers to strokes occurring in the territory supplied by the vertebrobasilar (*ver-ti-bro-baz-ee-lar*) system. Typical symptoms include vertigo, vomiting, and nystagmus (due to involvement of the vestibular system), diplopia (due to opthalmoplegia caused by ipsilateral third or sixth cranial nerve paralysis), dysphagia (due to palsy of the cranial nerves supplying the palate), and contralateral sensory or motor loss. Prognosis is variable and risk of recurrence is high.

Investigations

- **Blood tests**, including full blood count (polycythaemia?), glucose (diabetes?), erythrocyte sedimentation rate (ESR) (vasculitis?), and urea and electrolytes (degree of hydration?).
- **Electrocardiogram (ECG)**—myocardial infarction? atrial fibrillation?
- **Chest radiograph**—intracerebral metastasis rather than stroke?
- **Carotid duplex** (*due-plex*) is useful if your patient has had a stroke in the anterior circulation territory and would be fit for a carotid endarterectomy (*end-art-er-wreck-tummy*) in the future.
- A **cardiac ultrasound** may be useful (particularly if your patient has atrial fibrillation).
- **CT scanning** is useful in two situations: to rule out haemorrhage (if you are contemplating starting aspirin) and if you suspect a diagnosis other than stroke, for example, tumour or abscess.

Treatment

- Aspirin for thrombotic and thromboembolic infarcts if the patient is able to swallow.
- If the patient also has atrial fibrillation then warfarin is given after an interval unless there are contraindications.
- Risk factors are treated.
- Rehabilitation of the patient is undertaken via a multidisciplinary approach.
- Prevention of complications (bedsores and contractures, aspiration pneumonia, and depression).

Benign intracranial hypertension

This is also called pseudotumour cerebri (*serry-bry*) and idiopathic intracranial hypertension. This is a condition where intracranial pressure rises for reasons that are unclear. It affects females more than males, particularly those who are overweight. It has a peak onset between the ages of 20 and 40 years. It can occur suddenly or have a gradual onset. Symptoms are those associated with raised intracranial pressure, including headache, nausea, and vomiting. Fundoscopy will usually demonstrate papilloedema (unless the onset is sudden and the eyes have not had time to develop changes). A CT scan is required to rule out a SOL. Following a normal scan a lumbar puncture should be performed and the CSF pressure measured. If the pressure is raised this confirms diagnosis of BIH. Some cases resolve spontaneously. Others respond to diuretics or steroids. Treatment may also require repeated lumbar punctures to remove CSF in a bid to relieve the pressure. In refractory cases shunts may be used to divert CSF from the cerebral ventricles but these procedures have risks and complications of their own.

Epilepsy

To the lay public, epilepsy conjures up an unconscious person who convulses, jerking all four limbs rhythmically. Some believe people with epilepsy are likely to be mentally impaired or become that way as a result of a fit. The latter assertion is clearly untrue as the majority of people with epilepsy are of normal intelligence. The classical 'grand-mal' seizure is just one way in which an epileptic person might present and the definitions of epilepsy and seizures will give clues as to why this might be.

Epilepsy: what is it?

This is a pathological state where a person has a continuing susceptibility to seizures.

Seizures: what are they?

This is the physical manifestation of paroxysmal, uncontrolled discharges of neuronal activity occurring anywhere in the brain. Therefore a seizure can produce a variety of clinical presentations depending on the area of brain affected.

Classification

What follows represents a simplified classification based on the International League of Epilepsy recommendations. Seizures can be generalized or partial (local).

Generalized seizures

A generalized seizure is where the electrical discharge spreads to both cerebral hemispheres simultaneously. Consciousness is impaired and there may or may not be convulsions evident. If this occurs from the outset, the seizure is termed primary generalized. Generalized seizures may be atonic, tonic, clonic, tonic–clonic, myoclonic, or absences.

With **atonic seizures**, the person loses control of all voluntary muscles and falls to the floor. With **tonic seizures** these muscles contract leading to rigidity. Again the patient will fall to the floor because they are unable to make any postural corrections. With **clonic seizures** the person exhibits jerking of the limbs and trunk as the muscles contract and relax alternately. With **tonic–clonic seizures** this clonic phase will follow the period of tonic contraction. Tonic–clonic seizures are what the lay public recognize as fits and what used to be termed grand-mal seizures. **Myoclonic seizures** are seizures that are described as rhythmical, shock-like jerking movements that are less coarse and violent than clonic seizures. An **absence seizure** is a non-convulsive episode usually seen in childhood and is synonymous with 'petit-mal' seizure. This usually manifests as a period of vacant staring often attributed to day-dreaming and is usually short lived.

Partial seizures

Partial seizures (also called focal seizures) are those where the electrical activity is confined to a focal area of the brain. Partial seizures are further subdivided into simple and complex partial seizures. Simple partial seizures are those where consciousness is not affected and complex partial seizures are those where consciousness is impaired. Simple partial seizures produce effects depending on which area of the brain is affected. This could be motor, sensory, autonomic, disturbed memory, speech abnormality, and so on. The electrical disturbance may spread and consciousness may become impaired, that is, the seizure becomes a complex partial one. If this disturbance spreads to both hemispheres then it will become a secondary generalized seizure. One particularly dramatic demonstration of this spread of activity is the 'Jacksonian (*jack-sew-knee-an*) march' (John Hughlings-Jackson (1835–1911), UK neurologist). This is a focal seizure, which has progressive motor effects. It may start with the twitching of a hand before spreading up the arm to the trunk and lower leg. This form of seizure is uncommon. A complex partial seizure may commence from the outset or develop from a simple partial seizure. Many of these seizures originate in the temporal lobe and the phenomenon was therefore named temporal lobe epilepsy.

Presentation

A generalized seizure, whether primary or secondary, will present in the same manner. In a typical tonic–clonic seizure, the first phase is the tonic phase. All the muscles of the body contract and the body goes rigid. At this stage the patient may give out a cry as the contraction of the respiratory muscles forces air out of the larynx. In the tonic stage the person falls rigidly to the ground with the possibility of injury. The contraction of other muscle groups can lead to tongue biting and urinary and possibly faecal incontinence. During this phase there is no flow of oxygen into the lungs and the patient becomes rapidly cyanosed (this is the presentation for pure tonic seizures before recovery). This may last up to a minute before the clonic phase supervenes. There follows rhythmic jerking of the limbs and trunk, which may last several minutes. 'Frothing at the mouth' may be caused by the convulsing jaws churning up saliva that has pooled in the mouth (a purely clonic fit will exhibit these features only). A period of unconsciousness follows before recovery. When they recover from a fit an epileptic person is usually confused for a variable length of time, called the postictal period ('ictal' means fit).

For some elderly patients this can last several hours or even days (the possibility of epilepsy should always be considered in older patients with recurrent confusional states that evade diagnosis). Occasionally a series of seizures may follow each other concurrently (called status epilepticus) and this is a medical emergency. The patient is in danger of dying of cardiorespiratory failure and prompt treatment is therefore required. Some patients may experience an aura prior to a convulsion. This may be a smell, taste, or strange indefinable feeling. These auras represent simple partial seizures experienced as a prelude to a secondary generalized seizure. Some recognize their auras as harbingers of a fit and attempt to get to a place of safety before the onset of the seizure.

Simple partial seizures produce clear-cut symptoms depending on the area of the brain affected. It may not always be easy to attribute the more unusual manifestations of these seizures to epilepsy, for example, recurrent disturbance of mood, strange sensations, and so on unless the possibility is borne in mind. Complex partial seizures involve impairment of consciousness, which may be partial, so that the patient has some awareness of events happening around them. Things may seem unreal (a situation called jamais-vu (*jam-ay-voo*)) or there may be a sense of experiencing events over again (called déjà vu (*day-jah-voo*)). The patient may also experience hallucinations, which may involve any sense including visual, taste, or smell. Even with the total loss of conscious control, the patient may still be able to exhibit complex behaviour patterns without memory (called automatism). Following a seizure the patient may feel exhausted and confused and they may have a headache.

Causes

There are many causes of epilepsy, ranging from genetic syndromes, which are inherited, to acquired causes such as trauma or stroke. In addition there are circumstances where illness or antisocial behaviour can lead to seizures without the patient being epileptic, for example, electrolyte imbalance or alcohol or drug misuse. In some cases the cause of epilepsy is unknown and is called idiopathic epilepsy. What is increasingly clear is that with the refinement of diagnostic tools such as CT or MRI scanning, structural lesions have been found in cases that would have been labelled idiopathic in the past. The final point to make is that certain causes of seizures predominate at different stages of life.

Some epileptic people can find their seizures precipitated by stress, anorexia, alcohol, or lack of sleep. Some can have epilepsy triggered by flickering lights and even music (sometimes called reflex epilepsy). Those controlled on anti-convulsants may find they lose control because the addition of drugs can interfere with the metabolism of the anticonvulsant and lead to inadequate drug levels.

Treatment

The treatment of epilepsy is beyond the scope of this book. It involves the specialized knowledge of different age groups—children, adults, and elderly people—plus dealing with circumstances such as the treatment of women in pregnancy. Certain principles need to be followed including the following:

- Identify an underlying cause and remove or modify the cause if possible.
- If the cause cannot be cured the patient will need stabilizing with anti-convulsant therapy.
- The patient will also need educating about epilepsy and how to live with it.
- Families and carers also need education.
- Driving is an issue and patients cannot drive in the UK until they are seizure free for a year.

Migraine

Migraine is an episodic headache that usually lasts 4–72 hours. It affects females more than males. Migraine tends to be unilateral and may cause headaches of such severity that it disrupts the patient's life (many taking to their beds in a darkened room). The pain is usually described as throbbing or pounding and is usually associated with nausea, photophobia, phonophobia, or osmophobia (aversion to certain smells). Many sufferers endure one to five attacks per month although a small minority may have more frequent attacks. Some patients recognize triggers to their migraines including stress, diet, fatigue, loss of sleep, oversleeping, bright lights, and hormonal changes in women.

Migraine used to be described as classical if an aura was experienced and common if not. Now this is simply called migraine with or without an aura. Visual disturbances include photophobia and blurring of vision. A variety of visual aura can be experienced including flashing lights or colours (photopsia) and zigzag shapes (fortification spectra or teichopsia). Later scotomas or visual field defects may develop. Auras usually last about 30 minutes and rarely last more than 2 hours. More unusual manifestations of migraine include paraesthaesiae, numbness, paralysis (hemiplegic migraine), speech disturbances, vertigo, and ataxia. Many of these symptoms may precede the onset of headache by several hours and in some circumstances it can be difficult to determine whether the patient has suffered a transient ischaemic attack rather than a migraine attack.

The diagnosis of migraine is made through the history. Examination and investigations such as CT head scans are to rule out the possibility of other disease. Always be suspicious of anyone who develops migraines for the first time over the age of 40 years old. The treatment of migraine includes the use of analgesia and anti-emetics in the acute attacks. In those prone to more severe headaches there is ergotamine or 5-hydroxytryptamine (serotin) agonists, for example, sumatriptan, which are particularly useful during an acute attack. If a migraineur (*me-grain-err*) suffers frequent attacks every attempt should be made to unearth any triggers and failing this drugs such as pizotifen (*pies-hot-i-fen*), β-blockers, and methysergide (*meth-ee-surge-hide*) (resistant cases) can be used as preventatives.

Tension headache

This is the most common form of headache. It is usually bilateral and tends to get worse in the evening. It is usually associated with stress. It can be a generalized dull ache in the frontal or occipital regions and sometimes it can be experienced as a tight band or a feeling of pressure on the top of the head. It is unusual for it to be associated with photophobia or phonophobia. The underlying cause of tension headaches is not known although there

may be abnormal muscular contraction (hence the old term contraction headache). It does not respond readily to analgesics but some may respond to amitryptylline (an anti-depressant with analgesic properties). Occasionally patients who have chronic headache that has been assumed to be tension headache may respond to migraine treatment, suggesting some overlap between these two conditions.

Cluster headaches

Cluster headaches produce severe, excruciating pain and affect males more than females. They tend to affect people between the ages of 20 and 50 years. The pain is usually unilateral and experienced around and behind the eye. The pain has been described as sharp, stabbing, or burning in nature and is so severe that the patient can literally bang their head against the wall out of despair. The affected eye may become red and watery and there may be rhinorrhea (a runny nostril) on the ipsilateral side. There may also be an associated Horner's syndrome. In some cases the headache can be triggered by alcohol. Some may experience one to two attacks in the day but this can be as many as seven in a day for others. As the name suggests the headaches occur in clusters and there can be attacks spanning up to 2 months before symptoms abate. Treatments that are used for migraine are often used for cluster headaches with good effect. There is a tendency for cluster headaches to burn out in the fourth or fifth decade.

Benign paroxysmal positional vertigo

This is the hallucination of movement that is triggered by certain positions of the body. Our understanding of the condition is advancing. Knowledge of the vestibular apparatus will aid your understanding. Each inner ear has three semicircular canals (SCCs) that are orientated in perpendicular planes. Within each canal is fluid and the direction of flow can be detected by the cupula (*cup-you-la*), which is deflected by the fluid and generates an electrical signal that is transmitted to the brain. A recent theory, the canalithiasis (*canal-lith-i-ay-sis*) theory (meaning canal stones) proposes that calcium carbonate debris collects in the SCC. When the patient changes position, these particles, after a lag period, tumble down the canal and stimulate the cupula. These signals are not congruous with the motion of the patient's head and produce nystagmus, vertigo, and nausea. If the patient then reverses their position, these stones will roll back in the direction they started in but this time the direction of the nystagmus will reverse (think about pebbles in a tyre and visualize how they tumble around the inner tube as they roll in one direction and then in reverse). Once the motion has ceased, the stones settle and the nystagmus and vertigo abate. It is postulated that this debris can be created in young adults through head injury and develop in old age through degenerative changes in the labyrinths. A subclassification of BPPV can be made on the basis of the SCC affected, that is, posterior superior SCC, posterior inferior SCC, and lateral SCC. Clinically a patient may develop sudden vertigo when changing positions. The vertigo is intermittent and may last 30 seconds before wearing off. Examination is usually unremarkable and nystagmus may not be elicited while the patient is still. The Hallpike–Dix manoeuvre will confirm the diagnosis. Recently a treatment has been developed for the condition, the Epley (*ep-lay*) manoeuvre.

Acute labyrinthitis

Often acute labyrinthitis or sometimes the term acute vestibular neuronitis is used to describe a condition where a previously healthy patient develops a sudden onset of severe vertigo. There is no hearing loss or tinnitus and the acute attack can last several days. The patient may be bed bound for fear of falling and there is associated nausea and vomiting. The symptoms usually ebb away over a few weeks. Treatment is symptomatic relief with anti-emetics.

Ménière's syndrome

This is a syndrome comprising attacks of vertigo, hearing impairment, and tinnitus. The cause is unknown but the end result is the accumulation of excessive endolymphatic fluid in the endolymphatic sac of the inner ear. It affects females more than males and usually occurs between the ages of 35 and 55 years.

Hearing loss may precede an attack; it is sensorineural in origin and affects the lower frequencies preferentially. It is the vertigo that is debilitating and brings the patient to medical attention. There may be the sensation of pressure in the affected ear before the onset of vertigo. The vertigo may last several hours and may be accompanied by tinnitus. There may be several attacks of vertigo over several weeks but the natural history of the condition is one of gradual recovery.

The treatment is symptomatic with anti-emetics with or without sedatives. β-Histidine (*beater-hiss-ti-dean*) (serc) is often given, although its efficacy is limited. Occasionally in severe cases surgical decompression of the endolymphatic sac or surgical division of the vestibular nerve is undertaken.

Cerebellar syndromes

There is a range of diseases that can affect the cerebellum. They can be acute or chronic and may lead to incoordination and loss of balance. The causes are:

- MS (use the word 'demyelination' in front of patients until the diagnosis is confirmed)
- alcohol
- stroke (within the cerebellum or affecting its tracts)
- tumour (primary, metastatic, or paraneoplastic)
- Friedreich's ataxia and other inherited neurodegenerative syndromes.

Friedreich's ataxia

This neurodegenerative disease is one of the most common inherited ataxias. The usual mode of transmission is autosomal recessive, although other forms have been described. The median age of onset is 12 years. Clinical features relate to the neural tissue involved: cerebellum and spinocerebellar tracts (ataxia, nystagmus, dysarthria, and incoordination), corticospinal tracts (spastic paraparesis and extensor plantars), and peripheral neuropathy (sensory loss and pes cavus (*pes-cave-us*)). Other features include optic atrophy, kyphoscoliosis, and cardiomyopathy. The disease is progressive and irreversible; patients inevitably become wheelchair bound and usually die in the fifth decade from the associated cardiac disease.

Multiple sclerosis

MS is a disease of unknown aetiology characterized by two or more episodes of neurological dysfunction, which are separated both in time and site. These are attributable to multiple plaques of demyelination scattered throughout the CNS.

Findings in the arms

Cerebellar signs may be present, with or without UMN signs such as hyper-reflexia.

Features elsewhere

Eye movement testing may display nystagmus (due to cerebellar involvement) or ataxic nystagmus (due to involvement of the median longitudinal fasciculus), optic atrophy. There may also be a spastic paraparesis (*para-par-ee-sis*).

Treatment

Treatment of an acute episode is with steroids (a short course of high-dose intravenous methyl-prednisolone). Interferon (*interfere-on*) has more recently been shown to have a modest beneficial effect. Baclofen (*back-low-fen*) is useful for treating spasticity.

Optic atrophy

This is the irreversible degeneration of the optic nerve head and associated fibres leading to visual loss and a pale optic disc. There are a variety of causes of optic atrophy. Hereditary causes can be autosomal dominant (usually milder disease) or autosomal recessive. One particular form, Leber's (*leb-buzz*) optic atrophy (*Theodor von Leber (1840–1917), German ophthalmologist*), may be X-linked because it predominantly affects males. It usually presents around the age of 20–30 years. Acquired causes include

- compression of the optic nerve, for example, pituitary tumours
- central retinal artery occlusion
- trauma
- optic neuritis
- toxins, for example, alcohol or tobacco
- retinal degeneration, for example, due to retinitis pigmentosa.

The only hope for treatment is to intervene early in those cases with an underlying cause before irreversible visual loss.

Optic neuritis

This is the inflammation of the optic disc and optic nerve and the most common cause in the UK is MS. If the optic disc is affected this is called papillitis (*pap-ill-light-iss*) and this produces changes that can be seen on fundoscopy. If the optic nerve is affected this is sometimes called retrobulbar neuritis, inferring that the inflammation is behind the optic disc and as a result produces no visible changes on fundoscopy. Papillitis is the resultant swelling of the optic disc due to inflammation and the appearance on fundoscopy is indistiguishable from that of papilloedema. The term papilloedema should only be used if the cause is clearly due to raised intracranial pressure. The features that help distinguish papillitis from papilloedema are given in Table 6.23.

With papillitis there is a rapid loss of central vision over a few hours. There follows a gradual recovery over the following weeks. There are usually signs of optic atrophy months after the event. If all or most of the features described about papillitis are present without signs of a swollen optic disc, this suggests retrobulbar neuritis. In cases of papillitis or retrobulbar neuritis the possibility of MS should always be borne in mind.

Internuclear ophthalmoplegia (INO)

To enable both eyes to move as a coordinated unit, they need to be interconnected. This is achieved through the median longitudinal fasciculus. Among other functions this connects the nerve VI of one eye (controlling the lateral rectus) to the nerve III of the other eye (controlling the medial rectus). If there is damage to this pathway it disrupts conjugate movement in the horizontal plane. This usually manifests as nystagmus in the abducting eye and a failure of adduction of the other eye. However if the direction of gaze is reversed, the eye that failed to adduct can abduct fully and now has nystagmus. The other eye is unable to adduct. INO is unusual and occurs most often in MS. It may also occur with brainstem infarct, trauma, or syringobulbia.

Holmes–Adie pupil

This is a slowly reacting or myotonic pupil. If the pupil is exposed to light the pupil may remain dilated for a long period before finally constricting. Conversely in poor light the pupil may remain constricted for a long time before dilating. There are no other neurological complications

Table 6.23 Distinguishing papillitis from papilloedema

Papillitis	Papilloedema
Reduced visual acuity	No visual disturbance
± Central scotoma	May have an enlarged blind spot
Diminished pupillary light reflex (Marcus Gunn pupil)	Normal pupillary light reflex
May be pain on eye movements	No pain on eye movements

associated with this condition. There is no ptosis or any abnormal eye movements, which distinguishes it from cranial nerve abnormalities. There is an association with absent tendon reflexes.

Ramsay–Hunt syndrome

This is the combination of a LMN facial nerve palsy with herpes zoster infection (shingles). Initially there may be pain in the ear with nothing to find on examination. A few days later the characteristic vesicular eruption of shingles can be seen on the pinna and external auditory canal. The vesicles can contain pus (pustules) or become haemorrhagic, before crusting over to leave a scab and eventually a scar. There may also be nerve VIII involvement leading to sensorineural deafness and vertigo.

Bell's palsy

This is the cause of a LMN facial nerve palsy of unknown cause. The paralysis occurs suddenly and is complete within 24 hours. Symptoms are the result of swelling of the facial nerve within the restrictive facial canal of the skull. If the involvement is extensive the chorda tympani branch may be affected leading to the loss of taste on the anterior two-thirds of the tongue. There may also be hyperacusis due to paralysis of the stapedius muscle. As the eye cannot close it may be vulnerable to damage by foreign body or infection. Therefore a patch may be required temporarily to protect the eye. The condition usually resolves slowly over 2 months.

Parkinson's disease

This is caused by degeneration of the dopamine-containing cells in the substantia nigra of the basal ganglia.

Findings in the arms

- Resting tremor, which improves with action.
- Assessing tone will identify rigidity.
- Check for bradykinesia (*braddy-kine-easier*) (slowness of movement) by asking the patient to tap a hand on to their lap as fast as they can.

Features elsewhere

The face is expressionless ('mask-like') and the voice is often monotonous and of low volume. Ask the patient to walk to demonstrate the stooped posture, shuffling gait, and lack of arm swing. You could also ask the patient to write; the words are often small and spidery (micrographia)

(*my-crow-graph-ia*). Patients also have a tendency towards drooling (sialorrhoea) (*sigh-al-owe-rear*) and greasy skin (seborrhoea) (*seb-owe-rear*).

Treatment

L-Dopa and similar drugs help restore the dopamine within the brain and are particularly useful for treating bradykinesia and rigidity. Tremor responds less well, but if this is the predominant symptom, patients may benefit from anti-cholinergic drugs.

Parkinsonism

As well as the idiopathic form of the disease, other conditions may mimic Parkinson's because of their involvement of the basal ganglia. Examples include stroke disease, certain drugs (neuroleptics), Alzheimer's disease (*Alois Alzheimer (1864–1915), German psychiatrist/neurologist*), head injury, Wilson's disease (*Samuel Alexander Kinnier Wilson (1878–1937), British neurologist*), and heavy metal poisoning.

You should be alerted to the possibility of parkinsonism rather than Parkinson's disease if your patient has evidence of UMN signs (suggesting stroke disease) or dementia (suggesting Alzheimer's), although dementia is a late feature of Parkinson's. In addition, three syndromes exist that are known as the 'Parkinson plus' syndromes.

- **Steele–Richardson–Olszewski (*ol-chef-ski*) syndrome** (*John C. Steele (born 1934), Canadian neurologist, J. Clifford Richardson (1909–1986), Canadian neurologist, Jerzy Olszewski (1913–1966), Polish-born Canadian neurologist*). Parkinsonism plus failure of vertical gaze and pseudobulbar palsy due to degeneration of the upper brainstem. Also known as progressive supranuclear palsy (PSP).

- **Shy–Drager (*shy-dray-guh*) syndrome** (*George Milton Shy (1919–1967), American neurologist, Glenn Albert Drager (1917–1967), American neurologist*). Parkinsonism plus autonomic failure (postural hypotension and atonic bladder). Also known as multisystem atrophy.

- **Olivo-ponto-cerebellar syndrome**. Parkinsonism plus cerebellar and pyramidal involvement.

In general, parkinsonism responds poorly or even adversely to conventional anti-parkinsonian drugs.

Spinal cord

The spinal cord is the continuation of the brainstem as it passes through the foramen magnum of the skull and terminates approximately at the level of the L1 vertebrae in an adult. It runs down through the foramen of successive vertebrae and is protected by these and also the meninges as they maintain their original relationship during the descent. Even though the spinal cord terminates at L1, the dura mater continues downwards before terminating at the level of S2. Nerve roots originating near the termination of the cord pass vertically downwards to supply the lower body and limbs. Collectively they are referred to by the Latin term 'cauda equina' (cord-a-equine-a) because this sheath of nerves resembles a horse's tail. The subarachnoid space beneath the dura mater is filled with CSF which is in continuous circulation with the CSF of the brain and it is here that CSF can be removed by lumbar puncture for analysis in relative safety (there is a risk of damage to the spinal cord if this technique is performed at a level higher than L1). Lesions of the cord can be described by their level in the vertebral column eg. cervical, thoracic, lumbar and sacral. Their site can also be described in the same way as the brain with respect to their relationship with the meninges—epidural (or extradural), subdural, etc. There is another term to be familiar with whose use is restricted to the lower brainstem in the brain and that is medullary. In the spinal cord lesions can be intra and extramedullary and this simply means that the lesion is within the spinal cord or outside it. The terms intra-axial and extra-axial still apply to the spinal cord and can be used interchangeably with intramedullary and extramedullary respectively.

Spinal cord compression

This occurs due to any mass lesion in or around the spinal cord that compresses it. Causes include:

- Tumour
  - Secondary metastases (commonest form of tumour involvement)
  - Primary tumours (e.g. meningiomas, neurofibromas, ependymomas)
- Abscess formation
- Haematoma
- Spinal stenosis
- Bone (e.g. fractures or new bone formation)
- Herniated intervertebral disc.

Neurological deficits will occur because of compression of the adjacent cord causing damage to the nerve cells directly or possibly through ischaemia, due to the interruption of arterial blood supply or obstruction of venous drainage. The clinical signs will be determined by the level of the lesion (e.g. cervical, thoracic, lumbar); by the site of the lesion (e.g. extradural or intradural); or the speed of onset (e.g. haematoma vs slow-growing tumour). However, regardless of the variety of lesions and sites, some common patterns in presentation occur. It is imperative that you can recognize signs of spinal cord compression because if it is not recognized and treated, irreversible cord damage will lead to paralysis and possibly bladder and bowel disturbance. See 'Important clinical patterns' for clinical features.

Cauda equina syndrome

This is the collection of signs caused by damage to the bundle of lumbar and sacral nerve roots emerging from the termination of the spinal cord. See 'Important clinical patterns' for clinical features.

Causes

- Trauma
- Disc herniation
- Fractured lumbar vertebrae
- Spinal stenosis
- Spinal cord tumours
- Epidural abscess
- Iatrogenic (e.g. epidural haematoma following spinal anaesthesia)
- Spina bifida

Spinal stenosis

This is the narrowing of the central canal which transmits the spinal cord. This narrowing can be congenital or acquired. Acquired stenosis can be caused by diseased structures surrounding the canal. This can include osteophyte (os-tea-owe-fight) formation, new outgrowth of bone which can project into the canal, or expansion of the vertebrae itself in Paget's disease of the bone. There may be hypertrophy of the supporting ligaments of the spine (the ligament flavum and posterior longitudinal ligament) which can also encroach on the canal. These degenerative changes are seen commonly in older people and contribute to spondylosis. In addition a herniated intervertebral disc can also protrude into the spinal canal, or trauma can cause fractures or slippage of the vertebrae on each other called spondylolysthesis (spon-dee-lol-iss-thesis) which can impinge on the cord and compress it. NB: if the spinal canal is already narrow because of a congenital cause it will not take much to precipitate cord compression.

Clinical features

- It may be asymptomatic and be a chance finding while imaging the spine for a different reason.

- There may be symptoms and signs of spinal cord compression depending on the level of the lesion.

- Additionally in lumbar stenosis the patient may exhibit 'spinal claudication'. The symptoms are very similar to intermittent claudication of vascular origin, in that pain can be experienced in the buttocks or back of the calves on walking. However, whereas the pain is relieved by the cessation of walking in vascular claudication, the same is not true of spinal claudication. The pain will not abate unless the patient sits down or bends forwards (movements that open up the spinal canal and relieve the pressure on the spinal cord). The condition is diagnosed on MRI or CT scan and treatment depends on the underlying cause. Some patients will be treated conservatively if the patient has significant comorbidity or the surgery is judged as too risky. Otherwise a number of surgical approaches can be employed depending on the underlying cause.

Cervical spondylosis

This is a common disease, characterized by degeneration of the intervertebral discs, thickening of the ligaments surrounding the lower cervical spine, and osteophyte formation (new outgrowths of bone). These changes may result in compression of nerve roots as they exit the spinal cord, leading to LMN signs in the arms. C5, C6, and C7 are the roots most commonly involved. Encroachment on the spinal cord itself may also occur, involving the descending UMN tracts. The latter is sometimes known as cervical myelopathy (*mile-op-athy*). However, if these motor fibres are damaged due to cervical spondylosis impinging on the C5, C6 nerve roots then biceps contraction does not occur. Instead, the sensory impulses entering the cord at this level stimulate adjacent spinal cord fibres, for example, those supplying triceps and the finger flexors, resulting in contraction of these muscles. This is known as reflex inversion. There may be stiffness in the legs and other UMN signs in the legs if there is a cervical myelopathy. Sometimes Lhermitte's (*ler-meats*) phenomenon can be experienced (*Jacques Jean Lhermitte (1877–1959), French neurologist*). This is elicited or experienced when the head is bent forwards. This flexion of the cervical spine causes an electric, shock-like pain to shoot down the spine and into the arms (and occasionally the legs). It is sometimes called the barber-chair phenomenon because this is a common movement during a haircut and historically precipitated a few cases.

Syringomyelia

In this condition a fluid-filled cavity gradually expands within the central cervical cord. The spinothalamic fibres from the arms enter and cross the midline of the cervical cord, so these are the first tracts to be affected, leading to a loss of pain and temperature sensation in the arms. There is relative sparing of the dorsal columns because these are situated in the posterior part of the cord. This leads to a 'dissociated sensory loss' because proprioception and vibration sense remain relatively preserved.

Later features include LMN signs in the arms (via compression of the anterior horn cells in the cervical cord that supply the arms) and UMN signs in the legs (via involvement of the descending pyramidal tracts to the lower limbs). MRI is the imaging investigation of choice and treatment is via surgical decompression.

Motor neuron disease

This is a disease characterized by progressive degeneration of motor fibres. There are three clinical patterns based on the motor fibres involved:

- **Progressive muscular atrophy**. Anterior horn cell degeneration leading to LMN signs.

- **Amyotrophic (*ay-myo-trow-fic*) lateral sclerosis**. Lateral corticospinal tract involvement, hence the name.

- **Progressive bulbar palsy**. This affects the motor cranial nerves IX–XII. In practice, patients tend to have features of more than one of these clinical patterns.

Clinical features

There is often a mixture of UMN and LMN signs with a striking absence of sensory signs, for example, generalized wasting, fasciculations, with brisk reflexes. However pure LMN signs may be present. Dysarthria, dysphagia, wasted fasciculating tongue (bulbar palsy), and spastic paraparesis (*para-par-ee-sis*).

Peripheral nervous system

Hereditary polyneuropathies

HSMN I is also known as Charcot–Marie–Tooth disorder or peroneal muscular atrophy; it is inherited as an autosomal dominant and causes a symmetrical polyneuropathy in a glove and stocking distribution.

It causes a characteristic distal wasting of muscles of the arms and legs, which slowly progresses up the limbs. In the legs this gives the appearance of an inverted champagne bottle. It is also associated with pes cavus and kyphoscoliosis.

The diagnosis is suggested by a family history and the clinical features above and is supported by nerve conduction studies and chromosomal studies. HSMN II has the same features as HMSN I but has a slightly delayed onset (third to fifth decades). HSMN III or Dejerine–Sottas (*de-je-rin-sot-tas*) syndrome (*Joseph Jules Dejerine (1849–1917), French neurologist; Jules Sottas (1866–1943), French neurologist*) is the recessive form with an early onset in the first decade and could be associated with mental retardation.

Guillain–Barré syndrome

This is an acute inflammatory polyneuropathy. In over two-thirds of patients, a preceding acute viral illness is followed in 1–3 weeks by an ascending paralysis, areflexia with mild sensory involvement.

Diagnosis is usually made on the clinical features, supported by nerve conduction studies, showing evidence of demyelination and lumbar puncture showing raised CSF protein. Thirty per cent of patients may require ventilatory support for respiratory paralysis.

The prognosis is good with 75–80% recovering without any neurological deficit. Treatment with intravenous immunoglobulin or plasmapharesis commenced early in the course of the disease (within a week) is shown to be effective.

Mononeuropathy

This is where a single nerve trunk is affected leading to LMN weakness and sensory loss specific to the nerve trunk involved. An example of this in the leg is the common peroneal nerve palsy.

Mononeuritis multiplex

This is a simultaneous or sequential involvement of isolated nerves or nerve roots over a period of time. Vasculitis is the most common cause of this syndrome and includes multisystem disorders such as systemic lupus erythmatosus (*loo-pus-eryth-mat-owe-sis*) (SLE); polyarteritis nodosa (*polly-art-er-eye-tiss-no-dose-a*) (PAN), ANCA-associated granulomatous vasculitis (formerly known as Wegener's granulomatosis; *vague-ners-granule-owe-mat-owe-sis*), also known as granulomatosis with polyangitis (GPA);

sarcoidosis; Churg–Strauss syndrome, also known as eosinophilic granulomatosis with polyangitis (EGPA); systemic sclerosis; and other vasculitides (another collective name for disorders that cause clinical symptoms through an inflammatory process of blood vessels).

Diabetic amyotrophy

This is an asymmetric, femoral neuropathy affecting the thigh muscles causing severe wasting of the anterior thigh, pain, and weakness of knee extension. The knee jerk is absent but sensory impairment is minimal. This condition also reflects poor metabolic control in diabetes and improves with strict glycaemic control.

Duchenne muscular dystrophy

This is an X-linked recessive disorder due to mutation of the dystrophin gene. Pseudo-hypertrophy of the calves occur (this means that although the muscles are enlarged they are paradoxically weak) and progressive weakness of the girdle muscles commences early in the first decade leading to waddling gait and Gower's sign (*Sir William Richard Gower (1845–1915), English neurologist*); when asked to stand from a squatting position the patient raises themselves up by climbing up their legs with their hands (See Fig 14.9). Patients may become chair bound in the second decade and develop respiratory failure in the third. Sensory function and reflexes are preserved. The diagnosis is suggested by a family history, serum creatine kinase, electromyelograph (EMG), and muscle biopsy. Other variants of muscular dystrophy exist including Becker's muscular dystrophy, limb-girdle dystrophy, and fascio-scapulo-humeral dystrophy.

Proximal myopathy

There is wasting and weakness of the shoulder girdle with relative sparing of the distal musculature, that is, grip strength is preserved. There are usually no other abnormal neurological signs. In particular the reflexes are normal, in contrast to UMN and LMN pathology. The legs are similarly affected, with proximal weakness leading to difficulty standing from a sitting position and a waddling gait. The important causes include polymyositis (*polly-my-owe-site-iss*), myasthenia, osteomalacia (*os-tea-owe-mal-ay-sha*), alcohol, and steroids. Treatment is of the underlying cause.

Polymyositis

Polymyositis and dermatomyositis are autoimmune inflammatory conditions affecting the muscles (dermatomyositis is usually reserved for the additional involvement of the skin). There is a proximal muscle weakness affecting the thighs, shoulders, and neck and in addition the muscles can be tender due to the inflammatory process. Problems with swallowing may occur due to pharyngeal striated muscle involvement. Those patients with skin involvement may have a characteristic skin rash around the upper eyelids (described as a heliotrope rash), a vasculitic rash at the fingertips, and occasionally nailfold infarcts. Investigations such as elevated creatine phosphokinase (CPK) level, raised inflammatory markers, EMG, and characteristic muscle biopsy help make the diagnosis.

Myasthenia gravis

This is an autoimmune condition where the body's immune system produces antibodies against the postsynaptic receptors of striated (voluntary) muscles. In normal circumstances nerve impulses pass down the axon of a motor neuron to the motor endplate. Motor endplates are synaptic junctions which consist of the termination of the neuron and the commencement of the postsynaptic membrane of the target motor fibre/s and a small gap that separates the two. This is also called the neuromuscular junction or myoneural junction. For a muscle to contract this gap has to be bridged and this occurs by vesicles which are released from the presynaptic termination that contain acetylcholine.

The acetylcholine binds with receptors on the postsynaptic membrane of the muscle fibres and depolarization occurs leading to muscle contraction. Once the voluntary action has been performed the acetylcholine is broken down by the enzyme cholinesterase to render it inactive. In myasthenia gravis the antibodies to the muscle receptors are in competition with the acetylcholine to bind to the postsynaptic receptors. If there is insufficient concentration of acetylcholine available the muscle fibres may fatigue or fail to contract at all.

Most people with myasthenia will function well in the morning because they have usually synthesized sufficient concentration of acetylcholine overnight but as this becomes depleted they are unable to displace the competing receptor antibodies and start to tire as the day progresses.

Clinical features

The commonest muscles to be affected are the ocular muscles (including the eyelids) leading to ptosis and diplopia. In a small proportion of patients the ocular muscles are the only muscles affected and this is called ocular myasthenia.

- Fatiguability can be demonstrated in muscles (using repetitive tasks)

- Facial muscle involvement can lead to an expressionless face or a limited snarl when trying to smile
- There may be drooling, or difficulty chewing and swallowing with bulbar involvement and can lead to aspiration pneumonia
- Dysphonia

Respiratory involvement can lead to dyspnoea and is a dangerous development. This could lead to a *myasthenic crisis* where insufficient ventilation leads to respiratory failure. In this circumstance the patient needs to have assisted ventilation on an intensive care unit.

The main treatment is with cholinesterase inhibitors which increase the concentration of available acetylcholine to overcome the competitive blockade of the autoimmune receptor blockers. The usual agent is pyridostigmine. Prednisolone is also used to try to suppress the immune system and hence the manufacture of the receptor blockers. In serious situations intravenous gamma globulin can be used to diminish the activity of the condition although not all patients will respond to the therapy. Plasmapheresis can also be used to remove circulating antibodies and can have some short-term benefit.

Investigations

Electromyography

EMG is the recording of electrical activity of muscle fibres for diagnostic purposes. A small needle electrode is inserted into the muscle to be tested. The needle tip detects signals from the surrounding muscle fibres. These signals are amplified and recorded on an oscilloscope.

Characteristic findings may point towards a diagnosis, although in practice the findings are not always clear cut and the EMG should be used in conjunction with the clinical picture.

Nerve conduction studies

These also involve the use of electrodes, which are attached to the skin. The nerve under test is excited percutaneously by a stimulatory electrode; the impulse is carried along the nerve and detected at a recording electrode further along the nerve (for example, in the case of sensory neurons) or at the target muscle (in the investigation of motor neurons). Information gained includes action potentials (motor and sensory), motor latency, and conduction velocities (motor and sensory). Velocities are calculated by dividing the distance separating the two electrodes by the time taken for the impulse to travel between them. Nerve conduction studies are useful in differentiating between the different types of periph-eral neuropathies.

Electroencephalography

To put it simply, electroencephalolography (*elect-roe-en-kef-allo-graffy*) (EEG) is the brain's equivalent of an ECG. Multiple electrodes are put in strategic, internationally agreed positions. These record the electrical activity of the brain and deductions can be made, depending on the patient's characteristics, for example, age, medication, arousal, and so on.

Four main brain rhythms may be identified: alpha rhythms (frequency of 8–12 Hz), usually seen when the eyes are closed; beta rhythms (faster rate, frequency 20–22 Hz), seen in anxious individuals and with sedative medication; delta rhythms (slower waves 1–4 Hz), which can be found in children but are normally pathological in adults; and theta rhythms (5–7 Hz), found in children. Interpretation of the EEG should only be done in con-junction with the patient's history and examination. It can be used to investigate seizures, blackouts, confusion, and sleep disorders. Various physiological challenges can be used to try and unmask a latent condition (usu-ally epilepsy), for example, hyperventilation or the use of strobe light.

There are limitations to the use of the EEG and neuro-physiologists will take these into account when analysing any trace. For example, an epileptic may have a normal EEG between attacks. Also, large intracerebral lesions may not register any electrical abnormality, whereas small lesions (invisible on the CT scan) can cause widespread electrical changes.

Lumbar puncture

This is the introduction of a special lumbar puncture nee-dle into the spine to withdraw CSF. This is usually per-formed between the L3–L4 or L4–L5 vertebrae because the spinal cord terminates at L2 and this minimizes the risk of injury to it. The CSF circulates in and around the brain and spinal cord and therefore the fluid withdrawn from the lumbar spine approximates to the fluid around the brain. This feature is used in the diagnosis (or differ-ential diagnosis) of a central neurological disease. The CSF is examined for glucose, protein, white and red cells, and microorganisms (CSF pressure should be measured also but this is not often done). Any abnormalities in any of these parameters can suggest a diagnosis. Diseases that can be diagnosed include meningitis (the most

notorious), encephalitis, spinal cord tumours, Guillain–Barré syndrome, subarachnoid haemorrhage, and BIH. Care must be taken when doing a lumbar puncture. Physicians should always be aware of the possibility of raised intracranial pressure because if the procedure is done in this situation, the pressure difference gener-ated by the removal of CSF will force the brainstem down through the foramen magnum of the skull ('coning') and lead to a rapid death. If at all possible a CT scan should be performed before doing a lumbar puncture. In areas where CT is not readily available, the decision is a clinical one. The physician should always examine the eyes for papilloedema as a potential marker for raised intracra-nial pressure.

CT

This is a sensitive radiographic technique, which is a use-ful diagnostic aid. An X-ray beam is passed through the area to be imaged in consecutive horizontal 'slices', which are 2–10 mm apart. The information obtained is pro-cessed by a computer, which constructs two-dimensional images. Further information is obtained when intravenous contrast is administered at the time of scanning. CT has uses throughout the body. In the brain, unenhanced scans (no intravenous contrast) are useful in demonstrat-ing intracranial bleeds (which show up as abnormal white areas) or infarcts (provided the scan is performed after 24 hours; before this time the scan is usually normal). Cerebral atrophy is seen as shrinkage of brain tissue with corresponding enlargement of the sulci (*sul-sigh*) and ventricles. Enlargement of the ventricular system alone is termed hydrocephalus. Intravenous contrast will high-light vascular abnormalities such as tumours, abscesses (showing 'ring enhancement'), and arteriovenous malform-ations. However, CT may miss very small lesions and is less adept than MRI at demonstrating pathology in the brainstem.

MRI

This technique employs magnetism rather than radiation to produce images. An area of the body is exposed to a mag-netic field leading to excitation of hydrogen nuclei (remem-ber that the body is 70% water). The signals produced by this process are computed, resulting in transverse images similar to CT; in addition a midline sagittal (*saj-it-al*) image can be obtained, which is useful in the diagnosis of brain-stem and cervical cord pathology such as MS or syringo-myelia. The use of magnetism, however, precludes its use in patients who have cardiac pacemakers and the screening process is performed in a small, enclosed chamber, which is most unpopular with claustrophobics.

Finals section

For revision read the examination summary and the key points throughout the chapter and try the questions at the end of the chapter. See Tables 6.24 and 6.25 for day-to-day and Finals cases, respectively.

The most common neurological problem you will see is stroke, although these tend to be concentrated on designated stroke units rather than on general wards (as this improves survival and recovery). Other conditions include MS and Parkinson's disease. If you are lucky enough to have an attachment on a neurology ward you may see more exotic diseases. These may sometimes be used for Finals examinations because they are rich in neurological signs.

Key diagnostic clues

Perhaps this section should be called 'key localizing clues' because many of the signs you look for will point you to the site of the lesion rather than indicate the diagnosis. With motor loss, tone and reflexes give the most diagnostic information. With sensory loss, it is the pattern of loss that gives the most diagnostic information. It is helpful to categorize neurological signs into the following:

Motor

- **UMN**. Little wasting, increased tone, decreased power, hyper-reflexia (clonus, upgoing plantar, spastic or hemiplegic gait in the legs).
- **LMN**. Wasting, decreased tone, decreased power, decreased or absent reflexes (downgoing plantar in the leg).

- **Extrapyramidal**. Involuntary movements, increased tone, rigidity, (abnormal gait in the legs).
- **Cerebellar**. Intention tremor, past-pointing, incoordination, dysdiadochokinesis, nystagmus in the eyes, ataxic gait in the legs.

Sensory

Patterns of sensory loss:

- The whole limb (cortical lesion?)
- Dermatomal (root lesion? peripheral nerve lesion?)
- Distal arm greater than proximal arm (peripheral neuropathy?)
- Dissociated sensory loss (spinal cord lesion?)

Remember that the above classification of motor and sensory deficits is somewhat arbitrary and many of the categories can coexist.

Some advice relating to examination problems

General

Use the neurological examination routine given in this chapter.

Instructions

The OSCE examination will usually have a straightforward case with straightforward written instructions. Make sure you read this carefully so that you are clear what is required. Usually you will be expected to examine an aspect of the nervous system such as the motor system, sensory system, or cranial nerves. It is possible that

Table 6.24 Day-to-day cases

Stroke
Parkinson's disease
Cervical myelopathy
Multiple sclerosis

Table 6.25 Finals cases

Day-to-day cases
Cerebellar syndromes
Motor neuron disease

you may have to do a complete neurological examination of the arms or legs. If this is the case I recommend that you perform the motor system first.

General look

This is important so do not forget it. A quick glance at the face and the rest of the body may give you a vital clue; for example, an expressionless face and a hunched posture may suggest Parkinson's disease and this may alert you to look for a pill-rolling tremor and cogwheel rigidity.

Relax the patient

It is vitally important that your patient is relaxed throughout the examination (particularly when assessing tone and reflexes). It will help your cause if you can be as relaxed as possible too!

The neurological examination

The next dilemma you might face is which aspect of the neurological system to test first, that is, sensory or motor system (unless it is stated explicitly to do **only** one of these). In the absence of any leading clues I would advocate starting with the motor system as this is relatively quick to do (tone, power, reflexes, and coordination), whereas the sensory system (light touch, pin-prick, vibration, and proprioception), can be more time consuming and depends on subjective responses from your patient (you should get user-friendly patients in the exam). If you have not found any abnormalities during the motor assessment then it is highly likely that the problem will be in the sensory system.

Analyse as you go

As you examine do not simply elicit signs and then try to make sense of all of it at the end (in front of impatient and off-putting examiners). Try to analyse the significance of each sign as you go along. This will guide your subsequent examination, for example, looking for supplementary signs that may support a diagnosis as well as helping you to come to a conclusion more quickly (see Case 6.16).

Tone

Do not waste time agonizing whether or not the tone is increased. If it is increased it is usually obvious (so long as you have practised sufficiently). If you are unsure, work through the rest of your examination looking for further clues. If you find hyper-reflexia, then it is likely that the tone is increased.

Power

This is straightforward. Look for asymmetry of power (stroke? root lesion? nerve lesion?) and whether power is weaker proximally compared to distally (proximal myopathy?).

Reflexes

Make sure you are competent at eliciting reflexes in the left arm and left leg. Remember, if you cannot demonstrate reflexes then you must try to elicit them with reinforcement!

Sensation

Be systematic when assessing sensation. Aim to compare both arms or legs systematically. Compare proximal areas to the same proximal area on the other limb and likekwise distal to distal. Do the same with the medial

CASE 6.16

Problem: You have found hyper-reflexia (and hypertonia) and are unsure whether to demonstrate Hoffmann's sign, finger jerks, deltoid reflexes, and so on.

Solution: If hyper-reflexia is obvious it is probably not necessary, but you are in an examination and so you want to demonstrate that you know more than the average. If you are confident, then perform Hoffman's sign and the finger jerks as these will add weight to the findings of

hyper-reflexia (if you are not confident do not attempt them). I would draw the line at eliciting the deltoid and pectoral reflexes, as this could be seen as 'gilding the lily' and not adding too much more to your present state of knowledge unless you are suspicious that there could be a lesion at C5 in which case the deltoid will be absent (along with diminished biceps, supinator, and pectoral reflexes).

and lateral surfaces of each limb also. If you find a deficit try to elicit the pattern of loss. Is the whole arm affected (cortical lesion?)? Is the distal portion of both arms affected (peripheral neuropathy?)? A difference between the radial and ulnar borders of the arms, for example, may suggest a root lesion (radial border C6, ulnar border T1). Does it conform to a dermatomal distribution or to a peripheral nerve distribution? If you can answer these questions you are on the way to localizing where a lesion might be.

Presentation

Always mention that you would normally perform a full neurological examination and not just any system in isolation, as there may be clues elsewhere that could help pinpoint the source of a lesion. Try to be confident— avoid the words 'seems' or 'might'!

OSCE examples

History-taking station

You are an FY2 in neurology outpatients and you are asked to see a 38-year-old woman with headaches. Take a focused history and present your differential diagnosis to the examiners.

Remember:

- Introduce yourself to the patient.
- Ask questions about the pain (SOCRATES) with special emphasis on sudden/gradual onset: is it worse in the morning/when bending/coughing, exclude previous trauma.
- Associated features such as nausea, vomiting, flashing lights, other visual disturbance, tenderness of a local area of the scalp when combing the hair, fever and feeling generally unwell, paraesthesia, numbness, or weakness of the limbs.
- Ask about previous meical history and family history especially of migraines, tension headaches, subarachnoid haemorrhage, polymyalgia rheumatica, previous neurosurgery.
- Ask a drug history for analgesia, any new medications especially nitrates, calcium channel blockers.
- Social history—check smoking and especially alcohol. What occupation do they do? Is it stressful? Especially now? Any other stresses in their life.
- Thank your patient.

- Your differential diagnosis will depend on the responses you get but will include migraines, tension headache, SOL, subarachnoid haemorrhage, meningitis, temporal arteritis, etc.

Examination station

You are an FY1 on an admissions ward and you are about to see a new patient. He is a 69-year-old man who has had a fall. Examine his lower limbs neurologically and present your findings. There is no need to take a history.

Remember:

- Introduce yourself and gain consent for the examination.
- Wash your hands/use alcohol gel provided.
- Get your general look in and check to see if they have a facial nerve palsy, check their voice for dysarthria, check the posture of upper and lower limbs—is a stroke possible?
- Assess motor system, inspection, tone, power, reflexes including plantars. Don't forget cerebellar function.
- Assess sensory system, light touch, pin-prick, proprioception.
- Get the patient to stand and perform Romberg's test.
- Don't forget to get your patient to walk.
- Thank your patient and wash your hands/use alcohol gel provided.
- Finish by saying that you would normally check cranial nerves and the upper limbs neurologically to complete your examination.
- Present your findings and don't forget important negatives.

Good luck!

Questions

1 What are fasiculations? In which circumstances may they occur?
2 In stroke classification how would you differentiate a total from a partial anterior circulation infarct?
3 What are the causes of increased muscle tone?
4 What are the causes of a cerebellar syndrome?
5 What is sensory neglect? How does it affect a patient's recovery from stroke?

6 What are the key features of Parkinson's disease?

7 How would you differentiate between upper and lower motor neuron lesions?

8 Which drugs may cause a tremor?

9 What are the risk factors that predispose to a stroke?

10 What are the causes of a proximal myopathy?

Further reading

Crossman AR, Neary D. *Neuroanatomy, an illustrated colour text*, 4th edn. Edinburgh: Churchill Livingstone; 2010.

Donaghy M. *Neurology*, 2nd edn. Oxford; Oxford University Press; 2005.

Fuller G, Manford M. *Neurology, an illustrated colour text*. 3rd edn. Edinburgh: Churchill Livingstone; 2010.

Parsons M. *A colour atlas of clinical neurology*, 3rd edn. London: Wolfe; 1992.

Patten J. *Neurological differential diagnosis*, 2nd edn. London: Springer; 1995.

Perkin G. *Mosby's colour atlas and text of neurology*, 2nd edn. London: Mosby-Wolfe; 2002.

Ross RT. *How to examine the nervous system*. New Jersey: Humana Press; 2006.

7 Abdominal system

Introduction

The abdominal system includes the gastrointestinal tract from mouth to anus and the organs within the abdominal cavity. It is important because the abdomen is affected by several common (and some potentially serious) diseases, for example, peptic ulcer, gastro-oesophageal reflux disease, irritable bowel syndrome, inflammatory bowel disease, and cancer. Also, diseases from other systems may cause abdominal symptoms—diarrhoea, constipation, vomiting, weight loss, and so on. In this chapter, you will learn what to ask patients with abdominal diseases and how to examine the abdominal system.

Symptoms

There are many diseases that affect the gastrointestinal tract. To be able to diagnose these conditions you will need to learn about them and how they present. Although this chapter concentrates on common symptoms that affect the abdomen, it must be remembered that no one symptom is diagnostic. What you will learn to do is ask about a range of symptoms and the responses you get from your patients will help to build a picture of the disease, that with practice, will help guide you to a diagnosis.

Abdominal pain

Abdominal pain (particularly of the upper abdomen) is a common complaint. Pain in the epigastric region can often be mistaken for retrosternal pain and vice versa, leading to problems with diagnosis (see Case 4.1).

The approach to abdominal pain is similar to that of pain anywhere else in the body. However your questions will be modified to reflect this area of enquiry. Common causes of abdominal pain are given in Table 7.1.

- **Oesophagitis**. Inflammation of the oesophagus caused by the reflux of gastric acid back into the oesophagus.
- **Gastro-oesophageal reflux disease**. This is also due to reflux of gastric acid back into the oesophagus, but many patients do not exhibit the inflammatory changes of the oesophagus despite having similar symptoms.
- **Gastritis**. Inflammation of the stomach mucosa (*mew-cose-a*), which can be due to bile reflux, *Helicobacter pylori* infection, non-steroidal anti-inflammatory drugs (NSAIDs), or an autoimmune cause (pernicious anaemia).

Table 7.1 Common causes of abdominal pain

Oesophagus	Oesophagitis, gastro-oesophageal reflux disease
Stomach/duodenum	Gastritis, peptic ulcer
Hepatobiliary tract	Biliary colic, cholecystitis
Pancreas	Pancreatitis
Kidneys	Renal colic
Large bowel	Constipation, diverticulitis, irritable bowel syndrome
Appendix	Appendicitis
No cause found	

- **Peptic ulcer**. This is simply a deficit in the mucosa of the stomach or duodenum that penetrates the muscularis mucosa (*musk-you-lar-iss-mew-cose-a*) layer. The muscularis mucosa is a thin layer of muscle found throughout most of the gastrointestinal tract which forms the basal layer of the mucosa and separates it from the underlying submucosa.
- **Gallstones**. These are precipitates of cholesterol or bile pigments, which can occur in the gallbladder or bile ducts. The majority are asymptomatic but they can cause abdominal pain if they impact in a biliary duct, or jaundice (*jawn-dis*) if they lodge in the common bile duct. Stones in the ducts or gallbladder can act as a source of infection and cause ascending cholangitis (*coal-ann-jite-iss*) or cholecystitis (*coal-ee-sis-tight-iss*) respectively.
- **Pancreatitis**. Inflammation of the pancreas, which can occur acutely or chronically. Alcohol and gallstones are major factors in causing pancreatitis.
- **Kidney stones**. These can be made of a number of materials, for example, calcium oxalate. If they block a ureter they can cause severe pain, termed renal colic.
- **Constipation**. Definitions vary but a useful one is a bowel frequency of less than three per week or having to strain for more than a quarter of the time during defecation (usually because of hard stools).
- **Diverticulitis; diverticulae** (*die-ver-tick-you-lee*). In the context of the large bowel, these are outpouchings of the bowel due to an increased pressure within the lumen. They are common and asymptomatic in a large number of Western adults, if a diverticulum becomes inflamed it can become painful and is called diverticulitis.

- **Irritable bowel syndrome**. This is a condition that can exhibit a range of symptoms including constipation, diarrhoea, and abdominal pain. However, there is no obvious organic cause and all gastrointestinal investigations including colonic biopsies are normal. It is more common in Western society and particularly in people with anxiety or depression. One theory suggests that certain individuals are simply hypersensitive to normal gastrointestinal functions.

- **Appendicitis**. Inflammation of the appendix. The most common predisposing cause is a faecolith within the lumen of the appendix.

Tip

If there is any doubt that you could be dealing with a myocardial infarction arrange an electrocardiogram (ECG).

What to ask

This can be broken down into two sections: (1) questions about the pain itself and (2) questions about potential causes of the pain.

Questions about the pain itself

Begin with an open question, 'Tell me about the pain?' but as with chest pain, you need to establish certain key facts.

- Was this a single bout of pain or were there several bouts?

- Where was the pain? This is an important question, as the site of pain can give a clue to which organ is affected. Also ask about radiation (spread) of pain, e.g., through to the back (pancreatitis?) or around to the scapula (biliary colic?).

- What kind of pain is it (character?) Pain is always difficult to describe so give options—knife-like, burning, or aching. One particular character you should look for is the **colicky** pain. This is a squeezing pain that builds up and then eases off and usually comes in waves. This sort of pain indicates a blockage in a duct or hollow organ and represents the body's attempt to overcome the blockage.

- Onset? Was this a gradual build-up or was the pain severe at the start?

- Did anything bring it on? Ask specifically about certain foods, for example, gallstone disease exacerbated by fatty foods, peptic ulcer by spicy foods, or oesophagitis by hot tea.

- Did anything make it better? Ask about effect of treatments, for example, relief with antacids or milk for oesophagitis or peptic ulcer.

- How long did it last? You need an answer in seconds, minutes, hours, and so on. Reassure the patient that you only need an estimate and give options: 'Did it last seconds only, 5 minutes, about 12 hours?'

Try to get some indication of the severity of the pain. With acute abdominal pain the pain can be very severe. The pain of renal colic is so intense that the patient will roll around in agony. The pain of a perforated peptic ulcer is so bad that the patient dare not move. In each case there may be pallor and sweating.

The answers to the previous questions will offer some signposts to the cause of pain. The descriptions of pain for each condition detailed below will add further clues. Also see Table 7.2 to review the causes of acute and chronic abdominal pain.

Table 7.2 Causes of acute and chronic pain in the abdomen

Organ	Acute	Chronic
Oesophagus		Oesophagitis, gastro-oesophageal reflux disease
Stomach/duodenum	Perforated peptic ulcer, peptic ulcer	Peptic ulcer
Biliary tract	Biliary colic, cholecystitis	Cholecystitis
Kidneys	Renal colic	
Pancreas	Pancreatitis	Pancreatitis
Large bowel	Diverticulitis	Diverticulitis, irritable bowel syndrome

- **Oesophagitis** tends to result in a pain that is retrosternal and burning, is made worse by citrus fruits and spicy foods, and is eased by milk and antacids. It may last from a few minutes to several hours. It tends to be recurrent. It may occasionally be relieved by glycerine trinitrate (GTN), where this reduces oesophageal spasm through its muscle relaxant properties.

- **Peptic ulcer pain** is usually located in the epigastrium (*epi-gas-tri-um*) and is burning or gnawing in nature. It is said that the pain of gastric ulcer comes on after a meal while that of a duodenal ulcer is relieved following a meal. However, this distinction is not often true and is unhelpful. Sometimes the pain of duodenal ulcer can wake a patient from sleep. Often the pain is so localized that the patient can put a finger on where it is. One complication of a peptic ulcer is perforation leading to peritonitis. When this occurs the pain is severe and the patient can only lie still.

- **Gallstones**, when they obstruct a duct or the outlet to the gallbladder, cause **biliary colic**. The pain is experienced in the epigastrium or right upper quadrant and often radiates around to the back under the scapula. It occurs suddenly and builds up to a severe pitch lasting for several hours. The pain is severe and the patient usually rolls around in agony. Although the pain is labelled as colic the pain rarely fluctuates.

- **Pancreatitis**, when acute, can also cause severe pain in the epigastrium, which often radiates through to the back. It needs to be considered in any diagnosis of acute abdominal pain. The pain of chronic pancreatitis is usually less intense, if experienced at all.

- **Renal stones** can cause **renal colic** if they get stuck in the renal pelvis or the ureters. The pain is felt in the loins and is severe enough to cause the patient to roll around in agony also. The pain can radiate down the abdomen and can be felt in the testes in the male or labia in the female.

- **Constipation** may cause pain but usually in the elderly patient. The pain can be dull or sharp and may be constant or colicky. It tends to be diffuse and the patient has some difficulty pointing to a specific area. The pain may also move site (the elderly patient can sometimes be accused of being confused or lying because their story changes).

- **Diverticulitis** can cause pain, which can be severe and acute in onset. It may originate in the centre of the abdomen before localizing in the left iliac fossa (or be felt in the left iliac fossa immediately). The pain can behave like the mirror image of appendicitis and is sometimes called left-sided appendicitis.

- **Irritable bowel syndrome** can cause a variety of painful experiences. The pain can be dull, sharp, or burning in nature and can affect any part of the abdomen. The pain however is rarely severe.

- **Appendicitis**, during a classical attack, causes colicky, central abdominal pain before localizing to the right iliac fossa. However the appendix can occasionally lie in different positions within the abdomen and can lead to the pain localizing in more unusual places (which may lead to a delay in diagnosis).

Questions about the potential causes of the pain

You should always ask about the other abdominal symptoms—has the patient had nausea, vomiting, or a change in bowel habit? When did they last open their bowels? If it is longer than 48 hours (and unusual for them) the patient may have developed intestinal obstruction (especially if they are unable to pass wind (flatus) as well). With any luck, your previous questions will have given you some idea of what the diagnosis is, so obtain further information about what you think are the likely causes. Ask about **associated symptoms** and **risk factors** relevant to the condition(s) you suspect.

- **Oesophageal pain**. Associated symptoms—nausea, vomiting, abdominal pain. Risk factors—smoking, alcohol.

- **Peptic ulcer**. Associated symptoms—anorexia, nausea, vomiting, belching, waterbrash. Risk factors—*Helicobactor pylori* (*heli-co-back-ter-pie-lorry*) infection, NSAIDs, smoking, alcohol.

- **Gallstones**. Associated symptoms—anorexia, nausea, vomiting, belching, jaundice, fever (with cholecystitis or chalangitis). Risk factors—high cholesterol, age >40 years, female sex.

- **Pancreatitis**. Associated symptoms—anorexia, nausea, vomiting, fever, hypotension, weight loss (chronic pancreatitis). Risk factors—gallstones, alcohol, viral infections, drugs, for example, steroids.

- **Renal stones**. Anorexia, nausea, vomiting, urinary frequency, haematuria (*he-mat-you-rear* or *he-mat-chew-rear*). Risk factors—dehydration, immobility, hypercalcaemia (*high-per-cal-see-mia*), stagnant or infected urine, hyperuricaemia, for example, after chemotherapy.

- **Constipation**. Associated symptoms—anorexia, nausea, vomiting, flatulence, spurious diarrhoea. Risk factors—dehydration, lack of dietary fibre, drugs.

- **Diverticulitis**. Associated symptoms—anorexia, nausea, vomiting, diarrhoea or constipation, bleeding per rectum (PR), fever. Risk factors—poor dietary fibre, increasing age.

- **Irritable bowel syndrome**. Associated symptoms—nausea, constipation or diarrhoea, belching, heartburn, flatulence. Risk factors—anxiety, depression.
- **Appendicitis**. Associated symptoms—anorexia, nausea, vomiting, urinary frequency, constipation or diarrhoea. Risk factors—poor dietary fibre.

You may have noticed that the associated features of many of the acute causes of abdominal pain are very similar. In fact, many of the causes of an '*acute abdomen*' can be difficult to distinguish on history alone and you will have to consider them all in your differential diagnosis. An acute abdomen is an emergency and needs to be recognized. When dealing with one, the crucial decision is whether urgent surgery is needed. This is one instance when clinical examination is more important than the history. If during your examination you find signs of peritonitis, for example, abdominal rigidity, guarding, or rebound tenderness, you need to refer your patient to the surgeons immediately.

I have not mentioned less common causes of abdominal pain, such as bowel obstruction, mesenteric (*me-sent-eric* or *mez-ent-eric*) ischaemia, diabetic ketoacidosis (*key-toe-acid-owe-sis*), acute intermittent porphyria (*pour-firi-a*), and hypercalcaemia. These are described briefly at the end of this chapter.

Anorexia, weight loss, and weight gain

Anorexia

Anorexia means a loss of appetite. Most of us have experienced temporary anorexia, say after a short illness, or if we find a fly in our soup. A loss of appetite is only important if it is prolonged and associated with significant weight loss. Care must be taken not to take anorexia at face value. Dig a little deeper. Sometimes there are other symptoms that put your patient off eating, for example, vomiting, difficulty swallowing (dysphagia) (*dis-fage-a*), or loss of taste (ageusia) (*ay-goo-zia*), yet your patient may report all these as simply being 'off their food'.

Weight loss

Weight loss is an important symptom that can be difficult to evaluate. It needs to be assessed in two stages: (1) verify weight loss (and define amount and time scale) and (2) search for a cause.

- **Verify weight loss**. Unfortunately the degree to which a patient complains about weight loss does not always correlate with the true amount lost. Some may complain bitterly that they have lost weight but a flick through their notes (if available) may show that their weight is unaltered say after a year. Others may seem unconcerned but on further questioning will have lost gross amounts of weight. Therefore you must be diligent and try to confirm the presence of true weight loss. Some patients will be pretty accurate, for example, 'I have lost a stone in 2 months.' If they cannot be precise, try asking questions that might imply significant weight loss, for example, 'Are your clothes loose and ill fitting these days?' or 'Do you have to tighten your belt a further notch or two?' If your patient remains vague and looks well nourished, you may have to take their story with a pinch of salt. In this situation I would simply record their weight and do some baseline blood tests, for example, full blood count (FBC), urea and electrolytes (U&Es), liver function tests, and thyroid function tests.

- **Search for a cause**. If you are convinced that there is weight loss, you must search for a cause. The first question you should ask is about food intake. Some weight loss may be deliberate, in the case of dieting. Otherwise anorexia may herald a wide range of diseases. Less obvious causes of anorexia include depression. You may suspect this from the patient's demeanour (hunched posture, lack of eye contact, and so on). Sometimes it is less apparent and you need to ask about key symptoms: 'Do you have trouble sleeping?', 'Do you wake up early in the morning and have difficulty getting back to sleep?', 'Do you sleep excessively?', 'Have you lost interest in your work or hobbies?' Another condition that can be hard to spot is anorexia nervosa. You need to have an index of suspicion especially if you are dealing with a young girl with weight loss. It is a sign of the times that girls afflicted with anorexia are getting even younger and that boys are also being affected. Sometimes weight loss may occur despite a normal or increased appetite. This can occur in thyrotoxicosis (an overactive thyroid), diabetes mellitus, or some malignant conditions. Also ask about night sweats. What you are looking for are episodes that lead to drenching of their nightclothes or bed sheets. This symptom together with weight loss may be due to tuberculosis or lymphoma (*lim-foam-a*). Any further questions will depend on any further symptoms volunteered by your patient; for example, an elderly patient with alternating diarrhoea and constipation may suggest cancer of the colon and you should ask further gastrointestinal questions about bleeding PR, abdominal pain, tenesmus (*ten-ez-muss*) (a feeling that defecation is incomplete), and so on. An intolerance to a warm environment and irritability may suggest hyperthyroidism and you should ask about diarrhoea, excessive sweating, tremor, lack of periods in a woman (amenorrhea) (*ay-men-owe-rear*), or eye problems (Grave's disease). If no symptoms are forthcoming, you will have to screen the patient by asking questions from all of the systems review and seeing if any clues occur.

Weight gain

People do not often complain of weight gain. Some patients with depression, rather than lose their appetite, eat excessively for comfort and put on weight. Another important cause of weight gain is an underactive thyroid (hypothyroidism). Other symptoms include intolerance of a cold environment, constipation, dry skin, and heavy periods in women (menorrhagia) (*men-owe-rage-ia*). Rarely a lesion of the hypothalamus or pituitary can lead to hypopituitarism (*high-poe-pit-you-it-are-izm*) and sufferers may have an increased appetite and weight gain. If weight gain is rapid this may be due to fluid retention. This could be due to congestive cardiac failure or ascites (*a-sigh-tease*) (see later) or drugs such as non-steroidal pain-killers or steroids (steroids also stimulate appetite).

Key points

- Verify if weight loss has actually taken place
- Weight loss despite a good appetite suggests thyrotoxicosis (or malignancy)
- Ask about night sweats, which might indicate tuberculosis or lymphoma
- Weight gain may be due to fluid retention (as well as fat)

Heartburn

Heartburn is a common symptom and most of us will have experienced it at some point in our lives. It is a retrosternal burning pain, which can sometimes radiate into the neck. In most cases this is due to gastro-oesophageal reflux, or peptic ulcer disease. However, occasionally it is due to cardiac ischaemia or even infarction. With hospital patients, the proportion of people with a cardiac cause for heartburn is likely to be a lot higher than in the community. If patients say they have heartburn, get them to describe it, so you know you are both on the same wavelength. Also ask for accompanying symptoms, for example, nausea or fluid rising into the mouth (waterbrash). Heartburn aggravated by spicy or citrus foods,

or by lying flat, suggests a gastrointestinal origin. If the pain is relieved within half an hour by antacids, or within days by a proton pump inhibitor (a powerful acid suppressant) such as omeprazole, then this will strengthen the hypothesis that the heartburn is of gastrointestinal origin. Always check to make sure that heartburn is not related to exertion (that is, anginal in nature). If there are any doubts, do an ECG.

Key points

- Make sure you and your patient understand what is meant by 'heartburn'
- Ask about other gastrointestinal symptoms particularly those related to gastro-oesophageal reflux and peptic ulcer
- Always give a thought to cardiac disease

Dyspepsia

What is it?

This is an elusive term because it can mean different things to different doctors, for example, some use it to describe indigestion. Perhaps an easy way of describing dyspepsia (*dis-pepsi-a*) is that it is a collection of symptoms including epigastric pain, heartburn, nausea, upper abdominal bloating, and belching. Therefore dyspepsia is not a precise entity. Luckily you will not meet many patients who will complain they have dyspepsia; it is a term used predominantly by doctors. I find it a vague and unhelpful term. If I hear a patient has dyspepsia, all I can deduce is that they have some upper gastrointestinal pathology and nothing more. I prefer to concentrate on the individual symptoms such as heartburn or epigastric pain and investigate these accordingly. Peptic ulcers are a common cause of dyspepsia and because of this a distinction is sometimes made between this (as a cause) and non-ulcer dyspepsia. A patient must be investigated (usually by endoscopy) and have a peptic ulcer excluded before being categorized as having non-ulcer dyspepsia. The final thing to say is that you should always be alert to malignant conditions that can masquerade as dyspepsia. Danger signs include anorexia, weight loss, dysphagia, vomiting, haematemesis (*he-mat-emma-sis*), and constant abdominal pain. If a patient has these signs they should be thoroughly investigated.

Key points

- Dyspepsia is a collection of symptoms including epigastric pain, heartburn, bloating, belching, and nausea
- The distinction is usually made between ulcer dyspepsia (a common and important cause) and non-ulcer dyspepsia
- Beware of dyspeptic patients with anorexia, dysphagia, vomiting, haematemesis, constant abdominal pain, and weight loss; these need further investigation

Dysphagia

What is dysphagia?

Dysphagia means difficulty in swallowing. The problem usually resides in the oesophagus but you have to ask specific questions to exclude other causes that can affect swallowing. Other factors include (1) local factors in the mouth, (2) pain on swallowing (odynophagia) (*owe-die-no-fay-jah*), and (3) globus hystericus (*glow-bus-hysteric-us*).

- **Local factors in the mouth** include aphthous (*apf-thus*) ulcers, herpes simplex, and candida, which may cause pain when chewing food. This pain may be sufficient to put the person off eating. A lack of dentures can prevent a patient from chewing food sufficiently to be able to swallow anything other than a soft or pureed diet.

- **Pain on swallowing** may be caused by tonsillitis or pharyngitis or by inflammation of the oesophagus itself, for example, by candidal infection. The patient will experience a raw, painful sensation as food is swallowed and this is usually enough to put the patient off their food.

- **Globus hystericus** is a terrible name for this condition. The 'hystericus' label conveys the impression of some screaming, out-of-control patient, who is frankly mad. In fact, this is a recognized condition that affects anxious people who complain that they have a lump in their throat, usually at the level of the larynx. This sensation may be intermittent but the crucial thing is that the patient is still able to swallow normally despite its presence.

In **all** these cases the normal function of the oesophagus is retained. To exclude the above, ask if there is pain in the mouth or the throat on swallowing. Check elderly patients for dentures and ask if they fit well. The small number of patients with globus hystericus will normally volunteer this symptom. The term **globus pharyngeus** is being increasingly used.

The causes of dysphagia can be divided into mechanical and neurological causes (see Table 7.3). With mechanical causes a physical barrier to the passage occurs because of narrowing of the lumen. The dysphagia usually worsens in a progressive fashion, starting with difficulties with large boluses of food, then smaller pieces, until even liquids and the patient's own saliva cannot be swallowed in extreme cases. With neurological causes the normally coordinated contractions of the oesophagus are impaired. Patients tend to have difficulties swallowing liquids more than solids. Sometimes they may experience nasal regurgitation of fluids. With some neurological causes of dysphagia, the swallowing problem is just part of a bulbar or pseudobulbar palsy (a lower motor neuron lesion or upper motor lesion of the IX, X, and XII cranial nerves respectively). They may also experience dysarthria or dysphonia and you should be alert to this when you are listening to your patient.

In all cases of dysphagia, it is possible for regurgitation of food to occur. Sometimes your patient will mistakenly call this vomiting. The key feature here is the absence of retching and usually undigested food is brought back.

Table 7.3 Causes of dysphagia

Mechanical
Stricture
Carcinoma
Brown-Kelly–Paterson/Plummer–Vinson syndrome[a]
Neurological
Stroke
Motor neuron disease
Multiple sclerosis
Parkinson's disease
Achalasia (*ay-ka-lazier*) of the oesophagus

[a] *Adam Brown-Kelly (1865–1941), Scottish ear, nose, and throat surgeon; Donald Ross Paterson (1863–1939), Scottish ear, nose, and throat surgeon; H. S. Plummer (1874–1936), American physician; and P. P. Vinson (1890–1959), American physician; all described oesophageal stricture associated with iron deficiency anaemia.*

CASE 7.1

Problem. A 65-year-old man is admitted with a pneumonia. He has a 2-year history of Parkinson's disease and is on treatment to control his symptoms. He is an ex-smoker of 20 cigarettes per day for 40 years. He claims he has never had a bad chest until recently but he admits this is his third attack of pneumonia in the last 6 months. What is happening?

Discussion. To have three attacks of pneumonia in such a short time should ring alarm bells. You should be considering what could be predisposing your patient to repeated attacks of pneumonia. An ex-smoker may have developed lung cancer and this needs excluding. However, a patient with Parkinson's disease is at risk of aspiration pneumonia. Silent aspiration of food, particularly at night, can easily be missed. If you suspect this, a speech therapy assessment will be of great value. A therapist may identify problems with swallowing and can offer strategies that may help with dysphagia and reduce the risk of aspiration.

Key points

- Exclude local problems in the mouth or pain on swallowing before labelling a symptom as dysphagia
- Dysphagia may be due to mechanical obstruction or neurological diseases
- Mechanical causes of dysphagia usually lead to progressive problems with solids more than with liquids
- Neurological causes of dysphagia usually lead to greater problems with liquids than with solids
- Dysphagia may lead to aspiration pneumonia

Of more concern is that regurgitation can occur while the patient is asleep and can lead to aspiration of contents into the respiratory tract (see Case 7.1).

Nausea and vomiting

Everyone at some stage in their lives will have experienced nausea and vomiting, whether through a bout of food poisoning, travel sickness, the fear of medical exams, or the alcoholic celebrations (or consolation) following an examination. There are many causes of nausea and vomiting and it is easier to consider them in broad categories. Here, vomiting will be concentrated upon, as this is the more serious symptom of the two. See Table 7.4.

What to ask

Questions can be divided into (1) questions about the vomiting itself and (2) questions about the potential cause of vomiting.

Questions about the vomiting itself

Don't spend too much time finding out details about the vomit. Vomiting is a non-specific marker of disease

Table 7.4 Some causes of vomiting

Gastrointestinal
Peptic ulcer
Pancreatitis
Cholecystitis
Bowel obstruction
Non-gastrointestinal
Psychogenic (*sigh-co-jennik*)
Sepsis
Severe pain, e.g. myocardial infarction, aortic dissection
Endocrine, e.g. diabetes, Addison's disease, hyperparathyroidism
Central nervous system, e.g. meningitis, space-occupying lesion
Drugs, e.g. opiates, non-steroidals, digoxin, cytotoxic drugs

and it is ultimately the cause you are most interested in. Nonetheless, there are certain important features you need to look into.

- Is it acute or chronic?
- Is there nausea or retching preceding the vomit? Effortless vomiting may in fact be regurgitation and suggest oesophageal pathology.
- How much did they vomit? You only need a rough guide. Give suggestions such as an eggcupful, a cupful, a bucketful.

- What is in the vomit? Was it undigested food (for example, from a pharyngeal pouch)? Was it digested food (large quantities vomited in a projectile fashion may be pyloric stenosis)? Was it dark and did it smell faeculant (this could indicate a bowel obstruction)?

- Does it contain blood? Or did it contain elements that resembled coffee grounds (this is called haematemesis).

Questions about the potential cause of vomiting

As the causes of vomiting are so great it will provide a significant challenge to your history-taking skills. Sometimes your patient will help narrow your focus straight away by telling you about associated features unprompted. Otherwise you will need to be methodical and patient in your hunt for clues.

- Start by asking if there are any **precipitating factors**. Can they pinpoint the start of vomiting to eating suspect food? This usually occurs at social gatherings or at restaurants where food may be insufficiently prepared. The time to vomit following consumption of contaminated food can be as little as 6 hours with toxin-forming organisms, for example, *Bacillus cereus* (*ba-sill-us-serious*) to 12–24 hours for other organisms, for example, salmonella.

- **Pain** is another important feature to ask about. Severe pain anywhere in the body can cause nausea and vomiting. Ask specifically about chest pain, which could signify a myocardial infarction (MI) or epigastric pain, which could be due to a range of abdominal pathologies, for example, peptic ulcer, pancreatitis, and cholecystitis, not to mention MI again (see Case 7.2). Colicky abdominal pain with faeculant vomiting could indicate intestinal obstruction.

- From this point it is recommended that a review of gastrointestinal symptoms such as heartburn, dysphagia, and bowel habit be performed.

- Do not forget to check the past medical history for significant events such as previous operations (which can cause adhesions in the abdomen leading to bowel obstruction).

- Check for diabetes, renal problems, liver problems, and so on.

- A drug history is mandatory. Just about any drug can cause nausea and vomiting, whether in normal dosage, for example, antibiotics, cytotoxic (*sigh-toe-toxic*) drugs, and non-steroidal medication or in overdosage. Some drugs have a narrow therapeutic index, that is, the dose range that produces a beneficial effect is small and any further increase in dose can lead to toxic side effects. Drugs in this category include digoxin (*di-jox-in*), aminophylline (*am-in-off-i-lin*), and phenytoin

(*fen-it-toe-in*). Alcohol should be enquired about because it can cause vomiting following a binge or through chronic damage to other organs, particularly the liver.

- If no clear signposts have emerged with these questions then you will have to slowly review all the other non-gastrointestinal systems looking for clues. Do not discount the effect of emotions and be prepared to ask tactfully about stresses in a patient's life, for example, exams or bullying at work.

Key points

- There are a large number of causes of nausea and vomiting
- Severe pain and vomiting suggests a serious underlying condition
- Give a thought to food poisoning
- Always ask about travel
- Ask if there is blood in the vomit
- Always ask about drug treatment

Haematemesis and melaena

What are they?

Haematemesis and melaena (*muh-leaner*) are important symptoms, which should be taken seriously. The causes of these symptoms are given in Table 7.5.

Haematemesis

This is the vomiting of blood. This can be bright red blood from a fresh bleeding site; or, if the blood has been in the stomach for long enough, it is transformed by the stomach acid into a coffee-ground appearance.

Melaena

This is the faecal output from the anus following a bleed from the upper gastrointestinal tract. The stools look black and tarry. Melaena can occur because of bleeding anywhere from the oesophagus down to the right side of the colon. In general the bleeding has to be slow enough to allow time for the blood to be chemically altered during its transit through the bowel.

What to ask

Haematemesis

The questions follow a similar pattern to ordinary vomiting with some critical differences. You need to ask

CASE 7.2

Problem. A 72-year-old woman who is a type 2 diabetic is admitted to your ward. She has vomited four times at home and now looks clammy and unwell. How do you assess this woman?

Discussion. This woman is unwell and you need to get answers fast. You must modify your history-taking to reflect the urgency of the situation. Your first steps will include a cursory examination of your patient and the instigation of some preliminary investigations; all this must be done while taking a focused history. Ask the nursing staff to do some preliminary observations, for example, pulse, blood pressure, and temperature (this was 58/min, 80/40, and 36.8 °C in this case). Insert an intravenous cannula and withdraw blood for analysis (at least an FBC, U&Es, and random blood sugar (RBS)) and ask for an ECG and chest radiograph. Any patient with low blood pressure who looks clammy and unwell should initially trigger three important groups of causes in your mind: cardiac, sepsis, and haemorrhage. Ask if there is any pain anywhere, particularly the chest or epigastrium. Is there any breathlessness (could suggest pulmonary embolism or pneumonia)? Is there any blood in the vomit (suggesting gastrointestinal haemorrhage as a cause)? Have they passed any black, tarry motions (melaena) (again suggesting haemorrhage)? Have they felt cold and shivery then hot with bouts of uncontrollable shaking (rigors) (which may indicate underlying sepsis)? If these questions are negative then you need to ask detailed questions from your systems review. Record your clerking while you wait for the results of your investigations to percolate back to you.

This patient had no pain but was later found to have an inferior MI. This case also demonstrates the 'silent MI' and you need to be aware of such cases, particularly when you deal with high-risk patients like those who are elderly or have diabetes.

Table 7.5 Causes of haematemesis and melaena

Oesophagus	Stomach	Duodenum
Severe oesophagitis	Gastric ulcer	Duodenal ulcer
Mallory–Weiss tear	Gastric erosions	Duodenitis
Oesophageal varices	Gastic varices	
Oesophageal cancer	Gastric cancer	

because not all dark vomit is 'coffee-ground' in nature. It is also worth a quick question to see if the patient has drunk any port, red wine, or blackcurrant beverages beforehand, as this can be mistaken for haematemesis if vomited up.

- The next question to ask is whether the patient is haemodynamically stable or hypovolaemic (*high-poe-vol-ee-mick*). If blood loss is severe enough, the patient will complain of dizziness particularly on standing (see 'Haematemesis'). Your questions should be supplemented by a quick visual inspection and examination of the patient. Look and see if they are pale and clammy. Check the pulse for a tachycardia (>100 is serious) and the blood pressure, looking for hypotension (systolic <100 mmHg). If these signs are positive you have an emergency on your hands and you need to resuscitate and investigate your patient urgently. Other symptoms that might be experienced include palpitations, angina, and dyspnoea.

- Ask if there was any nausea or retching beforehand. The crucial observation is the timing of blood with the vomiting episodes. If a person has retched repeatedly before blood finally appears, this suggests a Mallory–Weiss (*mal-lorry-vice*) tear of the oesophagus (*George Kenneth Mallory (1900–1986); American pathologist, Soma Weiss (1898–1942), American physician*). Blood or coffee grounds found early in the vomit suggest another pathology, for example, peptic ulcer. Effortless vomiting of large amounts of bright red blood (often by the bucketload) suggests bleeding oesophageal varices (*va-ri-seize*). This is an emergency. Suspect this in a patient who is known to have varices, is an alcoholic, or has chronic liver disease.

- Ask how much blood they vomited, for example, eggcupful, cupful, or bucketful.

The causes of haematemesis are more limited than those of vomiting.

(1) questions about the haematemesis and (2) questions about the potential causes of the haematemesis.

There are four questions you need to ask about haematemesis: (1) What is the appearance? (2) Is the patient haemodynamically stable? (3) Is there nausea or retching? (4) How much did they vomit?

- The appearance of the vomit is all important in the diagnosis of haematemesis. Bright red blood is usually easy to spot but dark vomit can be misleading

- Ask about repeated retching, which could signify a Mallory–Weiss tear.

- Ask about pain, which may suggest peptic ulcer disease, gastritis, or duodenitis (*duo-de-night-iss*). It must be noted that these conditions can present with haematemesis without pain.

- Check the past medical history. Some patients will be well known and may be alcoholics or have chronic liver disease. Alarm bells should ring if these patients are admitted with haematemesis, and oesophageal varices or ulcers should be on the top of your list. There may be times when people known to have oesophageal varices are admitted with haematemesis. These people can bleed from lesions other than their varices and the cause of bleeding should always be looked for with an urgent gastroscopy.

- Check for other gastrointestinal symptoms, particularly danger symptoms such as anorexia, dysphagia, or weight loss, which may signify underlying malignancy.

- Ask about medication, for example, aspirin, NSAIDs, warfarin (*war-fa-rin*), and steroids. NSAIDs are a potent cause of gastric erosions and ulceration. Their use is widespread, particularly among older people. Do not just accept standard medications. Ask about 'over-the-counter' preparations that can be bought from the local chemist as some of these may contain aspirin or non-steroidal anti-inflammatory elements. Warfarin does not cause bleeding but it can cause significant bleeding from minor lesions or exacerbate a major bleed. I have also included steroids in this list because in the past many doctors have believed they also cause ulcers. Research has shown that this is not the case, but if they are combined with NSAIDs they markedly increase the risk of bleeding.

- Always ask about alcohol and the amount of units that are drunk in a week.

Melaena

The appearance of melaena is unmistakable. The only time there may be confusion is with a patient taking iron or bismuth compounds where the stools may also appear black (they usually lack the tarry consistency!). Also beware that patients on iron can still have melaena, so do not accept that black stools are solely due to iron until you have fully assessed the patient. All the causes of haematemesis can lead to melaena if sufficient blood passes through the bowel, therefore the questions you ask to define the causes of haematemesis are relevant for melaena also. In addition, lesions in the right side of the colon, for example,

Key points

- Haematemesis: confirm that haematemesis has taken place, for example, bright red blood or coffee-ground vomit
- Repeated retching or vomiting before blood appears suggests a Mallory–Weiss tear
- Melaena: confirm that melaena has taken place, that is, black stools are not due to iron or bismuth ingestion
- Melaena is due to bleeding in the upper gastrointestinal tract (or right-sided colonic lesions). See Case 7.3
- For both haematemesis and melaena ascertain whether the patient is haemodynamically stable (pulse <100/min, blood pressure >100 systolic)
- Is the patient on NSAIDs or warfarin?
- Always ask about alcohol consumption
- Always ask about preceding abdominal pain

cancer of the caecum (*see-cum*), can cause melaena and therefore questions relevant to the large bowel should also be asked, for example, change in bowel habit, tenesmus abdominal pain, and weight loss.

Bleeding per rectum

Bleeding can occur in two forms: (1) melaena (which has already been described) and (2) frank bleeding. The most common source of bright red bleeding is the anorectal region, although sources in the sigmoid and descending colon can also be responsible. The further proximally you go in the bowel the longer the blood takes to work its way to the anus and the darker it will look. The exception to this is torrential bleeding from an upper gastrointestinal source, where the blood can rush through the bowel and manifest as bright red bleeding. In these cases the patient is usually ill with a tachycardia and low blood pressure and will need urgent intervention. See Table 7.6 for causes of bleeding PR.

What to ask

The first question to ask is whether the patient is haemodynamically stable or hypovolaemic. If blood loss is severe enough the patient will complain of dizziness particularly on standing (see 'Haematemesis'). Your questions should be supplemented by a quick visual inspection and examination of the patient. Look and see if they are pale and

CASE 7.3

Problem. A 56-year-old man is admitted unconscious into casualty and you shadow the specialist trainee for medicine (ST2) ['2' denotes that they are in their second year of training] as she assesses the patient. The only history available is that he had been complaining about indigestion on and off for a month. He is normally fit and well except for hypertension, for which he takes atenolol (50 mg). He is pale and clammy, his pulse is 60/min, his blood pressure is 100/70, and he is apyrexial. The specialist trainee suspects that the patient has had an inferior MI leading to bradycardia and collapse; however, the ECG only shows left ventricular hypertrophy with lateral ischaemia. The ST2 now considers performing a head CT scan to find out why the patient is unconscious. Can you save her from making a mistake?

Discussion. The ST2's working diagnosis is a good one. The month's history of indigestion could have been unstable angina leading up to an inferior infarct, which can affect the conduction system of the heart and cause bradycardias and even complete heart block. Do not be put off a diagnosis of an infarct because of a normal ECG; if necessary repeat one a few hours later and follow up with cardiac enzymes as changes may develop later. Your priority in this case is to first check that the patient is breathing and that his airway is patent. An intravenous

cannula should be inserted for venous access and blood sent for analysis. An ECG and later a portable chest radiograph will be of value.

In this case, however, there are a number of catches. The first is that the patient's blood pressure of 100/70 might be dismissed as normal. However, as a hypertensive individual, his blood pressure might normally run at a higher level, for example, 190/110, and this new blood pressure could represent a significant drop. Another catch is that he is on a β-blocker, atenolol, which slows the pulse and can mask a tachycardia. Therefore you must be aware of these pitfalls. Re-evaluate the clues again. He is pale and clammy, suggesting that his circulation is under stress. Sepsis has not been demonstrated and a cardiac cause is still possible if not proven. Remember this patient has complained of indigestion and it is possible that he may have a peptic ulcer. It can bleed without obvious haematemesis and therefore if you suspect this as a possibility then you should perform a PR examination. In this case a PR examination revealed melaena and the cause of collapse became clear. He was resuscitated with fluids with further blood sent for cross-matching and once stable he was sent for urgent endoscopy, which revealed a bleeding gastric ulcer, which was injected.

Table 7.6 Causes of bleeding per rectum

Anus/rectum	Colon	Upper gastrointestinal tract
Haemorrhoids	Ulcerative colitis	Torrential bleed
Anal fissure	Crohn's colitis	
Carcinoma of rectum	Ischaemic colitis, carcinoma of colon, polyps, angiodysplasia (*an-ji-owe-dis-play-zia*)	

clammy. Check the pulse for a tachycardia (>100 is serious) and the blood pressure, looking for hypotension (systolic <100 mmHg). If these signs are positive you have an emergency on your hands and you need to resuscitate and investigate your patient urgently.

If the situation is not life-threatening you can take a more measured history. As the most common causes of bleeding PR are due to anorectal pathology, this is a good place to start.

- Ask if the blood is bright red or dark red. The more proximal the bleeding lesion is in the bowel, the darker red it will be.
- Ask if the blood is mixed in with the motion. You will have to ask supplementary questions here because most people will finish in the toilet and will see a mixture of blood and faeces and claim that the blood is mixed in. Therefore ask if any blood dripped in the toilet bowl after they finished defecation and if any blood was wiped off with the toilet paper. If the answer to both is yes, the likelihood is that you are dealing with haemorrhoids or occasionally an anal fissure.
- Now ask about pain on defecation. If it is painless when a motion is passed, the diagnosis is likely to be haemorrhoids. If it is painful, then an anal fissure is more likely (usually after constipation with the passage of hard faeces). Before accepting that rectal bleeding

is due to haemorrhoids, ask about other abdominal symptoms. More than one cause of bleeding PR can coexist and you may still have to investigate the large bowel even if you do demonstrate haemorrhoids or a fissure. If there are no other bowel symptoms you can be confident that bleeding PR is a local anorectal problem and you can spare your patient needless investigations.

- Ask about diarrhoea and constipation. Profuse diarrhoea may suggest inflammatory bowel disease, for example, ulcerative colitis (*ulcer-at-ive-coal-eye-tiss*) or Crohn's (*crones*) disease and constipation could herald an anal fissure (*Burrill Bernard Crohn (1884–1983), American physician*).
- Ask if there is any mucus passed as this also suggests an inflammatory cause of diarrhoea and bleeding PR.
- Do not forget to ask about recent travel because some infective conditions can cause rectal bleeding, for example, shigella (*shig-ella*) or amoebic (*am-ee-bic*) dysentery or schistosomiasis (*shis-toe-so-my-a-sis*).
- Abdominal pain may be a feature of a number of conditions. Ask about the nature of the pain, particularly if it is colicky and note its site, radiation, and relation to defecation; for example, pain with ulcerative colitis may be colicky or cramp like prior to defecation and is relieved by the act.
- Finally in some cases the blood loss may be chronic and occult and the patient may present to you with symptoms of anaemia, for example, dyspnoea, dizziness, or angina.

Key points
- Bleeding PR can be in the form of bright red, dark red blood, or melaena
- Bright red or dark red blood suggests a lower gastrointestinal source of bleeding
- Is the patient haemodynamically stable?
- Always ask about diarrhoea or constipation
- Painless bleeding following defecation with blood on the toilet paper suggests haemorrhoids (but you must still rule out other causes)

Jaundice

Jaundice is another challenge to your history-taking skills. There are many causes of jaundice and to help you understand these there is a section explaining the physiology of jaundice near the end of this chapter. The key to learning about jaundice is the liver because this is the focal point of bilirubin (*billy-rue-bin*) metabolism.

What is it?

Jaundice is the yellow discoloration of the skin and sclerae due to the deposition of the bile pigment bilirubin. Some old-fashioned textbooks call this icterus (*ick-ter-us*). Bilirubin is the breakdown product of haemoglobin and is modified in the liver (conjugated) before being excreted in the bile.

Causes

See Table 7.7. As the liver is the key organ in bilirubin metabolism it is useful to divide the causes into prehepatic, hepatic, and posthepatic causes. Sometimes you may read about a different classification of jaundice into **hepatitic** and **cholestatic** causes. Hepatitic causes simply mean those agents that damage the liver cells, interfering with their functions (including bilirubin metabolism). Cholestatic causes are those that obstruct the normal flow of bile into the small intestine and these are subdivided into intrahepatic cholestasis (*coal-ee-stay-sis*), where the disturbance occurs in the intrahepatic bile ducts and canaliculi (*can-a-lick-you-lie*) and the intrahepatic ducts

Table 7.7 Causes of jaundice

Prehepatic	Hepatic	Posthepatic
Haemolytic anaemia, e.g. autoimmune hereditary spherocytosis	Hepatitis, e.g. viral hepatitis A, B, or C	Gallstones in common bile duct
	Leptospirosis	Bile duct stricture
	Hydatid disease	Cholangiocarcinoma
	Drugs, e.g. halothane	Chronic pancreatitis
	Autoimmune, e.g. primary biliary cirrhosis	Cancer head of pancreas
	Alcohol	Sclerosing cholangitis
		Malignancy, especially at porta hepatis (*porter-hepat-iss*)

and extrahepatic cholestasis, where the disturbance is in the extrahepatic ducts, for example, the common bile duct. This distinction between hepatitic and cholestatic causes is somewhat artificial because elements of both may coexist in the same patient; for example, viral hepatitis or cirrhosis (*si-roe-sis*) may include damage to the liver cells as well as some intrahepatic cholestasis.

What to ask

- Ask how long the patient has had jaundice.
- Also ask about the colour of their stools and urine. In obstructive causes of jaundice, bilirubin in the bile does not reach the intestine where it contributes to the colour of the stools. Instead the faeces are a pale, clay colour. The excess bilirubin is excreted in the urine giving it a dark colour.
- Also ask about itching. Bilirubin deposited in the skin is an irritant and can cause itching (the mechanism is not known).
- Ask about pain. The pain of biliary colic may suggest gallstones. Dull pain in the epigastrium or right hypochondrium (*high-poe-con-dree-um*) may be due to hepatitis. Painless, progressive jaundice is supposed to be the hallmark of carcinoma (*car-sin-owe-ma*) of the head of the pancreas, although other conditions can sometimes mimic this.
- Ask about fever. Sweating and rigors may suggest ascending cholangitis, a condition where infection occurs in the bile ducts (usually with a gallstone as a source) and ascends up the biliary tree. The triad of jaundice, pain, and fever is known as Charcot's (*shark-owes*) triad.
- Also ask about travel. This usually means travel abroad where your patient may pick up exotic infections. Hepatitis A is common in certain areas and can be acquired through seafood. Don't forget about journeys closer to home, for example, hydatid (*high-dat-id*) disease can be picked up in Wales (if you spend your time among the sheep!).
- Occupation should be noted as certain jobs may occasionally put a person at risk of jaundice: sewage workers— leptospirosis (*lept-owe-spy-roe-sis*); sheep farmers— hydatid disease; doctors and nurses— hepatitis B and C.
- Review the patient's past medical history as this may be packed full of useful information. Relevant questions include past blood transfusions (hepatitis B and C) although the risks with modern screening techniques should be miniscule these days. Ask about

previous operations particularly around the biliary tree, which could lead to bile duct stricture. Ask if they have had jaundice before and medical conditions such as autoimmune disease, for example, systemic lupus erythmatosis (SLE), which may be associated with an autoimmune hepatitis or inflammatory bowel disease, which can lead to sclerosing cholangitis.

- Always ask about drugs. Many drugs can cause jaundice through a variety of mechanisms (usually liver cell damage). As the list is so large it is always worth consulting the *British national formulary* (*BNF*), the drugs 'bible' for doctors, nurses, and pharmacists, if you are unsure of a particular drug.
- Do not forget to ask about alcohol, which can lead to chronic liver disease.
- Enquire about a family history. Some haemolytic diseases may be inherited, for example, hereditary spherocytosis (*sphere-owe-site-owe-sis*)—autosomal dominant.
- Take a social history. You will need to be tactful with your enquiries here. You will be asking about high-risk activities that can lead to viral infections and you will have to probe gently into the patient's sexual activities. Some people may be affronted by your questions and others may respond with nervous silence. All will feel some measure of embarassment. So just explain calmly beforehand why you need to ask these questions and reassure them that their answers will be confidential. Questions to ask include a history of intravenous drug abuse and unprotected sex with multiple partners (see Chapter 9), particularly among bisexual people or men who have sex with men. All these activities increase the risk of infection with hepatitis B and C and HIV.
- Finally do not forget your systems review (especially if the cause is still not clear) because multisystem diseases, for example, autoimmune diseases, can affect any organ and malignancy in just about any system can lead to metastases in the liver.

Key points
- Ask about pale stools and dark urine (suggest an obstructive jaundice)
- Ask if there is pain associated with the jaundice
- Is itching or fever associated?
- Ask about travel and previous blood transfusions
- Ask tactfully about certain lifestyles, for example, homosexuality or drug abuse
- Always ask about drugs

Bowel habit

It seems there is no aspect of a person's life that cannot be probed by a doctor and their bowels are no exception. Questions about bowel habit are a real test of your ability to control the consultation. The British (of yesteryear) are obsessed with their bowels. The patient who is virtually mute while talking about their heart attack may suddenly come alive when you ask them about their bowels.

Constipation

What is it?

Many people have their own idea of what constitutes constipation and therefore you must be clear that you and the patient are on the same wavelength. A useful definition of constipation is a bowel frequency of less than three times per week or where the patient has to strain for at least a quarter of the time during defecation. See Table 7.8 for causes of constipation.

What to ask

- The important question is to ask how long the patient has suffered with constipation. Somebody with symptoms for more than a year is unlikely to have sinister pathology. If they have had constipation all their life then the constipation is likely to be idiopathic or just a normal variant. It might be worth asking why they have complained if they have tolerated the symptoms for so long. Sometimes patients develop painful anal fissures or they may be worried about the possibility of cancer.

- Ask about the patient's diet. Find out what they eat in a typical day. It is amazing how little some people eat, or the lack of fibre in their diet. Adequate fluid (at least 1.5 litres) is required along with exercise to maintain a regular bowel habit. Simple advice regarding adequate fibre, fluid, and exercise may be all that is required. It may also be worth checking a calcium level and carrying out thyroid function tests to rule out hypercalcaemia and hypothyroidism.

- Also check the patient's occupation. Some jobs might not allow for a regular bowel habit, for example, lorry drivers or salesmen and these people often get used to 'hanging on' until a more appropriate moment.

- Anyone who has recently developed constipation or is alternating between diarrhoea and constipation requires further investigation. The diagnosis to worry about is cancer of the bowel, although diverticular disease and inflammatory bowel disease can present this way.

- A patient presenting with absolute constipation (even to flatus) together with colicky abdominal pain and faeculent vomiting should make you think of acute bowel obstruction.

- Do not forget to ask about other abdominal symptoms such as vomiting, pain, and indigestion. One further symptom you may not have heard of is tenesmus. It is a sensation of incomplete evacuation following defaecation and often leads to the patient returning to the toilet repeatedly. This may be due to an obstructive lesion such as carcinoma of the rectum but may be experienced in other diseases such as inflammatory bowel disease.

- Constipation may be a feature of other disease even if it is not the presenting complaint. Enquiring about this symptom can be an opportunity for you to improve the patient's quality of life by tackling the constipation. In cases of spinal injury, stroke, Parkinson's syndrome, and so on, be aware of the possibility of constipation and always ask about it because although it has a low priority among healthcare workers it has the ability to cause great misery.

- Never forget about the role of medication in causing constipation; ask for details. Common culprits include the opiates (*owe-pee-ates*), anti-cholinergics (*anti-coal-in-err-jicks*) (including classes of drugs with anti-cholinergic side effects, for example, anti-depressants or oxybutinin (*ox-ee-beauty-nin*) for incontinence), and aluminium-containing antacids, for example, aludrox

Table 7.8 Causes of constipation

Idiopathic
Diet
Drugs, e.g. opiates, anti-cholinergics
Cancer of the colon/rectum
Diverticular disease
Acute bowel obstruction
Spinal cord disease
Parkinson's syndrome
Hypothyroidism

or algicon. Be especially sensitive to patients undergoing palliative care who may be on large doses of opiate analgesia. Even now doctors outside palliative care still forget to write patients up for laxatives even though it is inevitable their patients will become constipated.

Diarrhoea

What is it?

Diarrhoea is a condition that all of us will have experienced, yet it is difficult to define. We all recognize at one extreme, loose watery stools being passed up to 10 times per day as obvious diarrhoea, yet normal stools being passed more than five times a day could be diarrhoea according to some definitions. Some institutions have used the passage of 250 g per day of stool weight as a quantitative expression of diarrhoea. Although useful in a research setting, this definition has no practical value to a general practitioner faced with a patient in their surgery. The author's view is that if you are dealing with a patient with loose, watery stools, you are dealing with diarrhoea. You will have to make your own judgement on more borderline cases where there may just be a small increase in the frequency of bowel action or 'the motion is not quite as solid as it usually is.'

Causes

The causes of diarrhoea are great in number and here only some broad categories along with some examples will be given. See Table 7.9.

What to ask

- The first fact you need to establish is whether you are dealing with diarrhoea. Ask what the stool looks like, whether it is formed, semi-solid, or watery? You also need to know the approximate frequency of the bowel action: 2 times per day, 6 times per day, 15 times per day, and so on. Most people (understandably) do not scrutinize their stools in great detail and may be unable to give an accurate account of what they produce. If their diarrhoea is continuing, it may be helpful if they keep a 'diarrhoea diary', charting the appearance and frequency of their bowel action. The Bristol Stool chart is a useful guide with pictures showing the different consistencies of stool that can be produced.

- Ask if the diarrhoea is acute or chronic. Diarrhoea is usually regarded as chronic if it lasts longer than 3 weeks. This is important because acute causes are usually short lived by definition and are predominantly infective.

Table 7.9 Causes of diarrhoea

Diet	Curry, malnutrition
Stress	Tests/examinations, irritable bowel syndrome
Infection	Viral gastroenteritis, food poisoning, 'traveller's diarrhoea', dysentery
Chronic inflammation	Ulcerative colitis, Crohn's disease, ischaemic colitis, radiation colitis,
Endocrine	Hyperthyroidism, carcinoid syndrome, Zollinger–Ellison syndrome[a]
Malabsorption	Small bowel mucosal disease, e.g. coeliac disease, bacterial overgrowth, surgery, e.g. ilieal resection
Pancreatic disease	
Drugs	Laxative abuse, antibiotics, digoxin, theophylline, magnesium compounds
Spurious diarrhoea	

[a] *Robert Milton Zollinger (1903–1992), US surgeon; Edwin Homer Ellison (1918–1970) US surgeon.*

- Ask about recent attendances to parties, restaurants, or food outlets of dubious reputation. This may point to food poisoning as a cause of the diarrhoea. Although most causes of food poisoning are over within a week, some cases can last for several weeks, for example, campylobacter (*camp-ee-low-back-ter*), so an infective cause is still worth looking for in an apparently chronic case of diarrhoea.

- Ask about recent travels abroad. The causes of diarrhoea contracted abroad are many and some of them have notable names such as 'Montezuma's revenge' or 'Delhi belly'.

- You will need to find out more detail about the diarrhoea. Ask if there is any blood mixed in with the motion, which might suggest an infective colitis, diverticular disease, inflammatory bowel disease, or malignancy.

- Ask about associated mucus, which can also be found in inflammatory conditions.

- Find out if the stools are loose, pale, and bulky and float in the toilet bowl. Are they difficult to flush away? This form of diarrhoea is called steatorrhea (*stee-at-owe-rear*) and is caused by malabsorption. Malabsorption can occur for a number of reasons, that is, small bowel mucosal disease, for example, coeliac (*seal-ee-yak*) disease or pancreatic disease, where the nutrients in the small intestine cannot be absorbed. The high fat content in the stool gives it a loose, bulky foul-smelling quality and also makes it difficult to flush away. It is also important to realize that malabsorption can occur in the presence of normal-looking stools and you should still be suspicious if the clinical picture and blood tests suggest this.

- Check the patient's occupation. This is probably more important for counselling rather than for a clue to a cause. People with infectious diarrhoea who work in 'sensitive' jobs such as cooks, food preparers, teachers, doctors, or nurses should not work until they are no longer a risk.

- Do not forget to ask about drugs. Many drugs can cause diarrhoea and it is worth checking any medication you are unsure of in the *BNF*. A common cause of diarrhoea is the broad-spectrum antibiotics. If taken for long enough, the antibiotics kill off the useful commensal organisms in the gut allowing more resistant pathogens such as *Clostridium dificile* (*clos-trid-iium-de-fitch-ee-lee* or *de-fe-seal*) to thrive, causing diarrhoea and in severe cases 'pseudomembranous' (*sue-dough-mem-bren-us*) colitis. Also ask about the use of laxatives especially in older patients. In the past a regular bowel habit was deemed essential and everything from prune juice to laxatives were used to achieve this aim.

Key points

- Constipation: there are a number of causes of constipation
- Check diet for adequate fibre and adequate fluid intake
- Always check a drug history
- Diarrhoea: there are a large number of causes of diarrhoea
- Give a thought to food poisoning
- Always check a travel history
- Pale, bulky stools that are difficult to flush (steatorrhoea) suggest fat malabsorption
- Always check the drug history
- In the elderly patient do not forget spurious diarrhoea

Many older people omit this aspect of the history when they complain of diarrhoea.

Tip

If a nurse informs you a patient has diarrhoea (particularly someone who was previously constipated), quickly check the drug chart and see if they are still on laxatives because doctors and nurses are notorious for not reviewing medication (particularly bowel medication and night sedation).

- Other drugs that commonly cause diarrhoea are given in Table 7.9.

- If you still have no clear idea as to the cause of diarrhoea then you will have to review all the systems. Pay particular attention to conditions, for example, hyperthyroidism (diarrhoea, normal appetite, weight loss, and intolerance to warm environments), and rarer causes such as carcinoid (*car-sin-oid*) syndrome (diarrhoea, wheezing, and facial flushing), and Zollinger–Ellison syndrome (diarrhoea and recurrent peptic ulcers).

- One final point to make is that paradoxically, some patients with constipation (usually elderly) can present with diarrhoea, faecal soiling of underwear, or faecal incontinence. This is called spurious diarrhoea. How liquid stools are formed around impacted stools is not known but the situation has to be explained carefully, or your patient will think you are crazy prescribing laxatives for diarrhoea.

Genitourinary system

This section will concentrate on urinary tract symptoms; sexual history-taking is covered in Chapter 9. There are a number of symptoms you need to know.

Dysuria

What is it?

Dysuria (*dis-you-ria*) is pain on passing urine. It is often described as burning or scalding in nature and usually indicates a lower urinary tract infection.

What to ask

Ask if there is burning or stinging when passing water. Look out for smart replies such as, 'I'll check the next time I drive past the river.'

Frequency

What is it?

As the name suggests this is where people pass urine many times during the day. It is difficult to define a point when going to the toilet becomes pathological because of the renal response to a wide range of fluid intakes. Nevertheless if a patient is going to the toilet so often that it affects their life it deserves to be investigated. See Table 7.10 for causes of frequency.

What to ask

- Try to get some idea of how often the patient is going to the toilet; 'lots' or 'a million times' is inadequate. Ask whether it is 2 times a day, 5 times a day, 10 times a day, and so on. Or ask if it is frequent what the average interval between passing urine is, for example, 10 minutes, 30 minutes, 1 hour, and so on. Also try to get an idea of the amount of urine the patient is passing. Small volumes passed frequently might suggest prostatic disease, while large amounts might suggest diabetes mellitus, diabetes insipidus, or psychogenic polydipsia (polydipsia means thirst).

- Ask how much fluid they drink in a day. A person drinking gallons of fluid is likely to pass a lot of urine, for example, in psychogenic polydipsia (a condition where the patient always feels thirsty and drinks continually). Paradoxically, too little fluid (<1 litre) may lead to frequency because concentrated urine in the bladder is an irritant. Try to gauge the amounts by cupfuls or glasses of drink, for example, a cup of tea or coffee = 150 mL, a mug of tea or coffee = 250 mL, and a glass of drink = 250 mL.

- This form of questioning is fairly crude and the majority of people cannot give accurate estimations of what they drink and pee. A useful thing to do is to give a diary and two measuring jugs so that they can chart their fluid intake and output over a 3-day period (please point out that they should measure their fluid intake and urine output from the different jugs).

- Ask about past attacks of cystitis or kidney infections (which may cause kidney damage).

- Ask about drugs, particularly diuretics. Most people are acutely aware of the relationship of their frequency with their diuretics (although some still neglect to mention that they are on them). When they are reminded, you will soon learn how they plan trips to town, for example, via a succession of toilets (most simply do not take the tablet).

Oliguria

What is it?

Oliguria (*ollig-you-ria*) means a low urine output. Very few people will complain of a low urine output, so this tends to be a medical observation. People who are dehydrated will become oliguric because their kidneys will decrease the excretion of water to conserve the body's supply. Oliguria can also be a sign of renal failure. The rule of thumb is that your patient should produce at least 20 mL of urine per hour (if your patient is at risk of renal failure they will probably be catheterized to help measure the urine output accurately). Sometimes kidney failure may occur with a normal urine output and therefore the quality of urine produced must always be analysed. This is done by looking at the electrolytes in the urine and by comparing the concentration of urea and creatinine with the plasma urea and creatinine. The urine of a normal person will have its urea and creatinine concentrated at least 20 times that of the plasma concentration. The urine of a person in renal failure may almost be at the same concentration as plasma.

Anuria

What is it?

Anuria (*a-new-ria*) means no urine output at all. Even in established renal failure there is usually some urine produced and therefore you must consider an obstruction to

Table 7.10 Causes of urinary frequency

Fluid intake
Increased
Decreased
Alcohol ingestion
Kidney disease
Diabetes mellitus
Diabetes insipidus
Psychogenic polydipsia
Prostatic disease
Detrusor instability
Drugs, e.g. diuretics (*die-you-ret-ticks*)

the flow of urine. Such a person will need an emergency abdominal ultrasound to try and pinpoint a cause of obstruction or to rule it out.

Urgency

What is it?

This is the desperate need to micturate as soon as the desire is experienced. All the causes of frequency can cause urgency.

What to ask

'When you get the sensation to pee do you have to go to the toilet there and then or can you hold on?'

Incontinence

What is it?

One definition of incontinence is where there is the involuntary loss of urine, which can be objectively demonstrated and is a social or hygienic problem. As the definition of incontinence infers, it is a difficult and embarrassing symptom to cope with and patients often attempt to hide it. You should always ask about this in a tactful and sensitive manner and reassure your patient that there is a lot that can be done to improve the condition.

See Table 7.11 for causes of incontinence. The top two causes are **urge** and **stress** (the two can coexist). All the causes of urgency can lead to incontinence if the patient is not quick enough getting to the toilet. An overactive bladder (detrusor (*de-true-za*) instability) is the greatest cause of urge incontinence (the detrusor is the bladder muscle). It can develop for no obvious reason or it can be secondary to bladder outflow obstruction. Stress incontinence is commoner in women because of childbirth and the potential damage to the pelvic floor musculature. Typically

Table 7.11 Causes of incontinence

Urge
Stress
Overflow
Environmental
Giggle
Continuous

the patient leaks a small amount of urine, if they cough, sneeze, stand, lift, or exercise. All these activities raise the intra-abdominal pressure, which is also experienced within the bladder. Leakage occurs when the bladder pressure exceeds the pressure exerted by the urinary sphincter. Sometimes the environment is less than optimal for a patient to maintain continence, for example, a urine bottle is placed on the hemiplegic side of a stroke patient, or the toilet is too far away for a patient with Parkinson's disease to reach in time.

Overflow incontinence is a paradox (similar to spurious diarrhoea), in that the fundamental problem is retention of urine. For reasons that are not understood, the patient may pass small amounts of urine at times or may just become incontinent. An examination of the abdomen will reveal an enlarged bladder (or you can confirm it with a bladder scanner, a portable ultrasound machine).

What to ask?

Before launching into questions about incontinence it is best if you prepare your patient. Say, 'I am sorry but I have to ask you some personal questions. They are designed to help find out what the problem is and hopefully to help you. Everything you tell me will be kept confidential.'

- Ask about urgency as before but follow up the question with 'Do you find there are times you do not make it to the toilet and wet yourself?'

- Ask 'Do you wet yourself if you cough, sneeze, stand, exercise, or lift heavy objects?' (stress incontinence).

- Ask about fluid intake.

- Ask about caffeine intake and the amount of tea and coffee drunk in a day (caffeine is a weak diuretic).

- Ask about medications. Diuretics on their own may be enough to cause incontinence or can make an existing problem worse. Anti-cholinergics can cause urinary retention and may cause overflow incontinence.

- Check to see if the patient has recently developed constipation because this can also cause urinary retention.

- Ask about childbirth in women. You need to know how many children they have had. Were they all vaginal deliveries? Find out what size the babies were if possible and more importantly were instruments involved, for example, forceps (stress incontinence).

- Ask about previous surgery. Women may have had previous surgery for incontinence, for example, bladder repair. Men may have had previous prostate surgery and their prostatic symptoms may have returned.

Occasionally a small proportion of men, following a transurethral prostatectomy, may develop true stress incontinence as a result of damage to the internal urethral sphincter.

- Find out whether they suffer with diabetes mellitus, kidney, or bladder problems.
- On rare occasions young girls may become incontinent when they laugh or giggle (giggle incontinence).

Haematuria

What is it?

Haematuria is the passing of blood in the urine. If it is visible it is termed macroscopic haematuria, if it is detected by a dipstick test of the urine it is termed microscopic haematuria. This is an important symptom and needs prompt investigation. See Table 7.12 for causes of haematuria.

What to ask

- The first thing to do is to establish if haematuria has truly taken place. There are occasions where what you ingest can colour your urine red. The culprits include beetroot, tablets such as rifampicin (*riff-am-pi-sin*) (red-man syndrome), and laxatives such as codanthrusate or codanthromer (although these have been withdrawn) and stalevo (Parkinson's medication), so ask about these.
- Ask about pain. Colicky pain in the loin radiating to the groin may suggest renal or ureteric stones. Painless haematuria should make you think about malignancy in the urinary tract, for example, kidney or bladder.

Table 7.12 Causes of haematuria

Kidney	Tumours, infection, infarction, stones, trauma, nephritis
Ureter	Stones, tumour
Bladder	Tumour, infection
Prostate	Benign prostatic hypertrophy, cancer of the prostate
Urethra	Trauma

- Ask about recent trauma. Any blow to the loin may damage the kidney. The urethra can be damaged in a road traffic accident or in an 'astride' injury where a person falls astride a bar or beam. Trauma may occur due to instrumentation of the urethra, for example, catheterization. Some confused patients with a catheter *in situ* may tug at it and cause haematuria.
- Ask about other urinary symptoms, for example, dysuria and frequency may suggest a urinary tract infection or frequency and nocturia may suggest prostatic disease in a man.
- Check to see if the patient is on warfarin (or has any other bleeding tendency). This may exacerbate any bleeding problem even from a minor source.

Abdominal system examination summary

This summary contains many terms that you will not understand on first reading. These terms are explained in the next section 'Abdominal system examination in detail'.

1. Introduce yourself to the patient and ask for permission to examine.
2. Ask the patient to get on to the bed (if not already there). You may need to get help!
3. Wash your hands.
4. Ask the patient to strip to their underwear.
5. Lie the patient flat on one pillow (if they are elderly or have a kyphosis (*kye-foe-sis*) two pillows may be needed).
6. While doing 1–5, have a 'general look'. Is the patient in discomfort? Is the abdomen distended? Is there evidence of jaundice, wasting of muscles, scratch marks, and so on?
7. Inspect both hands for signs of chronic liver disease (DF 6/10), for example, clubbing, leuconychia (*loo-co-nick-ia*), koilonychia (*coil-o-nick-ia*), palmar erythema, Dupuytren's (*dew-pit-runs*) contracture, spider naevi (*knee-vie*) (make sure you blanch these), and purpura (*purr-pew-ra*).
8. Look for a flapping tremor (DF 8/10) only if you suspect liver failure (jaundice, spider naevi, and so on). Ask the patient to extend their arms and cock their wrists back.

9 Inspect the face for xanthelasmata (DF 2/10), spider naevi (DF 6/10), and other telangiectasias (DF 9/10); inspect the eyes for jaundice (DF 7/10); and inspect the conjunctivae for anaemia (DF 9/10).

10 Inspect the lips for pigmentation or telangiectasia (*tee-lan-jeck-tay-sia*) (DF 9/10).

11 Examine the oral cavity (DF 8/10). Inspect for telangiectasia, pigmentation, dentition, ulcers, angular stomatitis (*stow-ma-tight-iss*), and candidiasis (*can-did-eye-a-sis*). Also examine the tongue and tonsils and check for odours.

12 Palpate the neck for cervical lymph nodes (DF 6/10), particularly the left supraclavicular region.

13 Inspect the chest for further spider naevi (DF 6/10), gynaecomastia (DF 7/10), and loss of axillary hair in men (DF 6/10).

14 Observe the abdomen for distension, herniae, scars, striae (*stry-ee*), pulsations, peristalsis, and distended veins (DF 8/10).

15 Ask the patient if they have any tender areas before commencing light palpation. Palpate the abdomen lightly, mapping any areas of tenderness and note any masses (DF 4/10). Watch the patient's face for signs of pain!

16 Palpate more deeply and assess any masses felt in more detail (DF 7/10).

17 Palpate specifically for enlarged organs: liver—commence in the right iliac fossa and move upwards towards the right costal margin while getting the patient to take deep breaths; spleen—commence in the right iliac fossa and move upwards towards the left costal margin while getting the patient to take deep breaths; kidneys—commence in the flanks and 'bimanually ballot' them.

18 Percuss over any masses or organs felt. Check for ascites. If the percussion note is dull in the flanks, go on to demonstrate shifting dullness (DF 7/10) or a fluid thrill (DF 6/10).

19 Auscultate for bowel sounds (DF 8/10) (and for bruits and rubs if necessary) (DF 9/10).

20 Examine the groins for lymphadenopathy and herniae (ask the patient to cough) (DF 8/10).

21 Wash your hands.

22 Now say, 'I would like to examine the external genitalia and perform a rectal examination.' Present findings.

Abdominal system examination in detail

Getting started

1 Introduce yourself to the patient and ask for permission to examine

Put out your hand to shake the patient's hand. Say something like, 'Hello I'm Berkeley Moynihan, a third-year student. Do you mind if I examine your tummy and hands?' (some people do not understand 'abdomen' and 'belly' sounds a bit rough).

2 Ask the patient to get on to the bed (if not already there). You may need to get help!

Usually this will be no problem, but if the patient is unable to get on to the bed, find a friendly nurse to transfer them into bed.

3 Wash your hands

This is germ warfare.

4 Ask the patient to strip to their underwear

Traditionally it is said that the abdominal examination should be performed with the patient exposed 'from nipples to knees'. Mercifully, these days the patient's dignity can be maintained by covering the groin with a sheet (until this area is examined in detail). Women patients can be examined with their bra on. There is very little that can be missed under a bra in the abdominal examination. However, you must scan very carefully around the chest so as not to miss telangiectasia. These are dilated capillaries or small arterioles that look like thin red streaks or blobs. If you press on them, they disappear, or 'blanch' to use the correct medical term. This is because blood is forced out of the vessels and once the pressure is released the vessel refills and reddens again).

5 Lie the patient flat on one pillow (if they are elderly or have a kyphosis two pillows may be needed)

The abdominal system is examined with the patient lying flat on one pillow. Sometimes people with a kyphosis, usually elderly people, have difficulty lying flat because of the curvature of their spine. In these cases use two pillows

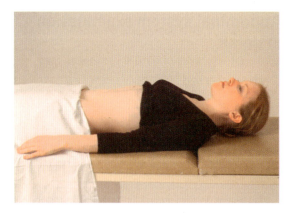

Figure 7.1 Abdominal examination position.

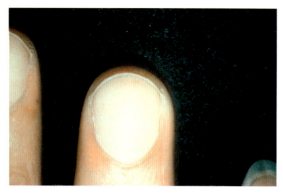

Figure 7.2 Leuconychia.

to maintain their comfort. Occasionally you may get a person who has orthopnea who becomes breathless when they lie flat. Try and get them as flat as their breathing will allow but sometimes you may be forced to examine them practically upright. In all cases the patient must be comfortable (see Fig. 7.1).

6 While doing 1–4, have a 'general look'. Does the patient look in discomfort? Is the abdomen distended? Is there evidence of jaundice, wasting of muscles, scratch marks, and so on?

Patient distress suggests severe illness. An intravenous cannula could suggest severe pain requiring analgesia, for example, acute pancreatitis or an infection requiring antibiotics and fluids, such as acute cholecystitis (an infection of the gallbladder). A yellow appearance of the skin could suggest jaundice and a distended abdomen could represent ascites. Also check to see if there is general muscle wasting or scratch marks.

Hands

7 Inspect both hands for signs of chronic liver disease (DF 6/10), for example, clubbing, leuconychia, koilonychia, palmar erythema, Dupuytren's contracture, spider naevi (make sure you blanch these), and purpura

Chronic liver disease is, by definition, liver disease that has lasted longer than 6 months. There are a number of

causes of which alcohol is the most common. What you are looking for are signs associated with a malfunctioning liver, including some which reflect the body's attempt to compensate. In addition some signs may be caused by malnutrition, particularly in alcoholic liver disease where a normal diet may be replaced by alcohol. These patients can show signs of anaemia and vitamin deficiency also. There are many signs to look out for. Each individual sign on its own is not diagnostic of liver disease and may have other causes. However the more signs you see in one patient, the greater the likelihood that you are dealing with chronic liver disease.

Clubbing

Clubbing (DF 8/10) is mainly seen in respiratory disease and therefore is discussed in detail in Chapter 5. It is seen occasionally in abdominal disease, particularly in cirrhosis of the liver. It can also occur in diseases such as ulcerative colitis, Crohn's disease, and coeliac disease.

Leuconychia

(DF 5/10.) See Fig. 7.2.

What is it?

White nails (compare with your own fingernails to help make the diagnosis).

Causes

Cirrhosis of the liver and nephrotic (*nef-rot-tick*) syndrome.

Significance

White nails are a marker for conditions causing low albumin.

(a)

(b)

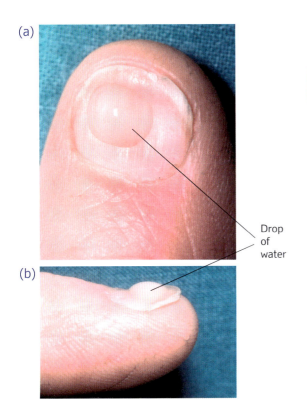

Drop of water

Figure 7.3 Koilonychia.

Koilonychia

(DF 8/10.) See Fig. 7.3.

What is it?

Koilonychia is a 'spoon-shaped' depression of the nail plate. In the early stages the convex curvature of the nail is lost as it becomes flattened. Later the nail edges curl up leaving a depression in the centre 'like a spoon'. In advanced cases it is said you can hold a drop of water in the central depression.

Causes

Chronic anaemia and rarely, exposure to strong detergents.

Significance

This indicates a chronic anaemia (most commonly due to iron deficiency). This finding should prompt a search for a cause of the anaemia.

Palmar erythema

(DF 5/10.) See Fig. 7.4.

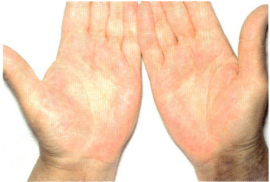

Figure 7.4 Palmar erythema.

What is it?

It is a redness of the palms. The redness is concentrated on the thenar (*th-ee-nar*) eminence (the muscular mound beneath the thumb), the hypothenar eminence (the muscular mound beneath the little finger), and the pulps of the fingers, with the centre of the palm being spared. This can be subtle and easily missed. It is always worth comparing with your own palms to appreciate the difference (unless you have palmar erythema too!)

Causes

Chronic liver disease, pregnancy, the contraceptive pill, and rheumatoid arthritis.

Significance

In the cases of chronic liver disease, the contraceptive pill, and pregnancy, the palmar erythema is due to increased levels of circulating oestrogens. In chronic liver disease (especially due to alcohol), there is gonadal atrophy and depressed testosterone production. A larger proportion of this testosterone is rapidly metabolized to oestrodiol (*east-roe-dial*).

Dupuytren's contracture

(DF 9/10.) See Fig. 7.5. Dupuytren's contracture is named after *Baron Guillaume Dupuytren (1777–1835), French surgeon.*

What is it?

This is the thickening and contracture of the palmar aponeurosis, a fibrous sheet that protects the tendons of the hand. It divides at the bottom of the fingers and attaches to the base of the proximal phalanges. The thickening usually occurs at the root of the ring finger causing it to curl in towards the palm. Later the little

finger is also affected. Early cases can be easily missed. If you look carefully at the palm especially in the region of the fourth and fifth fingers you can often see vertical furrows due to the thickening. Running your fingers over this region is also a good way of making the diagnosis. In advanced cases you might get a clue when you shake the patient's hand. They may tickle or scratch your palm with their flexed ring finger. So if you think that you are examining a mason with a funny handshake, make a quick visual check because it might just be a Dupuytren's contracture.

Causes

Alcoholism, chronic liver disease, diabetes mellitus, and heavy manual labour.

Significance

In advanced cases, the hand is unsightly and the contracture interferes with the function of the hand. The condition can be helped by an operation, which can be performed under local anaesthetic.

Spider naevi

(DF 6/10.) See Fig. 7.6.

What are they?

These are telangiectasia with a specific appearance. They consist of a central arteriole with tiny vessels radiating from it like 'spider legs'. This central arteriole feeds the spider legs with blood. You must demonstrate this by **blanching** it. Press on the central blob and very quickly remove your finger. If you are quick enough, you should see the blood rush back and the red spider legs reappear.

Causes

Chronic liver disease, pregnancy, and thyrotoxicosis; they can also be a normal finding.

Significance

One or two spider naevi can be found in normal people, in pregnancy, and in thyrotoxicosis. However, if more than five spider naevi are found then it is likely that you are dealing with chronic liver disease (especially if there are other supporting features).

Purpura

(DF 2/10.) See Fig. 7.7.

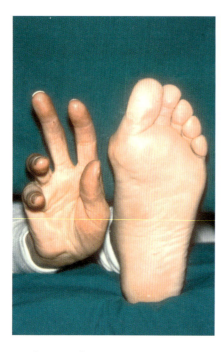

Figure 7.5 Dupuytren's contracture.

(a)

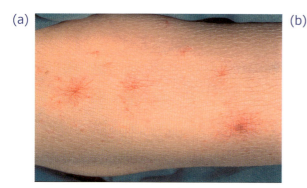

(b)

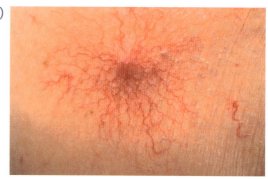

Figure 7.6 Spider naevi.

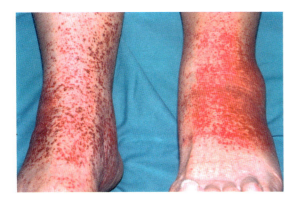

Figure 7.7 Purpura. Drug-induced purpura affecting the legs.

Table 7.13 Causes of purpura

Abnormal blood vessels

Steroid induced

Old age (senile purpura)

Abnormal platelets

Idiopathic thrombocytopenic (*throm-bo-sigh-toe-pee-nick*) purpura (translated this means bleeding due to low platelet count of unknown cause)

Malignant infiltration of the bone marrow, e.g. leukaemia, myeloma, secondary deposits

Abnormal clotting factors

Haemophilia (deficiency of factor VIII)

Anti-coagulation therapy, e.g. warfarin

What is it?

This is due to spontaneous bleeding into the skin. If the bleeding is localized to blobs less than 3 mm across they are called petechiae (*pet-ee-key-eye*). Very large areas of bleeding are called ecchymoses (*eck-ee-moe-seize*).

Causes

See Table 7.13.

Significance

In the case of chronic liver disease, bleeding may be caused because of a deficiency of clotting factors (II, VII, IX, and X).

Flapping tremor

8 Look for a flapping tremor only if you suspect liver failure (jaundice, spider naevi, and so on). Ask the patient to extend their arms and cock their wrists back

In some textbooks a flapping tremor is called asterixis (*ass-stir-ix-iss*). It is elicited in the same manner as the flapping tremor associated with carbon dioxide retention in respiratory failure (see Fig. 5.6). Sometimes people call it a 'liver flap' to qualify the cause of the tremor. Only look for it if you suspect liver failure (you may have spotted jaundice, spider naevi, or other signs described earlier). Get the patient to extend their arms, cock their wrists back, and spread their fingers. If liver failure is present the hands should start flapping rhythmically. In fact it is more of a flapping twitch than a tremor, with the twitching directed down towards the floor. There are other signs of liver failure to look out for. The patient may be confused and drowsy. In the context of liver failure this is called hepatic encephalopathy (*en-keff-a-lop-pathy*). One feature is the inability to reproduce a five-pointed star, which is termed constructional apraxia (*ay-pracks-ya*). Although an interesting sign, in practice it is more important to gauge the conscious level along with liver function tests and other blood measurements in the assessment of such a patient. In addition, patients have a characteristic odour on their breath (hepatic fetor (*feet-or*)), which is described as sweet and musty. You will only really appreciate this when you meet a patient with this problem.

Beware! In some patients with a very acute presentation of liver failure, for example, paracetamol overdose, the pace of liver damage can be so overwhelming that none of the above signs will have time to develop.

Face, eyes, and lips

9 Inspect the face for xanthelasmata (DF 2/10), spider naevi (DF 6/10), and other telangiectasia (DF 9/10); inspect the eyes for jaundice (DF 7/10); and inspect the conjunctivae for anaemia (DF 9/10)

Xanthelasma

See Fig. 7.8. These are little yellowish papules (fatty deposits) around the eye that signify hyperlipidaemia. In the context of an abdominal examination they suggest prolonged cholestasis (obstruction of bile drainage). The likeliest cause is primary biliary cirrhosis.

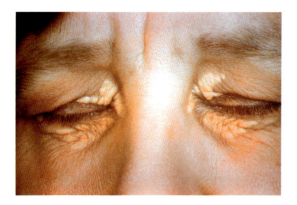

Figure 7.8 Xanthelasma.

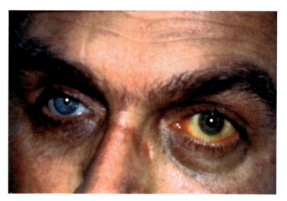

Figure 7.9 Jaundice. Note the prosthetic eye on the right is unaffected.

Spider naevi

See previous discussion.

Other telangiectasia

A different form of telangiectasia can be found in hereditary haemorrhagic telangiectasia (HHT), also known as (Osler–Weber–Rendu syndrome (*William Osler (1849–1919), Canadian physician; Fredrick Parkes Weber (1863–1962), English physician; Henri-Jules Louis Rendu (1842–1902), French physician*). These look like different sized red blebs, which can be seen on the face, the lips, the buccal mucosa, and both sides of the tongue (make sure you look at the underside of the tongue). Although rare, the importance of this condition lies in the fact that these telangiectasia can be found elsewhere, in the nose, gut, and lungs. They are prone to bleeding and cause epistaxis (*epi-stacks-sis*), gastrointestinal bleeding, and haemoptysis (*he-mop-ta-sis*) respectively. See Fig. 13.15.

Jaundice

See Fig. 7.9. The best place to check for jaundice is the sclera of the eyes. You may have already noticed yellow skin with your 'general look' but this can be misleading. You need to confirm the presence of jaundice by observing yellow sclera.

How to examine

Ask the patient's permission: 'Can I gently pull down your eyelid?' When you pull down the lower eyelid ask the patient to look down and observe the sclera.

Anaemia

Significance

Anaemia may be the result of blood loss due to a number of causes in the gastrointestinal tract. This loss can be obvious and spectacular, as in bleeding oesophageal varices, or insidious and occult from a colonic polyp. Anaemia can also be due to malabsorption of iron, folate, and vitamin B_{12} because of a variety of diseases or can simply reflect an inadequate dietary intake through illness, alcoholism, depression, and so on. Chronic anaemia can also cause signs that you should search for if you find pale conjunctivae. These include koilonychia, angular stomatitis (painful cracks in the corners of the mouth), and atrophic glossitis (*gloss-eye-tiss*), a smooth, painful tongue. Rarely, iron deficiency anaemia can lead to an oesophageal web, which can cause dysphagia (see 'Symptoms').

How to examine

While you are checking for jaundice, scan down and look between the eyeball and the margin of the eyelid that you are pulling. This aspect of the conjunctiva is usually pink. If it is pale this suggests anaemia. Do not worry if you are never sure. Keep practising seeing normal as well as abnormal conjunctivae and remember, this is a crude test and even experienced physicians are often wrong.

10 Inspect the lips for pigmentation or telangiectasia (DF 9/10)

Pigmentation of lips

Brown freckly pigmentation around the mouth and lips may herald a rare condition called Peutz–Jehgers (*perts-yay-gers*) syndrome (*Johannes Laurentius Augustinus Peutz (1886–1957), Dutch physician; Harold Joseph Jehgers (1904–1990), American physician*). This is associated with polyps in the bowel, which can cause bleeding or bowel obstruction (see Fig. 13.16).

Telangiectasia of lips

Telangiectasia here would be very suggestive of HHT.

Oral cavity

11 Examine the oral cavity (DF 8/10). Inspect for telangiectasia, pigmentation, dentition, ulcers, angular stomatitis, and candidiasis. Also examine the tongue and tonsils and check for odours

Important clues can be gained from inspecting the mouth, so you must not be tempted to skimp on this part of the examination. Make sure that you illuminate the inside of the mouth well with a torch.

Telangiectasia

(DF 9/10.) Lesions here may be further confirmation of HHT.

Pigmentation

(DF 9/10.) Brown freckly pigmentation could be further proof of Peutz–Jehgers syndrome (see Fig. 13.16). More diffuse pigmentation could represent Addison's disease (*Thomas Addison (1793–1860), English physician*), an endocrine disorder that can present with anorexia, vomiting, and diarrhoea (see Fig. 13.11).

Dentition

(DF 4/10.) Quickly examine the teeth and gums. Poor dentition and inflamed gums (gingivitis (*gin-ji-vie-tiss*)) may be markers of self-neglect. Elderly patients may have ill-fitting dentures, which can prevent them eating properly.

Ulcers

(DF 8/10.) Ulcers can have a variety of causes. One common form of recurrent ulceration is the aphthous ulcer (Fig. 7.10). They may be small or can be over 1 cm in diameter and can be sufficiently painful to deter the patient from eating. They have a yellow base with a surrounding rim of erythema. Some people with aphthous ulcers may have an increased risk of having ulcerative colitis. Patients with severe neutropenia (*new-trow-pee-nia*) (a decrease in a subset of white cells that normally fight infection) may develop similar-looking ulcers in the mouth and oropharynx. Herpetic ulcers are also recurrent and tend to occur in painful crops in and around the mouth. A painless ulcer should give cause for concern, as this may be the beginning of a squamous (*squay-muss*) cell carcinoma. Any

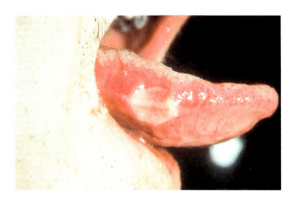

Figure 7.10 Aphthous ulcer.

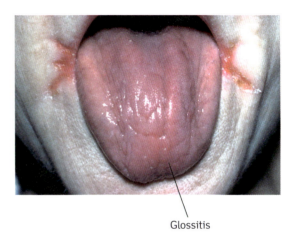

Glossitis

Figure 7.11 Angular stomatitis. The patient also has a smooth fissured tongue, indicative of a glossitis. The common causal feature is iron deficiency.

patient complaining of a long-standing ulcer or swelling in the mouth that is not healing or is increasing in size should have it biopsied to rule out cancer.

Angular stomatitis

(DF 2/10.) Do not forget to look at the corner of the mouth. Painful cracks in the corner suggest angular stomatitis. This may be due to candidal infection, chronic anaemia, or rarely vitamin deficiencies. See Fig. 7.11.

Candidiasis

(DF 8/10.)

What is it?

It is important to recognize the presence of candida (thrush). It is a fungal infection that can cause a sore mouth. In some cases, particularly in those who have a depressed immune system, the candida can spread into the oesophagus and cause a painful dysphagia. It can manifest in different forms.

Causes

Trauma, moist areas, antibiotic therapy, diabetes mellitus, steroid therapy (oral and inhaled), and other forms of immunosuppression.

How to examine

Look for whitish plaques in the oral cavity. Occasionally patients who have drunk some milk may leave some residue that resembles candida. You should scrape the plaque away with a spatula to reveal reddened mucosa (if you are unsure, you could send the scrapings to microbiology to identify). If you cannot remove the plaque after a number of attempts, you may be dealing with leukoplakia (*loo-co-play-kia*), a premalignant condition (a biopsy is required). A more difficult form of candidiasis to spot is a red inflamed mucosa, which may be erosive (particularly in denture wearers).

Tongue

(DF 7/10.) It is hard to miss the tongue during an inspection of the mouth but it is easy to miss vital clues without careful scrutiny. A furred tongue is supposed to signify illness or a fever but may be found in perfectly healthy people. In some patients, particularly after antibiotic therapy, this furring may be black in colour. This is a benign condition due to overgrowth of the papillae of the tongue together with infection due to *Candida nigricans* (*nigh-gri-cans*). You can reassure the patient that there is no serious disease but it can be a difficult condition to treat. A wasted tongue could signal a neurological cause (see Chapter 6). You should look for fasiculations (*fa-sick-you-lay-shuns*) (motor neuron disease) and observe the tongue movements for any lesion of the hypoglossal nerve. A large tongue is not always immediately obvious (unless very large). Possible causes include hypothyroidism (the commonest), acromegaly (*ack-crow-meg-alley*), and primary amyloidosis (*am-ee-lloyd-owe-sis*) (see Fig. 7.12).

Tonsils

(DF 8/10.) Now you need to view the tonsils. Get your patient to say 'Aaaah!' Quickly watch the central uvula (*you-view-la*), which should elevate in the midline. Then look down and to each side and inspect each tonsil. Are they obviously enlarged? Is there pus on them? Very rarely they may be involved in a lymphoma.

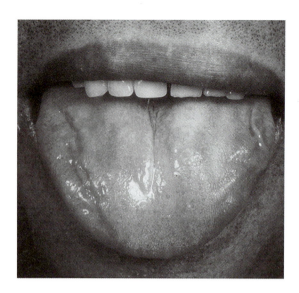

Figure 7.12 Large tongue due to amyloidosis.
Reproduced from *Rheumatology and the Kidney*, (2nd edn), eds. Dwomoa Adu, Paul Emery, Michael Madaio, 2012, with permission from Oxford University Press.

Odour

(DF 9/10.) The appreciation of smell on the breath is rarely ever taught because it is a difficult area to describe. Yet important information may be conveyed to your nose. Certain conditions have a characteristic odour, for example, the sweet musty smell of hepatic failure or the sickly sweet, acetone smell of diabetic ketoacidosis. The only real way of learning these smells is to find actual cases during your clinical attachment and memorize them (the odours are unmistakable). Alcohol on the breath is one smell that most medical students are acquainted with and is an important factor in many medical diseases. Foul-smelling breath (halitosis) may be due to poor dental hygiene, pathology of the nasopharynx, or bronchiectasis, or it may have no discernible cause.

Other

(DF 9/10.) Although beyond the scope of this chapter it is important to recognize that skin disease may also involve the oral mucosa. Sometimes this can be crucial in supporting a diagnosis, for example, lichen planus (*like-en-plane-us*) or pemphigus vulgaris (*pem-fig-us-vul-gar-iss*).

Palpation of the neck

12 Palpate the neck for cervical lymph nodes (DF 6/10), particularly the left supraclavicular region

When palpating the neck during an abdominal examination, pay particular attention to the left supraclavicular fossa. An enlarged lymph node here may be caused by spread from a gastrointestinal cancer, especially gastric cancer. This node is often called Virchow's (*ver-koffs*) node and is sometimes referred to as Troisier's (*twa-zee-ers*) sign. This node is preferentially involved because the lymph drains directly from the gut to this area. This area is readily felt with the fingertips with the patient lying flat. However, if you are palpating the rest of the cervical region, you must be aware that more traditional teachers believe that you can only examine this region properly from behind the patient as in the respiratory examination (see Chapter 5). (*Rudolph Ludwig-Karl Virchow (1821–1902), German pathologist; Charles Emile Troisier (1844–1919), French pathologist.*)

Inspection of the chest

13 Inspect the chest for further spider naevi (DF 6/10), gynaecomastia (DF 7/10), and loss of axillary hair in men (DF 6/10)

Spider naevi

Inspect and blanch as before.

Gynaecomastia

What is it?

Gynaecomastia is the enlargement of the breast tissue in men. See Fig. 7.13.

Significance

In the context of an abdominal examination, it usually occurs in chronic liver disease. Increased circulating oestrogens and decreased testosterone production lead to feminization in men. Other signs to look out for include loss of axillary hair and a female distribution of pubic hair.

Causes

See Table 7.14.

How to examine

Checking for gynaecomastia in a thin or cachexic man is relatively simple. In an obese man it can be much more

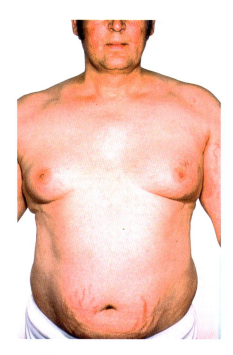

Figure 7.13 Gynaecomastia.

Table 7.14 Causes of gynaecomastia

Puberty
Thyrotoxicosis
Chronic liver disease
Klinefelter's (*kline-felt-hers*) syndrome[a]
Testicular disease/tumours
Pituitary disease
Hypothalamic disease
Drugs

[a] *Harry Fitch Klinefelter (1912–1990), US physician*: described the syndrome of feminization as a result of multiple X chromosomes linked with a solitary Y chromosome.

difficult to tell whether enlarged breasts are due to gynaecomastia or simply adipose tissue. Do not be satisfied simply looking at the breasts; you must also palpate them to check if glandular tissue is present. This too is not as easy as it sounds, so do not be put off if you are still unsure. Often, the patient is distressed about it and this can provide a vital clue.

Table 7.15 Other drugs causing gynaecomastia

Cimetidine (*sigh-met-a-dean*)
....

Digoxin
....

Cytotoxic drugs
....

Methyldopa (*me-thile-dough-per*)
....

Anti-androgens, e.g. cyproterone (*sigh-pro-ter-own*) acetate[a]
....

Oestrogens[a]
....

Gonadorelin (*go-nad-owe-rel-in*) analogue[a]

[a] These drugs are used in the treatment of prostate cancer. In addition, oestrogens may be administered to men who are preparing to become women as part of gender reassignment.

Loss of axillary hair

Another potential sign of increased oestrogen production in men with chronic liver disease. Make sure this has not been shaved off deliberately as a fashion statement or in men who may practice transvestism.

Other drugs causing gynaecomastia are shown in Table 7.15.

Inspection of the abdomen

14 Observe the abdomen for distension, herniae, scars, striae, pulsations, peristalsis, and distended veins (DF 8/10)

It seems that you have examined everything **but** the abdomen up to this point. As you get confident and slick you will find that it can take you less than a minute to get to this stage. But be patient! You still should not lay a hand on your patient. You need to focus your inspection on the abdomen itself and note any features. To help with your presentation the abdomen is divided into nine regions by a number of imaginary lines. A simpler version, dividing the abdomen into four quadrants, is also acceptable. Any abnormal findings should be mapped to any one of the nine regions (or four quadrants), for example, a 5 × 5 cm mass in the epigastrium or a scar in the left lower quadrant (see Figs. 7.14 and 7.15). At this point it is useful to stand at the foot of the bed and observe the abdomen. Check to see that it is roughly symmetrical and if it moves gently outwards with inspiration. If the patient has peritonitis and abdominal rigidity, there may be no visible movement with respiration.

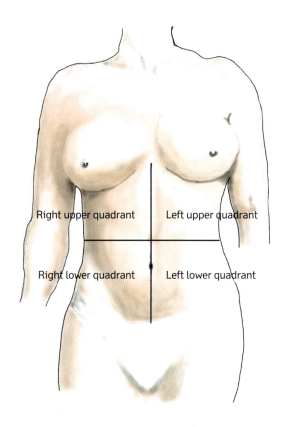

Right upper quadrant   Left upper quadrant

Right lower quadrant   Left lower quadrant

Figure 7.14 The abdominal quadrants.

Abdominal distension

(DF 2/10.) There is a range of normal appearances of the abdomen, ranging from the concave abdomen (scaphoid) (*scay-foid*) of the thin person (viewed from the side) to the more generous protuberance of the obese person. You will get a feel for these differences the more patients you examine. Any abdomen that appears swollen requires an explanation. A useful way of remembering the five causes of generalized abdominal distension is 'the five Fs': fat, foetus, fluid, flatus, and faeces. The first two are usually easy to identify. You will instinctively recognize the fatty abdomen of the obese patient and most women will tell you that they are pregnant (although you still hear stories of some women who are unaware of their pregnancy). The other three need further examination to distinguish between them. Sometimes you may notice more localized distension. The swollen area may give you a clue to the cause. If you have a good working knowledge of the anatomy of the abdomen you can make an educated guess, for example, a distended epigastrium could be due to gastric cancer, an enlarged left lobe of the liver, or a pancreatic

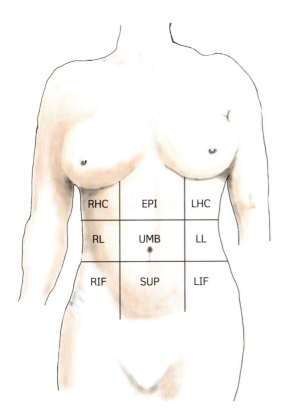

Figure 7.15 The abdominal regions: LHC, left hypochondrium; LL, left lumbar region (or loin); LIF, left iliac fossa; EPI, epigastrium; UMB, umbilical region; SUP, suprapubic (or hypogastric) region; RHC, right hypochondrium; RL, right lumbar region (or loin); RIF, right iliac fossa.

cyst or pseudocyst. Or a distended hypogastrium (suprapubic region) could indicate urine retention in an enlarged bladder or an ovarian cyst.

Herniae

(DF 8/10.)

What are they?

A hernia is defined as the protrusion of an abdominal organ through an abnormal opening. They can be internal, for example, hiatus hernia (the stomach protrudes upwards through the diaphragmatic opening) or external, where they can be viewed with the naked eye. Hernias are localized bulges, which occur in areas of weakness in the abdominal wall. They tend to be labelled according to their site, for example, epigastric hernia. One characteristic of

Table 7.16 Factors in the causation of a hernia

Weakness of abdominal wall
Congenital
Obesity
Cachexia
Multiparity
Surgical incision
Repeated rise in intra-abdominal pressure
Chronic cough
Respiratory disease
Constipation (straining)

hernias is that their bulging increases with a rise in intra-abdominal pressure. This feature is exploited when you get the patient to cough. Hernias may disappear when the patient lies flat (the contents return to the abdominal cavity under the influence of gravity). If this happens the hernia is described as reducible. You may have to push the contents back yourself. If the contents cannot be returned, the hernia is irreducible. This occurs if there are adhesions between the hernial contents and the inner wall of the sac. A hernia becomes life-threatening if it becomes strangulated. The likelihood of this happening increases the narrower the neck of the hernia. A narrow neck can constrict the blood supply of the abdominal contents leading to necrosis.

Causes

See Table 7.16.

Types

See Fig. 7.16.

- **Epigastric**. This is a small protrusion through the linea alba (*lin-ee-a-al-ba*) (the central part of the rectus (*wrecked-us*) abdominus muscle. It can occur anywhere along the linea alba above the umbilicus and usually contains extraperitoneal fat. For a small hernia it can be quite painful.

- **Umbilical** (*um-billy-cull* or *um-be-like-al*). The swelling here is localized to the navel and is common in babies.

- **Paraumbilical**. This occurs just above or below the umbilicus. It occurs in obese people and in women who

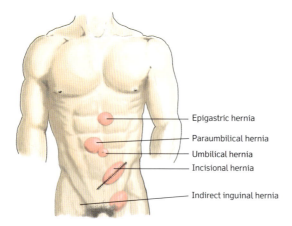

Figure 7.16 The different types of abdominal hernias.

Epigastric hernia
Paraumbilical hernia
Umbilical hernia
Incisional hernia
Indirect inguinal hernia

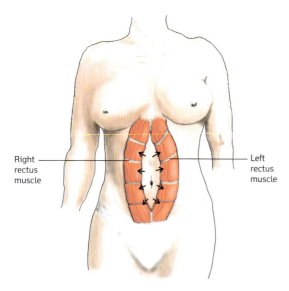

Right rectus muscle

Left rectus muscle

Figure 7.17 Divarication of recti. A rise in intra-abdominal pressure causes a characteristic bulge in the midline of the abdomen forcing the inner border of the recti muscles apart.

have had multiple childbirths (multiparity). It has a narrow neck and is therefore prone to strangulation.

- **Divarication of recti** (*die-varry-cay-shun-of-wreck-tie*). This is again common in obese people and in women who have had multiple childbirths. In each case the abdominal musculature is weak and the linea alba bulges in a vertical line between the rectus abdominus muscle (see Fig. 7.17).

- **Incisional**. Any surgical incision is a potential site of abdominal weakness. Sometimes a hernia can develop in a portion of a scar or along its whole length.
- **Direct inguinal** (see Fig. 7.36).
- **Indirect inguinal** (see Fig. 7.36).
- **Femoral**.

How to examine

You may notice a localized swelling on the abdomen as the patient undresses. As you do a general look, keep an eye on the swelling as the patient lies down. If the swelling enlarges (the act of lying down raises the intra-abdominal pressure) this can give you an early clue that you are dealing with a hernia. Do not worry if you miss this, as you will have the chance to check the swelling's response to intra-abdominal pressure in a little while. With any swelling you must assess it carefully, with regards to size, consistency, and so on. If you suspect that you are dealing with a hernia, then either get the patient to sit up or get them to cough. The rise in abdominal pressure will cause the swelling to bulge. Having diagnosed a hernia you must check to see if it is reducible. Do this by pushing the hernia gently with your fingers back into the abdomen. With any luck it should slide back. If it does not then the swelling is irreducible. You should then auscultate to see if you can hear bowel sounds over the swelling. If the hernia has become strangulated, the patient will be ill and in pain. The hernia itself will be tender and will lose its cough impulse.

Scars

(DF 3/10.) As in the cardiovascular examination, finding scars on the abdomen can be useful. Sometimes the information is just 'fodder' for interest but at other times it can be very relevant, for example, the patient with an appendectomy scar (gridiron incision) who has right iliac fossa pain. Their pain cannot be due to appendicitis and you need to think again.

Types of incisions

- **Median**. This type of incision gives access to most intra-abdominal organs. It is used in an emergency, especially if the cause of the surgical emergency is not clear (the operation is called a laparotomy (*lap-a-rot-tummy*)). Some surgeons dub this the 'incision of indecision'.
- **Paramedian**. This used to be the incision of choice for older surgeons for a laparotomy. However, it can lead to poor access to organs on the opposite side of the incision.

- **Kocher's (*cockers*)**. (*Emil Theodor Kocher (1841–1917), Swiss surgeon.*) This incision is found below and parallel to the right costal margin (aka right sub-costal incision). It allows access to the liver and biliary tract (on the left a similar incision allows access to the spleen).

- **Transverse**. This is used to gain good exposure of the upper abdominal organs. This is another incision that is not often used these days.

- **Gridiron**. This incision is used for access to the appendix.

- **Rutherford–Morrison**. This incision is used primarily for access to the kidneys.

- **Pfannenstiel (*fan-en-steal*)**. (*Hans Hermann Johannes Pfannenstiel (1862–1909), German gynaecologist*). This is a transverse incision just below the pubic hairline. It is used mainly for access to the uterus.

- **Umbilical**. Laparoscopy (note that small laparoscopic scars can be found almost anywhere on the abdomen because of the improvements in and desire to use laparoscopic techniques for certain operations). These laparoscopic operations require a good deal of skill and training to be effective.

How to examine

See Fig. 7.18. Scars may be difficult to see, especially old ones or those concealed in skin creases, for example, Pfannenstiel incision for caesarian sections or hysterectomy. You must look carefully and do not be afraid to get down close to look at scars. Also remember to lean over the patient and look at the left flank for a nephrectomy scar (Rutherford–Morrison). You can gain a rough idea of the age of the scar from its colour. A purply-red scar (in a white person) indicates a recent scar, usually within a year of operation. A silvery white scar indicates an older incision.

Striae

(DF 3/10). See Fig. 7.19. Striae are stretch marks. They indicate a recent decrease in the girth of the abdomen (especially a distended one). This can occur after pregnancy (striae gravidarum), following drainage of ascitic fluid, or in an obese person who has lost weight. They tend to be salmon pink in colour (older ones tend to be silvery white). Striae can also occur in Cushing's syndrome (*Harvey Cushing (1869–1939), American neurosurgeon*) except in this condition they are reddy purple in colour and are more substantial. Striae are not just seen in the abdomen but can be seen on the shoulders, upper arms, back, thighs, buttocks, and so on.

Pulsations

(DF 4/10.) Pulsations in the abdomen are usually due to the abdominal aorta. They are a normal finding in the epigastrium of thin patients. However, any pulsation, especially in an obese patient raises the spectre of an aneurysm (*an-your-ism*) of the abdominal aorta. Make a mental note of any pulsation you see as you will need to palpate the area more fully during your examination.

Peristalsis

(DF 9/10.) Peristalsis (*perry-stal-sis*) is the term used to describe the waves of contraction that propel food and gut contents along the bowel. Normally these waves are not visible (except in some thin patients). However, if a patient develops an obstruction in the stomach or intestine, the waves of contraction become more pronounced as the gut tries to overcome the blockage. In small bowel obstruction,

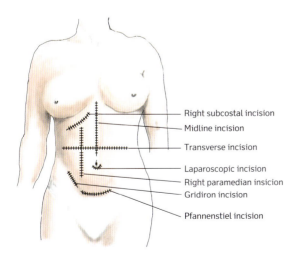

Right subcostal incision
Midline incision
Transverse incision
Laparoscopic incision
Right paramedian insicion
Gridiron incision
Pfannenstiel incision

Figure 7.18 Surgical scars.

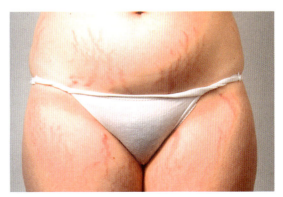

Figure 7.19 Striae.

waves of peristalsis can be seen in the centre of the abdomen. With pyloric (*pie-lor-rick*) stenosis, where the outflow to the stomach is blocked, a peristaltic wave can be seen rippling from the left hypochondrium to the right (if the stomach is distended the wave can travel down past the umbilicus before ascending to the right hypochondrium). To clinically confirm pyloric stenosis, it was said that you should perform a 'succussion (*suck-cushion*) splash', that is, if you grasped the patient by the lower chest bilaterally and shook them vigorously from side to side, a sloshing sound can be heard (due to the copious contents of the stomach). However, this sound can be heard in normal people up to 2 hours after a meal, and as it is not a very dignified test it is not recommended. If you have good clinical reasons to suspect pyloric stenosis, proceed with gastroscopy.

Distended veins

(DF 7/10.)

Significance

Normally there are very few distended veins on the abdominal wall. There are two important situations when distended veins are a prominent feature, portal hypertension in chronic liver disease and inferior vena caval obstruction (IVCO). In both cases the normal flow of blood back to the heart is impeded. To try to overcome this, blood is diverted through veins called collaterals to provide an alternative route back to the right side of the heart. As the volume of blood is large, the collaterals distend to accommodate the increased load. The abdominal veins represent a visible and important group of collaterals.

How to examine

First look at the distribution of the enlarged veins. Veins radiating from the umbilicus in a star-like fashion (termed the caput medusae) suggest portal hypertension (Fig. 7.20). Veins coursing vertically up the abdomen suggest IVCO. The next step is to work out the direction of blood flow, which is different in the two conditions. In portal hypertension the blood flow is away from the umbilicus and in IVCO the flow is upwards. To determine the blood flow, you need to press on a vein with the index finger of one hand. Place the index finger of the other hand next to it and milk the blood out of the vein by sliding your finger about 3–5 cm in any direction. Lift up the finger of the milking hand and if the vein refills, then the blood flow is opposite to the direction of milking. If you lift up the milking finger and the vein does not distend then the blood flow is in the direction of milking and is being dammed back by your non-milking finger. See Fig. 7.21.

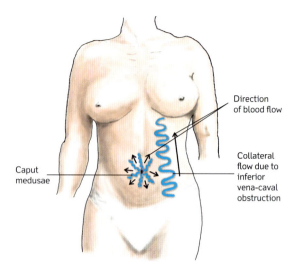

Figure 7.20 Caput medusae.

Direction of blood flow

Caput medusae

Collateral flow due to inferior vena-caval obstruction

Palpation of the abdomen

15 Ask the patient if they have any tender areas before commencing light palpation. Palpate the abdomen lightly, mapping any areas of tenderness and note any masses (DF 4/10). Watch the patient's face for signs of pain!

You are aiming to get a superficial overview of the abdomen and are looking specifically for tender areas and masses. There are varying degrees of tenderness, ranging from mild discomfort to the extreme pain associated with peritonitis. In addition, there are a number of phenomena that you need to be able to spot as they herald life-threatening complications. These are guarding, rebound tenderness, and rigidity.

Peritonitis

(DF 6/10.) This is inflammation of the peritoneum. The cause is usually a bacterial infection or irritation from bowel contents following leakage into the abdominal cavity. This can follow perforation of an organ, for example, perforated gastric ulcer. Other causes include penetrating injuries, for example, stabbing or after surgery, which will be obvious from the history, and rarely blood-borne sources, which may be difficult to spot. Peritonitis is life-threatening and must be recognized. The patient is usually ill and clammy with a rapid thready pulse and may exhibit guarding, rebound tenderness, or rigidity.

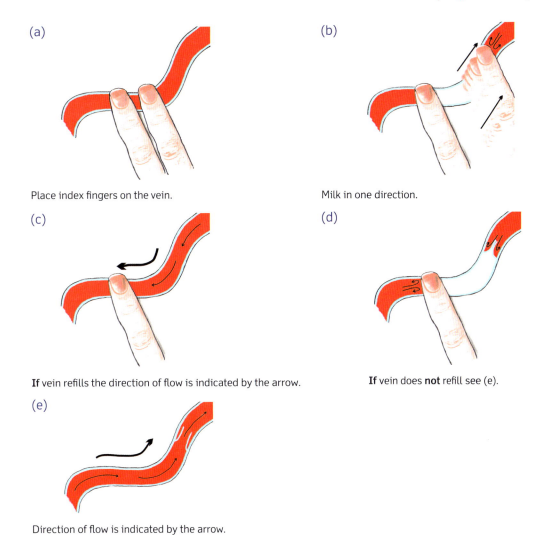

(a)

Place index fingers on the vein.

(b)

Milk in one direction.

(c)

If vein refills the direction of flow is indicated by the arrow.

(d)

If vein does **not** refill see (e).

(e)

Direction of flow is indicated by the arrow.

Figure 7.21 Sequence of drawings demonstrating direction of flow.

Guarding

(DF 7/10.) This is the instantaneous contraction of muscle overlying an inflamed organ or peritoneum. This reflex contraction attempts to guard the inflamed area from being prodded further. Guarding is usually associated with marked tenderness.

Rebound tenderness

(DF 7/10.) This is another sign of an inflamed peritoneum. This time the pain is experienced after quickly lifting your hand off the affected area. Sometimes the inflammation is so severe that rebound pain can be elicited in the affected area by lifting your hand off an area remote from it.

Rigidity

(DF 6/10.) Severe inflammation of the peritoneum can lead to generalized rigidity of the abdomen. The pain associated can be so intense that the patient can only lie still. Even breathing can exacerbate the pain, so that the abdomen is held totally rigid as the patient takes rapid shallow breaths using chest movements only.

How to examine

Always ask the patient if they have any tender areas before starting. You should also follow up by saying 'Let me know if anywhere is tender when I press' (it is amazing how many patients will wince in silence, so as not to cause a fuss). Make sure your hands are warm before touching the patient. If you touch a patient with cold hands (this is an unprofessional act!) they will tense up or shout out and you may have to conduct the rest of your examination on the ceiling! Begin by kneeling down by the bedside (you can stoop, but this can be tiring) (see Fig. 7.22). Place your hand flat on the abdomen away from any tender areas. Keeping your hand flat, press gently with the pulps of your fingers. Do this by flexing with straight fingers from your metacarpophalangeal joints (the knuckles). Watch your patient's face for signs of pain. Work your way around the abdomen palpating in this manner. Try to be systematic, so that you cover the whole abdomen efficiently. As a guide you can palpate each of the nine regions in turn. Any tender areas should be assessed for guarding or rebound tenderness. As well as checking for tenderness you should be on the lookout for any unusual masses. At this stage do not try to work out what the mass is. Simply note the region it is in.

16 Palpate more deeply and assess any masses felt in more detail (DF 7/10)

Now you need to palpate more deeply. If there is marked tenderness, guarding, rebound tenderness, or rigidity this is unnecessary (and unkind). Palpation is done using the same technique as light palpation but by pressing down more firmly (some people achieve this by placing their free hand on top of the palpating hand).

If there were no abnormalities found on light palpation then retrace the areas you felt, pressing more deeply this time. There are potential pitfalls when palpating the abdomen. There is the possibility of missing any abnormal structures and there is also the possibility of misinterpreting normal organs as abnormal (see Fig. 7.23). Normal structures you may encounter include the descending

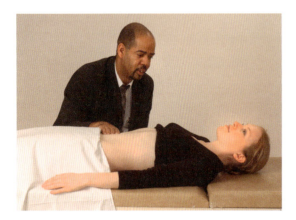

Figure 7.22 Position of examiner for abdominal examination. Crouch or kneel beside the patient and do not forget to observe the face for signs of pain.

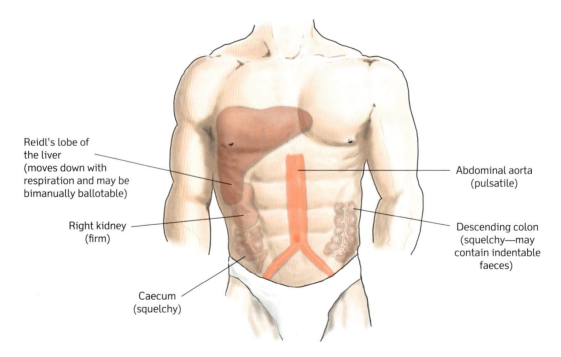

Reidl's lobe of the liver (moves down with respiration and may be bimanually ballotable)

Right kidney (firm)

Caecum (squelchy)

Abdominal aorta (pulsatile)

Descending colon (squelchy—may contain indentable faeces)

Figure 7.23 Normal palpable structures.

colon (this feels like a tube you can roll under your hand in the left lower quadrant) and the caecum in the right iliac fossa (this feels soft and ill defined and often squelches when pressed). The abdominal aorta is sometimes prominent in thin people (a pulsating tube found in the epigastrium). It is sometimes possible when palpating the epigastrium to be fooled into thinking that a contracting rectus muscle is a swelling. Be aware of this and if you are suspicious, try to get your patient to relax. The swelling should disappear with relaxation. In all cases you need to be aware of these pitfalls before you classify any mass as abnormal. If you do encounter an abnormal mass, you need to assess it in more detail. All the features listed below need to be examined.

Assessment of an abdominal mass

- **Site**.
- **Size**. Measured with a tape measure.
- **Border**. Hard, irregular? This suggests cancer.
- **Consistency**. Hard, irregular? This suggests cancer. Nodular? This suggests cancer or, in the liver, possibly cirrhosis.
- **Tenderness**. Suggests inflammatory process or distended capsule of an organ.
- **Mobility**. Parts of the bowel are attached to mesentery and are mobile. Bowel tumours may become fixed if they spread and invade adjacent organs or skin. Some organs are permanently fixed, for example, the pancreas.
- **Movement with respiration**.
- **Percussion note**.
- **Pulsatility**. This suggests a vascular cause (beware transmitted pulsations).
- **Overlying temperature**. Warm? May suggest underlying inflammation, for example, abscess or infected cyst.
- **Bruit**. Suggests a vascular cause.

This information will help you to build an identikit picture of the mass and enable you to make a reasoned guess as to what it is. A knowledge of the anatomy of the abdomen will also help you in working out the potential origins of the mass.

Epigastric mass

See Table 7.17 and Fig. 7.24.

Right iliac fossa mass

See Table 7.18.

Table 7.17 Causes of an epigastric mass

Stomach	Cancer, pyloric stenosis
Liver	Enlarged left lobe
Pancreas	Pancreatic cysts, pancreatic pseudocyst (fluid in the lesser sac), cancer head of pancreas
Gallbladder (distended)	Mucocoele/empyema

Left iliac fossa mass

See Table 7.19.

Hypogastric mass

See Table 7.20 and Fig. 7.25. The most common cause of a hypogastric mass is an enlarged bladder and it usually occurs in elderly men with enlarged prostates that obstruct the flow of urine (see Fig. 7.26). The bladder can extend upwards as far as the umbilicus. If it occurs acutely it is an intensely painful condition. It can occur chronically over many weeks in the absence of pain. As it arises out of the pelvis you cannot get below it to feel its lower margin. It is also dull to percussion. These features are also shared by ovarian cysts and uterine fibroids. If you encounter an enlarged bladder you need to pass a catheter to drain the excess urine (in the acute situation this is accompanied by great relief for the patient). Sometimes if you are unsure about a hypogastric mass, passing a catheter may help. If urine drains and the mass decreases in size you can be sure you are dealing with an enlarged bladder. If little urine drains and the size of the mass is unaffected then the mass is not a bladder.

Other masses

Aortic aneurysm

(DF 7/10.) This is the dilatation of the aorta, which usually occurs because of atherosclerosis. It is found in the midline in the centre of the abdomen. As an aneurysm enlarges, the risk of it rupturing increases with possible catastrophic consequences. Therefore it is important that you are able to detect one. To do this you use a key feature of any artery, that is, its expansibility. If you find a pulsatile mass, place both your hands on either side of it and let your fingers rest gently against both borders. With each pulsation your fingers should be pushed up and outwards if it is an aortic aneurysm. This is important because a mass overlying the aorta can transmit its pulsation and give the illusion that it is a vascular structure.

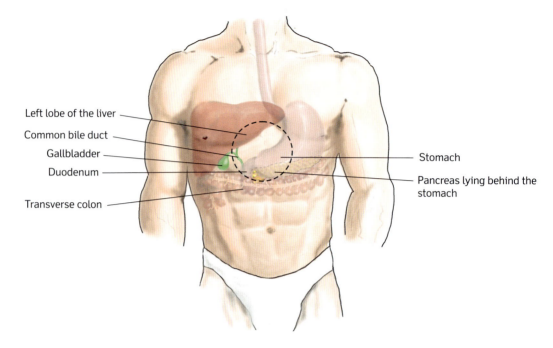

Left lobe of the liver

Common bile duct

Gallbladder

Duodenum

Transverse colon

Stomach

Pancreas lying behind the stomach

Figure 7.24 Epigastric structures.

Table 7.18 Causes of a right iliac fossa mass

Caecum	Carcinoma, Crohn's disease, tuberculosis
Appendix	Appendix abscess
Ovary	Cyst, carcinoma
Psoas muscle	Psoas abscess
External iliac artery	Aneurysm
Pelvic kidney	

Table 7.19 Causes of a left iliac fossa mass

Sigmoid colon	Cancer, diverticular abscess
Ovary	Cyst, carcinoma
Psoas muscle	Psoas abscess
External iliac artery	Aneurysm
Pelvic kidney	

Table 7.20 Causes of a hypogastric mass

Enlarged bladder
Ovarian cyst
Uterine fibroids/pregnancy
Tumour of sigmoid colon

In this case, if you straddle the mass with your hands as before, your fingers will be lifted upwards but not outwards. See Fig. 7.27.

Gallbladder

(DF 9/10.) The gallbladder is only palpable occasionally. Gallstones are the commonest pathology to affect the gallbladder and this usually leads to a thickened fibrotic organ, which is impalpable. This observation is the basis of Courvoisier's law (*Ludwig Georg Courvoisier (1843– 1918), French surgeon*). This states that in the presence of jaundice a palpable gallbladder is unlikely to be due to a gallstone (exceptions do occur). If a gallbladder is palpable, other causes are more likely, for example, carcinoma of the head of pancreas, where the common bile duct is

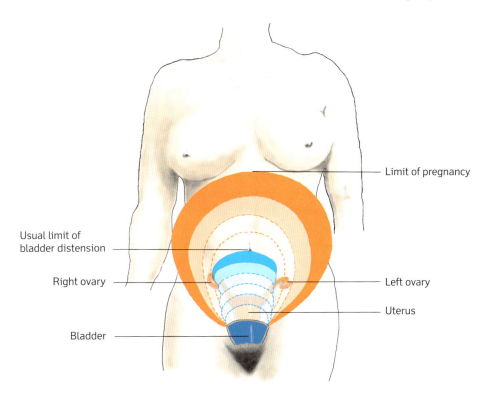

Limit of pregnancy

Usual limit of
bladder distension

Right ovary

Left ovary

Uterus

Bladder

Figure 7.25 Hypogastric structures.

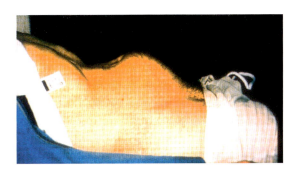

Figure 7.26 Distended bladder. This is acute retention and requires immediate catherization.

obstructed leading to distension of a normal gallbladder. A palpable gallbladder in the absence of jaundice can be due to a gallstone obstructing the cystic duct. The flow of bile is obstructed and in time the bile pigments trapped in the gallbladder are absorbed. Mucus is continually secreted by the gallbladder epithelium leading to distension. This is called a mucocoele (*mew-co-seal*) of the gallbladder. If this material becomes infected this creates an empyaema (*em-pie-ee-ma*) of the gallbladder.

17 Palpate specifically for enlarged organs: liver—commence in the right iliac fossa and move upwards towards the right costal margin while getting the patient to take deep breaths; spleen—commence in the right iliac fossa and move upwards towards the left costal margin while getting the patient to take deep breaths; kidneys—commence in the flanks and 'bimanually ballot' them

The liver, spleen, and kidneys are always routinely examined for. They are the most common organs to become palpable following disease and they have unique features that identify them. You must know them and be able to recognize them in your patient. In medical speak an enlarged organ has the suffix 'megaly' added to it, for example, hepatomegaly (enlarged liver) and splenomegaly (enlarged spleen).

Liver

(DF 7/10.) The liver is normally found under the right costal margin and is not normally palpable (a liver edge can

(a)

(b)

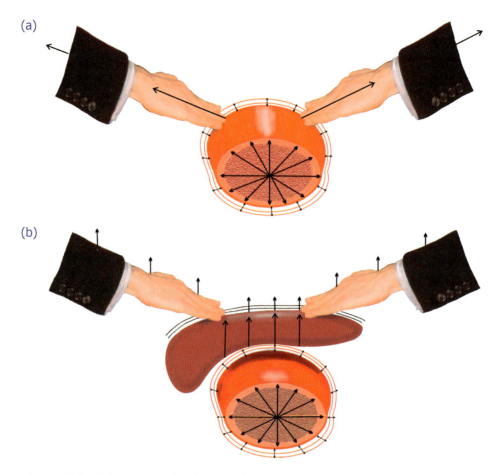

Figure 7.27 Differentiating between expansile pulsation and transmitted pulsation of an aortic aneurysm. (a) The expansile nature of an aortic aneurysm: the fingers are pushed out laterally; (b) transmitted pulsation from an aortic aneurysm: in this case an enlarged liver transmits the pulsations upwards, elevating the hand.

sometimes be felt at the right costal margin). As it enlarges the liver edge can be felt in the right hypochondrium. With some diseases the liver can become massively enlarged and descend right down into the right iliac fossa. See Fig. 7.28.

How to examine

See Fig.7.29. Remain kneeling down. You should always start off in the right iliac fossa so as not to miss massive hepatomegaly. Place your hand flat on the abdomen with your fingers angled up towards the patient's head. You will need to exert firm but gentle pressure into the abdomen while keeping your hand flat. It is the tips of the second and third fingers that are seeking the liver edge. Some people prefer to use the distal half of their index finger and the liver edge is felt against the radial border (the edge facing the thumb) of the digit.

The key to palpating for a liver is that it descends in the abdomen with inspiration. Ask your patient to take a deep breath and hold your hand still. You need to apply some pressure so that your hand is not displaced with the respiratory effort. You are feeling for an 'edge' that should descend to meet your fingers. This 'edge' is not always sharp but may be a feeling of a 'fullness' or 'something' bumping into or running under your fingers. If you do not feel anything, as the patient exhales, move your hand a few fingerbreadths up towards the right costal margin and then hold your hand steady. Ask your patient to take another deep breath. Repeat this until you feel a liver edge or you reach the costal margin. A common mistake to make is to move your hand up towards the costal margin 'seeking' a liver during inspiration. If a mass is encountered, this movement of the hand may give the illusion that it is the mass itself that has moved to meet the fingers, so keep your hand still.

If you palpate a liver, feel its substance all the way to the costal margin. You should not be able to feel an upper border of the liver as it is under the lower ribs. It is said that you cannot get above the mass. This is a second very important characteristic of the liver. If you do feel an upper margin to a swelling then you are not dealing with a liver. Assess the liver and note if it feels smooth or irregular and whether it is tender or not. Also get some idea of the size of the liver. You can do this accurately by using a measuring tape from the costal margin to the liver edge or crudely by using fingerbreadths below the costal margin. Finally you need to percuss for both the upper and lower border of the liver, as occasionally in emphysema a normal liver can be pushed down by a hyperinflated lung. The liver is usually dull to percussion and therefore first percuss below the liver in an area that should be resonant. Percuss upwards and when the liver is encountered the note should become dull. Now percuss for the upper margin of the liver (this is normally in the sixth interspace). Start percussing just above the nipple on the right side of the chest (in a man) and percuss downward. The resonant note should become dull in the sixth interspace. If it remains resonant then suspect emphysema (look for other features) and downward displacement of the liver.

Causes of hepatomegaly

See Table 7.21.

Spleen

(DF 8/10). The spleen lies under the left costal margin along the ninth, tenth, and eleventh ribs and does not extend beyond the midaxillary line in the adult. As it enlarges it can be felt in the left hypochondrium. In some diseases it can become massively enlarged and cross the midline into the right iliac fossa. See Fig. 7.30.

How to examine

You will need to stand to examine the spleen. You should always start off in the right iliac fossa so as not to miss massive splenomegaly (the identical position to Fig. 7.29a). Place your hand on the abdomen with your fingers aimed towards the patient's left shoulder. This time only the tips of your second and third fingers can be used to feel a splenic border. Now reach over with your non-palpating hand and pull up on the left lower ribs. This manoeuvre is meant to accentuate a spleen that is only just palpable. The key to palpating the spleen (like the liver) is that it descends in the abdomen with inspiration. Use exactly the same technique you used for the liver, but this time work your hand towards the left costal margin. If

Figure 7.28 Sequence of hepatic enlargement.

(a) 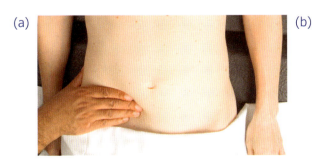 (b)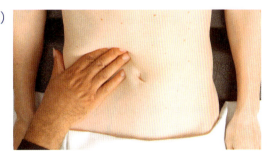

Figure 7.29 Examining for a liver (see text for a full explanation).

Table 7.21 Causes of hepatomegaly

Cardiac	Congestive cardiac failure, tricuspid incompetence, hepatic vein thrombosis (Budd–Chiari syndrome[a])
Infective	Viral (e.g. hepatitis A, B, or C, glandular fever), bacterial (e.g. brucellosis), parasite (e.g. hydatid disease), protozoal (e.g. amoebic abscess)
Haematological	Lymphoma, leukaemia (especially chronic granulocytic leukaemia), myelofibrosis, haemolytic anaemia
Infiltrative	Gaucher's disease[b], amyloidosis

[a] *George Budd (1808–1882), UK physician; Hans Chiari (1851–1916), Austrian pathologist.*
[b] *Philippe Charles Ernest Gaucher (1854–1918), French dermatologist.*

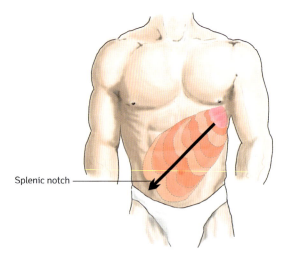

Figure 7.30 Sequence of splenic enlargement.

Splenic notch

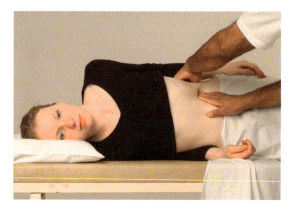

Figure 7.31 Position for tipping the spleen (see text).

you palpate a spleen feel its substance all the way to the costal margin. You should not be able to 'get above it', to feel its upper border. This is the second distinguishing feature of the spleen. If you can get above it, you are not dealing with a spleen. Now feel the consistency of the spleen, note if it is tender and pay close attention to the splenic border. If you find a notch in it, this is the third unique feature of the spleen. Measure the size of the spleen with a tape measure or by gauging the number of fingerbreadths below the costal margin. Finally percuss the lower border of the spleen starting well below the edge from an area of resonance. The percussion note should be dull when the spleen is encountered.

There may be times when the spleen may only just be palpable. A technique called 'tipping the spleen' may help in this circumstance. Get your patient to roll onto their right side, with their left knee bent upwards. Ask the patient to reach over with their left arm and to rest it on your left shoulder. Put your hand right up to the left costal margin and get the patient to take a deep breath. If the spleen is just palpable you may be able to 'tip' it in this position (see Fig. 7.31). Sometimes you cannot palpate the spleen and the only clue to its enlargement is a dull percussion note in Traube's space (*Ludwig Traube (1818–1876), German physician*). This is the region in the ninth intercostal space that lies anterior to the anterior axillary line. Normally this area is resonant but as the spleen enlarges it occupies this space and the percussion note becomes dull.

Causes of splenomegaly

See Table 7.22.

Kidneys

(DF 9/10.) The kidneys can prove very difficult to palpate especially if your technique is not spot on. In normal

Table 7.22 Causes of splenomegaly

Infective	Viral (e.g. hepatitis A, B, or C, glandular fever), bacterial (e.g. subacute bacterial endocarditis (SBE)), protozoal (e.g. malaria), parasite (e.g. hydatid disease)
Haematological	Leukaemias (especially chronic granulocytic leukaemia), myelofibrosis, lymphoma, haemolytic anaemias
Cirrhosis of the liver	
Infiltrative	Gaucher's disease, amyloidosis

(a)   (b)

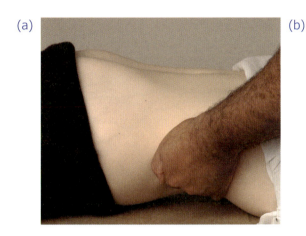
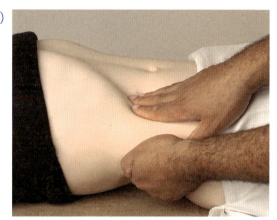

Figure 7.32 Examining the right kidney (see text).

people they are impalpable (very occasionally the right kidney can be felt in thin people).

How to examine

See Figs. 7.32 and 7.33. You need to stand up to examine the kidneys and you will need both hands to palpate (bimanual palpation). To examine the right kidney you must place your left hand under the patient in the renal angle. This is below the twelfth rib, above the posterior iliac crest and not as far in as the spine and paravertebral muscles. If you are too near any of these positions the area will feel hard and firm. You may have to move your hand around until you feel the right area, which should feel soft and yielding under your fingers. Now place your right hand flat on the abdomen on the right flank, lateral to the rectus muscle. This hand should be lying over the lower hand, with the patient's flank sandwiched between the two. Now press down with your right hand while flexing upwards with the fingers of your left. If the kidney is large enough you can feel it bumping against the right hand. This is called ballotting. As this movement is very

(a)   (b)

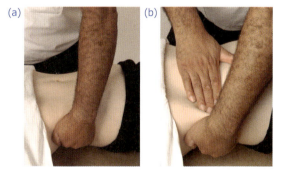

Figure 7.33 Examining the left kidney (see text).

brisk there may not be enough time to gauge the consistency and size of the kidney, unless the kidney is very large. In polycystic disease of the kidneys, they can be large and irregular and these features are readily appreciated and unforgettable. Now percuss over the kidney. It should be resonant over the kidney because of overlying gas-filled bowel.

Palpating the left kidney can be very tricky. Remain standing and lean over your patient so you can slide the palm of your left hand around and then under the patient into the left renal angle. This may feel awkward at first so keep persevering. Check that the area above your fingers is soft and yielding to indicate that you are in the renal angle. Now place your right hand on the left flank aiming to overlap the fingers of both hands and produce the sandwich of the left flank. Now ballot the left kidney. This will need a lot of practice before you will feel comfortable doing it. It is interesting to note that the kidney does move downwards with respiration (just at the end of inspiration) but this property is not used in palpating for the kidneys.

Causes of an enlarged kidney

See Table 7.23.

Table 7.23 Causes of an enlarged kidney

Polycystic kidneys
Tumours
Hydronephrosis
Amyloidosis

Percussion

18 Percuss over any masses or organs felt. Check for ascites. If the percussion note is dull in the flanks, go on to demonstrate shifting dullness (DF 7/10) or a fluid thrill (DF 6/10)

The general principle here is that any solid organ will sound dull and any gas-filled structure (usually bowel) will sound resonant. If any enlarged organ lies beneath bowel the percussion note above it will be resonant, for example, kidney. Usually your percussion will follow automatically if you find an enlarged organ or mass (as above). Even if you do not find anything you should still percuss carefully below the costal margins as a dull note can inform you of a liver edge or splenic border that you may have missed on palpation. Percussion has an additional role in differentiating between some causes of abdominal distension. It is used particularly for eliciting ascites.

Ascites

What is it?

Ascites is the abnormal collection of free fluid in the abdominal cavity. Traditionally it is divided into a transudate or an exudate depending on the protein content. If it is less than 30 g/L it is a transudate and if it is greater than 30 g/L it is an exudate (you may read different figures in other textbooks, for example, 20 g/dL or 25 g/dL, but the principle of high protein–exudate and low protein–transudate remains the same). Recently it has been recognized that the concentration of protein can vary with respect to the plasma protein and hence a modified definition states that ascitic fluid is a transudate if it is less than 10 mg/L **less** than the plasma albumin. Therefore if a patient has a plasma albumin of 25 mg/L and has ascitic fluid with a concentration of 19 g/L, this is still an exudate (despite being in the transudate range in the original definition). Ascitic fluid (like any liquid) will flow to the most dependent levels in a patient (see Fig. 7.34). In the supine patient this will be the flanks. Also loops of bowel will float uppermost in the centre of the abdomen. This distribution of fluid and bowel is exploited by examining the percussion note from the centre of the abdomen to the flanks.

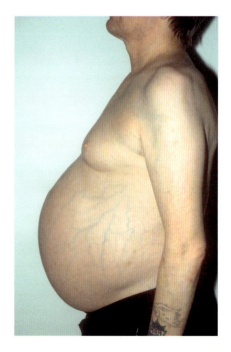

Figure 7.34 Patient with ascites.

Causes

See Table 7.24.

How to examine

See Fig. 7.35. Percuss the centre of the abdomen. The note should sound resonant. Now percuss in steps out towards the left flank. If abdominal distension is due to flatus the flanks will remain resonant. Sometimes the distension is so great that the percussion note is termed tympanitic (like a kettledrum). If the percussion note is dull in the flanks (and there is no splenomegaly) then it is likely that ascites is present. This requires confirmation by looking for shifting dullness. Having elicited a dull note in the flank, keep the percussed finger firmly on the flank and ask your patient to

roll towards you (making sure your finger does not move). Allow the patient about 20 seconds to settle on their right side (this allows time for the fluid to redistribute and to shift down to the right). Now percuss your finger again. This time the note should be resonant. Some people prefer to make a mark on the flank with a pen to denote the area of dullness (get the patient's permission first) and to percuss over the mark once the patient has turned on their side.

Another method of demonstrating ascites is to elicit a fluid thrill. This technique is particularly good in the presence of large amounts of ascitic fluid. The aim here is to tap a flank with your fingertips (flicking with your finger can be painful) and the resulting impulse is conducted through the fluid to the opposite flank where you can observe or palpate it. As this wave can also be transmitted along the subcutaneous fat of obese patients you should get the patient (or any help-ful person handy) to place a hand vertically in the midline so that the ulnar border is pressed firmly into the abdomen.

One final method that you might be taught is the pud-dle sign. This is performed with the patient kneeling on all fours. In this position the fluid gravitates to the centre of the abdomen. This area should sound dull to percussion. It was said that this particular technique was sensitive and could detect small amounts of fluid. However, this has been shown not to be the case. As this is an undignified test for both patient and examiner it is not recommended.

An important point to note is that a large amount of ascites can obscure masses or enlarged organs within the abdomen. In these circumstances a technique called dip-ping may be useful. Rather than palpating with the flat of your hand you dip your fingers into the abdomen with a sharp, rapid movement. If a mass is present you may feel something impact on your fingers for a brief moment. This technique can only alert you to the presence of something

Table 7.24 Causes of ascites

| **Transudate** |
| Congestive cardiac failure |
| Chronic liver disease |
| Nephrotic syndrome |
| Constrictive pericarditis |
| Hypoproteinaemia |
| **Exudate** |
| Intra-abdominal malignancy |
| Bacterial peritonitis |
| Tuberculous peritonitis |

(a) 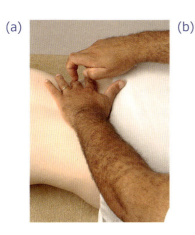 (b)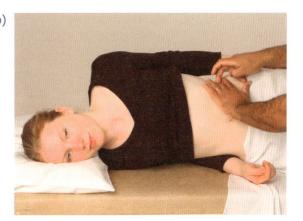

Figure 7.35 Percussing for ascites (see text).

unusual within the abdomen because there is little opportunity to assess the features of any structure in such a brief instant. Many people are baffled as to how this technique works. It works on the principle of inertia. If the same force is applied to objects of different masses in the same direction, the one with the lighter mass will move first, followed shortly by the heavier one (because of its greater inertia). When you dip your hand into an abdomen with ascites, the object with the lighter mass will move first, that is, the fluid. The fluid flows away from your fingers (and around any underlying mass). A heavier object such as a bowel cancer may remain motionless long enough (due to inertia) for your hand to feel it before it moves away also.

Auscultation

19 Auscultate for bowel sounds (DF 8/10) (and for bruits and rubs if necessary) (DF 9/10)

The first time you hear bowel sounds you will instantly recognize them. They are gurgling sounds that can be heard approximately every 10–20 seconds. If bowel sounds are absent (you sometimes have to auscultate for up to 1 minute), this can represent a paralytic ileus or if the abdomen is rigid, peritonitis. These sounds usually become more plentiful after a meal. Bowel sounds are even more exaggerated with diarrhoea and can become loud enough to be audible to the unaided ear. Audible bowel sounds are called borborygmi (*bor-be-rig-me*). In mechanical obstruction of the bowel, the distended bowel can add a tinkling quality to the bowel sounds, which is pathognomonic (they are called tinkling bowel sounds, funnily enough). Other sounds to listen for include renal artery bruits, which can be heard just above and lateral to the umbilicus in either flank. Bruits can sometimes be heard over an enlarged liver in alcoholic hepatitis or a hepatoma. Very rarely rubs (like a pleural rub) can be heard over the liver and spleen due to infarcts (these are so rare the author has yet to find someone who has heard one).

20 Examine the groins for lymphadenopathy and herniae (ask the patient to cough) (DF 8/10)

Now is the time to expose the groins. Take some time to inspect before you launch into palpation. Note any swellings in the groin and observe the testicles in men. In chronic liver disease there is loss of pubic hair (or change to female distribution in men) and testicular atrophy. Now feel along the inguinal ligament. A small amount of irregularity is normal, as are small shotty lymph nodes that are less than 1 cm in diameter. Large lymph nodes should make you suspicious. Unilaterally enlarged nodes may herald skin malignancy of a leg. Unilateral or bilateral lymph nodes may be due to a lymphoma (look for nodes elsewhere and hepatosplenomegaly).

Herniae

The principles of herniae have been described earlier. There are three main types of herniae to be found in the groin; the indirect inguinal hernia, the direct inguinal hernia, and the femoral hernia. The knowledge of the anatomy of this region is crucial to understanding the difference between them. See Fig. 7.36. The inguinal canal is an oblique canal that runs from the internal ring (a hole in the transversalis fascia) to the external ring (a defect in the external oblique aponeurosis). It allows the passage of the spermatic cord in men and the round ligament of the uterus in women, together with the ileoinguinal nerve. The femoral canal runs beneath the inguinal ligament, under its medial aspect. On its lateral aspects lies first the femoral vein, then the femoral artery, and then the femoral nerve. The femoral canal only contains a lymph node and some fat.

Indirect inguinal hernia

This is the most common hernia in the groin. The hernial sac and contents pass through the internal ring into the inguinal canal. If the hernia is large enough it can pass through the external ring and descend into the scrotum or labia majora. As the internal ring is narrow there is potential for the hernia to strangulate.

Direct inguinal hernia

This hernia bulges forward directly through the posterior wall of the inguinal canal. As the hernial neck is wide this hernia rarely strangulates. See Fig. 7.36 for a diagram showing the relationship of indirect and direct inguinal hernia.

Femoral hernia

A femoral hernia passes down the femoral canal into the upper thigh. If large enough the hernial sac can emerge through the canal and turn upwards sometimes extending beyond the inguinal ligament. Because of the very narrow canal this hernia is very prone to strangulation.

How to examine

You may have already noticed a swelling in the groin. Even if you do not see one, get your patient to cough. A bulging may betray the presence of an occult hernia.

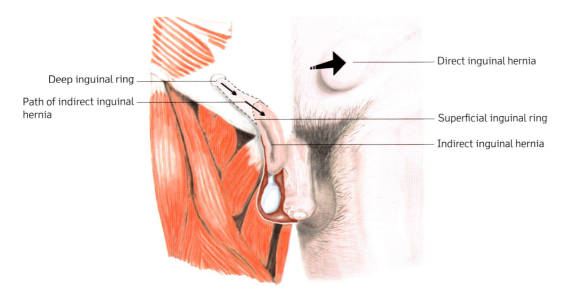

Deep inguinal ring

Path of indirect inguinal hernia

Direct inguinal hernia

Superficial inguinal ring

Indirect inguinal hernia

Figure 7.36 The inguinal region demonstrating a direct and indirect inguinal hernia.

Get your patient to repeat the cough and this time place your hand over the swelling and feel the impulse. If you still have not found a hernia ask your patient to stand up before coughing again. Look and palpate as before. To distinguish between the different hernias you need to identify the pubic tubercle. Place your index finger in the crease of the groin at the beginning of the pubic hair. If you press firmly you should feel the inguinal ligament. Run your finger medially towards the scrotum or labium until you feel the bony knub of the pubic tubercle (do this quickly and professionally, or you could get some worried looks from your patient). If the neck of the hernial sac is above and medial to the pubic tubercle it is an indirect inguinal hernia. If it is below and lateral to the pubic tubercle, it is a femoral hernia. You should now try to reduce the hernia with firm pressure. This manoeuvre will help you distinguish between an indirect inguinal and direct inguinal hernia. Once reduced an indirect hernia can be controlled by a finger over the internal ring (this can be found approximately half an inch (1 cm) above the pulse of the femoral artery). As the direct inguinal hernia is a forward bulge through the abdominal wall a finger will be unable to control it.

Wash your hands

21 Wash your hands

Be obsessive or develop the insanity of the insanitary.

Presentation of findings

22 Now say, 'I would like to examine the external genitalia and perform a rectal examination.' Present findings

Having felt for lymphadenopathy in the groin stand up straight and say, 'I would like to examine the external genitalia and perform a rectal examination.' The examiner will usually indicate that this is not necessary.

Then start the presentation. The exact style of presentation depends on your findings. If your findings point to an exact diagnosis, then be confident and mention this up front. For example,

'This man has chronic liver disease. He has hepatomegaly, which is three fingerbreadths below the costal margin and I could just tip a spleen. He has, in addition, jaundice, leuconychia, palmar erythema, and Dupuytren's contracture. There was no abdominal distension and I could not demonstrate any ascites.'

If your findings are inconclusive, detail them, give a differential diagnosis, and if you are unsure of an abdominal mass or organ or its aetiology suggest an abdominal ultrasound. For example,

'This man is jaundiced and has a mass in the right upper quadrant. It moves downward with inspiration

and is dull to percussion. This man therefore has hepatomegaly, which could be due to liver metastases, lymphoma, cirrhosis of the liver, or congestive cardiac failure. Ultrasound will be helpful to confirm hepatomegaly and in defining its cause.'

Here the student has missed the subtle signs, which would have clinched the diagnosis. They were also less certain as to the identity of the right upper quadrant mass but by listing its properties (and remembering the jaundice), quickly deduced that this had to be a liver. They then put together a reasonable differential diagnosis.

Other abdominal signs

Grey-Turner's sign

(DF 9/10.)

What is it?

Grey-Turner's sign (*George Grey-Turner (1877–1951), English surgeon*) is a subtle discoloration in the flanks that looks like a faint bruise. See Fig. 7.37.

Significance

Caused by bleeding into the abdominal cavity, with blood tracking into the subcutaneous layer of skin. Causes include haemorrhagic pancreatitis, a ruptured aortic aneurysm, or a ruptured ectopic pregnancy.

Cullen's sign

(DF 9/10.)

What is it?

Cullen's sign (*Thomas Stephen Cullen (1868–1953), American gynaecologist*) is a discoloration, similar to Grey-Turner's sign, that occurs around the umblicus. See Fig. 7.38.

Significance

Same as for Grey-Turner's sign.

Murphy's sign

(DF 5/10.)

What is it?

Murphy's sign (*John Benjamin Murphy (1857–1916), American surgeon*) is the sudden pain elicited when palpating in the region of the gallbladder.

Significance

It denotes an inflammatory process of the gallbladder such as cholecystitis.

How to examine

You need to locate the area where the gallbladder normally lies (on the underside of the liver). Its position is located where the lateral border of the rectus muscle intersects with the right costal margin. As you get the patient to take a deep breath you slip your finger under the costal margin at this point. If the sign is positive the patient will cry out in pain or freeze in mid-breath in obvious discomfort. You can look for this sign deliberately if you suspect

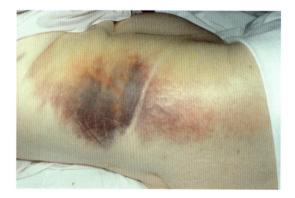

Figure 7.37 Grey-Turner's sign.

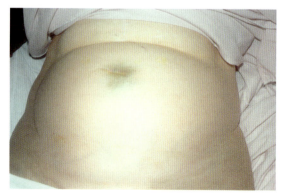

Figure 7.38 Cullen's sign.

gallbladder disease but sometimes you may elicit this sign incidently when you are palpating for a liver.

Abdominal diseases and investigations

In the earlier parts of this chapter, various medical conditions have been mentioned. In this section I now describe these. In general these descriptions are brief, though certain aspects not well described in other textbooks are discussed in some detail.

Pharyngeal pouch

In old textbooks, this is sometimes referred to as Zenker's diverticulum (*Friedrich Albert Von Zenker (1825–1898), German pathologist*). This is an outpouching of the oesophagus that develops most commonly in elderly men. It causes dysphagia, sometimes accompanied by noisy gurgling sounds. At night there is often the regurgitation of undigested food, which may lead to aspiration pneumonia. Treatment is by excision, either by surgery or by endoscopic means.

Mallory–Weiss tear

This is a tear in the mucosa of the oesophagus, which occurs after repeated retching or vomiting. Bright red blood is seen in subsequent vomits.

Achalasia of the oesophagus

This condition is a cause of dysphagia. It can be primary (cause unknown) or secondary to conditions such as malignancy of the oesophagus. The primary condition is thought to be due to the degeneration of nerve cells in the myenteric plexus of the oesophagus. Dysphagia is caused through a combination of factors: decreased or absent peristalsis and increased resting pressure of the lower oesophageal sphincter, which fails to relax when food is swallowed.

Oesophageal varices

Varices (dilated veins) are found in chronic liver disease (of any cause) when portal hypertension develops. Normally blood flows from the gut along the hepatic portal vein to the liver (portal circulation) and from there to the inferior vena cava and hence to the heart (systemic circulation). When portal hypertension develops, blood flow is reversed away from the liver and has to find another way back to the systemic circulation. This occurs via collaterals (these are minor blood vessels that carry only a small proportion of blood in the same direction as the main blood supply). If blood flow is blocked in the main vessel, the body compensates by diverting the flow along these minor channels, which dilate with the increased blood volume. In portal hypertension there are four main clinical collaterals, called portasystemic anastomoses (see Table 7.25). The most important of these are the ones that form oesophageal varices. Clinically if they rupture they can be the site of torrential bleeding.

Pancreatitis

This is a painful inflammatory condition of the pancreas, which can be acute or chronic. The most common predisposing causes are gallstones and heavy alcohol ingestion. The inflammation is caused by the pancreas's own enzymes. This can set off a sequence of metabolic events, which can have systemic effects and possibly lead to

Table 7.25 Portasystemic anastomoses

Portal circulation	Systemic circulation	Clinical result
Oesophageal branch of left gastric vein	Oesophageal veins draining middle third of oesophagus to azygous vein	Oesophageal varices
Paraumbilical veins	Superficial veins of anterior abdominal wall	Caput medusae
Superior rectal veins	Middle and inferior rectal veins	Haemorrhoids
Veins of ascending colon, descending colon, pancreas, duodenum, and liver	Renal, lumbar, phrenic veins	

multiorgan failure. An acute attack is suggested by a rise of serum amylase to three times the upper limit of normal (a lower level does not exclude it). A chronic pancreatitis may result from repeated acute attacks (the serum amylase rise may be slight or non-existent). Malabsorption may result with chronic pancreatitis.

Gallstones

These can be made from cholesterol, bile pigments, or both. Most are asymptomatic and are found by chance on radiographic or ultrasound examination. If a stone impacts in the common bile duct it can cause biliary colic, jaundice, or ascending cholangitis. Stones in the gallbladder can provoke cholecystitis. The definitive treatment for symptomatic gallstones is surgery. It is also possible to dissolve certain gallstones with bile acid or to shatter them with lithotripsy (focused sound wave therapy).

Cholecystitis

This is inflammation of the gallbladder and is a complication of gallstones in the gallbladder. If a stone impacts in the gallbladder outlet, the gallbladder wall becomes inflamed by the increasing concentration of bile. A secondary bacterial infection may occur. Repeated attacks of inflammation can cause fibrosis of the gallbladder (chronic cholecystitis). Occasionally cholecystitis can occur in the absence of gallstones. This is termed acalculous cholecystitis.

Jaundice

Knowledge of bilirubin metabolism will help you understand jaundice (see Fig. 7.39). The liver is the key because it is at the centre of bilirubin metabolism and all the causes of jaundice can be related to it, for example, prehepatic, hepatic, and posthepatic jaundice. Bilirubin is formed by the breakdown of old or damaged red blood cells in the reticuloendothelial system. It is not soluble in water and is therefore bound to plasma protein and transported to the liver (at this stage bilirubin is described as unconjugated). The bilirubin is taken up by the liver and made water soluble by conjugating it with glucuronide. This process is facilitated by the enzyme glucuronyl transferase (you may see its full name, UDP-glucuronyl transferase, in other textbooks). The conjugated bilirubin is secreted in the bile and eventually passes into the duodenum. In the gut bacteria convert

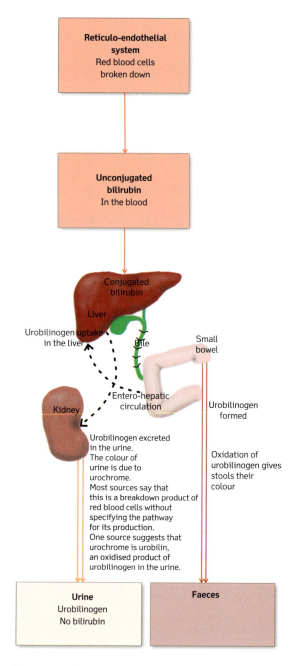

Figure 7.39 The normal production and metabolism of bilirubin.

bilirubin to urobilinogen, which is later converted to stercobilins, which give faeces their characteristic brown colour. Some urobilinogen is absorbed by the ileum into the portal blood, which transports it to the liver. Here the majority of urobilinogen is secreted into the bile and back into the gut. This recycling of urobilinogen is termed the enterohepatic circulation. Small amounts of urobilinogen escape into the general circulation and are eventually filtered by the kidney and excreted in the urine.

Prehepatic jaundice

Overall prehepatic causes are not common. The two circumstances you should know about are haemolytic anaemia and Gilbert's syndrome (see Fig. 7.40).

Haemolytic anaemia

There are various forms of haemolytic anaemia but in all cases there is the premature destruction of red blood cells. This leads to a greater amount of bilirubin being formed and causes jaundice when the concentration exceeds 30 µmol/L. The bilirubin is conjugated in the liver as normal but the liver is overwhelmed by the excess amount produced by haemolysis and hence the build-up of unconjugated bilirubin in the blood. The jaundice is usually mild and rarely exceeds 100 µmol/L. All the other aspects of bilirubin metabolism continue as normal, for example, the secretion of conjugated bilirubin in the bile, the formation of urobilinogen in the gut, the recycling of urobilinogen through the enterohepatic circulation, and the passage of urobilinogen in the urine. The only difference is that larger quantities of bilirubin are processed leading to greater quantities of urobilinogen in the gut and urine. As a result the colour of the stools and urine are unchanged.

Gilbert's syndrome

Gilbert's syndrome (*Nicolas Augustin Gilbert (1858–1927), French physician*) is one of the familial hyperbilirubinaemias. It is the most common and can affect 2–7% of the population. A number of minor defects in bilirubin metabolism cause mild unconjugated jaundice. These are a decrease in uptake of bilirubin by the liver, decreased activity of glucuronyl transferase, and mild haemolysis. The key fact is that the liver is normal, which is reflected in normal liver function tests and the prognosis is excellent. The jaundice becomes more noticeable following alcohol ingestion, starvation, or intercurrent illness. Otherwise Gilbert's syndrome is usually found by chance when liver function tests show a mildly elevated bilirubin with normal levels of liver enzymes (should be confirmed by ruling out haemolysis as a cause of jaundice). A rare form of familial hyperbilirubinaemia is Criggler–Najjar syndrome (*John Fielding Crigler (born 1919), American paediatrician; Victor Assad Najjar (born 1914), Lebanese-born American*

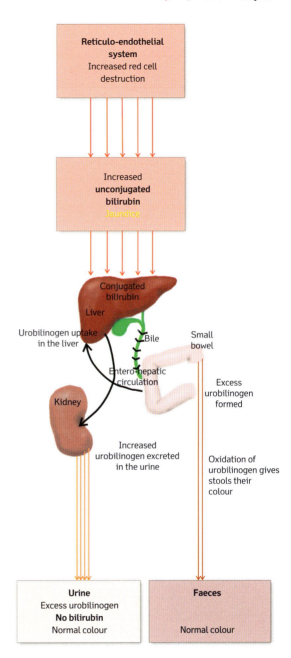

Figure 7.40 Prehepatic jaundice due to haemolysis (unconjugated bilirubin).

paediatrician). This is due to an absence of glucuronyl transferase (fatal in childhood); a milder form with reduced activity of glucuronyl transferase is compatible with survival into adulthood. The only treatment for this condition is liver transplantation.

Hepatic jaundice

There are many hepatic causes of jaundice. In this context, it can also be called hepatitic or hepatocellular jaundice. The causes can be acute, for example, drugs and viruses or chronic, for example, alcohol and other drugs and viruses. Any damage to the liver cells can interfere with their ability to take up bilirubin, to conjugate it, or to secrete it into bile. In addition, there is sometimes a cholestatic phase to the jaundice, that is, conjugated bilirubin is not secreted into bile but refluxes back into the blood stream. This is called intrahepatic cholestasis and the mechanism for this is not known. This cholestatic phase can be recognized clinically by pale, clay-coloured stools and dark orange/brown urine (see Fig. 7.41).

Posthepatic jaundice

The causes of posthepatic jaundice are easy to understand. There is obstruction to the flow of bile beyond the liver. This is often termed extrahepatic cholestasis and can occur anywhere in the biliary system from the liver to the duodenum. The bilirubin is unable to reach the small intestine and as a result, little or no bilirubin is converted to urobilinogen and hence the stools become pale (clay-coloured). In addition, excess conjugated bilirubin refluxes back into the bloodstream (levels can reach >100 µmol/L) and is deposited in the skin (yellow colour and itching) and sclera (yellow colour) and is also excreted in the urine, which becomes a dark orange colour (see Fig. 7.41)

Chronic liver disease

This is simply any liver disease that is present for more than 6 months. Some patients have acute attacks, which then go on to become chronic, for example, hepatitis B. Others are asymptomatic and are only discovered on blood tests. When followed up they may remain well for years before exhibiting symptoms, for example, primary biliary cirrhosis. Other patients may be asymptomatic until they present with a complication such as ascites or bleeding oesophageal varices when portal hypertension supervenes.

Cirrhosis of the liver

Cirrhosis is strictly a pathological diagnosis. Although it can be suspected clinically, it can only be confirmed following histological examination of a biopsy specimen. It

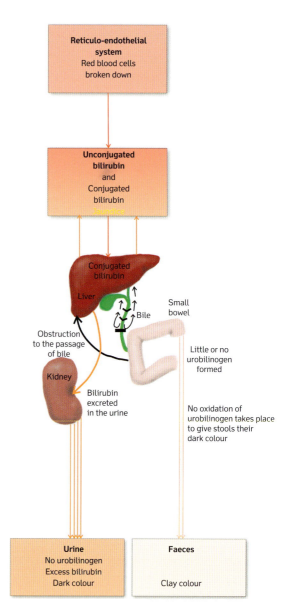

Figure 7.41 Posthepatic jaundice due to cholestasis (conjugated bilirubin).

is the irreversible endpoint of a variety of insults; alcohol is the most common cause in the UK. Sometimes students make the mistake of using cirrhosis and chronic liver disease interchangeably. Cirrhosis is one form of chronic liver disease (other examples include hepatitis B and malignancy) although it may be the final endpoint for many causes of chronic liver disease.

Primary biliary cirrhosis

This form of cirrhosis is more common in females. The cause is unknown although an immunological mechanism is strongly suspected. More than 95% of sufferers have anti-mitochondrial antibodies.

Cholangiocarcinoma

This is an adenocarcinoma that arises from the biliary ducts. It is a rare cancer that usually presents with cholestatic jaundice. It may also cause abdominal pain, anorexia, and weight loss. It has a poor prognosis and treatment is usually palliative, that is, placing a stent by endoscopic retrograde cholangiopancreatogram (ERCP) (a stent is a hollow structure placed within the lumen of an obstructed vessel to allow the free flow of fluid through it).

Sclerosing cholangitis

This is an inflammatory process of the biliary tree resulting in fibrosis and narrowing of the tract. It can be primary or secondary to other causes such as previous bile duct surgery, gallstones, or AIDS. Although there is no known cause for primary sclerosing cholangitis, there is a strong association with inflammatory bowel disease.

Inflammatory bowel disease

This term is used to describe a family of diseases that have in common an inflammatory infiltrate of the bowel of unknown cause. It is often used to describe ulcerative colitis or Crohn's disease although microscopic colitis is also embraced by the term. There are other causes of an inflammatory infiltrate in the bowel, for example, infection, radiation, and ischaemia, but these are not classified as inflammatory bowel disease.

Ulcerative colitis

This condition primarily affects the large bowel. The inflammatory infiltrate usually affects the mucosa. It usually presents with bloody diarrhoea. Other symptoms include anorexia, weight loss, fever, and abdominal pain relieved by defecation. A rare complication is toxic megacolon, where the gut dilates and eventually perforates in a severe attack. It also has complications outside the gut, including (1) in the joints—arthritis, ankylosing spondylitis; (2) in the eyes—episcleritis; (3) in the skin—erythema nodosum and pyoderma gangrenosum; and (4) in the

biliary tree—sclerosing cholangitis. There is a risk of cancer developing in some patients (usually those with extensive disease involving the whole of the large bowel—pancolitis) and in those who have had the disease a long time. The risk is quoted as 5–10% at 15–25 years in those with a pancolitis. These people are kept under surveillance by colonoscopy.

Crohn's disease

This condition can affect any part of the bowel from mouth to anus. The inflammatory infiltrate usually affects the submucosa. It also commonly presents with bloody diarrhoea and has similar symptoms to ulcerative colitis. The unusual feature with Crohn's disease is that it can affect some areas of the bowel and have normal bowel in between (the affected areas are called skip lesions). It can also lead to fistula formation (a fistula is an abnormal connection between two epithelial surfaces, for example, between small bowel and large bowel or between bowel and skin). Ileal involvement may lead to malabsorption. It can also lead to similar extraintestinal manifestation as ulcerative colitis although the frequency of complications differs.

Microscopic colitis

This is a form of inflammatory bowel disease where the bowel looks normal on colonoscopic or barium enema examination. However if biopsy samples are examined with microscopy they have characteristic histological appearances. Patients usually present with watery diarrhoea (bleeding PR is unusual).

Mesenteric ischaemia

This can be acute or chronic. It is difficult to diagnose, as there are few clinical signs and no diagnostic tests (plus doctors do not often think about the possibility). The acute form is usually caused by an embolus or thrombosis occluding the gut supply (although it can occur due to decreased perfusion in cardiogenic or hypovolaemic shock). With infarction of the bowel peritonitis may develop, leading to increased abdominal pain with the signs of peritonism. Chronic ischaemia leads to abdominal pain up to an hour after a meal (this has been called intestinal claudication or angina, the analogy being drawn from coronary heart disease or peripheral vascular disease). Always think of this diagnosis in elderly patients, smokers, and those who have atrial fibrillation or other cardiovascular pathology, for example, stroke, ischaemic heart disease, and peripheral vascular disease.

Ischaemic colitis

This is a form of inflammatory disease of the bowel due to ischaemia that usually afflicts older people. It usually presents with left-sided abdominal pain and diarrhoea. Bleeding PR is unusual. It can be diagnosed on colonoscopy (biopsies may be needed to clinch the diagnosis) and changes tend to centre around the splenic flexure (the splenic flexure is the watershed between the superior mesenteric artery supply and the inferior mesenteric artery supply).

Acute intestinal obstruction

There are four main symptoms with intestinal obstruction: colicky abdominal pain, abdominal distension, faeculant vomiting, and absolute constipation (even to flatus). It can occur because of an obstruction in the lumen of the bowel, for example, tumour; because of an obstruction in the wall of the bowel, for example, stricture; or because of compression from outside the bowel, for example, adhesions following previous surgery.

Diverticular disease

A diverticulum is an outpouching of the bowel wall. It occurs because of the high pressures created within the lumen of the bowel during muscular contraction. This forces pockets of bowel through areas of weakness (usually where blood vessels enter the bowel via the mesentery). The presence of diverticulae scattered throughout the bowel is called diverticulosis. If inflammation occurs within a diverticulum, this is called diverticulitis. The whole spectrum of presentations associated with diverticulae is called diverticular disease. Other complications include diarrhoea and constipation, bleeding PR, abscess formation, and fistulae formation. If diverticulae occur in the jejunum, bacteria may multiply in the pockets in sufficient numbers to cause malabsorption of fat (the bacteria deconjugate bile salts preventing the absorption of fat).

Polyps

Polyps are small outgrowths from a mucous membrane surface. In the gut they can be sessile (flat and slightly elevated from the gut surface) or pedunculated (attached to the gut by a stalk). The majority of polyps are found by chance following bowel investigations. Others cause bleeding or iron deficiency anaemia. The importance of polyps lie in the malignant potential that some possess. These include some adenomas and inherited conditions such as Peutz–Jehgers syndrome, Gardner's syndrome, and familial polyposis coli.

Haemorrhoids

Internal haemorrhoids are also known as 'piles'. They are varicosities of the superior haemorrhoidal veins (also called the superior rectal veins). With your patient in the lithotomy position (think of the (undignified) position that women get into for a cervical smear), if you were to view the anus from the front (this gets worse) and you were to regard it as a clock, then haemorrhoids appear at 3, 7, and 11 o'clock. There are three categories of haemorrhoids:

- **first-degree haemorrhoids** (confined to the anal canal)
- **second-degree haemorrhoids** (prolapse from the anus following defecation but return spontaneously or can be replaced with a finger)
- **third-degree haemorrhoids** (prolapse from the anus and cannot be replaced).

All three categories are painless unless thrombosis occurs. They usually cause bright red bleeding PR following defaecation or on the toilet paper. Predisposing causes include constipation, compression by a pregnant uterus, compression by other pelvic tumours, and rarely, portal hypertension.

Angiodysplasia

Angiodysplasia ('angio'—blood, 'dysplasia'—loss of differentiation of cells) are malformations of blood vessels in the gut that are susceptible to bleeding. They are more common in older people. The best investigation to identify them is colonoscopy, where the lesions can be cauterized. Rarely, if bleeding is excessive or the lesions extensive, the patient may need resection of the affected bowel.

Endoscopy

This is a test using a flexible fibreoptic instrument, which can be passed within the body cavities to visualize the internal organs. Modern equipment has evolved to enable a variety of procedures to be undertaken via the endoscope. These include:

- biopsy (taking a sample of tissue for histological analysis)
- diathermy (passing an electric current to control bleeding)
- suction for removing secretions or washings for analysis
- inserting stents
- using a variety of baskets for removing foreign bodies or unwanted material.

Endoscopy is a generic term that covers all the medical fibreoptic procedures (the prefix 'endos' means inside). Often the prefix is changed to denote the organ being investigated, for example:

- gastroscopy—stomach
- colonoscopy—colon
- sigmoidoscopy—sigmoid colon
- cystoscopy—bladder
- hysteroscopy—uterus.

Try to work out the organs that are visualized from the following:

- bronchoscopy
- laparoscopy
- mediastinoscopy
- arthroscopy
- proctoscopy.

Endoscopic retrograde cholangiopancreatogram

The ERCP is a special form of endoscopy where the instrument is passed into the second part of the duodenum. The ampulla of Vater is cannulated (the common exit point of the common bile duct and the pancreatic duct). Radio-opaque dye is introduced into the duct system and the patient screened under radiographic control. This allows the diagnosis of biliary and pancreatic disease. The instrument can also be used therapeutically, for example, to remove stones or introduce stents.

Carcinoid syndrome

Carcinoid syndrome is a collection of symptoms due to high levels of circulating 5-hydroxytryptamine (5-HT) secreted from tumours of neuroendocrine origin. The symptoms include flushing, wheezing due to bronchospasm, hypotension, tachycardia, and diarrhoea. Tumours can be found in the gastrointestinal tract, bronchus, thyroid, and testis. Gut tumours only manifest their symptoms if there are liver metastases because the 5-HT is normally metabolized in the liver. The rare bronchial carcinoid does not need this prerequesite as the 5-HT is secreted into the general circulation. Diagnosis is aided by finding the breakdown product, 5-hydroxyindoleacetic acid (5-HIAA), in the urine.

Zollinger–Ellison syndrome

This condition is due to a gastrinoma (a tumour secreting the hormone gastrin), which is usually found in the pancreas. The gastrin causes a hypersecretion of acid in the stomach, which causes severe peptic ulceration in the stomach, duodenum, and even jejunum. Diarrhoea is also a common feature and the increased acidity in the small intestine can be sufficient to inactivate the pancreatic enzymes and precipitate malabsorption. Occasionally this tumour can be associated with multiple endocrine neoplasia type 1 (MEN-1), which also includes pituitary tumours and hyperparathyroidism.

Acute intermittent porphyria

This is a rare disorder of haem synthesis (the haem part of the haemoglobin molecule). An enzyme porphobilinogen deaminase involved in the formation of haem has reduced or no activity, leading to a build-up of by-products in the blood. This causes severe abdominal pain (sufferers have been known to have undergone surgery in the mistaken belief that they have had an acute abdomen). Other features include hypertension, tachycardia, peripheral neuropathy, encephalopathy, and coma.

Hypercalcaemia

(The prefix 'hyper' means increased or excessive.) Hypercalcaemia may be caused by a number of conditions. The most common are hyperparathyroidism (the parathyroids glands are tiny glands within the substance of the thyroid, which are responsible for calcium metabolism) and malignancy. Hypercalcaemia can cause abdominal pain, constipation, thirst, polyuria, and urinary stones. This has led to the expression 'moans, groans, and abdominal stones' with respect to the symptoms of hypercalcaemia.

Diabetic ketoacidosis

This is a serious complication of diabetes mellitus. It can occur due to sepsis, starvation, or a diabetic failing to take insulin. Occasionally a person may present with this complication for the first time. Ketoacidosis occurs because the patient is unable to use glucose for energy (as occurs normally). Instead they use fat as an alternative energy source, which leads to the production of ketones (acetoacetate and hydroxybutyric acid) in the blood and urine, where they can be detected. The patient suffers thirst (polydipsia), polyuria, and weight loss due to excessive dehydration. The acidosis stimulates an increase in the breathing rate called 'air hunger' or 'Kussmaul's respiration' and the sweet acetone smell of ketones can be detected on the breath. The condition is insidious and if undetected can lead to confusion, coma, and death. Abdominal pain is an unusual method of presentation. Initial treatment involves fluid replacement and intravenous insulin.

Urinary tract infection

This is a non-specific term describing an infection anywhere in the urinary tract (it includes cystitis—infection of the bladder and pyelonephritis—infection of the kidneys). A patient may experience a fever, dysuria, and urinary frequency (older people may be non-specifically unwell or become confused).

Finals section

In this section, as with the previous chapters, issues dealing with Finals will be discussed. For revision read the examination summary and the key points throughout the chapter, and do the questions at the end of the chapter.

If the cardiovascular system is at the heart of general medicine then the abdominal system is the guts of the specialty (sorry!). Many of the more common gastrointestinal pathologies, for example, gastro-oesophageal reflux disease, peptic ulcer, and irritable bowel syndrome, produce minimal signs and do not present a serious challenge for the short cases. Most Finals short cases will involve a palpable mass or organ, jaundice, or ascites. Each one will present a challenge to your clinical skills. Some masses can be difficult to identify even with the 'perfect' clinical technique, so do not panic if you do not know the answer. As long as your technique is sound and you can come up with a reasonable differential diagnosis, then you will be given credit. Common cases are shown in Tables 7.26 and 7.27.

Table 7.26 Finals cases

Jaundice
Hepatomegaly
Splenomegaly
Chronic liver disease
Hepatosplenomegaly
Ascites
Abdominal mass/palpable kidney

Table 7.27 Day-to-day cases

Abdominal pain
Dyspepsia
Diarrhoea/constipation
Inflammatory bowel disease
Any of the Finals cases

Key diagnostic clues

In real life many of the common conditions do not produce diagnostic signs. However with all abdominal conditions and in particular those associated with pain, **palpation** is the key. Signs of acute surgical complication, for example, guarding, rigidity, and rebound tenderness, constitute an emergency. With regards to short cases, where masses and organomegaly predominate, **palpation** again provides the most important clues.

Key signs of common palpable abnormalities

- **Hepatomegaly**. Enlarges into the RHC (massive hepatomegaly can reach the RIF), moves downward with inspiration, a hard irregular edge suggests malignancy (rarely a polycystic liver), dull to percussion. **Always percuss down the right side of the chest to rule out displacement of the liver by emphysema**.
- **Splenomegaly**. Enlarges into the LHC (massive splenomegaly can reach the RIF), it has a notch in its border, moves downward with inspiration, dull to percussion.

- **Chronic liver disease**. Leuconychia, palmar erythema, Dupuytren's contracture (alcohol), spider naevi, purpura, jaundice, loss of axillary hair, testicular atrophy, caput medusae, hepatomegaly, splenomegaly, ascites.

- **Ascites**. Abdominal distension, everted umbilicus (sometimes), fluid thrill, dull percussion in flanks, demonstrate shifting dullness.

- **Enlarged kidneys**. Palpable in flanks using bimanual technique, moves down minimally with inspiration, resonant to percussion.

Some advice relating to examination problems

General

Use the abdominal system examination routine described in this chapter. Cases 7.4–7.9 give useful tips you might encounter in an exam setting.

The instruction

The examiner will usually ask you to 'examine the abdominal system' or to 'examine the abdomen'. With the second command students feel obliged to dive straight on to the tummy. Resist this! Both commands mean the same thing so be thorough and start with the hands (following your inspection). Sometimes the examiner is more specific and may say 'palpate the abdomen.' Do exactly this. However, be vigilant and keep your eyes peeled for other clues such as jaundice or spider naevi. These may help you to a final diagnosis. The instructions in an OSCE tend to be straightforward and standardized (see 'OSCE examples').

General look

Fit this in while you introduce yourself to the patient and get them into position. It is recommended that the first thing

CASE 7.4

Problem. You are still unsure whether to do a full examination or to concentrate on the abdomen.

Solution. If there is any doubt, do the full examination. This at least shows that you are thorough and if the examiners want you to concentrate on the abdomen, they will stop you and direct you to it (do not be upset by any irritation they might display, just concentrate on your performance).

checked for in an abdominal case is jaundice. If you spot this, you know immediately there is a problem in the hepatobiliary system (this is usually the case in a Finals examination but do not forget haemolytic jaundice, drugs, and so on). Check for lesions that may be spider naevi, for bruising, and for abdominal distension (you could make a diagnosis of chronic liver disease before you even start examining the patient, but make sure you are methodical and find **all** the features).

Positioning

Whatever position the patient is in make sure you lie them flat. Ask the patient's permission before doing so. If the patient is already flat, quickly check they are comfortable (older people or those with musculoskeletal problems of the neck may need two pillows).

Hands

CASE 7.5

Problem. You always miss leuconychia and palmar erythema.

Solution. You must be **aware** of their possibility, particularly in an abdominal case. If you keep thinking about them, you are less likely to miss them.

Face

CASE 7.6

Problem. You have seen red spidery marks on the hands and face and told your examiners they are spider naevi, yet they seem dissatisfied.

Solution. You must always demonstrate blanching before your examiners will accept the diagnosis of spider naevi. Your clinicals are like a driving test; you must be **seen** to do the right things no matter how obvious they seem.

The abdomen

Now you have got to the abdomen do not rush to get your clammy hands on it. Step back and inspect it from a distance. Does it move quietly with respiration? Is it distended? Does it have distended veins on its surface? Never rush into palpation and when you do start, be methodical.

CASE 7.7

Problem. You have missed the lesions of Peutz–Jehgers or HHT syndromes.

Solution. Do not fret if you miss these. These conditions are rare and if you get a case you are more likely to be up for an honours mark. Your examiners are more concerned that you do not miss common and easy signs that could put a life in jeopardy. The answer here is the same as for leuconychia. You must be aware of the syndromes. Pay particular attention to the lips. If you are suspicious, get your patient to open their mouth and inspect the buccal mucosa (with HHT inspect their tongue, including the underside, for lesions).

Palpating the abdomen

CASE 7.8

Problem. After getting permission to palpate, the patient winces when you touch them. Should you continue?

Solution. It depends. It could have been a surprise or your cold clammy hand that could have provoked them. So apologize to the patient for causing discomfort and ask them if the area is normally tender. If it is, ask if you can feel the area, albeit gently (the same applies even if it is not normally tender). If the patient still flinches with pain despite the gentlest of touches, again apologize and abandon the examination. State to your examiners that you cannot proceed because of the obvious pain the patient is experiencing. For extra credit, also add that you would normally check for guarding or rebound tenderness to make sure the patient is not developing a surgical complication.

Presentation

Always offer to check the external genitalia and perform a rectal examination. Try to be confident and avoid the words 'seem' or 'might'.

OSCE examples

History-taking station

You are an FY1 working in the emergency department. A 31-year-old woman presents with abdominal pain

CASE 7.9

Problem. You always find you forget one or two small but relevant features during your presentation (especially the numerous signs of chronic liver disease).

Solution. There are two possible solutions. The first is to know all the signs like the back of your hand so that you are less likely to forget them when you recite your findings to the examiner. The second is to give a running commentary as you go along: 'On examining the hands I have noticed leuconychia and palmar erythema. I have just noticed red spidery lesions on the arms, face, and upper trunk that are reminiscent of spider naevi. I shall now attempt to blanch them . . . and yes they do blanch; they are spider naevi.' It is up to you to find the technique you prefer.

accompanied by vomiting. Please take a history from her and present your findings afterwards. You have 10 minutes in which to do this.

Remember:

- Introduce yourself to the patient.

- Take a comprehensive history of the patient's pain. Remember SOCRATES and ensure you enquire about whether the patient has had this pain before, and what cause was identified then.

- Enquire about past medical and past surgical history, especially relating to the abdomen. Has the patient had investigations beforehand and what did they show? Has she had any operations in the past?

- How much has been vomited, over how long, and what colour is the vomit? Remember to ask about 'red flag' signs—is there any haematemesis/coffee-ground vomit?

- Ask about a change in bowel habits, and blood in the motions/malaena, unintentional weight loss, appetite, dysphagia and urinary symptoms.

- Could the patient be pregnant?

- Ask about any medications that the patient is taking. Specifically ask about NSAIDs and anti-platelet medications such as warfarin and aspirin, especially if there is haemetemesis.

- Ask about smoking and alcohol and screen briefly for infectious causes—recent travel, infected contacts, etc.

- Thank your patient.

- Present your findings succinctly, and offer a differential diagnosis.

Examination station

You are an FY1 working on the gastrointestinal (GI) ward. A 68-year-old man presents with a month-long history of general malaise and fatigue, and a week-long history of confusion. He is known to have a history of excessive alcohol consumption. Please perform an examination of his gastrointestinal system and present your findings. You have 10 minutes.

- Introduce yourself to the patient and gain consent to examine him.
- Wash your hands/use alcohol gel provided.
- Generally inspect the patient from the end of the bed. Ensure he is suitably exposed but maintain dignity. Look for scars, muscle wasting, jaundice, spider naevi, and bruising.
- Inspect the hands and face and neck for stigmata of GI disease such as clubbing, palmar erythema, anaemia, gingivitis, dehydration, and supraclavicular nodes.
- Ensure he does not have a flapping tremor, which in this context would suggest liver failure.
- Inspect the abdomen carefully, looking for distension, dilated veins and organomegaly.
- Ask if the patient has any pain before lightly and then more deeply palpating the nine abdominal regions. Do so at the patient's level, continually looking at the patient's face for evidence of discomfort.
- Specifically palpate for the liver, spleen, and kidneys and a pulsatile abdominal aortic aneurysm. Try to practise your palpation technique as much as possible so that when you do it in the examination, you feel comfortable with it. Practice makes perfect!
- Percuss the liver and splenic areas, and for ascites/ shifting dullness.
- Auscultate for bowel sounds and then for bruits over the aorta and renal arteries.
- Thank your patient and wash your hands/use alcohol gel provided.
- Suggestions for further bedside investigations that you may like to offer are: to take a stool sample, to check the hernial orifices, perform a PR examination, test the urine and examine external genitalia.

Good luck!

Questions

- How many signs of chronic liver disease can you name?
- What are the causes of a right iliac fossa mass?
- What are the causes of hepatomegaly?
- How do you differentiate between an enlarged kidney and a spleen?
- What are the 'five Fs' that cause abdominal distension?
- How do you distinguish between a reducible hernia and an obstructed hernia?
- How do you confirm an abdominal mass is an aortic aneurysm?
- What six properties does an enlarged spleen possess?
- How do you assess an abdominal swelling found on palpation?
- What are the symptoms of intestinal obstruction?

Further reading

Cline DM, Stead LG. *Abdominal emergencies*. McGraw-Hill Medical, New York, 2008.

Dawson C, Nethercliffe J. *ABC of Urology*. BMJ Publishing Group/ Wiley-Blackwell, Chichester, 2012.

Rhodes JM, Tsai HH. *Clinical problems in gastroenterology*. Mosby-Wolfe, London, 1995.

Sewell DP, Chapman RGW, Mortenson N. *Ulcerative colitis and Crohn's disease, a clinician's guide*. Churchill Livingstone, Edinburgh, 1992.

Silen W. *Cope's early diagnosis of the acute abdomen*, 2nd edn. Oxford University Press, Oxford, 2000.

Smith ME, Morton DG. *The digestive system, basic science and clinical conditions*. Churchill Livingstone, Edinburgh, 2001.

Talley NJ. *Clinical gastroenterology: a practical problem based approach*, 3rd edn. Elsevier Australia, Chatswood, NSW, 2011.

8 Rectal examination

Introduction

The rectal examination (per rectum (PR) examination) is a test that is guaranteed to send shudders through any student (and their patient). Unfortunately it is not the kind of thing, like brain operations, which only qualified doctors are allowed to do. Students are not only allowed but are expected to do PR examinations. Many of our hang-ups about this examination revolve around our fear of contact with faeces or subjecting our patient to such an invasive and embarrassing test. Even today, some qualified doctors and nurses fail to think of performing the test or devise excuses to get out of doing it. In a recent national audit of continence in England the results showed that digital rectal examination was performed for faecal incontinence in only 53% of cases in acute care, 29% in primary care, 19% in mental health care, and 15% in care homes. Some of this reluctance may be linked to inadequate training and experience. In a number of national studies of medical schools, including Africa, Canada, Australia, Ireland and the UK, there were some students who had no experience of performing rectal examination on patients. Those that performed the test had limited experience and the unifying theme in all the studies was that they lacked confidence in interpreting findings. Clearly there is still a lot of work to be done by medical schools to improve this aspect of medical training.

Yet a PR examination is quick and easy to do and is usually painless. In fact, the hardest part of the examination can be putting your gloves on. Because of the intimate nature of this examination you will be unlikely to perform this on a real patient in a Finals examination. Although rectal examinations are not common in Finals, more medical schools are using manikins to address this deficiency.

The importance of the rectal examination

A great deal of information can be gained from a PR examination. The more common reasons for doing one are as follows.

- Assessment of gastrointestinal disturbance, for example, constipation, diarrhoea, tenesmus, or bleeding PR.
- Assessment of the prostate in men.
- Assessment of the acute abdomen.

Occasionally a PR examination can be used for unusual reasons such as searching for a cause in a pyrexia of unknown origin or the assessment of anal tone in a neurological examination. As with any test, a doctor has to weigh up the advantages of doing the test against the potential harm it may cause. If there is any doubt about the need for a PR examination it might be useful to remember the old surgical saying, 'Put your finger in it before you put your foot in it.' There is no point sparing the patient's feelings if in the long run you have missed a potentially treatable lesion such as an early rectal carcinoma.

Rectal examination summary

1 Introduce yourself to your patient and explain why you want to perform a PR examination.

2 Ask for permission to perform the PR examination.

3 Get a chaperone/helper.

4 Ensure equipment is at hand and ready.

5 Position the patient.

6 Wash your hands.

7 Put on gloves.

8 Put lubricant on your index finger.

9 Warn the patient that you are about to perform the test.

10 Inspect the perianal region.

11 Introduce your finger into the anal canal.

12 Examine the rectum in a logical sequence.

13 Take your finger out and inspect the glove for faeces, blood, and so on.

14 Clean the perianal region.

15 Tell your patient you have finished and allow them to get dressed.

16 Wash your hands.

17 Report your findings.

Rectal examination in detail

1 Introduce yourself to your patient and explain why you want to perform a PR examination

Say, 'Hello, I'm Marjory Warren, a fifth-year student.' Extend your hand for shaking. Explain why you are doing the test. Communication is essential in preventing a mildly uncomfortable procedure from becoming a traumatic one. There are still instances where patients are bewildered because they went to their doctors with what seemed a trivial complaint and end up with a finger rampaging up their rear end. **You** might see the logical need for a PR but a patient has not shared your training. For example, a patient goes to his GP and complains, 'I feel tired, doctor'. The GP quickly notices the patient looks clinically pale and knowing that gastrointestinal blood loss is the most common cause of anaemia, rushes to do a PR examination. Under pressure to see a large number of patients he does not fully explain his motives. Later, in the pub, the

man recounts his tale of horror to his mates. 'I was only feeling a bit tired and the next thing the doctor is sticking his finger up my ****.' One of his mates replies, 'He sounds like a pervert, I would complain if I were you'. There are two messages here. Always give a full and frank explanation of why you are doing things and, no matter how busy you are, make sure that you have access to a chaperone who can back you up in case of complaints.

2 Ask for permission to perform the PR examination

This will follow on from your explanation. Say something like, 'Do you mind if I examine your back passage?' Hopefully your patient will understand what you mean. If however they wonder why you have taken an interest in their house, you may have to elaborate further by using another word such as anus, rectum, or tail end. At this stage you need to alleviate any anxiety. Ask 'Have you had this done before?' If the answer is no, resist the temptation to say 'Me neither.' Be reassuring and say something like, 'Don't worry! I am just going to examine with a finger. It will be over in seconds and it is not normally painful'. If the patient has had it before and it was uncomfortable, try saying, 'I **will** be quick!'.

3 Get a chaperone/helper

The General Medical Council (GMC) in the UK in its guidance on intimate examinations does not give explicit instructions with regard to the gender of a chaperone. However, for a male doctor examining a female patient, it is highly advisable that you provide a female chaperone. Most local policies will recommend a chaperone of the same gender as the patient if at all possible. There are some patients who might object to a chaperone. In these cases gently try to persuade them the reasons why a chaperone is necessary (for both parties). If they are still insistent, it may be better to postpone the examination for another time (or another person) rather than run the risk of litigation.

4 Ensure equipment is at hand and ready

The equipment is usually kept on a tray. You should have lubricating gel, disposable gloves, and some tissues or swabs to clean your patient afterwards. There is nothing more embarrassing than being stranded with your finger up a patient's bottom and realizing that you have nothing to clean them with and no means of getting to it (especially if you have no chaperone handy).

5 Position the patient

There are four main positions that can be used to perform a PR examination:

- left lateral position (see Fig. 8.1)
- standing position (usually leaning over a support such as a bedside table)
- modified lithotomy position (see Fig. 9.16)
- knee–elbow or crouching position (see Fig. 8.2)

The position used varies from country to country; for example, many United States physicians prefer the standing position while in the UK the left lateral position is preferred. Even within countries, different medical specialties may use different positions. There are a handful of small studies which have looked at patient preference but they tend to be underpowered and reach differing conclusions. In this chapter I will concentrate on the left lateral position as I find it is particularly useful for frail, elderly patients and those with limited mobility (see Case 8.1). I also perceive it to be the least embarrassing of the above positions. Regardless of the position you choose, the subsequent technique is the same. Ask your patient to lie on the bed on their left side with their back facing you (see Fig. 8.1). It is helpful if they are near the edge of the bed, close to you. Pump the bed up to a height that will not put a strain on your back. Now ask your patient to bend their knees up towards their chest. It is helpful if you have an assistant, particularly for an elderly patient. They can be supervising the positioning of the patient and keeping them calm while you go off to wash your hands.

6 Wash your hands

Wash those mitts, it's a microbe blitz.

7 Put on gloves

This is not as easy as it sounds. The big disposable gloves are the easiest to put on. The surgical-type rubber gloves can be difficult. Often there is only one size available (a nightmare for those of you with large hands) and they can be hell to put on if your hands are sweaty (a usual occurrence with your first few attempts) or incompletely dry after washing your hands.

8 Put lubricant on your index finger

Just a small blob on the tip of your finger will do. Avoid the temptation to swamp your finger with the lubricant and get it everywhere.

9 Warn the patient that you are about to perform the test

Prepare your patient by saying, 'You are going to feel some cold jelly and then my finger'.

10 Inspect the perianal region

Before doing the digital examination, get your head down close to the perianal area, 'cheek to cheek' as it were, and inspect. If the bed cannot be raised high enough, then bend at the knees and keep a straight back. Use the fingers of your left hand to separate the buttocks. Your inspection

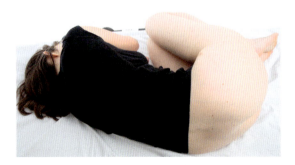

Figure 8.1 The left lateral position for the rectal examination.

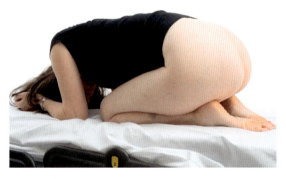

Figure 8.2 The knee–elbow position for rectal examination prior to elevation of the buttocks.

should be brief so that there is little delay between your warning and the PR examination itself. You need to look for skin tags, prolapsed haemorrhoids (piles), or rarely evidence of fistulas (*fist-you-las*) (see Fig. 8.13). A raw, excoriated area may be found in someone with diarrhoea due to frequent wiping with toilet paper and in older people who are bedbound you may notice pressure sores.

11 Introduce your finger into the anal canal

See Fig. 8.3. If the anal sphincter is tight (your patient may be anxious) this manoeuvre can be aided if you ask your patient to take a deep breath or ask them to bear down or strain as if they are going to the toilet (see Case 8.2) The passage of your finger might feel a little uncomfortable but if your patient shouts out in pain, **stop the examination**. Such a painful rectum may indicate the presence of an anal fissure (*fisher*).

12 Examine the rectum in a logical sequence

Once your finger is in the rectum you need a strategy for your examination. It does not matter what order you do things in so long as you are thorough and do not miss

pathology. Knowing the anatomy of the region is essential (see Fig. 8.4). Developing a set routine will also stop you ferreting with your finger in a random and hopeful manner and decrease the likelihood of raised eyebrows from your anxious patient. The routine adopted by the author is to feel the posterior wall first (see Fig. 8.5). This is because the posterior wall of the rectum naturally faces your finger following insertion. Simply flex your wrist and curl your index finger and you will soon feel the back wall.

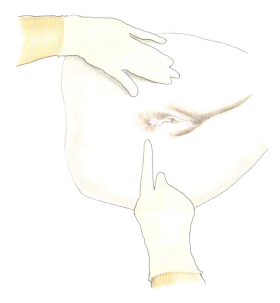

Figure 8.3 Preparing to introduce finger through the anal sphincter.

CASE 8.1

Problem. What is the point of showing these different positions if you do not describe how to examine in these situations also?

   Discussion. The point is to make you aware that other positions exist so that you have an alternative to turn to if problems crop up. Sometimes we get locked into the 'traditional' mindset that dictates that the way we have been taught is the only way to do things. For example, the standing-up technique is perfectly fine for most circumstances but will be inadequate for a patient with paraplegia. Or in a specialty like gynaecology if you are examining a patient in the lithotomy position and you feel a rectal examination is required, all you have to do is to get your patient to tilt their pelvis up and complete your examination rather than making them stand up, roll onto their left side or crouch. As mentioned before, the technique is exactly the same for all positions although you will have to reorient yourself to the anatomy depending on the position they adopt. However, if you think bottom 'posterior' and genitalia 'anterior' everything falls into place very readily.

CASE 8.2

Problem. You attempt to insert your finger in the rectum of your patient but are having great difficulty.

   Discussion. The likeliest explanation is that your patient is anxious and has a 'tight' sphincter. Try the manoeuvres outlined above, for example, get the patient to take a deep breath or push down as if going to the toilet. The resistance to your finger should lessen and your finger should slide into the anal canal (the sphincter should have an elastic feel around your finger). Occasionally difficulties can arise due to an anal stricture, a tumour near the anal verge, or with an anal fissure. With an anal fissure, the associated pain may be so great that the sphincter can go into spasm.

(a)

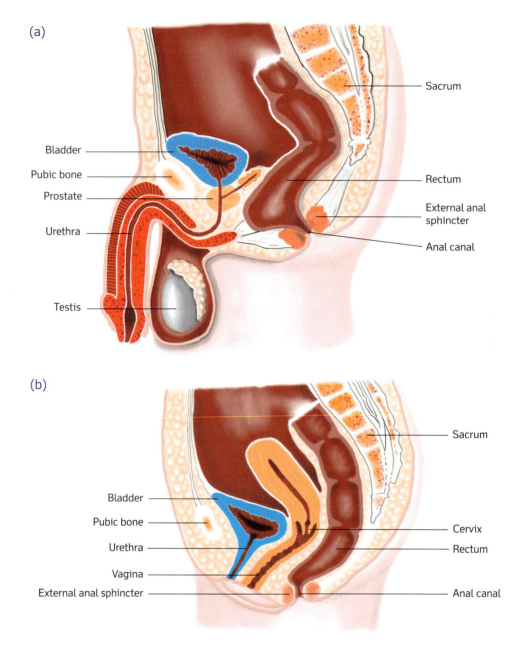

Sacrum

Bladder

Pubic bone

Prostate

Urethra

Rectum

External anal
sphincter

Anal canal

Testis

(b)

Sacrum

Bladder

Pubic bone

Urethra

Vagina

External anal sphincter

Cervix

Rectum

Anal canal

Figure 8.4 (a) Normal male pelvic anatomy; (b) normal female pelvic anatomy.

It usually feels hard because of the sacrum (*say-crumb*) and coccyx (*cock-sicks*) directly behind it. Nevertheless, if you sweep your finger along the surface of the wall it should feel smooth. Next, rotate your finger by pronating your wrist. Now your finger will be lying against the left lateral wall of the rectum (the pulp of your finger will be facing down to the couch). Again run your finger over the mucosal surface. Now supinate your wrist fully. Your finger should travel back in the direction it came and rotate a full 180°. You will now be examining the right lateral wall (the pulp of your finger should now be facing up to the ceiling). Finally, rotate your finger back in the direction you have just come as if you were going to re-examine the left lateral wall but this time you need to continue to rotate your finger through a further 90°. To achieve this, you will naturally have to bend your trunk down to the left while rotating your right elbow up so that it lies above your examining wrist. This is an awkward position but the only way to examine the anterior wall (Fig. 8.6). Through the anterior wall you can assess the prostate in a man (see Fig. 8.7) and appreciate the cervix in a woman (this is not a standard means of assessing the cervix).

The most likely diagnoses are a normal examination, faecal loading (see Fig. 8.8), benign prostatic hypertrophy (BPH), prostatic carcinoma, or rectal carcinoma (see Fig. 8.9).

- **Normal examination**. This is the most common finding. Only by doing plenty of PR examinations will you be able to appreciate this (as well as knowing when something is abnormal).

- **Faecal loading**. This may be found particularly in older people. Your finger may pass easily through soft faeces or may impact upon hard faeces. A patient in this situation may complain of constipation or paradoxically complain of diarrhoea (called spurious diarrhoea) with bouts of faecal incontinence of which they have no sensation. The exact mechanism why liquid faeces are produced around a hard faecal mass is not known. The treatment required includes adequate hydration, increased fibre in the diet, exercise, and laxatives. In the case of impacted faeces a stool softener is recommended. Faeces may mimic a rectal tumour. However, you will be able to indent a faecal mass and separate it from the rectal wall. You will not be able to do this with a rectal tumour.

- **Benign prostatic hypertrophy**. BPH is not easy to appreciate at first. You have to do plenty of PR examinations to be familiar with the dimensions of the normal prostate. In a normal young man you will feel a rubbery swelling with a groove in the centre. On either side of this groove are the lateral lobes of the prostate, which should feel smooth and firm. In BPH these lobes can be very large and pronounced but the median groove usually remains palpable. It is important to note that a normal-sized prostate can still cause obstruction to the flow of urine, and conversely a large prostate may cause little in the way of obstruction to the flow of urine.

- **Prostatic carcinoma**. Any hard lump felt in the substance of the prostate is highly suggestive of a prostatic carcinoma. Another clue to the possibility of cancer is the obliteration of the median groove due to tumour growth.

- **Rectal carcinoma**. This is usually readily apparent to the finger and often protrudes into the lumen (some can ulcerate through the mucosa). Always check that the mass is part of the rectal wall and not adherent faeces.

13 Take your finger out and inspect the glove for faeces, blood, and so on

Do not simply take your finger out thinking your ordeal is over. Your examination is not complete until you observe your index finger. You are looking for traces of faeces so

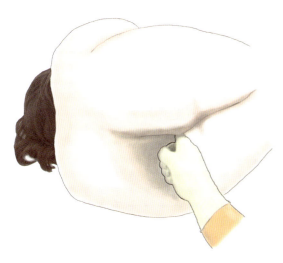

Figure 8.5 Palpating the posterior wall of the anal canal.

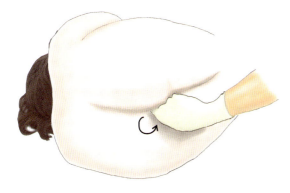

Figure 8.6 Palpating the anterior wall of the anal canal.

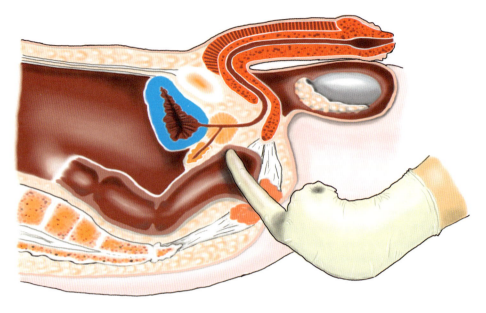

Figure 8.7 Palpating the prostate and the anterior anal canal in a male (in cross-section).

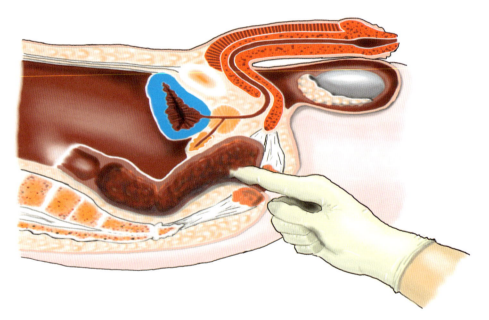

Figure 8.8 Faecal loading.

that you can check the colour. A black residue might suggest a stool due to iron consumption or, if it looks tarry, melaena. Is there bright red blood or mucus on the glove? (see Case 8.3).

14 Clean the perianal region

It is only courtesy for you to clean your patient of any smears, stains, or excess lubricant.

15 *Tell your patient you have finished and allow them to get dressed*

This will be their cue to pull up their underwear and to get dressed while you reflect on your findings.

16 *Wash your hands*

This is the most under-rated clinical skill.

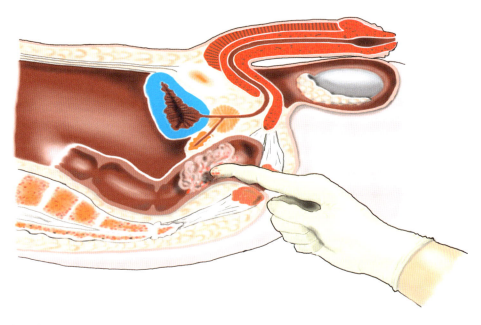

Figure 8.9 Rectal carcinoma.

CASE 8.3

Problem. You perform a PR examination, which is uneventful until you withdraw your finger and notice some bright red blood. What is the cause?

Discussion. The likeliest cause is haemorrhoids (piles). Typically they cause bright red bleeding which can be seen in the toilet or on toilet paper. However, before accepting that they are the cause of bleeding you must take a full gastrointestinal history, particularly asking about features such as diarrhoea, constipation, tenesmus, and so on because there are many causes of bright red bleeding PR (usually from the left side of the large bowel such as the descending and sigmoid colon). Some causes of bleeding PR include

- anal fissure
- carcinoma of the colon
- inflammatory bowel disease
- diverticular disease
- angiodysplasia (*an-jio-dis-play-zia*) of the colon
- upper gastrointestinal bleeding, for example, from a peptic ulcer (can cause fresh bleeding PR if it is a large bleed with rapid transit through the gut).

17 *Report your findings.*

After you have subjected your patient to this examination they will be keen to know what you have found. In most cases you can reassure them that everything is normal. You should also document your findings in the case notes. As a student you should never be put in the position where you find something abnormal without a qualified doctor present. Usually you will be told to do a PR examination on someone who is already aware of their diagnosis.

You will need to report your findings to a doctor for feedback. They will want to know about the following:

- external abnormalities (see Figs. 8.10, 8.11, 8.12, 8.13, and 8.14)
- rectal masses
- prostate in men
- faeces.

Here is an example:

'On rectal examination there is a small anal tag externally. There are soft faeces in the rectum but no evidence of masses. The prostate is enlarged and firm.'

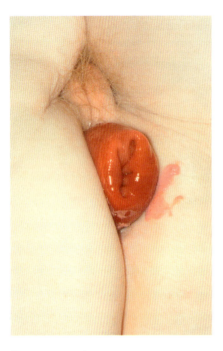

Figure 8.10 Rectal prolapse.

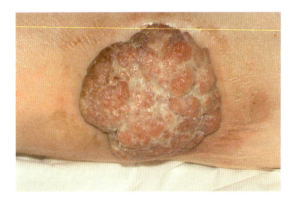

Figure 8.11 Squamous cell carcinoma of the anus.

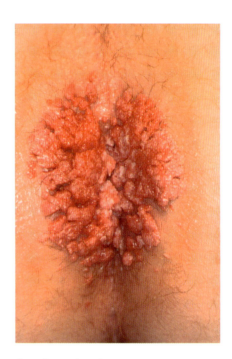

Figure 8.12 Perianal warts.

A further point to make once you begin your practice after passing your Finals is that you should always record in the notes if you do **not** perform a PR examination following an examination of the abdomen. In some cases this will not be relevant, for example, in a patient with a simple chest infection. However, if a PR examination is relevant and not performed you must give a good reason why it was not performed; for example, patient refused consent.

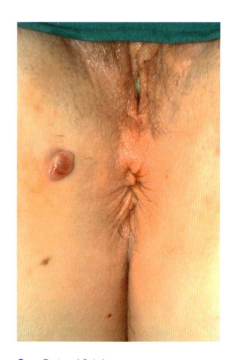

Figure 8.13 Perianal fistula.

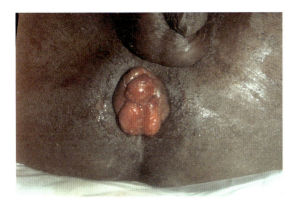

Figure 8.14 Thrombosed haemorrhoid.

....

Tip

Haemorrhoids can be confirmed as the source of bleeding by performing proctoscopy. This instrument allows a visual inspection of the rectum. If haemorrhoids are not seen or there are potential doubts about the source of bleeding (for example, other symptoms in the history) then you must go on to investigate the rest of the large bowel.

....

Key points

- Always explain why you are doing a PR examination and ask permission
- Always have a chaperone present (particularly male doctors)
- Examine a logical sequence, check for masses and faeces, and assess the prostate in men
- Stop the examination if it is painful for the patient
- Always inspect the glove after withdrawing your finger
- Always record your findings in the patient's notes

Finals

As stated earlier, this examination is rarely done in Finals although this will change. The use of manikins makes it easier to test your proficiency at the procedure. However, unlike some of the major systems this is relatively simple to do with very few possible outcomes.

So do not be afraid if you get this in an OSCE, just make sure that you treat the dummy (the manikin, not the examiner) as a normal patient and make sure you gain consent and offer a chaperone.

OSCE example

Examination station

You are an FY1 attached to a GP's surgery and you have been asked to perform a rectal examination on a 62-year-old woman who has been passing blood PR. Treat the manikin provided as if it is your patient.

Remember:

- Introduce yourself and gain consent to examine.
- Make sure the patient fully understands what is to be expected and try to put her at ease.
- Offer a chaperone before proceeding with the examination.
- Wash your hands and put on gloves.
- Use the routine described above to perform the examination.
- Don't forget to wipe the perineum clean of gel etc. once finished.
- Don't forget to thank the patient and ask her to get dressed again.
- Wash your hands.
- Despite the history the examination could be normal, so do not be afraid to say this if that is what you find.
- However, be warned that many pathologies can be simulated, so be on the lookout for signs of a rectal carcinoma.

Questions

1 What are the common indications for doing a rectal examination?
2 What positions can be used to perform a rectal examination?
3 What structure can normally be felt anteriorly in the male?
4 What structure can sometimes be felt anteriorly in the female?
5 Does the patient have the right to refuse a chaperone?

6 Are there any neurological indications for performing a rectal examination?
7 What structures can normally be felt posteriorly on rectal examination?
8 Name six causes of PR bleeding.
9 What are the features of a malignant prostate on rectal examination?
10 Have you performed more than five PR examinations?

References and further reading

Eziyi AK, Ademuyiwa AO, Eziyi JA, et al. Digital rectal examination for prostate and rectal tumour: knowledge and experience of final year medical students. *West African Journal of Medicine* 2009; **28**(5):318–22.

Fitzgerald D, Connolly SS, Kerin MJ. Digital rectal examination: national survey of undergraduate medical training in Ireland. *Postgraduate Medical Journal* 2007; **83**(983):599–601.

Forlan AB, Kato R, Vincentini F, et al. Patient's reactions to digital rectal examination of the prostate. *International Braz J Urol* 2008; **34**(5):572–5.

General Medical Council. *Maintaining boundaries— guidance for doctors*. GMC, London, 2006.

Kyle G. Why are nurses failing to carry out digital rectal examination? *Nursing Times* 2010; **106**(48):8.

Lawrentschuk N, Bolton DM. Experience and attitudes of final-year medical students to digital rectal examination. *Medical Journal of Australia* 2004; **181**(6):323–5.

Nensi A, Chande N. A survey of digital rectal examination training in Canadian medical schools. *Canadian Journal of Gastroenterology* 2012; **26**(7):441–4.

Turner KJ, Brewster SF. Rectal examination and urethral catheterization by medical students and house officers: taught but not used. *BJU Int* 2000; **86**(4):422–6.

9 Genitourinary system

Introduction

The prospect of taking a sexual history and performing a genital examination can fill medical students with dread. Despite the growing acceptability of screening for sexually transmitted infections (STIs) patients are also likely to be anxious about the process and gaining trust is paramount.

When taking a sexual history we ask people to divulge personal and sensitive information which they may not have shared with anyone else. An empathic approach in a confidential setting is crucial to enable you to elicit a frank and complete history.

The examination itself can also be intimidating for patients as well as clinicians. This anxiety may be due to a variety of reasons including; embarrassment, fear of the examination process itself, stigma surrounding STIs, or lack of knowledge regarding normal variants. As well as being affected by sexually transmitted conditions the external genitalia can also be affected by a variety of non-infective skin and systemic diseases which can be a source of great anxiety. With experience and a sensitive approach a genital examination can be informative and reassuring for a patient.

In this chapter you will learn how to take a sexual history and how to perform a genital examination. You will learn about normal genital variants and how to perform investigations to diagnose STIs and other disorders that can affect the genitalia. These skills will be useful for hospital specialties as well as general practice. This chapter also gives background information covering a range of common sexually transmitted and non-sexually transmitted conditions that can affect the genitalia.

Symptoms

The key symptoms to elicit in men are dysuria (see Chapter 7), the presence of any urethral discharge, testicular pain, and any genital skin changes. In women the important symptoms are any change in discharge, dysuria, pelvic/abdominal pain, pain during intercourse, unscheduled bleeding, and genital skin changes. Rectal symptoms of pain, bleeding, and discharge are also important for either sex, depending on sexual activity.

Symptoms in women

Discharge

The vagina naturally contains lactobacilli bacteria from the age of puberty to menopause. These keep the vaginal environment healthy. It is normal for women to experience some discharge, which they will describe as coming from the vagina; however, the source of the discharge may be either the vaginal walls, or the endocervix. Women may note a change in their normal discharge; this should prompt a search for a cause.

What to ask

See Table 9.1.

Tip

Always ask about any associated symptoms such as pelvic pain, rash, conjunctivitis and joint pain.

Dyspareunia

What is it?

Dyspareunia (*dis-par-oon-i-a*) is the word used to describe pain during sexual intercourse. Although both men and

women can complain of dyspareunia, it is a very rare presentation in men. Dyspareunia is, however, a common complaint in women.

When women complain of dyspareunia you need to establish the location of this pain, as dyspareunia is broadly divided into two categories: superficial and deep. Superficial dyspareunia is pain that occurs around the entrance to the vagina, usually during initial penetration. Deep dyspareunia is pain that is felt deeper within the pelvis during sexual intercourse. The two different categories have different causes and most women are able to easily identify the difference when asked.

Superficial dyspareunia

Causes

Superficial dyspareunia is most often due to inflammation of the vulval skin. This has many causes including infection, such as candida or herpes simplex virus, or skin conditions such as eczema, lichen planus or lichen sclerosis.

Other causes of superficial dyspareunia include:

- Inadequate sexual stimulation or foreplay (the use of lubricants may overcome this).
- Previous surgery, for example following childbirth, causing tightening of the vaginal opening.
- Vulval vestibulitis (vestibulodynia) (*vest-tib-you-low-din-ia*). This is pain confined to a specific area of the vaginal vestibule on touch or attempted penetration, the underlying cause of which is unknown.
- Vaginal atrophy following the menopause.
- Vaginal or rectal malignancy (a very rare presentation).

Deep dyspareunia

Causes

One of the main causes of deep pelvic pain on sexual intercourse is pelvic inflammatory disease (PID). This is when bacterial infections of the vagina and endocervix ascend to the upper genital tract and peritoneal cavity causing inflammation and pain in these areas (endometritis (*endo-me-try-tis*), salpingitis (*sal-pinj-eye-tis*), pelvic peritonitis, and perihepatitis). In sexually active women the usual cause is a sexually transmitted infection such as chlamydia or gonorrhoea.

Other causes of deep dyspareunia include:

- **Endometriosis**. Endometrial tissue that is usually only found within the uterus is found elsewhere within the pelvis.

Table 9.1 Questions to ask about discharges in women

	Has there been a change in amount of discharge?	What colour is the discharge?	Can you describe the consistency?	Have you noticed any smell?	Have you had any discomfort or itching?	How long has this been going on?
Infective causes						
Cervical infections						
Chlamydia	May notice increase	Clear or white. May be blood stained after sex	Mucus-like	Not usually	May have pain (dyspareunia)	Short history
Gonorrhoea	May notice increase	White, yellow or green	Thick	Not usually	May describe vaginal soreness or dyspareunia	Short history
Herpes infection of the cervix	Increase	Watery, may be blood stained	Thin	Not usually	May have painful external herpetic lesions	Short history, or may describe recurrent symptoms
Vaginal infections						
Trichomonas vaginalis (see Fig. 9.1)	Increase	Yellow	Frothy	Fishy smell may be present	Itching or soreness. External skin may be red or raw	Short history
Bacterial vaginosis	Typically increase	White or watery	Homogenous (all the same texture)	Fishy smell may be present	Not associated with discomfort or itch, but may complain of 'wetness'	Typically long history over weeks to months, may be recurrent
Candidiasis	May be an increase, not always	White or yellow	Thick and lumpy ('cottage cheese')	No smell	Itch may be the only symptom. Skin may be red or raw	Short history but may be recurrent
Non-infective causes						
Foreign body, e.g. retained tampon	Increase	White or yellow or green	May be thicker	Offensive smell	Internal discomfort or pelvic pain	Short history

(*continued*)

Table 9.1 (*continued*)

	Has there been a change in amount of discharge?	What colour is the discharge?	Can you describe the consistency?	Have you noticed any smell?	Have you had any discomfort or itching?	How long has this been going on?
Non-infective causes						
Hormonal influences, e.g. contraception, pregnancy	Increase	Clear or white	Non-specific	Not usually	No	Related to hormone use/ change
Physiological, e.g. cervical ectropion or polyp	Increase	Clear or white. May be blood stained after sex	Non-specific	Not usually	No	Variable

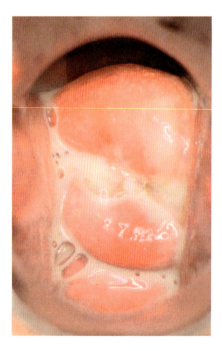

Figure 9.1 Cervical discharge in *Trichomonas vaginalis* infection.

- **Urinary tract infection**. Always ask the patient about urinary symptoms including dysuria, urinary frequency and nocturia.
- **Some sexual positions** may be uncomfortable for the female partner in the absence of any pathology and may be related to penis size in the male partner.

Pelvic pain

What is it?

Pelvic pain is pain in the suprapubic region, or the right or left inguinal fossa, an important cause of which is PID. PID can result in acute, subacute or chronic pelvic pain. Untreated infection and inflammation can cause scarring and future fertility problems, especially if the fallopian tubes are involved.

Other causes of pelvic pain to consider in your differential:

- **Suprapubic pain or loin pain**. May suggest a urinary tract infection.
- **Cramping dull pelvic pain**. Often felt 1–2 days prior to menstruation ('period pains') and is usually recognized as such by the woman.
- **Colicky pain**. May originate from the bowels.

Any acute severe pain in the pelvis should be investigated promptly for a possible ectopic pregnancy or ruptured ovarian cyst, particularly if there are signs the woman is systemically unwell (fever, tachycardia or low blood pressure).

What to ask

Ways to explore pelvic pain:

- 'Have you had any pain in the lower tummy? Point to where you feel it.'
- 'When did it start?'
- 'How would you describe the pain?' (sharp, dull, constant, intermittent, etc.)
- 'Does the pain go anywhere else?'

- 'Does anything make the pain worse?' (e.g. sex, micturition, not opening bowels).
- 'Does anything make the pain better?'
- 'Can you find a pattern to the pain?' (Is it 'cyclical' or every month, suggesting the pain is related to the menstrual cycle?)
- 'Have you felt unwell in yourself?'

....

Tip

An ectopic pregnancy is a pregnancy occurring outside the uterus, for example in the fallopian tube. This should be excluded in any woman of reproductive age who presents with abdominal pain. This is easily done with a urinary pregnancy test. If the pregnancy test is positive and the patient is complaining of abdominal or pelvic pain or is otherwise unwell, urgent referral to gynaecology for further assessment is required.

....

Intermenstrual bleeding

What is it?

This is bleeding which occurs in between the normal pattern of menstruation for a woman.

Causes

See Table 9.2.

Table 9.2 Causes of intermenstrual bleeding

Cervicitis secondary to STIs such as chlamydia or gonorrhoea
Hormonal contraception (ask about any missed pills or the use of emergency contraception)
Pregnancy related, including ectopic pregnancy
Following a midcycle fall in oestrogen
Recent insertion of intrauterine device (IUD)/ intrauterine system (IUS) for contraception
Endometrial fibroids or polyps.
Cervical, endometrial, or ovarian carcinoma—this must always be considered, particularly in an older woman

Key points

- With a discharge in women find out about the volume, consistency, colour, smell and any other associated symptoms
- Superficial dyspareunia is usually due to inflammation of the vulval skin
- Deep dyspareunia may herald PID
- Severe acute pelvic pain in a woman who is systemically unwell could be due to an ectopic pregnancy or a ruptured ovarian cyst
- Intermenstrual and postcoital bleeding should always be investigated

Postcoital bleeding

What is it?

Postcoital (*coy-tal*) bleeding (PCB) is bleeding that occurs after sex.

Causes

See Table 9.3.

Table 9.3 Causes of postcoital bleeding

Trauma
Cervical ectropion
Cervical/endometrial polyps
Cervicitis due to STIs (consider chlamydia, gonorrhoea, and *Trichomonas vaginalis*).
Cervical, endometrial, or vaginal carcinoma must be considered in an older woman

An examination and an STI screen is a useful starting point for the investigation of PCB but if this is negative and if symptoms persist, further investigation is required to establish a cause.

Symptoms in men

Discharge

Men will not normally have any discharge from the urethral opening (termed the meatus [*me-ate-us*]). However, they may notice that under the foreskin (also called the sub-prepuce [*sub-pre-puce*]) is relatively moist due to the protective covering of the foreskin and secretions coming

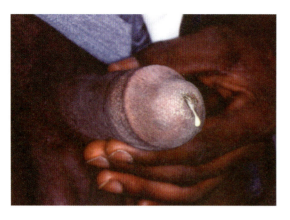

Figure 9.2 Urethral discharge in a male.

from underlying sebaceous glands known as smegma (*smeg-ma*). Discharge from the meatus should always be investigated for infection (see Fig. 9.2 and Case 9.1). Subpreputial discharge can be related to infection or hygiene.

What to ask

See Table 9.4.

....

Tip

Always remember to ask about any associated symptoms such as epididymal or testicular tenderness, joint pain, rash and conjunctivitis.

....

CASE 9.1

Problem: A 19-year-old student has a 3-day history of a clear penile discharge. He has a regular girlfriend but also had sex with a girl he met at a party 2 weeks ago. He has since had unprotected sex with his girlfriend. He has been treated for a non-gonococcal urethritis (NGU) and subsequently his gonorrhoea and chlamydia tests have come back negative. He has not told his girlfriend about this episode and does not plan to, saying it is not necessary as he has not been found to have an infection.

Discussion: Negative chlamydia and gonorrhoea tests do not exclude an STI as the cause of his discharge (see 'Non-gonococcal urethritis vs non-specific urethritis' in the 'Genitourinary diseases and investigations' section). It is important that his girlfriend is treated as this will prevent reinfection.

Table 9.4 Causes of discharge in men and how to ask about it

	What colour is the discharge?	Have you had any discomfort or itching?	Any other symptoms?	How long has this been going on?
Urethral discharge				
Chlamydia or non-specific urethritis (NSU)	Clear or milky	Stinging during micturition	Ask about joint pain, conjunctivitis, pain in epididymis and rash	Short history
Gonorrhoea	Yellow or green, purulent	Stinging during micturition	Disseminated gonorrhoea is rare (rash, joint pain)	Short history
Subpreputial discharge				
Anaerobic infection	Typically white, thick	May complain of soreness over glans	May be an odour	Chronic or recurrent
Candidiasis	Typically white	Soreness and itching over glans	Prepuce may be cracked and dry	Short history. May be recurrent in diabetics or immunocompromised

Testicular pain

Testicular pain is a common presenting symptom. In the absence of trauma, it is useful to establish whether pain is unilateral (one testis) or bilateral (both testes), of sudden or gradual onset, and to ascertain the severity of the pain; for example, is it an ache or is it disabling pain? Associated symptoms such as discharge, dysuria, swelling, overlying scrotal skin changes, fever, or systemic upset are also helpful in forming a differential diagnosis. NB: Any sudden onset of severe testicular pain is testicular torsion until proven otherwise. It can be accompanied by nausea, vomiting and abdominal pain in approximately one-third of patients. The testicle is enlarged and exquisitely tender. This is a surgical emergency and requires urgent specialist assessment.

Causes

See Table 9.5.

Table 9.5 Causes of testicular pain

Inflammation of the epididymis and testicle (epididymo-orchitis)
Trauma
Torsion
Tumour

Epididymo-orchitis can be caused by STIs such as chlamydia, urinary tract infections, or more rarely other infections such as mumps.

Haematospermia

What is it?

Haematospermia is the presence of blood within the ejaculate (or semen). Although this is alarming for the patient it is usually not serious. It is important to establish true haematospermia from haematuria (blood within the urine; see Chapter 7) or urethral bleeding. The commonest cause of haematospermia in younger men is trauma to the genital tract, which may be minor, but always ask the patient about any possible injuries. If trauma is the cause then the haematospermia usually spontaneously resolves.

Other causes include:

- infection, either of the prostate, seminal vesicles or occasionally the testes or epididymis
- disorders of blood clotting, including the use of anticoagulant drugs such as warfarin

- prostate malignancy—usually in men over the age of 40 (haematospermia is a rare symptom).

Key points

- With a discharge in men, find out about the colour and any other associated symptoms
- Any sudden onset of severe testicular pain (in the absence of trauma) is testicular torsion until proven otherwise

Symptoms common to men and women

Dysuria

What is it?

Dysuria can be defined as pain just prior to, during or just after urination and is often described as a stinging or burning. It is associated with both STIs and non-sexually-transmitted infections. Dysuria can be felt internally due to urethritis (inflammation of the urethra) or externally due to urine contacting broken skin. Other urinary symptoms are described in Chapter 7, but useful symptoms which may point to a non-sexually transmitted cause of dysuria include urinary frequency, urgency, and nocturia.

Genital skin changes

Lumps

Any change in the genital skin, real or perceived, can be a source of anxiety to a patient. It is common for people to present seeking reassurance that they 'look normal'. It is helpful to think about genital lumps as either physiological or pathological in origin. The most common causes are given in Table 9.6.

On examination you should be able to describe the anatomical position of the lumps, and use appropriate descriptive words for the skin change.

Ulcers

An ulcer is defined as a complete break in any epithelial surface, for example skin or mucosa. Ulcers or sores on the genital area can be a source of much distress for patients. Aside from the appearance, the pain can be significant as this area rubs on clothes or is in contact with urine or faeces. The most common cause of genital ulceration in the

Table 9.6 Causes of genital lumps

Cause	Description
Physiological lumps	
Pearly penile papules OR coronal papillae (Fig. 9.3) (also found in vagina)	Small, regular soft lumps under the glans penis (the coronal area) OR the inner walls of the vagina (usually symmetrical)
Epidermal inclusion cysts	Arising from the dermis of the scrotal skin or skin on the penile shaft OR the outer labia in women. Firm on palpation, may be yellow, or white if calcified
Fordyce spots	Small, superficial, enlarged sebaceous glands which can be white, yellow or skin-coloured in appearance
Pathological lumps	
Genital warts (Fig. 9.4)	Appearance varies depending on where they are growing. Soft if found on mucosal surfaces e.g. glans penis, vaginal walls, perianal; keratinized if on stratified squamous skin; may also be smooth in texture. Often multiple and various sizes
Molluscum contagiosum (Fig. 9.5)	Smooth papules with indented centres (central 'punctum'). Often multiple, on any genital skin or on thighs

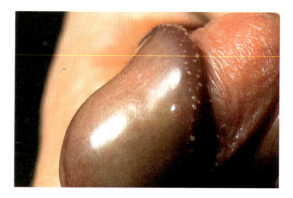

Figure 9.3 Penile pearly papules.

(a)   (b)

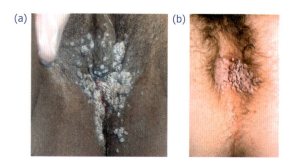

Figure 9.4 Appearance of genital warts in different ethnic groups.

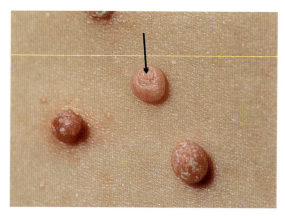

Figure 9.5 Close-up of molluscum contagiosum.

UK is herpes simplex (HSV) (see Fig. 9.6), but don't forget about primary syphilis (see Fig. 9.7), and rarer causes such as tropical ulcer diseases and systemic illnesses. Ask if the patient has had anything similar before and if they suffer with any mouth ulcers as HSV and some systemic conditions can affect both the mouth and genitals.

Rash

As with any skin complaint, the words used by a patient to describe the problem to you may not match words you would use as a trainee doctor. For example, patients may describe a crop of genital warts or herpetic ulcers as a 'rash', whereas we think of a rash as a reaction within the skin itself to a local or systemic trigger. Because of this, establish as much as you can about the symptom early in the history. The following list gives some possible causes for a rash.

- **Friction**. From sexual intercourse, or from rubbing of clothing.

- **Atopy, or dry, sensitive skin**. Ask about change in shower gel or washing powder, or history of eczema.

- **Fungal infection**. Candida can cause an erythematous rash over the vulva in women (see Fig. 9.8) and glans penis in men. Erythema in the groins with an advancing border suggests tinea infection.

- **Drug reaction**. Genital skin can be involved in a generalized reaction. Fixed drug eruptions can cause a localized rash anywhere on the body and may occur only on the genitals where it can also present as an ulcer. Ask about new medications in the last month.

- **Syphilis**. The secondary stage of syphilis can present with a widespread erythematous rash.

- **Shingles (varicella zoster)**. The vesicular rash of shingles can appear on the thighs or buttocks if these dermatomes are affected.

Genital itch

Itch is a very common symptom and has many causes. Always ask about any skin problems elsewhere on the body and if there is anything to see on the skin. In a woman, ask if the itch is inside the vagina or outside on the skin. Think about:

Skin

- Dry skin conditions, for example, eczema, psoriasis (see Fig. 9.9).

- Lichen simplex (a physiological reaction in the skin after repeated trauma from scratching; the skin becomes lichenified and dry which then causes the patient to scratch more).

- Scabies (can be just on the genitals and may appear as discrete lumps, but always examine the rest of the skin, in particular finger webs and forearms) (see Fig. 9.10).

- Early stages of ulcerating infections such as herpes simplex can be itchy.

- Inflammatory skin conditions, for example, lichen sclerosis (*liken scler-owe-sis*), lichen planus (*liken play-nus*).

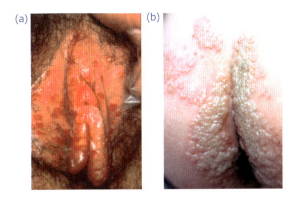

Figure 9.6 Herpes simplex infection: (a) first episode, affecting the vulva; (b) secondary bacterial infection infecting the natal cleft.

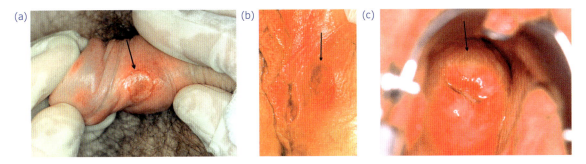

Figure 9.7 Primary chancre (painless ulcer of syphilis): (a) affecting the penis; (b) affecting the vulva; (c) affecting the cervix.

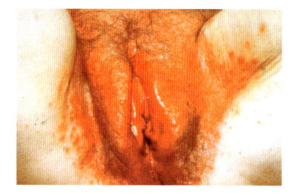

Figure 9.8 Vulval candidiasis.

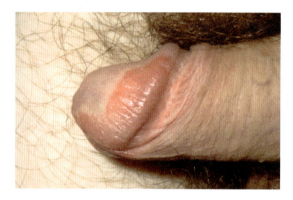

Figure 9.9 Patch of psoriasis on the glans penis.

Pubic hair

- Folliculitis or ingrowing hairs.
- Infestations such as pubic lice ('crabs').

Vaginal/urethral infections

Some vaginal infections can be itchy, classically candida, but itch is also described as a symptom of *Trichomonas vaginalis*. Any vaginal infection (or urethral infection in a man) that produces a lot of discharge may give a sensation of itching on the skin.

Other symptoms

STIs and skin disorders can affect other organs or areas of the body as well as the genital tract. It is always worth asking about any other symptoms. The following is a list of the commonest that might be associated with an STI.

Eyes

Infectious organisms such as chlamydia and gonorrhoea can also cause eye conditions such as conjunctivitis (see Fig. 9.11) and uveitis. These are often caused by autoinoculation (the patient transfers the infection themselves from a genital source).

Joints

STIs can cause inflammatory reactions in joints, particularly knees and ankles, known as sexually acquired reactive arthritis (SARA).

Other skin areas.

Some skin conditions affect the genital skin as well as other areas. For example, eczema also affects the flexor surfaces (inner aspect of the elbow and the backs of knees) and psoriasis affects extensor surfaces (backs of elbows and fronts of knees).

Mouth

Some skin conditions that affect the genitals also commonly affect the oral cavity. An example is lichen planus. It is always worth a look inside someone's mouth as part of an examination of a patient with a genital skin complaint to see if there are any changes within the oral cavity, such as candida (see Fig. 9.12).

(a)

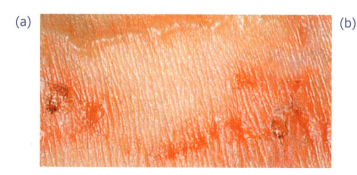

(b)

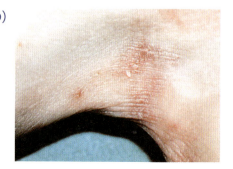

Figure 9.10 Magnified view of the finger web space demonstrating the burrows of the scabies mite.

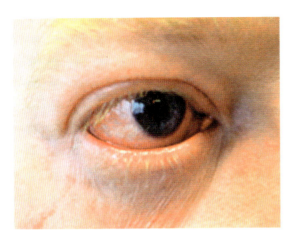

Figure 9.11 Conjunctivitis due to chlamydia.

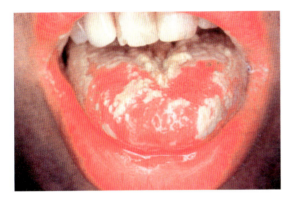

Figure 9.12 Oral candida.

Key points

- Genital lumps can be physiological or pathological
- With genital ulcers also check the mouth as some conditions can affect both
- With a rash you should check the rest of the skin surface as a number of skin conditions such as eczema and psoriasis can also affect the genitals
- Be alert to eye, joint and skin involvement with STIs

What else to ask?

Sexual history

It is important to establish a patient's sexual history in order to ensure that appropriate testing is done from appropriate sites at an appropriate time. It also helps to establish an individual's risk of specific infections such

as HIV. This enables the practitioner to give the patient meaningful information and to identify if recall is needed at a later date for further testing. It is helpful to explain that you are going to ask some personal questions and why you are doing so. Use language that both you and your patient understand. Not everybody knows the anatomical terms for various parts of their genitalia, or knows the official name for a particular sexual act. Never make assumptions about somebody's sexuality, sexual behaviour, or the presence or absence of concurrent partners.

Tip

When asking difficult questions during the sexual history the patient will feel more comfortable if you explain why you need to ask the questions. It is also polite to check that the patient is happy for you to continue. When asking about sexual practices try 'Because you can get STIs in different places it's important that we ask about the sort of sex that you have, is that OK?' Then give the patient the opportunity to simply answer yes or no to the following questions: 'Was that vaginal sex?', 'Was there any oral sex?', 'Was there any anal sex?' In a male patient, investigate further whether the patient was giving anal sex (insertive partner) or receiving anal sex (receptive partner).

You should ask the patient when their most recent sexual contact was. This is important as different infections have differing incubation periods. The incubation period of a disease is the time it takes from transmission of infection to the infected person displaying symptoms or signs of the disease. A screen for chlamydia, for example, if carried out 2 days after sex will not reliably exclude chlamydia. It may therefore be necessary to arrange further screening at a later date. A suggested time frame for screening for common bacterial infections is at least 14 days after unprotected sex.

Having established when your patient last had sex, go on to establish the sex of their partner and whether this was somebody they have had sex with on a single or multiple occasions, and over what period of time. The type of sexual contact is important in order to identify what sites have been exposed. Patients should be specifically asked if there has been any anal or oral contact, as this information may not be spontaneously volunteered (see Tip above). It is also important to ask if a condom was used, and if so was it used for all sexual contact and were there any problems such as breakages. The same questions should then be asked about the last time the patient had sex with a different partner. It is helpful to establish how many sexual partners the patient has had over a 3-month period, as this gives an idea of risk behaviour and guides when a patient should be tested for blood-borne infections.

Contraception

All women of childbearing age should be asked whether they are using any contraception. If they are not, this is an opportunity to give advice. The overall risk of pregnancy in every menstrual cycle is approximately 20%, but the risk is highest around the time of ovulation (midcycle) when it can be up to 40%.

In the UK, a wide variety of forms of contraception is now available free to all women through the NHS. An easy way to break this down is to think of hormonal contraception vs non-hormonal contraception (see Table 9.7).

With any hormonal contraception there may be an effect on the menstrual cycle, so this is an important area to explore when a women presents with abnormal bleeding.

Table 9.7 Hormonal and non-hormonal contraception

Hormonal contraception
Combined oestrogen and progesterone
Tablets ('The pill')
Skin patch ('The patch')
Vaginal ring
Progesterone only
Injection
Implant
Intrauterine coil (Mirena© coil)
Progesterone-only tablets ('mini-pill')
Non-hormonal contraception
Copper intrauterine coil
Fertility awareness methods
Barrier methods
Condoms
Diaphragm
Cervical cap
Female condom

Risk assessment

The idea of risk assessment is to identify patients who might be at a higher risk of blood-borne viruses such as HIV and hepatitis. These are not easy topics to discuss with a patient so it is important to explain to your patient why you need to ask them. It is easiest to start with 'Is it all right if I ask you some questions about risk factors for HIV and hepatitis?' and also to reduce the possibility of offence 'We ask these questions routinely'. The important areas to cover are

- **Sexual intercourse with people from areas of the world with a high background prevalence of HIV and hepatitis**. 'Have you ever had sex with anybody born outside the UK or were you yourself born outside the UK?'
- **Sex with men who have sex with men**. People often find this the most difficult question to ask: to men try, 'Have any of your sexual partners ever been male?' and to women, 'Have any of your male partners ever had sex with other men that you are aware of?'
- **Intravenous (IV) drug use**. 'Have you or any of your partners ever injected drugs?'
- **Commercial sex work**. 'Have you ever paid or received money for sex?'

If you identify any risk factors this may indicate that the patient needs further information about HIV to prepare for testing. Blood tests for HIV and syphilis are routinely offered to all patients in the sexual health clinic, regardless of risk factors. If a patient is at increased risk of hepatitis B or C (IV drug use, commercial sex work, men having sex with men) these tests should also be offered.

Men who have sex with men, women who have sex with women

It is important to establish what sexual practices people participate in to ensure that the appropriate anatomical sites are examined and sampled, as well as to guide what information is given to the patient regarding their personal risk of sexually transmitted infection. Rather than using the term 'gay' or 'homosexual', it is preferable to use 'men who have sex with men' (MSM) and 'women who have sex with women' (WSW) as this avoids any connotation of 'gay culture', which people may not identify with. In MSM it is necessary to ask if they are the penetrative or non-penetrative partner (or both) as this establishes which anatomical sites need sampling for infection, and helps to assess their risk (for example, receptive anal sex carries

CASE 9.2

Problem: A 40-year-old man presents with a single painless penile ulceration. He has a long-term male partner of 3 years and always uses condoms for anal sex. You suspect a diagnosis of syphilis but are unsure how he acquired this.

Discussion: It is important not to forget to ask about other partners. This patient also had anonymous oral sex with several men in a sauna 2 months ago. He did not use a condom for oral sex as he believes this is a low-risk activity. However, syphilis can easily be transmitted through oral sex.

the highest risk of HIV). When recording this information rather than describing intercourse as 'active' or 'passive', use the terms 'insertive' and 'receptive'. Other sexual practices such as ano-oral contact can be a route of transmission and should be asked about (see Case 9.2). Remember that WSW may have previously had sex with men, and are therefore still at risk of infections associated with penetrative sex. They may also use penetrative sex toys which, if shared, can be associated with STI transmission.

Transgender individuals

When an individual identifies their gender as different from their physical appearance/genetic sex, they are said to be transgendered. Transgender individuals may take hormones or undergo surgery to correct their appearance. It is important to ask if any surgery has taken place before you proceed with genital examination, to enable accurate sampling for infection. Do not make any assumptions

Key points
- Never make assumptions about somebody's sexuality, sexual behaviour or the presence or absence of concurrent partners
- Patients should be specifically asked if there has been any anal or oral contact
- Establish when the patient's most recent sexual contact was, as different infections have differing incubation periods
- All women of childbearing age should be asked whether they are using any contraception

about which anatomical sites have been exposed, or the gender of their partner(s). A transgender individual must be referred to as, and treated as, the gender they identify themselves as being.

Male genital examination summary

1 Introduce yourself to the patient and ask permission to carry out the examination.
2 Explain the examination procedure.
3 Offer a chaperone.
4 Ask the patient to lie on a couch with clothing removed to expose the genital area; allow him privacy to undress.
5 Wash your hands and put on gloves.
6 Perform a general inspection, in particular noting skin rashes and oral lesions, and then a closer visual inspection of the genital skin.
7 Palpate for the superficial inguinal lymph nodes on both sides.
8 Inspect the skin of the scrotum and perform a testicular examination.
9 Inspect the genital skin in a systematic way: pubic hair area, dorsal shaft of penis, ventral shaft of penis, foreskin (if present) and subprepuce, glans penis, meatus. Take samples for infection testing as appropriate.
10 Examine the perianal and rectal areas if appropriate and take samples.
11 Consider additional examination of other body systems if relevant.
12 Wash your hands and allow the patient to dress in private before discussing findings.
13 Offer blood tests for HIV and syphilis. Consider screening for Hepatitis B and C if appropriate.
14 Report your findings.

Male genital examination in detail

1 Introduce yourself to the patient and ask permission to carry out the examination

As a medical student you should not be performing genital examinations without a supervising doctor present;

always make sure the patient is happy with you undertaking the examination.

2 Explain the examination procedure

Explain the purpose for the genital examination. Give as full a description as possible so the patient can understand why the examination is needed and what to expect.

Even if a man has no symptoms of infection it can be worth examining the skin and performing a testicular examination as an opportunity to reassure him he is 'normal', and to show him how to examine his own testicles. An examination can also identify unnoticed disease, for example genital warts. Some signs, such as the discharge of urethritis, will not be visible if the patient has recently passed urine. If the patient has symptoms of discharge it is advisable to perform the examination when he has held his urine for at least 1–2 hours.

3 Offer a chaperone

Always offer a chaperone for genital examinations. This should be done regardless of your gender and that of the patient. The chaperone is there to provide support and reassurance for patients, as some can find genital examinations embarrassing and even distressing. In addition, a chaperone is an independent observer who can be called on to give an account of events if necessary in the future.

4 Ask the patient to lie on a couch with clothing removed to expose the genital area; allow him privacy to undress

There should be a curtain or screen provided for this purpose. The genital area should be fully exposed and it is best to explain this before leaving the patient to undress, for example 'Push your trousers and underwear down to your knees, then lie down on your back'. The patient should be resting comfortably on his back on an examination couch.

5 Wash your hands and put on gloves

Do this for any genital examination.

6 Perform a general inspection, in particular noting skin rashes and oral lesions, and then a closer visual inspection of the genital skin

Note his general health, and any obvious skin rashes. Next look closer at the skin of the genital area. In particular note any abnormalities in the skin or pubic hair, such as balanitis (*ba-la-night-tis*) (infection of the glans and subprepuce) (see Fig. 9.13), fungal infection, infestation, ulceration, or warty lesions. Normal anatomical variations may be a source of worry for the patient and it is worth asking if they have any particular concerns to show you.

7 Palpate for the superficial inguinal lymph nodes on both sides

In a thin person the superficial inguinal nodes may be palpable but they should be soft and non-tender, and typically no more than 1 cm in size. Enlarged or painful superficial inguinal nodes on one or both sides should prompt you to inspect the skin very closely for signs of ulceration or infection (see Table 9.8). All the penile and scrotal skin and the superficial structures underneath the skin drain to the superficial inguinal nodes, as does anal and perianal skin. The collective term for this area is the perineum (*perry-knee-um*). Remember that the testicles

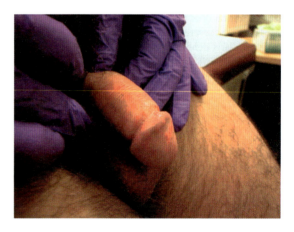

Figure 9.13 Balanitis due to candida.

Table 9.8 Causes of superficial inguinal lymphadenopathy in both men and women

Genital herpes
Other superficial genital skin infections
Syphilis
Lymphogranuloma venereum
Malignancy (e.g. lymphoma)
Mycobacterium infection

drain to the para-aortic lymph nodes which are not palpable. Other deeper structures in the penis, such as the urethra, drain to the deep inguinal and iliac nodes which are not palpable.

8 Inspect the skin of the scrotum and perform a testicular examination

Examine both groins by gently moving the scrotum to each side. Inspect all the skin of the scrotum before moving on to examine the testicles.

···

Tip
A good way to start this aspect of the examination is to ask the patient whether they examine their own testicles; if not, you can advise self-examination once a month in all men aged 20–40 years.

···

On inspection it is normal for the left testis to hang slightly lower than the right. Check with the patient if they have any pain in the testicles or if they have found any lumps they are worried about. Use the pads of your first two fingers and thumb on both hands to examine each testis in turn. Roll each testis gently between your fingers and thumb checking for a smooth texture, tenderness, and any swelling or lumps. Next palpate the epididymis and the spermatic cord on both sides. If a lump is found, further examination is necessary. Firstly, check if the lump is confined to the scrotum or extends upwards into the abdomen by seeing if you can get above the swelling. If you cannot, the lump may well be a hernia (see Chapter 7). Next, establish if a swelling or mass in the scrotum is part of the testis or separate from it. Swellings which are separate from the testis may include a hydrocele (a collection of fluid in the tunica vaginalis which can be transilluminated using a pen torch) or a varicocele (enlargement of the pampiniform plexus within the spermatic cord). Varicoceles are essentially varicose veins and on palpation feel like a 'bag of worms', best appreciated when the patient is standing upright. A mass which feels separate from the testis, but attached to it, may represent the normal epididymis or an epididymal cyst. If the epididymis is swollen and tender, this can indicate epididymitis. A lump within the body of the testis must be assumed to be a malignancy until proven otherwise, and an urgent ultrasound scan is required. A diffusely swollen testis may be due to torsion or due to orchitis/epididymo-orchitis. Consider malignancy in a non-tender diffusely enlarged testis. However, the seemingly enlarged testis may in fact be

normal with the smaller testis being abnormally small following atrophy due to previous infection or maldescent. A testis which was previously undescended carries a higher risk of malignancy and should be carefully examined. If only one testis is palpable and there is no history of orchidectomy (surgical removal of a testis) this should prompt investigations to search for the ectopic testicle.

9 Inspect the genital skin in a systematic way: pubic hair area, dorsal shaft of penis, ventral shaft of penis, foreskin (if present) and subprepuce, glans penis, meatus

Although it may feel intrusive and uncomfortable, it is important to look very closely at the skin in this area. A good light source is important and for small skin lesions a magnifying glass can be helpful. As long as you are considerate and maintain a professional manner, this part of the body can be examined much like any other.

Describe what you find in terms of type of lesion (warty, ulcerated, patch), number and distribution, and colour. In the pubic hair there may be signs of infestation or infection around the hair follicle.

Examine all the skin on the penile shaft. NB. The anatomical position of the penis is erect. Hence the dorsum of the penis is in fact the front of a flaccid penis as you look at it.

Now retract the foreskin gently, and always return it to the original position afterwards.

···

Tip
Retracting the foreskin isn't always easy for the examiner, but will be second nature for the patient who is likely to be very practiced at retracting and replacing his own foreskin. Don't be afraid to ask the patient to do it for you. The patient would much rather do it himself than watch you become more uncomfortable as you struggle with his foreskin and risk causing him pain.

···

Examine the glans penis and then look for the urethral meatus. If the meatus is not obvious, the patient may have hypospadias (*hype-owe-spade-ius*). This is a condition where the urethral opening in the male is not in the expected position in the middle of the glans penis. It is relatively common and caused by a failure of fusion during fetal development. It can also be associated with an incomplete prepuce or foreskin, and curvature of the penis (chordee [*cord-ee*]). The failure of fusion causes the meatus to open on to the ventral surface of the glans penis, and there may be an indent or a blind opening in the expected position. No action is needed in mild cases but it should be noted on examination, and if you are taking a sample for investigation both meatal openings (even if blind) need to be swabbed.

Now gently pinch the meatus at 6 o'clock and 12 o'clock to look inside for warts, ulcers, or strictures. Describe any urethral discharge, noting particularly its colour and volume. If required a urethral swab can now be taken (see 'Specimen collection'.

10 Examine the perianal and rectal areas if appropriate

If a man has any rectal symptoms, or reports sexual contact involving the rectum (including oro-anal) you should also examine this area as part of the full genital examination.

Explain clearly what you need to do and ask the patient to adopt the left lateral position on the couch (see Fig. 8.1).

Wash your hands and change your gloves. Inspect the perianal skin by gently parting buttocks looking for fissures, ulcers, and warts. Use a proctoscope (see Fig. 9.14) with plenty of lubrication to look inside the rectum at the mucosa. You will always need supervision to do this as a student. Take swabs as needed (see 'Specimen collection'). Continue examining the anal canal for lesions when withdrawing the proctoscope.

11 Consider additional examination of other body systems if relevant

Some areas to think about include:

- **Mouth**. Ulcers associated with syphilis and Behçet's disease; Wickham's striae of lichen planus. Consider taking samples from the **oropharynx** for investigation of STIs if a patient reports receptive oral sex with a man.

- **Rest of skin**. The rash of secondary syphilis (see Fig. 9.15) is a generalized rash which unusually can affect

---

CASE 9.3

Problem: A man with a urethral discharge requires a swab but refuses as he has heard about 'the umbrella' from his friends and is convinced that the swab will be very painful.

Discussion: The 'umbrella' refers to an instrument which has not been used in genital examination for decades but has become something of an urban myth. Reassure your patient that while sampling may be briefly uncomfortable it is very quick and a very slender swab is used.

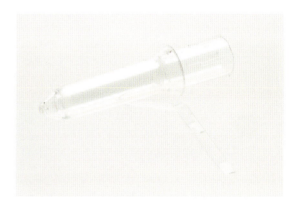

Figure 9.14 A proctoscope.

(a)

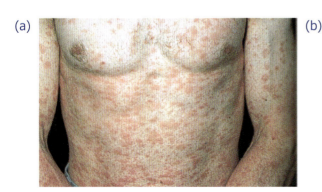

(b)

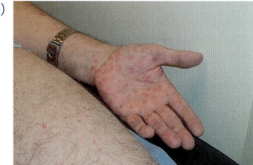

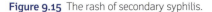

Figure 9.15 The rash of secondary syphilis.

the palms and soles; patches of eczema / psoriasis, skin burrows of scabies (finger webs and forearms); keratoderma blennorrhagica (*ke-rat-owe-derm-a blen-owe-ra-jick-a*) which is a rash on the palms and soles associated with SARA.

- **Eyes**. Conjunctivitis, uveitis, optic neuritis in syphilis; pubic lice in eyelashes or eyebrows.

- **Joints**. Swelling and pain in SARA.

12 Wash your hands and allow the patient to dress in private before discussing findings

13 Blood tests for HIV and syphilis are routinely offered in the sexual health clinic

If the patient is at increased risk of hepatitis B or C (intravenous drug use, commercial sex work, MSM) offer testing for these also.

....

Tip

It is important when performing a genital examination to be sensitive to the patient's feelings, and leave the genital area exposed for the minimum amount of time necessary. This does not mean you should rush through the examination so quickly that you miss things. Try and save your discussion for when the patient is dressed. This will also give you time to get your thoughts together.

....

14 Report your findings

For example:

'This 19-year-old man gives a 3-day history of urethral discharge with associated dysuria. He has no testicular pain or genital skin changes. He describes no additional features suggestive of a urinary tract infection (UTI). His last sexual contact was 2 weeks ago with an unknown female partner. He had vaginal and oral, but no anal, sex. A condom was not used. On examination there is no inguinal lymphadenopathy and no genital skin changes. Both testes are normal on palpitation as are the epididymides. However, there is a copious green discharge. This is suggestive of gonorrhoea which may be confirmed on microscopy and culture.'

Female examination summary

1 Introduce yourself to the patient and ask permission to perform the examination.

2 Explain the examination procedure.

3 Offer a chaperone.

4 Ask the patient to prepare for the examination by changing into a gown.

5 Position the patient correctly.

6 Wash your hands and put on gloves; ensure speculum is prepared.

7 Inspect the external genitalia and palpate for inguinal lymphadenopathy.

8 Pass the speculum.

9 Inspect the vagina and cervix.

10 Cervical cytology sampling.

11 Specimen collection.

12 If necessary, perform a bimanual examination.

13 Additional examinations and investigations if required.

14 Wash your hands and allow the patient to dress in private before discussing findings.

15 Offer blood tests for HIV and syphilis; consider screening for hepatitis B and C if appropriate.

16 Report your findings.

Female examination in detail

1 Introduce yourself to the patient and ask permission to perform the examination

Introduce yourself to the patient. Explain the purpose for the genital examination and gain the patient's permission. As a medical student you should not be performing intimate examinations without a supervising doctor present; always make sure the patient is happy with you undertaking the examination. An uncomfortable patient will make for an uncomfortable examination for everyone.

2 Explain the examination procedure

Explain the procedure to the patient so she knows what to expect.

3 Offer a chaperone

Always offer a chaperone for genital examinations, regardless of your gender and that of the patient. The same principle applies as for the male examination.

4 Ask the patient to prepare for the examination by changing into a gown

The patient should be offered a private area to undress and put on a gown. It is necessary for her to remove all of her lower garments including her underwear but it is not necessary for her to remove all of her clothing; she can put the gown on over her upper garments if she is more comfortable with this.

5 Position the patient correctly

To make the examination easier for you and more comfortable for the patient, it is worthwhile spending a short period of time correctly positioning the patient. The position of the patient will depend on the equipment and type of couch that you have available. A couch with leg rests is ideal as you will be able to examine more easily in the 'semilithotomy position'. If you only have a standard couch or bed for examination ask the patient to lie on her back with her head on a pillow, then ask her to flex her hips and knees and abduct her thighs apart while keeping her ankles together (see Fig. 9.16). Don't forget to ensure that there is adequate lighting.

6 Wash your hands and put on gloves; ensure a speculum is prepared

Now wash your hands and put on gloves. Ensure that any equipment required for taking swabs is easily available. If

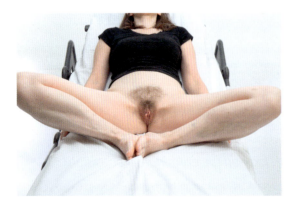

Figure 9.16 The semilithotomy position.

the speculum is metal, make sure it is warmed by placing it in warm water beforehand. The water will also act as a lubricant. If you are using a plastic speculum, use water-based lubricant.

7 Inspect the external genitalia and palpate for inguinal lymphadenopathy

Inspect the skin and hair over the pubic area. Once you have done this, gently feel with your fingertips within both inguinal regions for the presence or absence of lymphadenopathy. It is normal to be able to feel the presence of some small lymph nodes in slim women. Larger swollen lymph nodes palpable in the inguinal region are suggestive of an infectious or inflammatory process (see Table 9.8).

After palpating the inguinal region, move on to examining the external genitalia—the labia majora and minora. Gently separate the labia minora with your fingers and closely inspect this genital skin, including the clitoris. You are looking for any abnormal skin changes, for example, sores or breaks that could be suggestive of genital herpes. If there are any breaks in the skin, swab these areas for the presence of herpes simplex virus. Also look out for any changes to the colour of the skin which may be suggestive of skin conditions such as lichen sclerosis, dermatitis, or other genital dermatoses.

Occasionally you may come across appearances which suggest that female genital mutilation (FGM) has taken place. FGM refers to any procedure which removes, partially removes, or alters female external genitalia for non-medical reasons. It is sometimes called female circumcision. It most commonly occurs in females of African descent. Procedures may include clitoridectomy (partial or total removal of the clitoris) with or without removal of the labia minora and majora and infibulation (narrowing of the vaginal opening). FGM is recognized as a breach of human rights and, if seen, should prompt questions about any female children in the household who may be at risk of similar procedures. These procedures are most commonly carried out between infancy and age 15 years. If seen this must be reported to a senior promptly so they can take action.

8 Pass the speculum

Using the speculum can seem daunting for both the patient and the doctor. The most important thing to remember is the comfort of the patient. Preparation is key.

1 Reassure the patient using plain language, for example: 'This is a very common examination to check that the vagina and the neck of the womb (cervix) are healthy'.

CASE 9.4

Problem: I have tried to pass a speculum just as you describe but I still have difficulty viewing the cervix. What am I doing wrong?

Discussion: The most common reason is not going in far enough before opening the blades. The blades should advance easily, so let them advance as far as you can before trying to open the blades and the cervix should fall into view. Another tip is tilting the pelvis by asking the women to make her hands into fists before placing these under her buttocks. Asking the woman to cough can also help the cervix fall into view.

2 Take the speculum in your dominant hand. If the patient is positioned in the semi-lithotomy position with her legs elevated on leg rests then the handles of the speculum may be pointing either upwards or downwards. If the patient is on an ordinary bed then the handles of the speculum will need to be held pointing upwards.

3 With your non-dominant hand, gently part the labia minora to expose the vaginal opening (introitus) (*in-troytus*) and introduce the speculum slowly into the vagina.

4 Ensure the speculum is fully inserted into the vagina before gently opening the blades of the speculum to visualize the cervix. The cervix should easily come into view; if you are unable to see the cervix there are a few tricks to try (see Case 9.4).

5 Once the cervix is visible you can either tighten the screw to secure the blades in the open position, or hold it in place with your non-dominant hand.

6 When removing the speculum, ensure you hold the blades open until the end is well clear of the cervix to avoid clamping it when the blades close.

Remember that all women are slightly different shapes, and speculums do come in different sizes. A woman who has had children may need a speculum with wider blades to hold the vaginal walls out of view. Women who are tall may need a speculum with longer blades.

9 Inspect the vagina and cervix

Once the cervix is in view inspect it closely looking for any endocervical discharge, abnormalities to the mucosal surface and any evidence of inflammation (cervicitis). Also inspect the vaginal walls for the presence of any discharge or any mucosal abnormalities. See Case 9.5.

CASE 9.5

Problem: I've seen a patient with very swollen labia but little discharge. Could this still be candida?

Discussion: Candida commonly causes inflammation and swelling of the vulva, sometimes associated with pain. This can occur even if there is not much vaginal discharge to see. It is important to sample any discharge, however small, to try to identify candida with either microscopy or culture.

A common examination finding is a cervical **ectropion** which appears as a red ring around the cervical os. An ectropion is an extension of the columnar epithelium of the endocervix on to the squamous epithelium of the ectocervix. This occurs under hormonal influence and can be seen in puberty, pregnancy and when the combined oral contraceptive pill is used. Columnar epithelium is glandular and so an ectropion can be associated with increased mucus production. It is also more delicate than squamous epithelium and can be prone to bleeding.

Nabothian cysts are another common finding on the cervix, and can be singular or multiple. These are harmless mucus retention cysts, and appear as well-defined, shiny, pale yellow, circular lesions.

10 Cervical cytology sampling

If a cervical smear (cytology) sample is required, this should be the first sample that is taken. There is a specific brush designed for cervical smear sampling. Gently insert the end of the sample brush into the endocervical os and rotate it in a clockwise direction five times. Ensure that the brush ends of the swab remain in contact with the cervical surface as you rotate. After five rotations remove the brush and, depending on the sampling system used, dip the brush into the preservative pot or remove the head of the brush and place it into the pot.

11 Specimen collection

The exact choice of swab will vary from centre to centre, so check with your seniors which samples are required before undertaking genital examination. Always ensure that all samples are correctly labelled. In general, specimen collection in women will include one or more vaginal swabs and endocervical swabs (see Fig. 9.17).

Before taking endocervical swabs clean the surface of the cervix using a large cotton swab to ensure a true endocervical sample is taken.

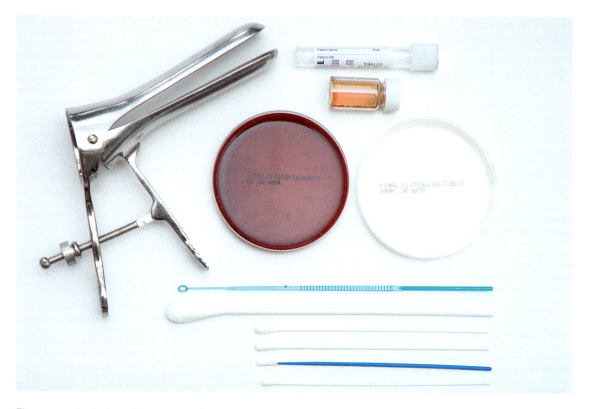

Figure 9.17 A selection of equipment including speculum, swabs, agar plates, and other storage media.

12 *If necessary now perform a bimanual examination*

This is indicated if a woman complains of pelvic pain or deep dyspareunia.

1 Ensure that the patient understands why this examination is necessary and what it involves, and obtain her consent.

2 Place some lubricating jelly on the index and middle fingers of your right (dominant) hand and gently insert your fingers inside the vagina, turning your palm upwards.

3 Make sure that you part the labia first with your left (non-dominant) hand and then press your left hand over the suprapubic area (just below the umbilicus but above the pubis bone).

4 Locate the cervix with your internal fingers and feel for any hardness or irregularity. Commonly the cervix points downwards and slightly backwards when a patient is supine (indicating an anteverted uterus).

5 Gently move the cervix with your fingers a little from side to side to assess for any tenderness. This is known as cervical excitation or cervical motion tenderness and is suggestive of PID.

6 Then palpate the uterus by pushing it upwards with your internal hand towards your external hand and catching it. (This manoeuvre is similar in technique to bimanually balloting a kidney.)

7 Initially, continue to hold the cervix while you locate the uterine body. Then use your internal hand to feel around the uterus while your external hand stabilizes the uterus. Assess its size and position and identify any tenderness.

8 The uterus should be palpable with your internal fingers in the anterior fornix but if the uterus is retroverted it will not be palpable here and you will need to move your fingers to the posterior fornix to locate it.

9 Then move your internal hand into each lateral fornix in turn while palpating above the same area with your external hand to identify any masses or tenderness.

CASE 9.6

Problem: My patient has a discharge from the rectum. Do I need to examine her?

Discussion: It is important to explore any symptoms of abnormal discharge. With a discharge from the rectum you need to establish if it is likely to be an STI by taking a sexual history, or discern if an alternative cause is more likely. (For example, a mucus discharge with acute diarrhoeal illness, chronic inflammatory bowel conditions, malabsorption, perianal fistulas; bloodstained discharge from fistulas or haemorrhoids). Once you have established the symptoms, examine this area externally and use a proctoscope to examine the anal canal and rectum (see Chapter 8). Samples can be taken for investigations.

13 Additional examinations and investigations

If the patient has any rectal symptoms, for example, rectal discharge or the presence of perianal warts, you should examine the rectal area following your speculum examination. Also consider the examination of other body systems if relevant (as in the male examination). See Case 9.6.

14 Wash your hands and allow the patient to dress in private before discussing findings

Thank the patient and ensure that she feels well. Cervical excitation either during a bimanual examination or through taking endocervical samples can occasionally cause a woman to feel faint or nauseous. If the patient feels unwell advise her to remain lying down until she feels better. Allow the patient to dress in private and then wash your hands, disposing of any used equipment before you remove your gloves.

15 Blood tests for HIV and syphilis are routinely offered in the sexual health clinic

If the patient is also thought to be at increased risk of hepatitis B or C (intravenous drug use, commercial sex work) offer the patient testing for these also.

Tip

While carrying out a genital examination you may become suspicious that the person has been assaulted, by the presence of bruising, injury, or the patient's demeanour. It is important to ask about non-consensual sex and question the reason for any injury. You can ask simply, 'Has somebody hurt you?' This is crucial, as the patient may feel unable to volunteer this information without prompting. If you do see someone following a sexual assault, always ask if they want the police involved before examining as a forensic examination must be performed before the medical, non-forensic examination. For patients reluctant to approach the police, a forensic examination may still be available through sexual assault charities and can be useful if the patient wishes to pursue prosecution at a later date. Always remember that men can also be sexually assaulted, so ask if you have any suspicions.

16 Report your findings

Present your findings as in the male examination section.

Genitourinary diseases and investigations

In the earlier parts of this chapter, various medical conditions and investigations have been mentioned. In this section I now describe these. In general these descriptions are brief though certain selected topics are discussed in more detail.

Non-gonococcal urethritis vs non-specific urethritis

These terms can be confusing and you will hear them used interchangeably. NGU refers to a male urethritis where gonorrhoea has been excluded as the cause. The most common cause of NGU is chlamydia; initial treatment of NGU should therefore always cover for chlamydia. The term NSU is used when both chlamydia and gonorrhoea have been excluded. The list of underlying causes of NSU is long and includes *Mycoplasma genitalium*, *Ureaplasma urealyticum*, *Trichomonas vaginalis*, herpes simplex virus, adenovirus, and non-infective causes (e.g. inflammatory skin conditions). Often no cause is found but symptoms will settle with empirical antibiotic treatment. An initial diagnosis of NGU is made in a genitourinary clinic following sampling of male urethral discharge and then Gram staining and light microscopy.

Chlamydia

This is a common bacterial infection caused by *Chlamydia trachomatis* (up to 10% of under-25-year-olds may be infected). It is spread through oral, vaginal, or anal sexual intercourse. *C. trachomatis* is a Gram-negative intracellular organism too small to be seen on standard light microscopy and is difficult to culture, but is now easily tested for using nucleic acid amplification tests (NAATs). It infects the epithelial cells of mucus membranes in genital tissue, and can also infect the conjunctiva. Left untreated, chlamydia can lead to complications from the spread of infection such as PID and epididymo-orchitis. Chlamydia is one cause of SARA.

Over half of those infected will be asymptomatic. Women with chlamydia may report one or more of a mucopurulent discharge, postcoital bleeding, intermenstrual bleeding, dysuria, or pelvic pain. Men may present with dysuria, a clear or milky discharge at the meatus, and epididymal or testicular tenderness. MSM may complain of pain in the rectum and there may be a discharge from the rectum.

When examining women look for a mucopurulent discharge coming from the endocervix. There may be evidence of contact bleeding if you swab the surface of the cervix or the endocervical canal. Perform an abdominal examination and a bimanual examination if there is any history of pelvic pain. In men, a discharge may be visible at the urethral meatus. Always check for epididymal and/or testicular tenderness. In both sexes check for signs of conjunctivitis (often due to autoinoculation in adults) and examine large joints (e.g. knee) for reactive arthritis if there is a history of new pain or swelling. As well as treating the patient it is also important to ensure that the patient's partners are treated to prevent reinfection.

A particular strain of chlamydia causing lymphogranuloma venereum (LGV) is currently increasing in prevalence among MSM in the UK. The rectal mucosa appears to be the main site of infection, and most men present with symptoms of proctitis. A longer course of treatment is required to eradicate LGV and prevent lasting damage to the gut.

Gonorrhoea

Gonorrhoea is caused by the organism *Neisseria gonorrhoea*, an intracellular Gram-negative diplococcus. *N. gonorrhoea* is a highly infectious organism and can be spread from person to person through oral, vaginal, and anal sexual intercourse. Over 50% of infected women have no symptoms, but if they do these tend to present

within 10 days of acquiring the infection. The symptoms include an increase in vaginal discharge, lower abdominal pain, and pain on urination. Intermenstrual bleeding is an unusual symptom. On examination of women there are commonly no abnormal findings. There may be a purulent cervical discharge, easily induced cervical bleeding, or pelvic or lower abdominal tenderness.

Men are more likely than women to present with symptoms with a similar incubation period of approximately 10 days. The majority of men with symptoms complain of a urethral discharge which may be accompanied by pain on urination. On examination the urethral discharge is typically yellow or green and copious, and there may be associated inflammation of the urethral meatus. If *N. gonorrhoea* infection is left untreated it can cause local sequelae including abscess formation in both sexes and PID in women. *N. gonorrhoea* can rarely spread systemically and cause a disseminated gonococcal infection with joint and skin involvement.

Although gonorrhoea can be effectively treated with antibiotics, antibiotic resistance is causing increasing concern. It is therefore important to identify antibiotic sensitivities using culture to ensure adequate treatment. It is also important that the patient's partners are treated to prevent reinfection.

Herpes

Herpes simplex virus (HSV) type 1 and 2 are common causes of genital ulceration. They are spread by genital to genital or oral to genital contact. Classically when first acquired the virus causes the formation of multiple genital vesicles which break down to form painful shallow ulcers. These can be accompanied by lymphadenopathy and constitutional symptoms. The skin changes may go unnoticed, particularly in women, where the presenting complaint may be external dysuria (due to urine coming in contact with the genital sores). This may be so painful that it leads to an inability to pass urine. Urinary retention may also occur due to sacral nerve involvement. Perianal, anal and cervical ulcers can also occur as well as extragenital sores around the groin and buttocks.

Infected patients may report a history of genital sores or oral cold sores in a partner, but many cases occur in the absence of any obvious contact. This is due to asymptomatic viral shedding in a partner who may or may not be aware of their HSV infection. Once acquired, HSV cannot be eradicated and lies dormant in the dorsal root ganglia of the nerves supplying the area in which the lesions appeared. The virus may sporadically reactivate, leading to either the asymptomatic presence of virus on the skin or the appearance of new skin lesions. These lesions tend to be less numerous and less troublesome than those associated with the initial acquisition of the virus. Type 1 herpes results in fewer recurrences (approximately one in the first year, then less often) than type 2 (approximately four in the first year, then fewer).

The diagnosis of herpes is based on clinical suspicion and is confirmed by viral swab taken from a lesion and polymerase chain reaction (PCR). Treatment with antivirals such as aciclovir should not be delayed while waiting for the swab result. Local and systemic analgesia is often also required. Without treatment, lesions will spontaneously heal, and antivirals are generally not required in herpes recurrences. A diagnosis of herpes can cause marked psychological morbidity and a full explanation of the condition and what to expect should be given to the patient.

Warts

Genital warts are a common STI caused by certain strains of the human papillomavirus (HPV), in particular strains 6 and 11. HPV is transmitted by skin to skin contact with microabrasions of the skin surface. This can occur even if penetrative sex has not taken place. The infection can be subclinical or latent, resulting in ongoing spread of virus from those without visible warts. Most genital warts are benign and are treated for cosmetic reasons only. Treatment, which can be the application of creams or physically ablative methods such as cryotherapy or curettage, does not eradicate the virus and recurrences can occur until the body naturally clears the infection.

Patients present with lumps on the skin in the genital area, in the pubic hair or perianally. These can be itchy and can bleed if traumatized. They are painless and flesh coloured or white with an irregular surface. When examining a patient for warts, check carefully in places where the patient may not have looked, for example inside the vagina and inside the urethral meatus. Any persistent (despite treatment), atypical, or ulcerating warts should be investigated with a biopsy to exclude malignancy.

Molluscum contagiosum

The molluscum contagiosum virus (a poxvirus) is a benign, self-limiting skin virus that causes lesions that clinically can look very similar to warts. Like HPV, the molluscum virus is spread through skin to skin contact and is presumed to be sexually transmitted if the lesions are present on the genital skin. However, non-sexual transmission (particularly among children) is well known to occur. The lesions of molluscum contagiosum can be distinguished from genital warts by their clinical appearance. 'Molluscum' are described as pearly white smooth papules that have a central punctum or umbilicus. As the lesions will regress by themselves over a period of 2–3 months they do not usually need treatment. However, physically ablative treatment can be offered for cosmetic reasons.

Trichomonas

Trichomonas vaginalis is a flagellated protozoan roughly the same size as a white blood cell, which infects the urogenital tract. It is sexually transmitted and presents more commonly in women as many men are able to spontaneously clear their infection. It can be asymptomatic in both sexes, particularly in men. This makes it difficult to estimate prevalence. When symptomatic, women classically present with a frothy, malodorous vaginal discharge and vaginitis. Dysuria may be present if the urethra is infected. A 'strawberry cervix' (small, punctuate cervical haemorrhages) is often described in textbooks but is a rare clinical finding. The diagnosis is based on culture and direct microscopy. The organism has a distinctive appearance being flagellated and can be seen 'swimming' on a wet slide. The presence of trichomonas may also be commented on in a cervical smear report but this should always be confirmed by culture or microscopy. Treatment is required for both the patient and their partners.

Bacterial vaginosis

Bacterial vaginosis (BV) is a vaginal infection caused by an overgrowth of the healthy vaginal flora (lactobacilli) by anaerobic organisms. It is a common cause of altered discharge in women and is not classed as an STI, although sex may be a trigger. Other triggers can be menstruation, vaginal 'douching' (washing inside the vagina with a jet of water), bubble baths, and washing with antiseptic products. All of these factors potentially alter the pH balance of the vagina, which allows the anaerobic bacterial overgrowth. Women may complain of an increase in the volume of their discharge which might be smelly (typically 'fishy'). Symptoms of itch and soreness are not associated with BV. Many women will not have any symptoms (approximately 50%). On examination a thin white, homogenous discharge is seen on the vaginal walls and may be visible on the vulva prior to passing the speculum. BV is diagnosed on a sample of vaginal discharge by Gram staining and light microscopy. The absence of lactobacilli and the presence of other mixed flora (which may be stuck to epithelial cells, termed 'clue cells') are required to make a diagnosis. Normally only symptomatic women require treating.

Candidiasis

Commonly referred to as 'thrush', candidiasis is the term used to describe infection with any candida species of which *Candida albicans* is the most common. The candida species are yeasts and occur as skin commensals (organisms that live on the surface of the skin but are not necessarily harmful). Only when the yeasts multiply and penetrate the skin mucosa do people develop symptoms. This happens much more commonly in women than men. Women with vulval or vaginal candida infection complain of itching and burning around these areas. Candida can cause local inflammation, and a change in vaginal discharge which is typically white and thick but can be watery or purulent. Like women, men with genital candidiasis also complain of burning and itching often with inflammation of the glans penis or the foreskin. On examination this inflammation may be visible as redness over the glans or the penis or there may be a white discharge over the glans. The presence of candida species can be confirmed by direct microscopy of a sample of any discharge in women or from skin scrapings in men. It can also be cultured from a vaginal swab in women and a swab from the glans penis in men. As candida occurs naturally it should only be treated if the patient is symptomatic.

Syphilis

Syphilis is caused by the spirochaete *Treponema pallidum* which can be acquired by sexual contact (including oral sex), needle inoculation, and from mother to fetus (transplacental).

   The natural history of syphilis is divided into an early stage (infectious) and a late stage (non-infectious). This is further subdivided based on the presence or absence of symptoms. Within early syphilis, the first symptoms present within 9–90 days of infection (primary syphilis) and occur at the site of inoculation. Classically this is a painless papule which ulcerates to form a chancre (*shan-cruh*), 1–2 cm in diameter. This may be accompanied by lymphadenopathy. The primary stage of syphilis may pass unnoticed and the patient may first present with symptoms of

secondary syphilis, typically 6–12 weeks after infection. Secondary syphilis symptoms are many and diverse and may take the form of skin lesions (including a rash affecting the palms and soles), mucous membrane lesions, systemic disease including organ involvement, alopecia, and eye involvement. Early latent syphilis, in which there are no signs or symptoms, is detected by positive serology in sexual health, antenatal, or blood donation screening. Late syphilis may also be asymptomatic (late latent) or be symptomatic with gumma formation, cardiovascular, and neurological signs. Congenital syphilis can present with failure to thrive, skin and mucosal lesions, or with specific malformations. Syphilis is diagnosed by dark ground microscopy (see 'Investigations'), PCR of a swab taken from an ulceration, and through serology.

HIV

The first patients with HIV were identified in 1981 in America. Since then there have been rapid developments in our knowledge and treatment options, but the numbers of people infected with HIV continues to rise. The main route of HIV transmission in the UK is through unprotected sex, so anyone who presents with an STI should be risk assessed and offered an HIV test as routine. The presence of ulceration or skin fissures on the genital skin can increase the risk of HIV transmission, as can the presence of other STIs. The initial stage of HIV infection (primary infection or 'seroconversion') can give vague symptoms of sore throat, fever, lymphadenopathy, or a rash. This commonly occurs within 6 weeks of infection and often goes either unnoticed, or is misdiagnosed as a mild viral infection. Following this, HIV can become asymptomatic for a period of time varying from months to years. Advanced HIV can present with general symptoms such as weight loss, lymphadenopathy, malaise, or it may present with the direct consequences of immunosuppression (i.e. infections not found in those with healthy immune systems) and malignancies. There are no specific genital symptoms or signs. Many general signs are possible in late disease. Some to look out for include:

- **General**. Wasting of muscles, lymphadenopathy (often in multiple sites).

- **Skin and mouth**. Orophayngeal candida, Kaposi's sarcoma (small pigmented skin lesions), severe psoriasis, severe seborrhoeic dermatitis, multidermatomal or recurrent herpes zoster (shingles).

- **Other**. Splenomegaly, peripheral neuropathy, retinal changes.

Scabies

Scabies is a skin infection caused by the mite *Sarcoptes scabiei*. The mite is spread by skin to skin contact, although this contact needs to be for several minutes, for example when holding hands. When found in the genital area it is likely that the mites have been transferred during sexual contact. Once on the skin the mite burrows underneath the surface where it lays eggs; the eggs then hatch into further mites. An intense itch develops only when the human host develops an immune response to the presence of the mite, which can take several weeks. A rash may be found, commonly on the hands, especially the web spaces between the fingers, as well as wrists, buttocks, armpits, and elbows. However, in genital infection, the genital area may be the only place affected, classically presenting as itchy lumps or papules on the scrotum or vulva. Once scabies is suspected the mites or eggs can be extracted from burrows with a needle and viewed under the microscope. It may take several weeks after treatment for the itching to resolve as the inflammatory reaction settles down and this may need treatment with antihistamines. The patient's household contacts and sexual partners should also receive treatment.

Pubic lice

Pubic lice (*Pthirus pubis*) are usually sexually transmitted through skin to skin, and therefore hair to hair, contact. The presenting complaint is normally intense itching in the pubic area, and the lice and their eggs can be seen attached to the pubic hair with the naked eye. Pubic lice can also infest any other coarse body hair including eyelashes, eyebrows, and axillary hair.

Genital dermatoses

Common skin conditions such as eczema and psoriasis can affect solely the genital skin, or can appear on the genitals in addition to other skin surfaces. Less common inflammatory skin conditions such as lichen sclerosis and lichen planus can also affect the genital skin. An example of a genital dermatosis confined to the genital area would be plasma cell balanitis or vulvitis. Atypical skin changes should always be biopsied to check for cancerous or precancerous cells.

Patients often worry that genital skin changes are caused by an STI so it is important to be able to identify common skin disorders in order to reassure them and treat them appropriately. It is worth asking the patient if they have any skin problems elsewhere on their body, including the mouth, or if they have a history of conditions that are associated with eczema (known as atopic conditions which include hay fever, asthma, and allergic rhinitis).

Specimen collection

In a non-medical setting such as a community chlamydia screening programme, a first-pass urine can be used to screen for chlamydia and gonorrhoea in both males and females using NAATs. A self-taken vulvovaginal swab is, however, preferable in women because of its better sensitivity and specificity. In a medical setting, these minimally intrusive sampling techniques can be supplemented by practitioner-taken swabs. As already mentioned, the number and type of swabs can vary depending on the setting, genitourinary medicine vs gynaecology for example, and within a speciality from clinic to clinic. Always remember to check what swabs are needed before starting. The following describes specimen collection from a genitourinary medicine point of view.

1 In a genitourinary medicine setting, there is the luxury of near-patient microscopy; urethral, vaginal, cervical, and if indicated rectal swabs can be used to prepare slides for microscopy. This allows an initial diagnosis to be made, partner notification to begin (the process of identifying sexual partners who may also be at risk of a specific infection and require treatment) and treatment to commence prior to the patient leaving clinic. The equipment and links with the microbiology lab in a genitourinary setting also allow samples to be inoculated directly on to culture plates (for gonorrhoea and candida), increasing the success rate of isolating these organisms.

2 In addition to a first-pass urine, all MSM and symptomatic heterosexual men require a urethral swab. Take a sample using a plastic loop or cotton swab inserted approximately 2 cm into the urethra. This sample can be inoculated on to a culture plate for gonorrhoea or transported in a charcoal medium for culture in the laboratory. A slide can also be prepared from this sample to be assessed using light microscopy.

3 Rectal swabs should be taken in men who have a history of receptive anal sex and are either taken under direct vision using a proctoscope or are taken 'blind' by inserting a swab 2–4 cm blind into the anal canal using lateral pressure to avoid any faecal mass. A gonorrhoea culture plate should be inoculated and if the patient has a suspicious rectal discharge a slide can be

prepared. Rectal swabs can also be sent for chlamydia and gonorrhoea NAATs.

4 Pharyngeal samples are also taken from men with a history of receptive oral sex and are obtained by wiping a cotton swab over the posterior pharynx, tonsils and tonsillar crypts. Depending on local policy swabs may be used to inoculate a gonorrhoea culture plate and be tested for gonorrhoea and chlamydia by NAATs.

5 Women may be screened for chlamydia and gonorrhoea by an endocervical or vulvovaginal NAATs swab. A vulvovaginal swab is performed by rubbing the swab around the external urethral area and then sliding it approximately 5 cm into the vagina and rotating it for 5–10 seconds. Additionally, gonorrhoea culture plates can be inoculated from both endocervical and urethral swabs and microscopy slides prepared if indicated.

6 In addition to chlamydia and gonorrhoea, symptomatic women will also receive swabs looking for BV, candida and trichomonas. Swabs are taken from the lateral vaginal wall for microscopy looking for BV and candida. Additionally a candida culture plate can be inoculated. A further swab is taken from the posterior fornix for microscopy and culture of trichomonas.

7 Rectal and pharyngeal swabs as described above may also be taken from selected female patients.

8 In both sexes swabs are also taken from any ulcer or skin break suspicious of herpes and are simply obtained by rubbing the swab over the affected area.

Light microscopy

Samples from urethral, vaginal and endocervical fluid are Gram-stained and examined using the light microscope. Rectal samples can also be used but can be more challenging to interpret.

Potential diagnoses are:

- **Urethral slide**. Presumptive gonorrhoea (Gram-negative diplococci within pus cells), NGU in men (indicated by the presence of five or more pus cells per high-power field, in five or more fields).
- **Vaginal slide**. Candida, BV.
- **Endocervical slide**. Presumptive gonorrhoea (Gram-negative diplococci within pus cells).

A sample of vaginal fluid mounted in saline ('wet mount') can also be examined down a light microscope for the presence of *Trichomonas vaginalis*.

Dark ground microscopy

Dark ground or dark field microscopy is a form of microscopy that can be used to identify the organism that causes syphilis, *T. pallidum*. This organism is not seen with a normal light microscope because the difference in contrast between the specimen and the background is too small. In dark ground microscopy the specimen is lit from the side, rather than from underneath, and the only light that is visible through the lens is that which is scattered by the specimen itself. *T. pallidum* appears as brightly illuminated spirals against the dark background.

If syphilis is suspected from a sore or ulcer, a small sample of fluid is taken from this and placed on a microscope slide. If you can see *T. pallidum* by using dark field microscopy then this confirms the diagnosis of syphilis. It is not always possible to identify the organism on dark ground microscopy and so if syphilis is suspected blood tests should always be taken even if the organism is not seen. In some centres it is also possible to swab the ulcer for PCR testing.

Pregnancy test

Urine pregnancy tests detect the hormone β-human chorionic gonadotrophin (βHCG) and become positive from the first day of a missed menstrual period. They cannot distinguish between ectopic and uterine pregnancies. They can also be positive in trophoblastic disease. If a test is negative but pregnancy is suspected, the test should be repeated in 7 days.

Laboratory tests

NAATs are biochemical techniques that are used to detect a virus or bacterium. When the amount of DNA present within the clinical sample would otherwise be insufficient for diagnosis, NAATs amplify the amount of DNA present, enabling detection and therefore diagnosis. This technique can be used to detect chlamydia and gonorrhoea as well as HSV, and is more sensitive and specific than culture of these organisms. The PCR is one such amplification test. PCR uses the enzyme polymerase to amplify the DNA sequence for detection.

Vaginal pH

Vaginal pH in a woman of menstruating age should be less than 4.5. The presence of menses (menstrual blood) or semen will raise the pH (i.e. it will become more alkaline); cervical pH is also higher. A higher vaginal pH in the absence of these can indicate BV, but this alone is not diagnostic. This is a simple test that can be done in genitourinary clinics or GP surgeries by putting litmus paper on to the vaginal walls while the speculum is in place and noting the colour change.

Skin biopsy

A skin biopsy is a procedure where a small sample of tissue is removed from the skin either to help with the diagnosis of a skin condition or to remove a skin lesion completely. The commonest type of biopsy used on the genital skin is a punch biopsy: a small sample of skin is taken (between 2 mm and 8 mm in diameter) which samples the full thickness of the skin. The skin is first numbed using local anaesthetic, and then the sample is taken using a punch biopsy tool. Small punch biopsies generally do not require suturing, and silver nitrate can be used to achieve haemostasis. The sample of skin is then sent to the laboratory in a preservative liquid, usually formaldehyde, and examined using staining and microscopy techniques to give a diagnosis.

Ultrasound

Ultrasound examination is the key imaging modality in genitourinary medicine and is used in the identification of scrotal and pelvic masses, and the investigation of pelvic pain. In the acute setting it is used in the evaluation of potential testicular torsion and ectopic pregnancy. In women, ultrasound may be transabdominal or transvaginal.

Cervical smear

Cervical smears should only be taken in accordance with the national screening programme. This starts at the age of 25 in England and Northern Ireland, but at the age of 20 in Scotland and Wales. Smears are repeated every 3 years until the age of 49, after which they occur every 5 years until age 64. However, if a woman has had an abnormal result she will require more frequent smears for a period of time and may be followed up beyond the age of 64. If a woman is HIV positive yearly smears are recommended due to increased rates of cervical intraepithelial neoplasia (CIN). A cervical smear test samples the transformation zone of the cervix: the junction between the columnar epithelium of the endocervix and squamous epithelium of the ectocervix.

A smear is not an appropriate test for an abnormal looking cervix, where a colposcopy and biopsy are required, but is designed to identify CIN, the preinvasive phase of cervical cancer.

Finals section

It is extremely unlikely that you would be expected to undertake a genital examination on a patient during a Finals examination. You may, however, be asked to explain to a patient what a genital examination would involve. It is therefore important that you are able to do this. Additionally you may be asked to demonstrate your skills using a male or female model pelvis. It is a good idea to visit your clinical skills lab to familiarize yourself with the types of models used locally. A 'patient' could also be in the station if there is additional history to be elicited, or if you are required to explain the examination procedure as you go along.

Table 9.9 provides a few ideas to focus your preparation and learning. Exact timings and formats of any examinations will depend on your own medical school. Remember that taking a sexual history will be relevant in stations which do not appear to be about sexual health; for example, a gynaecological station, a urological station, and any woman with pelvic pain.

OSCE examples

History-taking scenario

You are an FY1 in primary care. A 19-year-old man comes to see you with pain in his left testicle. This has been present for 1 week and is getting worse, which is causing him some anxiety. Take a focused history from him and discuss possible diagnoses and further management. You are not required to examine the patient. You have 10 minutes.

Remember:

1 Introduce yourself to the patient.

2 Cover a pain history as well as a sexual history, and ask about any associated genital symptoms, for example discharge or dysuria.

3 When taking the sexual history put the patient at ease and explain why you are asking sensitive questions (see Case 9.7).

Table 9.9 Common Finals cases

History-taking topics

Male

Testicular pain

Urethral discharge

Dysuria

HIV risk assessment

Female

Pelvic pain

Abnormal bleeding (intermenstrual, postcoital, postmenopausal)

Change in vaginal discharge

HIV risk assessment

Examinations

Male

Testicular examination

Female

Demonstration of speculum and swab taking

Bimanual examination

Smear taking

Information-giving/Explanation

Explain how a genital examination would be performed in a male or female patient

Explain the need to undertake screening for STIs in those who have symptoms suggestive of an STI and their partners

---

4 Recent unprotected sex in this patient's age group makes a STI the most common cause of epididymitis, but be prepared to discuss other possibilities.

5 Thank your patient.

6 Further management would include examination, investigations for STIs (chlamydia and gonorrhoea) and exclusion of a urinary tract infection with a mid-stream urine specimen. Epididymitis is treated by antibiotics—see your local guidelines.

CASE 9.7

Problem: How do I start asking about sexual history without offending the patient?

Solution: As long as you explain why you need to ask the questions, and approach the matter professionally and sensitively this will not be a problem. Simulated patients may have been instructed to only give this information if asked, and there are likely to be marks available for tackling it well. Examples: 'Is it all right to ask you about your sexual history? It may be relevant to the symptoms you are having'. Or 'These are questions I always ask when somebody has pain/abnormal bleeding.'

Examination scenario

You are an FY1 working in the emergency department. A 26-year-old woman presents with pelvic pain and postcoital bleeding over the last week. Her last period was 3 weeks ago and a pregnancy test is negative. She had a negative smear test last year with her GP. Perform a speculum examination to visualize the cervix and demonstrate a bimanual examination on the pelvis provided. You are not required to take swabs, or take any further history. You have 10 minutes.

Remember:

1 Introduce yourself and gain consent for the examination.

2 Ask for a chaperone and ensure the patient is happy to proceed with the examination.

3 Ensure that the patient knows what to expect during the procedure.

4 Demonstrate the required skills on the model pelvis, ensuring that the examiner can clearly see that you have found the cervix (see Case 9.8).

5 Thank the patient once you have completed the examination.

6 Report any findings, even negative findings (e.g. 'There is no tenderness on cervical motion').

7 Be prepared to give some differential causes for this presentation.

Information-giving/explanation scenarios

You are an FY1 working in primary care and have been asked to see a 21-year-old woman who presents with mild lower abdominal pain. Take a focused history from her,

CASE 9.8

Problem: What if I can't find the cervix with the speculum?

Solution: Practice, practice, practice. Even if you have done plenty of speculum examinations on your placements it can feel quite different on a model pelvis. Ensure you are familiar with the models and the speculums used locally. If you really can't find it, explain to the patient/examiner that you are not quite in the right position, remove the speculum, take a deep breath and try again.

and once you have completed the history explain to the patient what the possible diagnoses are and what investigations you would like to do next. You do not need to examine the patient. You have 10 minutes.

Remember:

1 Introduce yourself to the patient.

2 Take a pain history and check if there are any associated symptoms—for example, a change in vaginal discharge or dysuria (pain on urination).

3 Find out if there is a risk of pregnancy or STIs.

4 Explain that in a young female patient with abdominal pain, pregnancy should always be excluded using a urinary pregnancy test.

5 Explain that the main differential diagnosis in a young sexually active woman with lower abdominal pain and dyspareunia is PID.

6 Describe what an examination will entail, trying to put the patient at ease. This should include an explanation of screening for STIs.

7 Discuss that empirical treatment with antibiotics may be appropriate if pregnancy has been excluded and there is a high suspicion of PID. If treatment for PID is given, any current or recent partners should also be treated.

8 Be prepared to address the patient's concerns about future fertility.

You are an FY1 working in genitourinary medicine. Your next patient is a 19-year-old man who is complaining of pain on passing urine and has been diagnosed with chlamydia via a community screening programme. Take a focused history from the patient. Once you have completed the history, explain your management plan to the patient. You do not need to examine the patient. You have 10 minutes.

Remember:

1 Introduce yourself to the patient.

2 Check for any associated symptoms such as testicular pain, conjunctivitis, or arthritis.

3 Take a full sexual history including HIV risk factors.

4 Recommend an examination and full screen to check for other infections.

5 Discuss what chlamydia is, how it is acquired, and how it is treated.

6 Explain the need for all recent partners to be treated as contacts and the need for abstinence until both he and his partner have completed treatment.

7 Discuss safer sex and condom use.

8 Ask if the patient has any questions, then thank him for his time.

Questions

1 Name three causes of a urethral discharge in men.

2 What is the microscopic appearance of gonorrhoea?

3 When do women first receive cervical screening in the UK?

4 What are the microscopic appearances of BV?

5 How is chlamydia diagnosed?

6 Give four causes of intermenstrual bleeding.

7 Give three examples of STIs which affect extragenital sites.

8 List four questions that should be used to assess someone's HIV risk.

9 Name three genital 'lumps' which are in fact normal variants.

10 Give three causes of testicular pain.

References and further reading

GMC. *Maintaining boundaries—guidance for doctors*. General Medical Council, London, 2006.

Pattman R, Sankar N, Elawad B, Handy P, and Ashley Price D. *Oxford handbook of genitourinary medicine, HIV, and sexual health*, 2nd edn. Oxford University Press, Oxford, 2010.

Rogstad K. *ABC of sexually transmitted infections*, 6th edn. Wiley-Blackwell, Oxford, 2011.

10 Breast examination

Introduction

The breast or mammary gland is a modified skin appendage situated on the front of the chest. It is common to all mammals and its primary function is the production of milk (lactation) to nourish the young following birth. In humans the breast is also a secondary sexual characteristic and is a potent symbol of femininity. This important feature means that any examination of this organ has to be performed with great sensitivity. In medicine the most powerful driver for referral is the fear of breast cancer. Therefore any clinician must be able to differentiate benign disease from potential cancer and how to manage those situations that are not clear cut. This chapter will help you to perform a systematic and thorough examination of the breast and also introduce you to the more common diseases that you are likely to encounter.

Symptoms

Symptoms can arise from normal physiological processes affecting the breast during the patient's lifetime or may be due to pathological disease processes. In recent years a new classification called ANDI (**a**berrations in **n**ormal **d**evelopment and **i**nvolution in the breast) has been devised to encompass the range of benign diseases of the breast which are due to normal physiological processes.

Involution

In medical terms this is the decline or degeneration in function of an organ as a result of non-use or ageing. This is often accompanied by shrinkage of the organ or tissue. A more specific definition that applies to the breast is the process by which the breast returns to a non-lactating state. This can occur following weaning of a child after breastfeeding and more gradually with ageing particularly after the menopause.

Therefore, ANDI can be seen as any problem that can affect a female throughout the lifetime of breast development from puberty to old age. It must be noted that although the symptoms experienced by a patient reflects sensitivity to their normal physiological processes, some patients can still experience severe distress as a result.

Breast pain (mastalgia)

Unlike the major systems like the cardiovascular or gastrointestinal system there are few characteristics of pain that can point to any particular diagnosis when assessing breast pain. One important exception is the relationship of the pain to your patient's menstrual cycle. This has led to the concept of cyclical mastalgia (*mast-al-ja*) and non-cyclical mastalgia).

Cyclical mastalgia

Some element of breast pain or discomfort is a normal occurrence in women during their menstrual years. Frequently patients will complain of pain in one breast or one area of the breast, such as the upper outer quadrant. This usually commences in the second half of the menstrual cycle and gradually builds up in intensity and can become constant until menstruation begins. As menstruation finishes the pain eases off, sometimes completely, before returning again during the next cycle. The pain may radiate towards the nipple or towards the axilla in keeping with the sensory nerve distribution. For some women the pain is very severe and unremitting over long periods of time. Associated breast tenderness and a sensation of an extremely swollen breast are commonplace. See Case 10.1.

Non-cyclical mastalgia

Less frequently, patients present with a history of breast pain which does not show the classical relationship to the menstrual cycle. In this situation the pain may be more constant throughout the menstrual cycle and the decrease in pain after the onset of menstruation seen with cyclical

CASE 10.1

Problem: You are asked to take a history from a patient who has had repeated episodes of pain and tenderness in the outer half of her right breast which initially responded to antibiotics but these are no longer helpful.

Discussion: Breast pain and tenderness are extremely common symptoms. The most important fact to determine is the relationship of the symptoms to the menstrual cycle. There is usually an increase in the frequency and severity of the symptoms in the week leading up to her period and often continuing into the first day or two. Then the symptoms diminish and may disappear completely before returning again approximately 10–14 days later. If this pattern is confirmed then you are most likely dealing with cyclical mastalgia. As antibiotics have been prescribed it is prudent to check if there was ever any redness of the skin of the affected breast and if the patient has had symptoms of shivering or fever. If these symptoms and signs are absent it would mean an infective process of the breast is unlikely. Often your patient may credit the antibiotic with curing her symptoms when the pain resolves and may expect further prescriptions; however, it will soon become clear that the pain always reappears. Patients can be encouraged to take their temperature during a bout of pain and this should show no increase in temperature. Once it is clear that you are dealing with cyclical mastalgia you can reassure your patient that there is no sinister cause for the pain. Your efforts can then focus on finding the most symptomatic relief for her.

mastalgia does not occur. This can make the diagnosis trickier to obtain and other conditions will have to be excluded before accepting this. If non-cyclical mastalgia is finally confirmed it is not associated with any increased risks of infection or future cancer development.

Other diseases that can mimic non-cyclical mastalgia, include referred pain from musculoskeletal disorders affecting the back or rib cage, infections of the breast, and breast cancer. See Case 10.2. With musculoskeletal disorders the pain may be exacerbated by movement or posture. With infections there may be associated erythema, swelling of the breast together with constitutional features, such as a fever or malaise. Finally, a small percentage of patients with breast cancer can present with localized breast pain but it is rarely if ever the only symptom.

CASE 10.2

Problem: You have seen a 29-year-old woman who complains of pain in the left breast and you are wondering if you could be dealing with non-cyclical mastalgia. How can you be sure of the diagnosis?

Discussion: Unfortunately there is no shortcut to this diagnosis as it remains a diagnosis of exclusion. You need to be thorough in your history-taking and examination. If there is no obvious relationship to her periods, you need to build up a picture of the pain. When did it start? Is it constant or intermittent? Is it related to movement, inspiration, exertion etc.? It may be that you have to organize investigations to exclude certain conditions such as blood tests, chest radiograph, ECG, depending on what you uncover. It is not a diagnosis to rush and you may need to see the individual on a number of occasions before you can be sure that you are dealing with non-cyclical mastalgia.

Table 10.1 Questions to ask in a menstrual history

When was the first day of your last menstrual period (LMP)?

How long do your periods last?

What is the length of a typical/average cycle?

Are they regular or irregular?

At what age did your periods start (called menarche [*men-ark*])?

If relevant, ask 'When did the menopause start?'

What to ask

When asking about breast pain you need to ask the questions that you would in any other system, asking about the onset, site, radiation, duration, etc. (see Chapters 4 and 7).

- Ask, 'Is the pain related to your periods?' If it is, investigate the relationship closer. You should also take a relevant menstrual history (see Table 10.1).
- 'If you are on contraceptive medication, have you changed type or dose recently?'
- If relevant, ask, 'Are you breastfeeding?'
- Also ask, 'Have you noticed any redness of the skin?' as this could indicate an infective process.
- 'Does the skin rather than the underlying breast sting or smart when pinched?'
- 'Have you noticed any other skin changes?' This is to determine if they have noticed any dimpling or tethering that could point towards a cancer.

Benign breast nodularity

Sometimes your patient will complain of a 'lumpy' breast or breasts. Benign breast nodularity is a term used to describe lumpiness within the breast which has a physiological origin and again comes under the umbrella of ANDI. It is frequently associated with mastalgia,

particularly cyclical mastalgia, and most often located in the upper outer quadrant of the breast. It tends to be most prominent in the second half of the menstrual cycle. This condition has been referred to as fibrocystic disease in the past but the term is to be discouraged now as it has no informative meaning and merely describes the fibrosis and cystic changes found in the breast tissue on histological examination. Pathologists sometime use the term fibroadenosis but again this has little clinical value and benign breast nodularity is the current term to use.

Breast infection

Breast infection can occur when microorganisms gain entry to the breast either through the nipple and ducts, by trauma, through cracked skin, or other skin disorders, for example, eczema. If the skin and subcutaneous tissues of the breast are predominantly affected this is a cellulitis but if the deeper breast tissue is also affected this is called a mastitis (*mass-tie-tis*). Untreated the mastitis can develop into a breast abscess. Breast infections can be classified as lactational infection and non-lactational infection depending on the reproductive status of your patient. Lactational infection is more common because pressure and moisture from the baby's mouth can cause small cracks in the skin of the nipple or breast allowing entry of the microorganisms (see 'Breast diseases and investigation' section).

Breast lumps

Breast swellings are one of the commonest presentations of breast problems to the NHS. There are a variety of causes of a breast lump but the overriding concern

Key points

- The classification ANDI (aberrations in normal development and involution in the breast) covers the range of benign diseases that are due to normal physiological processes in the breast
- Physiological breast pain is common and is termed cyclical mastalgia when there is a clear relationship with menstruation and non-cyclical mastalgia when there is not
- Breast pain tends to be at its maximum in the week leading up to a period
- Breast pain associated with erythema and swelling of the breast may indicate a breast infection
- Breast infection is commoner in breastfeeding women

for your patient will be the fear of breast cancer. It must also be noted that occasionally breast lumps can occur in men. They can also suffer with breast cancer; in the UK 1 man develops breast cancer for approximately every 150 women who do.

Causes

See Table 10.2. Many of these causes are described in more detail in the 'Breast diseases and investigation' section.

What to ask

First of all ask:

- 'Is there a definite lump you can feel or is it just a tender area you are aware of?'

If they confirm the presence of a lump then ask:

- 'When did you first notice the lump?'
- 'Has it increased in size?'

Then determine if there are any associated symptoms or signs:

- 'Is there any pain in the breast?'

If there is pain, then ask the questions above.
Also ask:

- 'Have you noticed any discharge from the nipple?' (see 'Nipple discharge' section).
- 'Have you injured your breast in the past?' and if the answer is yes ask, 'How did it happen?' Trauma may cause a lump acutely as a result of haematoma formation and later due to fat necrosis as part of the body's

Table 10.2 Causes of a breast lump

Fibroadenoma (young women)
Cyst (35–40 year olds)
Physiological breast change
Hamartoma (soft discrete lump, softer than fibroadenoma)
Lipoma
Breast cancer
Breast abscess (smokers and postpartum)
Trauma (recent injury e.g. seatbelt)
Scarring from previous surgery
Leaking silicone implant

attempt to heal the injury. Sometimes, however, the patient may not recall any previous trauma which will make this possibility impossible to determine from the history alone.

Past medical history

Now investigate the patient's past medical history:

- 'Have you had breast lumps in the past?'
- If the answer is yes, ask, 'How did they treat it?'
- Also ask, 'Have you had any breast surgery in the past?'

Previous surgery can lead to lumpiness of the tissues near the scar site as there will be a dip in the breast contour where tissue was removed, making the edges seem lumpy. Operations and subsequent healing can also cause fat necrosis which makes the fat feel firmer than the surrounding breast. Your patient may volunteer that they have silicone implants, in which case you should consider the possibility of them leaking. Sometimes this will be obvious from the distortion of the breast but sometimes leakage can be insidious and not suspected.

Drug history

A drug history should be taken although the only relevant medications here are the contraceptive pill or hormone replacement therapy. If the patient is taking these establish which type they are on and the duration they have taken them as they may be relevant as a cause of breast pain and there is a small increased risk of developing breast cancer over time (see 'Breast diseases and investigations'). A history of antidepressant or antipsychotic medication is relevant for the presentation of copious nipple discharge (see 'Galactorrhoea' section). The drug history is also often informative for a man presenting with gynaecomastia (see Table 7.15).

Family history

A family history should be taken. For most women the biggest risk factor will be increasing age. However, a small proportion of women will have inherited genes that put them at a substantial risk of developing cancer. These are the *BRCA1*, *BRCA2*, and *TP53* genes among others (see 'Breast diseases and investigations' section). You can begin by asking, 'Is there anyone in your family who has had breast cancer?' You are most interested in first-degree or second-degree relatives who have developed breast cancer at an early age (see Table 10.3). You must also ensure that these relatives are from the same side of the family as your patient. You will also be looking for unusual patterns of cancer in the family, 'Is there anyone who has had cancer in both breasts?' 'Are there any male members of the family who developed breast cancer?' 'Is there anyone in the family that has had ovarian cancer (or other unusual cancers)?' A yes to all these questions substantially increases the possibility that your patient may be at risk of having or developing cancer. The risk stratification and management of these patients are documented in recent NICE guidelines. Ultimately a small percentage of patients may require genetic testing and counselling and may require annual surveillance with MRI scanning.

Review of systems

Finally do not forget your review of systems. In someone healthy this will be relatively quick as they will answer no to all of your questions. However, someone who has anorexia and weight loss and/or breathlessness, and/or bone pain with no other medical condition to explain the symptoms could have distant spread from a breast cancer.

Your history may have helped to point to some of the causes listed in Table 10.2 but the majority of breast swellings will require further investigation to classify them. The cornerstone of diagnosing breast lumps is the process called triple assessment (see 'Breast diseases and investigations' section).

Table 10.3 Classification of relatives

First-degree relatives	Mother, father, daughter, son, sister, brother
Second-degree relatives	Grandparent, grandchild, aunt, uncle, niece and nephew; half-sister and half-brother
Third-degree relatives	Great grandparent, great grandchild, great aunt, great uncle, first cousin, grand-nephew and grand-niece

Key points

- Breast lumps are the commonest presentation of breast disease to the NHS
- One man develops breast cancer for every 150 women, in the UK
- Do not forget to ask about the contraceptive pill or hormone replacement therapy
- A family history of first-degree relatives with breast cancer contracted at an early age, or in both breasts, affecting male relatives or ovarian/unusual cancers, strongly points to the possibility of an inherited form of breast cancer

Nipple discharge

A fluid discharge from a nipple, either spontaneously or following stimulation is a common occurrence for many women and is not usually associated with any significant breast problem. Ask, 'What colour is the discharge?' If the response is green, grey, or white then it is likely to be of benign origin.

Other features that point to a benign source include a toothpaste-like consistency and its isolation from more than one duct opening or from both nipples. There may be some associated crusting of the nipple when the discharge dries. In these situations further investigation is not indicated and your patient can be reassured.

If the response is bloodstained, this is a more worrying feature. Other features that suggest a pathological cause include a spontaneous discharge, a discharge from one nipple, and in particular from one duct of that nipple. This situation will require further investigation.

If the response suggests that the discharge is copious and milky or milk-like then you may be dealing with galactorrhoea.

Galactorrhoea

What is it?

Galactorrhoea (*ga-lack-toe-rear*) is the secretion of milk from the breast that is not associated with breastfeeding following childbirth. It can also occur in men and occasionally in neonates (an old-fashioned term for this is 'witch's milk').

In the months following the cessation of breast feeding some milky discharge from one or both nipples is a common occurrence and can occur for up to several years. As with other physiological types of nipple discharge the patient is encouraged not to express the breast as this habit is frequently associated with the provocation of further discharge.

If there is spontaneous and copious milky discharge bilaterally, this is more likely to represent galactorrhoea.

Causes

Lactation is normally controlled by the hormone prolactin secreted by the anterior pituitary gland. If the level of circulating prolactin in the blood becomes high (hyperprolactinaemia [*high-per-pro-lack-tin-knee-mia*]), this can lead to galactorrhea. See Tables 10.4 and 10.5.

Many of the non-drug causes are rare and in most cases the cause of the galactorrhoea is not found. The causes listed in Tables 10.4 and 10.5 only represent some examples as there are many other causes listed in the literature.

What to ask?

- Ask 'Is the discharge from one or both nipples?'
- Try to get a rough estimate of the amount, 'Is it just a few drops or does it keep pouring from the nipple?'
- 'Can it occur without warning (spontaneously) or does it only occur if the nipples are squeezed or the breast is manually expressed?'

Take a menstrual history and find out if the patient has had any children and if she has breastfed. Note that some women with hyperprolactinaemia can have an absence of periods (amenorrhoea [*ay-men-owe-rear*]), scanty periods, (oligomenorrhoea [*olly-go-men-owe-rear*]), hypogonadism, and infertility.

These initial questions are applicable to any nipple discharge.

Table 10.4 Non-drug causes of hyperprolactinaemia

Idiopathic (no cause known)
Prolactinoma (a tumour in the pituitary secretes excess prolactin)
Other pituitary tumours
Hypothyroidism
Head trauma
Encephalitis/basal meningitis

Table 10.5 Some drug causes of hyperprolactinaemia

Anti-depressants, e.g. selective serotonin reuptake inhibitors (SSRIs) such as fluoxetine
Anti-psychotics, e.g. chlorpromazine, haloperidol, risperidone
Anti-hypertensives, e.g. verapamil, methyldopa
Oral contraceptive

Also take a drug history, looking particularly for drugs in Table 10.5. If you are unsure of the side-effect profile of a drug, check in the British National Formulary (BNF) or a reputable internet source as you may find that the drug could be a cause.

If there are no obvious precipitating causes it is useful to ask if the patient has suffered with headaches or visual disturbance as this could herald the rare occurrence of a pituitary tumour. There is no single diagnostic feature of the headache associated with pituitary tumours: they can be unilateral, bilateral, migrainous in character, or resemble cluster headaches. Some cases can defy classification. The visual disturbance associated with some pituitary tumours is said to be a bitemporal hemianopia but this will only occur if the tumour enlarges sufficiently to compress the optic chiasma. In reality different visual deficits occur according to how the optic nerves, chiasma, or tract are affected.

It must be noted that many cases of pituitary tumours may be asymptomatic but if you are presented with a patient with galactorrhoea, especially if she has menstrual abnormalities and suffers with headache and visual disturbance, she should be investigated for the possibility of a pituitary tumour.

> **Key points**
> - A spontaneous uniductal bloodstained discharge from a nipple needs urgent investigation
> - In most cases of galactorrhoea no cause is found
> - Always consider drug causes in cases of hyperprolactinaemia
> - Hyperprolactinaemia may lead to hypogonadism, impotence (in men), amenorrhoea, and infertility
> - In rare cases, patients with hyperprolactinaemia, headaches and visual disturbance may have a prolactinoma

Accessory nipples/accessory breast tissue

Occasionally you may be faced with a patient who is concerned about a lesion that looks like a nipple or what looks like a lump that may resemble an extra breast.

What are accessory nipples?

The breast develops from ridges of specialized adapted skin on the chest wall as occurs with other mammals. These ridges (sometimes called the 'milk line') run vertically from the midclavicular point to the groins. Normally the excess tissue along the milk line that does not form breast tissue atrophies and disappears (in other mammals it persists as functioning pairs of glands on their ventral surface). However, if tissue persists, it can manifest as extra nipples anywhere along this milk line. These can also be called supernumerary nipples and the process polythelia (*polly-th-ee-lia*). They can be very rudimentary in nature and may give the appearance of just a skin lesion or they can be well developed with or without an associated areola. Their location vertically in line with the nipple provides the clue to their nature. They do not require any specific treatment as there is no extra risk of developing cancer.

What is accessory breast tissue?

Breast tissue can develop anywhere along this milk line also, and this process is called polymastia. More frequently accessory breast tissue presents as excess folds of tissue superficially in the medial axilla. As these folds contain breast tissue they will become more prominent during pregnancy and breastfeeding. Axillary accessory breast tissue can be excised, although some patients complain of pain and tenderness postoperatively. There are case reports of breast cancer arising in accessory nipple and breast tissue but the

current conclusion is that the cancer rate reflects the normal risk for breast cancer developing in any breast tissue.

Breast implants

It is increasingly common for women who have previously had breast augmentation for cosmetic reasons to present with breast complaints. The presenting complaint may or may not be related to the presence of the breast implant. In breast augmentation the most commonly used implants are silicone based with silicone gel in a silicone wrapper. The implants are placed deep to the breast tissue lying on the underlying pectoralis major (subglandular) or placed deep to the pectoralis major muscle lying on the ribcage (submuscular).

Patients may complain of feeling something abnormal. When examined this could represent a fold or edge of the silicone implant. This fact will be readily apparent as the abnormality will feel like a fold and indent under pressure of the examining fingers.

Gynaecomastia

See Chapter 7. The presence of excess breast tissue in a male can give rise to embarrassment as well as distress if they are worried about breast cancer. In the majority of adolescent males reassurance is all that is required as breast development may be a transient response to the hormonal changes they experience through puberty and should recede. In older men you will need to perform a thorough history and examination to identify any medical causes. Any discrete breast lump in a man is investigated by the same triple assessment process used for women (see 'Breast diseases and investigations' section).

Abnormalities of breast development

Young women can present with a discrepancy in breast size. Often the size differences are minor and no further action except reassurance is required. In other circumstances a breast may initially show signs of normal development but that growth is arrested, resulting in one breast being considerably smaller than the other and of a different shape. Some breasts do not develop at all and remain very rudimentary. Usually this occurs only in one breast. Such patients need to be seen by a specialist breast surgical team who can discuss all the issues and options available. Usually the developmental abnormalities are not associated with other significant medical problems.

Breast examination summary

1 Introduce yourself to the patient and ask permission to carry out the examination.

2 Explain the examination procedure and gain informed consent.

3 Offer a chaperone.

4 Ask the patient to undress.

5 Wash your hands.

6 Initially ask the patient to sit up on the couch/bed to face you.

7 Perform your general look.

8 Ask some preparatory questions.

9 Inspect the breasts for shape and contour; for erythema; for scars and dimpling; for ulceration; check the nipples.

10 Examine the neck.

11 Ask your patient to elevate both arms and inspect the breasts again.

12 With the arms still raised vertically, or alternatively placed behind the head, palpate the breasts systematically.

13 Examine the axillae for lymphadenopathy.

14 Ask your patient to lie supine and to place both hands behind her head.

15 Repeat the inspection of the breasts.

16 Repeat the palpation of the breasts.

17 Assessment of nipple discharge if relevant.

18 Examine other relevant systems if applicable.

19 Ask your patient to dress again.

20 Wash your hands.

21 Report your findings.

Breast examination in detail

Getting started

1 Introduce yourself to the patient and ask permission to carry out the examination

Say something like 'I am James Paget, a fourth year medical student. In view of your problem, is it all right if I examine your breasts?' Hopefully you may have had the opportunity to have taken a history and have therefore built up a rapport with your patient. However, do not feel slighted if she refuses as this is clearly a sensitive area to be examining as a student. Ask if it is acceptable to be present when the senior doctor examines so that you can learn from their approach and technique. Do not be disheartened, because there will be further opportunities for you to learn.

2 Explain the examination procedure and gain informed consent

If your patient agrees for you to conduct the examination then you must explain what you are about to do so that there are no surprises and you will gain her confidence. Increasingly it is becoming important to demonstrate that consent has been gained in all physical examinations and it is mandatory in intimate examinations. Only when you have explained why you are doing the examination and what she can expect, can you say that you have obtained true informed consent. If she is still agreeable for the examination to proceed then the consent obtained should be written clearly in the medical notes. Explain that it will be necessary for her to remove the clothes from the upper half of her body and that the breasts will be inspected and palpated. In the majority of cases you will be assessing any swellings in the breast but make sure she is aware that you need to check the other breast as well to ensure there are no other lumps (and also allow you to gauge the consistency of the 'normal' breast tissue with the affected side).

3 Offer a chaperone

A chaperone should always be present at the time of a breast examination. Ideally this should be a female chaperone. Should a patient decline the offer of a chaperone, it is sensible for you as a student to abandon the examination. Inform the supervising doctor who will have to make a judgement whether to proceed with the examination depending on the clinical necessity. Most patients appreciate the presence of a chaperone and understand that it is part of best practice. They can be a valuable source of support for the patient and can also reassure them if any anxieties surface during the examination.

4 Ask the patient to undress

The patient should be left to undress in private. In a clinic situation a suitable gown should be available as necessary.

5 Wash your hands

While your patient is getting undressed you can be washing your hands.

6 Initially ask the patient to sit up on the couch/bed to face you

The height of the couch or bed should be elevated so that the patient is almost making direct horizontal eye contact with the examiner (see Fig. 10.1).

7 Perform your general look

Although this aspect of the examination is put here, as your confidence and experience grows you will be doing this as soon as you are introduced to your patient. Observe their mood: are they anxious? A little anxiety is expected but it could also betray a more deep-seated fear of cancer. Are they low in mood? Do they look cachexic? suggesting the possibility of advanced cancer. Does one of their arms look much bigger than the other? This could suggest the possibility of lymphoedema. This could be as a result of infiltration of the lymphatic system by cancer preventing the drainage of fluid and leading to swelling of the arm. It can also be as a result of radiotherapy damaging the lymphatic vessels for treatment of breast cancer.

8 Ask some preparatory questions

Ask the patient. 'Is there any part of the breast that is painful or tender?' If there is a painful area it would be sensible to examine this last. Also ask, 'Have you noticed a lump or anything unusual with your breasts?'

If the patient has presented with a breast lump ask, 'Can you point with a finger to where the lump is?'

....
Tip
It can be helpful to put a small mark on the skin overlying the breast lump with a pen so that you can find it more readily later in the examination.
....

Examination of the breasts

9 Inspect the breasts

If the patient has a gown on at this point, ask them politely to remove it.

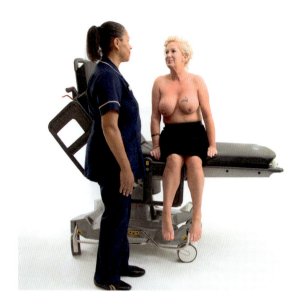

Figure 10.1 Starting position for examination.

Carefully inspect both breasts, both from an anterior view and from the side to ensure that there is no obvious distortion or abnormality in the contour of either breast. Make a note of the size and symmetry of each breast. There is usually a small degree of asymmetry between breasts. Be aware that your patient may have breast implants. See Case 10.3. The breasts may sit higher on the chest, seem rounder and appear unusually pert. Some women may not always volunteer straight away that they have had breast augmentation surgery. They may have bilateral transverse healed scars inferiorly under their breasts.

Check for erythema

Check the skin colour and look in particular for any signs of erythema. It is normal to see some linear reddening as a result of bra straps or underwiring. This can be more pronounced if the individual wears an ill-fitting bra. However, more confluent erythema, together with pain and warmth could suggest inflammation secondary to mastitis. Redness under the breast could be due to candidal infection as this site can get sweaty and together with poor hygiene can create the ideal condition for this fungal infection. Erythema can also be due to a more generalized skin condition such as psoriasis or eczema and there may be evidence elsewhere on the body. Occasionally the redness is due to radiation treatment for breast cancer and this possibility should be obvious from your history.

CASE 10.3

Problem: You have been told to go and examine a woman with bilateral silicone breast implants and you are concerned that you might be asked many difficult questions about implants and that examining the breast may be very difficult because of the presence of implants.

   Discussion: You should not attempt to answer the difficult questions about the implants should they arise. These are for the trained doctor to answer. Your patient may have implants as a result of four different situations: (1) She may have had previous breast cancer and required removal of her breasts with reconstruction using implants. (2) She may have had implants inserted as a cosmetic procedure. (3) She may have had breast implants inserted as one or both of her breasts did not develop normally. (4) The procedure may be part of the transformation of a patient who is transgender. In many of these situations you need to be sensitive to the fact that the patient may have some feeling of guilt or regret that they have implants as they may have received confusing advice and believe that the implants are hazardous to their health. It is very important not to be in any way judgemental and to stick to the facts. It should be explained that silicone implants have been used for about 50 years and there is considerable research evidence available. It is well known that silicone can escape from the implant into the surrounding tissue or migrate to the draining lymph nodes, for example, to the axilla. There is no convincing proof that leakage of this silicone causes any overall health problems. There is no evidence of additional cancer risk, that it leads to unusual illnesses such as connective tissue disorders, or that it interferes with the patient's immunological system. Silicone leakage can lead to firmness in the breast area or distortion, which can be uncomfortable or painful.

   Be reassured that it is just as easy to palpate a breast lump in a patient with implants as it is in any other woman. Also be aware when examining an augmented breast that you may encounter a palpable fold of the implant. This can be confirmed by exerting pressure on it with your palpating finger. It should return to its original position once the pressure is removed. It is essentially a herniation of the implant because there is insufficient breast tissue to cover it. Implants that have leaked silicone can produce surrounding fibrosis which can give rise to distortion and unusual palpable abnormalities.

Check for scars and dimpling

Having inspected the breasts quickly, now is the time to focus more closely to identify any subtle changes. Look to see if there are any scars that may suggest previous surgery. Surgeons are now more adept at hiding scars in skin creases and around the edge of the areolae to preserve the appearance of the breast. You may have to wait until you start palpating to ensure that you do not miss a scar hidden underneath the breast tissue. Look to see if there is any dimpling. Dimpling is where the normal surface appearance is disturbed and an area of skin appears to be pulled inward. In the absence of previous surgery this could indicate the presence of underlying cancer. Then look at the texture of the skin. In rare situations the texture can resemble orange peel (called 'peau d'orange' [*p-oh-duh-ronj*]). This can occur if there is localized infiltration or damage to the lymphatics leading to poor drainage of fluid and subcutaneous oedema. This localized swelling accentuates the skin pores (which do not swell); hence the resemblance to orange peel. This can be seen in some breast cancers or after radiation treatment with breast lymphoedema or with marked inflammation.

Look for ulceration

As with all ulcers seen elsewhere on the skin surface, make a note of the size of the ulcer and its general appearance. See Case 10.4. This will be useful when it comes to monitoring the effect of any intervention.

Causes

See Table 10.6.

Inspect the nipples

Finally, inspect the nipples. Are they symmetrical, or is one of the nipples flat or even inverted? Check with the patient if the inversion is long-standing or more recent. Women may worry that a recent inversion of the nipple is a feature of cancer. However, research has shown that an inverted nipple on its own even when of recent origin is unlikely to be due to cancer especially if the woman is under 50 years old, but the likelihood of cancer will increase if there is an association with a bloody discharge or palpable mass.

   Very occasionally there may be a scaly plaque or ulcer on the nipple and/or the surrounding areola. This may be associated with a weepy area that bleeds easily. This could

CASE 10.4

Problem: You see an older woman in a breast clinic who has been persuaded to attend by her family. She does not give any useful history and is very reluctant to be examined. However, when she does remove her gown, you are overwhelmed by a nasty smell coming from the breast and see a nasty fungating ulcer at 12 o'clock. The contour of the breast is clearly distorted by what looks like a large mass beneath the skin and the ulcer. You are astonished that the patient has allowed the situation to get this bad and you do not know where to start.

Discussion: First of all you should not be judgmental about your patient and try not to show any revulsion at the smell that is emanating from her breast. She will be all too aware of the smell herself and this may be one of the reasons that she has not presented herself for medical help. There may be many reasons why she has not accessed health care. People from certain ethnic groups, who may be recent immigrants, or asylum seekers, may not know how to access the health service. There are other transient groups such as gypsies or travellers who also traditionally do not engage with the health service. Some people are afraid to stop work because they are afraid of losing their jobs and have dependents. Other people may have learning difficulties; others have mental illness such as schizophrenia, depression, or dementia and cannot or will not see a doctor. Some people are just plain frightened of what might be found or are scared of doctors and hospitals. It would be useful to explore why this patient was reluctant to come to the breast clinic with the family who have accompanied her. In terms of her examination you will still need to be systematic and thorough despite your initial suspicions, while trying to be as sensitive as possible to your patient. One useful way of documenting the ulcer would be to take a picture, with the patient's consent. Otherwise record its dimensions, the appearance of the margins, any surrounding erythema and describe if slough is present in the base. If the ulcer smells, it suggests that there is an infection and this should be swabbed. Follow the routine below with regards to inspection and palpation of the breast and if you confirm a breast lump then record it as you would a lump found elsewhere in the body. Also assess its mobility. Check the axilla for lymphadenopathy and if you have reason to believe that you are dealing with an advanced cancer, assess other systems such as the abdomen for a liver, the respiratory system for a pleural effusion, etc.

Table 10.6 Causes of breast ulceration

Mastitis
Breast abscess
Trauma
Radiotherapy
Breast cancer invading skin
Paget's disease of nipple/breast

Key points

- Always begin with inspection and check for symmetry and for any distortion of the contour of the breasts
- Erythema of the breast can be caused by candidal infection, skin diseases or breast infection
- Look carefully for scars which may indicate previous surgery, especially around the margin of the areolae and inferiorly under the breast
- Do not forget to inspect the nipples for any abnormality including inversion, scaling or tell-tale crusting that may indicate a recent discharge

represent eczema especially if there is more widespread involvement of the skin elsewhere. It could also be Paget's disease of the nipple/breast, which is an uncommon form of breast cancer (see Fig. 10.2).

10 Examine the neck

With the patient sitting at the end of the couch or bed, go behind them in preparation to palpate the neck. Warn them that you are feeling for any lumps or bumps in the neck.

This aspect of the examination is optional so early in the examination but I find it useful for a number of reasons. The patient is already in the optimal position to perform the examination. Also I find that it helps the patient to get used to my touch on a less 'sensitive' part of the body before palpating the breasts. Use the distal pulps of the flat of your hand to examine the neck and supraclavicular region (see Chapter 11).

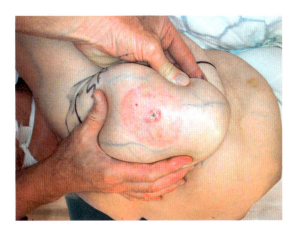

Figure 10.2 Paget's disease of the nipple.

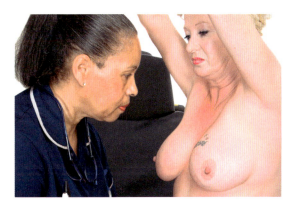

Figure 10.3 Inspection of the breasts.

11 Ask your patient to elevate both arms and inspect the breasts again

Get your patient to lift both outstretched arms vertically and to look forwards (see Fig. 10.3). Again if, there is no previous surgery or trauma there are very few benign causes for an abnormal breast contour or distortion of the breast (see Fig. 10.4). At this point the breast can be lifted or moved in order to gain a view of the entire breast surface (see Fig. 10.5); just warn your patient before you do so. Doing this will allow you to find surgical scars or rashes that may have been hidden under breast tissue.

12 With the arms still raised vertically or alternatively placed behind the head palpate the breasts systematically

It is often best to start with the normal breast and to palpate the area of concern last in case there is some associated

(a)

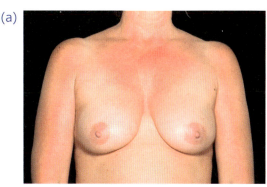

(b)

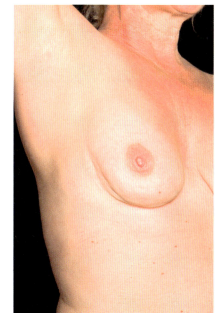

Figure 10.4 (a) The breasts appear normal in this relaxed position. (b) Dimpling of the lateral surface of the right breast only becomes obvious on elevation of the arms.

tenderness which may make the patient more tense. Use the flat of the fingers and press gently on the breast, making small circular movements (see Fig. 10.6). The consistency of the breast tissue should be appreciated by the distal pulps of the index and middle fingers as it presses the breast substance against the chest wall. The aim is to be systematic so that the entire breast is checked. There are a number of strategies that can be used to achieve this (see Fig. 10.7). Now palpate the affected breast and pay particular attention to the area of concern indicated by the patient. Make a mental note of any areas that appear different on

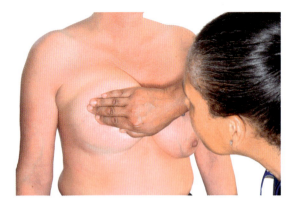

Figure 10.5 Displacement of the breast for inspection of hidden areas.

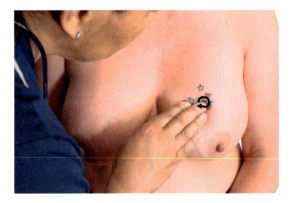

Figure 10.6 Palpation of the breast.

palpation. Is there any thickening or a discrete swelling with a distinguishable border? Sometimes you may have to vary the pressure and depth of your palpating hand to locate small lesions. Whatever strategy you adopt make sure the nipple is carefully inspected and the area directly behind the nipple is also palpated. It must be remembered that the breast continues towards the medial part of the axilla and this part of the breast should also be carefully examined. See Cases 10.5 and 10.6.

How to examine a breast lump

If you do find a lump or abnormality, then you need to be able to describe it as you would any other swelling in the body (see Chapters 7 and 11). It is also important to describe its location so that other healthcare professionals can find it. There are two main ways of noting your findings: either by mapping the lump to quadrants or to a clock face (see Fig. 10.8). If you are working in a breast clinic that integrates investigations as part of the overall assessment, then the pen-mark you made earlier may help when the patient is undergoing ultrasound.

Assess the mobility of the lump

The mobility of a breast lump is an important feature. Grasp the lump between the index finger and thumb and try to move it in different planes. If you can move the lump within the breast more than 2 cm it is unlikely to be a cancer and is likely to be a fibroadenoma. If there is restriction of the lump's mobility then this could indicate a cancerous lump. See Case 10.7.

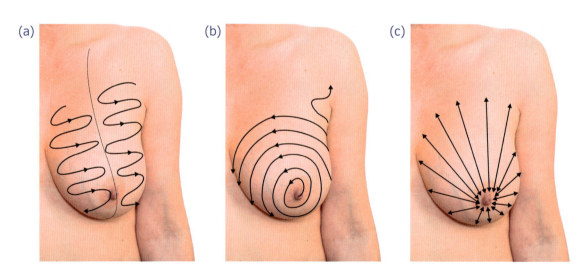

Figure 10.7 (a) Strategy for breast palpation; top to bottom for each half of the breast. (b) Spiralling outward from the nipple. (c) Wedge or spokes pattern.

CASE 10.5

Problem: You are asked to examine a woman who has reported that she has 'lumpy breasts' and you are uncertain if you are feeling a true lump or perhaps just fibrous tissue.

Discussion: Remember that most lumpy areas do not represent any pathology and are common findings in a breast examination. Also once you have completed your examination you should have a feel for the natural consistency of the breasts. So you are trying to pick up an abnormality or area which is out of the ordinary. It is perfectly reasonable to conclude that you have not found a definitive lump within the breast but in your description or with a diagram you can illustrate areas where you felt a thickening or firmness within the breast. In these circumstances you may need help from your diagnostic tests.

CASE 10.6

Problem: You are asked to examine a patient who has very large breasts and you are concerned that you might miss a clinical abnormality.

Discussion: The examination of large breasts is difficult for all clinicians, even those who are very experienced at breast palpation. Also you must be sensitive to your patient who may be embarrassed by the size of them. Ensure you follow your structured routine and examine each breast systematically and carefully in a professional manner. It is perfectly acceptable to ask your patient to lift their breast to one side or the other in order to facilitate your palpation. When the patient is lying supine you can use your non-palpating hand to lift the breast from out of the axilla so you can examine all of it more easily. Finally, you should remember the incidence of cancer is no greater in a large breast than in a smaller one.

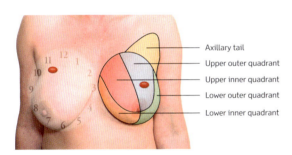

Axillary tail
Upper outer quadrant
Upper inner quadrant
Lower outer quadrant
Lower inner quadrant

Figure 10.8 Describing the position of a breast lump using the clockface method (right breast) or the quadrants method (left breast). The lump on the right is at 11 o'clock and the lump on the left is in the upper outer quadrant.

Demonstrating fixity of the breast lump to overlying skin

Gently pinch the skin overlying the lump in a few areas. If the skin moves freely over the swelling then there is no infiltration of the skin. If it does not move then this suggests that the breast lump has infiltrated and become fixed to the skin.

Demonstrating skin tethering

As you assess the mobility of the breast lump, if the skin puckers inwards on movement of the lump this suggests that the lump has infiltrated the supporting ligaments (of Astley-Cooper). If this has occurred then movement of the lump will pull the ligament, which in turn will cause

indrawing of the skin to which it is attached. If the lump is large enough, dimpling of the skin can be seen readily without movement of the lump or the dimpling may be seen when elevating the arms.

Demonstrating fixity to the pectoralis major muscle

If a cancerous lump is large and aggressive enough it can invade the pectoralis major muscle that lies behind the breast. Grasp the lump as before and move it around in different planes. Note how mobile the lump is. Now ask your patient to put her hands on her hips and to push into her waist. This should cause contraction of both pectoralis major muscles (see Fig. 10.9). Now try to move the lump again. If the movement is restricted compared to when the muscle was in its relaxed state this confirms that the breast lump is fixed to the pectoralis major muscle. Note that there will always be some movement because of the elasticity of the muscle fibres. Also you may notice that you cannot get your fingers behind the lump.

Tip

If you are unsure if the pectoralis major muscle is contracting or not, you can confirm it by palpating the anterior axillary fold between your thumb and index finger. This anterior axillary fold is predominantly the insertion of this muscle as it attaches to the humerus.

CASE 10.7

Problem: When you examine a woman and find a lump in the breast you are not able to decide from your clinical examination if it is malignant or benign and you wonder what you should say to the patient.

Discussion: There is no absolutely reliable means of knowing whether a breast lump is malignant or benign purely on physical examination. This is the reason why the process of triple assessment is so important. Nevertheless there are certain features that will point you in one direction or the other. If the lump is highly mobile it is less likely to be a cancer. If the lump is very firm and has an indistinct border to it, and particularly if there is some distortion of the surface or appearance of the overlying skin, then it is more likely to be a cancer.

However, you can only make a precise diagnosis with a combination of imaging with ultrasound (and mammography depending on age) along with obtaining a tissue diagnosis. In reality you should not have to deal with tricky questions like this and you should pass it on to a trained doctor and watch how they deal with the situation. The best approach is to be open and frank with the patient and confirm that a lump was found in the breast and that further investigations are now needed to try and determine the nature of that lump. If the patient asks directly whether the lump could be a cancer it is best to say that that is possible but there are also other possibilities and that they need to wait for the results of the investigations.

Demonstrating fixity to the chest wall

On rare occasions a cancer can invade posteriorly through to the chest wall and become fixed to the ribs and intercostal muscles. If the lump is large you may have to recruit your third and fourth fingers to hold it. Again try to move it in different planes. If it is fixed to the chest wall there will be no movement of the lump at all or you may succeed in moving the patient. Also you will be unable to get your fingers behind the lump.

Tip

A useful feature to help you anticipate the possibility of fixity of a lump to the pectoralis major muscle or the chest wall is to get your patient to bend forwards. Normally both breasts should swing forwards freely in unison; however, if there is invasion into the posterior structures the affected breast will lag behind the normal one. (You may notice this as your patient changes position during the examination!)

13 Examine the axillae for lymphadenopathy

The patient can relax their arms and palpation of the axilla can be performed (see Fig. 10.10). Follow the routine described in Chapter 5.

Small lymph glands are a normal finding. Significantly enlarged lymph nodes (approximately more than 15 mm in diameter) are of greater concern. The characteristics of the lymph glands should also be noted (see Chapter 5). If lymph glands are hard, irregular, and demonstrate

Key points

- If a breast lump is found make sure you document its location
- Make sure you assess the lump as you would any mass found in the body
- Assess the mobility of the lump and ensure there is no fixity to skin or to underlying structures
- The only sure way of determining the nature of a lump is through triple assessment

minimal or no mobility this would strongly suggest spread of cancer to those lymph glands.

14 Ask your patient to lie supine and to place both hands behind her head

This stretches the skin of the breast and the inferior half of the breast becomes more visible and easier to palpate.

15 Repeat the inspection of the breasts

(See Fig. 10.11)

16 Repeat the palpation of the breasts

17 Assessment of nipple discharge if relevant

If a patient complains of a nipple discharge and there is no ulceration or laceration of the nipple, the nipples should

(a) (b)

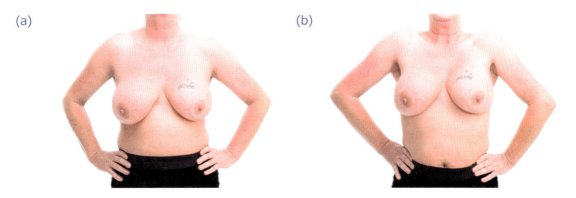

Figure 10.9 (a) Hands on hips prior to contraction. (b) Hands squeezing the waist to produce contraction of pectoralis major.

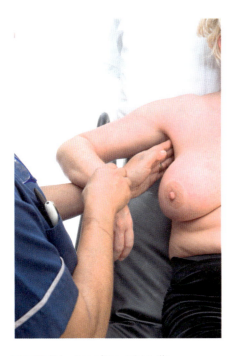

Figure 10.10 Palpation of the right axilla.

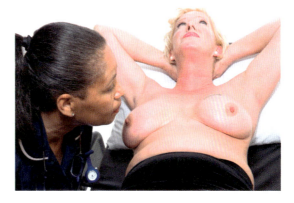

Figure 10.11 Further inspection in the supine position.

....

Tip

If the discharge looks bloodstained it can be useful to express a drop on to a white tissue. This is because sometimes a green discharge on the nipple surface can resemble a bloodstained discharge, especially in poor lighting.

....

be wiped clean with an alcohol steret and then carefully inspected to see if there is any visible discharge. If a green or grey/white discharge is seen no further action is required as this is a normal physiological phenomenon. However, if you confirm a bloodstained discharge, then this is a serious development and could herald cancer. A senior doctor may place some of the discharge on glass slides for a pathologist to examine for the presence of malignant epithelial cells (the investigation of nipple discharge for cytology). There is controversy in the literature whether this test is a reliable and worthwhile investigation.

After the breast examination

18 Examine other relevant systems if applicable

If you have a strong suspicion that you are dealing with an advanced cancer (i.e. a hard irregular lump with lymphadenopathy) then it may be prudent to check other systems in case there is evidence of more distant spread. An examination of the respiratory system may demonstrate a pleural effusion, or there may be hepatomegaly on abdominal palpation.

19 Ask your patient to dress again

Conclude the examination by asking your patient to get dressed.

···
Tip
It is very useful to get the chaperone to ask your patient if the examination has been satisfactory and has not caused any undue anxiety or concern. This can help to flag up any problems early and to clear up any misunderstandings.
···

20 Wash your hands

While your patient is getting dressed in private take this opportunity to wash your hands.

21 Report your findings

Say something like,

> **'This is a 62-year-old woman who presents with a lump in the right breast. There is no associated pain but she has noticed a bloodstained discharge on some occasions. She has also lost 6 kg in weight in the last 2 months. On examination she has a hard irregular lump in the upper outer quadrant (10 o'clock) of the right breast, with some associated skin tethering. She also has significant lymphadenopathy in the right axilla which is enlarged, hard, and irregular. The lungs are clear and there is no hepatomegaly. The most likely diagnosis is breast cancer with spread to axillary lymph nodes.'**

This report conveys the essentials of the case and also demonstrates that this student was alert to possible spread beyond the breast by the important negatives displayed towards the end.

Breast diseases and investigations

Earlier in this chapter, I have mentioned various medical conditions and investigations. In this section I now describe them. In general these descriptions are brief though certain selected topics are discussed in some detail.

Cyclical mastalgia

The cause of cyclical mastalgia is unknown but it appears that some areas of breast tissue can be more sensitive to normal circulating levels of hormones and therefore experience an exaggerated response during hormonal flux. It is this localization of pain that may lead patients to conclude that there must be a sinister problem at that site. Examination of the breast is best conducted in the first half of the menstrual cycle when hormonal influences are least evident. Once confident that you are dealing with ANDI and cyclical mastalgia then you will be able to reassure your patient that they do not have a life-threatening illness. You can inform them that it is a self-limiting condition of unknown cause and does not confer any increased risk of current or future breast cancer development. Treatment includes simple physical measures such as a well-fitted support bra, simple analgesics, or taking oil of evening primrose. Oil of evening primrose medication is available over the counter and needs to be taken regularly over a number of weeks before any relief is experienced. Although oil of evening primrose is recommended by certain adherents, the evidence for its efficacy beyond a placebo effect is weak. Regardless of what treatment is used, patients are encouraged to fill in a pain diary before starting medication to try to determine whether the treatment is beneficial.

Benign breast nodularity

When investigating the possibility of benign breast nodularity it is very helpful to re-examine the patient early in the first half of the menstrual cycle when the lumpiness may be least prominent. This will often coincide with the breast tissue being less tender, to permit a more thorough examination. As for mastalgia, the management of benign breast nodularity includes reassurance and simple supportive measures. In the past, excision of affected areas caused scarring and distortion of the breast and did not always abolish symptoms.

Lactational infection

Infection of the breast is more commonly associated with breastfeeding, when it is called lactational infection. Breastfeeding can create the ideal environment for infection as pressure and moisture from the baby's mouth can cause small cracks in the skin of the nipple or breast allowing entry of the microorganisms. Women who are diabetics or are immunosuppressed will be more susceptible. Breast infections like infection/inflammation at other sites, present with skin erythema, stretching and swelling of the skin, with pain and tenderness over the affected area. They may also exhibit constitutional symptoms, from a feeling of being 'off-colour' to being feverish and very unwell.

The management of lactational infection is to encourage the mother to continue to breastfeed including from the affected breast. There is no risk to the baby from this practice. The local application of heat and gentle massage may help the flow of milk and simple analgesics such as paracetamol will help the discomfort and are safe for the baby. Most of these infections are due to staphylococcus bacteria and are sensitive to the antibiotic flucloxacillin. If the complaint does not respond to the antibiotics and the pain and localized physical signs become more prominent with a swinging pyrexia then a breast abscess may have developed. The management of a breast abscess has changed in recent years and now consists of aspiration of the abscess, either blind or under ultrasound guidance. This process can be repeated over the following days until the abscess is eradicated and the patient is maintained on antibiotics during that time. If the breast skin overlying the abscess becomes unhealthy, thin, and loses its viability then that skin will require incision and the underlying abscess is drained through that incision. Once the abscess is drained and any associated cellulitis has disappeared then antibiotics are no longer required.

Non-lactational breast infection

This type of breast infection is uncommon although it is present more frequently in smokers. The infection tends to be centred around the nipple/areola complex and in this context is termed periductal mastitis. Frequently the infection will be situated superficially in the breast and can be slow to heal after intervention. Sometimes a mammillary fistula can occur (a fistula is a persistent track between two epithelial surfaces), for example, between the nipple duct and the breast skin in this instance (see Fig. 10.12). The successful eradication of non-lactational breast sepsis can be very difficult. In the acute phase patients are treated with antibiotics. If there are recurrent bouts of infection there may be other organisms involved with staphylococcus such as Gram-negative bacteria. Send any swabs for culture and seek guidance from your microbiology department. If the abscess is amenable to percutaneous aspiration then this is the preferred method of management. The patient is advised that if they continue to smoke it is likely that they will have repeated bouts of infection and that the problem may not

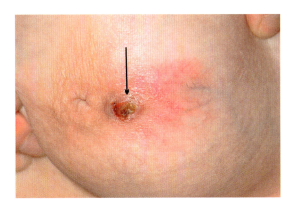

Figure 10.12 Mammillary fistula.

resolve. They should also be warned that they could still be affected even after they stop smoking. Surgery to disconnect all of the milk ducts from the back of the nipple can be employed in specific instances to try and reduce the frequency of non-lactational breast sepsis. The outcome from this type of surgery is variable.

Benign breast lumps

Fibroadenoma

Fibroadenomas are a definite discrete circumscribed mass or lump which occurs frequently in younger women. It is commonest in the 15–25-year age group. On palpation they are firm with a well-defined border and characteristically are mobile within the breast such that on palpation they can be moved more than 2 cm from their initial position by the palpating fingers. They are sometimes called breast mice because of their mobility. The cause for the development of fibroadenomas is unknown. Most reach a certain size and do not grow any further. Some women may have multiple fibroadenomas in one or both breasts.

As well as the characteristic clinical signs the diagnosis is confirmed by their appearance on ultrasound examination and usually a biopsy is obtained for the histopathologist to confirm that it is a fibroadenoma. There is no extra risk of developing breast cancer but there is an increased risk of developing further fibroadenomas in either breast in the future. The fibroadenoma may occasionally be symptomatic if it catches on a bra strap but most fibroadenomas are no longer removed from patients.

Cyst

A cyst is a fluid-filled swelling. They are a common finding in the breasts of women usually between the ages of 35 and 50. Other glands that are also subjected to hormonal influences, such as the thyroid and ovary, form similar swellings. They have a thin-walled envelope and feel smooth on palpation. Some will feel firm and others may be more yielding with a consistency similar to a grape. They are also slightly mobile. Patients may have multiple breast cysts. Cysts can be aspirated with a needle and syringe, and if the lump resolves and there is no old blood in the aspirate no further analysis is required.

Sometimes cysts are found incidentally on imaging of the breast but are not clinically significant and do not require any treatment. Some patients produce multiple cysts which can be distressing, but unfortunately there is no medical intervention that can reduce cyst formation. Cysts are less common after the menopause. Cysts do not have malignant potential but beware the breast swelling that demonstrates cyst-like characteristics but does not empty completely when aspirated or contains old blood in the aspirate. This situation requires further investigation because some cancers can be partially cystic.

Hamartoma/neurofibroma/lipoma

These are a variety of tumour-like growths that can arise in other parts of the body. A hamartoma is an overgrowth of mature cells and tissue that occur in the area that they arise from. With respect to the breast the hamartoma will consist of fibrous tissue fat and associated breast ductules. A hamartoma is softer in consistency than a fibroadenoma. A neurofibroma is a lump of tissue derived from nerve origin. Some people have a congenital condition, neurofibromatosis (see Chapter 6), where they have multiple neurofibromas at many body sites including the breasts. A lipoma is a fatty lump and its characteristic feature is that it feels as if it is slipping away from the palpating fingers (the 'slipping edge' sign of lipomas). All of these diagnoses can be suspected on clinical examination and confirmed on investigations which would include ultrasound and biopsy.

Pathological nipple discharge

Patients who are suspected of having a pathological discharge require very careful examination of the breast along with appropriate breast imaging to determine if there is evidence of a cancer within that breast. It is important to note that it is possible for the causative cancer to be a good distance away from the nipple. About 15–20% of women with a history of a pathological nipple discharge will have an associated malignancy within that breast. Analyses of samples of the discharge for their cellular content (nipple

discharge cytology) are not a sensitive or helpful investigation. Opinion is divided in the medical literature as to whether testing the nipple discharge for microscopic red blood cells is of assistance in confirming whether the discharge is indeed bloodstained. In recent years thin fibreoptic devices (fibreoptic breast duct endoscopy) have been developed to try and inspect these breast ducts but this method of investigation has not been universally adopted. It is not always technically straightforward and may not always provide an accurate diagnosis.

If a cancer is found then its management is as below (see 'Breast cancer' section). If no malignancy is diagnosed then a woman with a pathological nipple discharge will require excision of the relevant breast ducts to determine if there is any neoplastic process within them on histological examination. If there is no neoplastic process then one common cause is duct ectasia. This can occur following previous breastfeeding or infection. A duct can get blocked, which leads to a dilatation of the duct and thickening of the walls. Later fibrosis may occur which can shorten the ducts and lead to nipple inversion.

Another common cause of a pathological nipple discharge is the presence of a wart-like lesion in a breast duct, which is called a papilloma and is not a cancerous lesion. Papillomas are frequently excised in order to confirm the diagnosis.

Prolactinoma

A prolactinoma is a benign pituitary tumour. Pituitary tumours can be regarded as functioning tumours or non-functioning tumours depending on their activity. Functioning tumours are those that produce excessive amounts of one or more hormones and prolactinomas produce excess prolactin hormone. This is the hormone that stimulates breast milk secretion and its concentration is naturally higher during pregnancy and during breastfeeding. Therefore one of the effects of a prolactinoma is the production of breast milk in a non-pregnant female (and rarely in a male). Prolactin has other effects and so can lead to other symptoms and signs. Patients will have scantier periods (oligomenorrhea) or will not have periods at all (amenorrhoea) and a prolactinoma can therefore be a cause of infertility. It will also diminish libido and in men can cause impotence. It can also be a cause of hypogonadism, where there is a decrease in the function of sexual organs and the loss of secondary sexual characteristics.

Another means of classifying pituitary tumours is according to their size: tumours that are less than 1 cm in size are called microadenomas and those that are larger than 1 cm are called macroadenomas. As the tumour increases in size it can also produce other effects such as headaches or, with encroachment on the optic chiasma above, lead to bitemporal hemianopia. It can also interfere with the normal secretion of other hormones such as adrenocorticotropic hormone (ACTH) also called corticotropin, thyroid stimulating hormone (TSH) also called thyrotropin, gonadotrophins (luteinizing hormone [LH] and follicle-stimulating hormone [FSH]), and growth hormone (GH), leading to their deficiencies.

When investigating for a prolactinoma care must be taken with the interpretation of serum prolactin levels because they can vary considerably in the normal population. It may be increased by stress or with certain drugs, although if very high concentrations are found it may make the diagnosis of a prolactinoma more likely. If you suspect a prolactinoma then the patient requires assessment in a specialist endocrine clinic. The work-up should include an assessment of pituitary function looking at the various hormones produced and the target organs that they stimulate. If the patient's vision is impaired they should be assessed by an ophthalmologist including assessment of their visual fields. The investigation of choice for making the diagnosis is an MRI scan which has superseded CT scanning.

Treatment for small uncomplicated tumours is with bromocriptine, a dopamine agonist which inhibits the action of prolactin. In those who do not respond to bromocriptine, cabergoline can be tried. If there is a failure of medical treatment or there is a large tumour then surgery will be required. Sometimes a combination of surgery and bromocriptine is used. Other complications such as hypopituitarism or visual disturbance may need to be addressed.

Breast implants

The first recorded breast augmentation using a silicone prosthesis occurred in 1962 in the United States. There are two main types of implants in current use: the silicone implant that has a silicone shell filled with silicone gel, and the saline implant that has a silicone shell filled with saline solution. Early implants have been prone to leaking silicone into the surrounding tissues, giving rise to an irregular firm shell-like texture known as capsule formation. This is associated with distortion of the surrounding breast tissue and irregular lumpy areas on palpation of the breast. It can be very difficult to exclude the presence of a coexistent cancer within these areas and more direct investigations including tissue biopsies are required.

The presence of breast implants can give rise to technical difficulties in performing mammography and can

diminish the sensitivity of the test. There is no increased risk of developing breast cancer with breast implants, nor with leakage of silicone into the tissues. There is also no evidence that the leakage of silicone is associated with connective tissue disorders.

Gynaecomastia

Commonly presents in the teenage years after the onset of puberty, or in older men. The cause of gynaecomastia is unknown in the majority of individuals. The condition may only be present in one breast. In the younger male a testicular examination should be performed as part of the clinical examination. If there is any doubt then blood estimation of markers for testicular tumours can be performed as well as ultrasound of the testes to look for any abnormality. In older men, medical causes and drugs have to be ruled out as discussed in Chapter 7.

Triple assessment

The foundation for the accurate determination of the cause of a breast complaint is a process called triple assessment. This consists of clinical findings (history and physical examination), appropriate breast imaging, and cytopathology. The appropriate breast imaging is determined for each individual patient. If the patient has localized symptoms, particularly if they complain of a lump in the breast or if the clinician finds discrete abnormalities on palpation, then those sites are subjected to an ultrasound examination (targeted ultrasound).

Over the age of 40 all symptomatic patients will have mammography which will assess both breasts including the area of concern. Mammography provides further information regarding the surrounding breast tissue, local extension of that cancer, as well as the possible presence of other cancer sites in either breast. If a cancer of the breast is strongly suspected the axillary area on that side should have an ultrasound examination to detect any abnormal lymph glands, which can then be biopsied. The third component of triple assessment is cytopathology, where a needle is inserted into the abnormal area following the application of local anaesthetic and a sample of that area is removed. Negative pressure on a needle attached to a syringe will provide cell samples and this is called fine needle aspiration for cytology. This method of sampling is now less commonly used. More frequently the clinician will use a device that removes small cylinders of tissue from the abnormality; this is performed under local anaesthetic either by palpation of the lump or with ultrasound guidance and is known as core biopsy.

Triple assessment ensures that a breast cancer diagnosis is not overlooked because each component of the assessment can miss cancers when used individually. It is best practice that the results of these investigations are discussed at regular meetings by a multidisciplinary team of expert health professionals to optimize the management of patients and to minimize the risk of missing a breast cancer diagnosis.

Breast cancer

The following section is intended to provide a broad outline on breast cancer and is not intended to be comprehensive. Breast cancer is the commonest cancer in women and its incidence rises with age. It will affect approximately 1 in 10 of all women over their lifetime. It is very uncommon for breast cancer to occur under the age of 30 and rare under the age of 25. Most breast cancers are sporadic, which means that there is no discernible reason why the patient has developed the disease. Approximately 5% or less of breast cancer is familial, due to the presence of a gene abnormality that has been handed down through either the maternal or paternal blood line. There are a number of gene abnormalities that have been sequenced but the ones that are more publicized are the *BRCA1*, *BRCA2*, and *TP53* genes. It is important when taking a family history of breast cancer to establish an accurate picture of involvement. In general the involvement of a first-degree relative is of much greater significance than that of a third-degree relative (see Table 10.3). The risk of breast cancer increases (1) as more relatives are involved, particularly first-degree relatives; (2) if their cancer occurred at a young age (especially <40 years); (3) if they occur in both breasts; (4) if male relatives are involved; and (5) if relatives have had ovarian or other unusual cancers. The Ashkenazi Jewish population also have an increased incidence of breast cancer of the familial type. See NICE guidance about determining risk in familial breast cancer (see 'References and further reading').

The strongest risk factor for the development of a primary breast cancer is a past history of a cancer diagnosed in either breast. Another risk factor is the use of hormone replacement therapy. There is a small but definite increased risk of future breast cancer when receiving hormone replacement therapy and this risk increases the longer a woman is exposed to the medication. A rare but proven risk factor is having received extensive radiotherapy at an earlier age for lymphoma.

Patients with breast cancer are traditionally divided into two broad categories with respect to treatment: operable breast cancer and locally advanced–metastatic breast cancer.

Operable breast cancer

Patients with operable breast cancer have a tumour that is contained within the breast without ulceration of the overlying skin of the breast or marked inflammation of the breast and without involvement of the underlying rib cage. There may be spread to the axillary lymph glands but the cancer will still be considered operable if those lymph glands are mobile and not fixed to skin or muscle. The treatments for these patients consist of a combination of surgery, radiotherapy, and systemic treatment (the administration of drugs which will then circulate in the bloodstream to the whole body).

The surgical component of treatment consists of an operation to remove the malignancy. The extent of that surgery is determined by the width of the cancer within the breast and whether it is located in only one part or in multiple sites within the breast. A large cancer or cancer in multiple sites in the breast would require removal of the entire breast (called a mastectomy). Removal of part of the breast that contains the cancer (called wide local excision) is the most common surgical operation for breast cancer and requires postoperative examination of the excised specimen by the pathologist to ensure that no cancer extends to the edges. Later radiotherapy is administered to the rest of the breast. Radiotherapy is also given to approximately one-third of patients who have had a mastectomy.

A proportion of operable breast cancers (approximately 30–40%) will have tumour spread via the lymphatic vessels to the lymph glands in the axilla. This is a poor prognostic sign. These patients are more likely to have future cancer spread identified at other body sites as the cells clearly have the capability to migrate and this may have already occurred before diagnosis. They will also have an increased risk of death from the disease. Traditionally all the lymph glands in the axilla were removed for the pathologist to determine whether spread had occurred. Currently the axilla is investigated before surgery, particularly with ultrasound to check for spread. If no spread has been demonstrated by this test, then during breast surgery the first one or two lymph glands that drain the affected part of the breast (called the sentinel node/s) are removed and are sent for examination by the pathologist. If the sentinel node does not contain malignancy the other lymph glands do not need to be removed. This is important because it spares the patient from developing lymphoedema of the arm, which is an important complication of axillary lymph node clearance.

Systemic treatment

The systemic drug treatment component of breast cancer management is provided in order to treat any breast cancer cells which may have spread to other organs within the body prior to breast cancer excision. As these are only cells or small collections of cells they will not be visible on any body scans or detectable by any blood tests (known as occult metastatic disease). The purpose of the drug treatment is to try and eradicate these cancer cells when they are comparatively small in volume. This concept is known as adjuvant systemic treatment. The drugs used fall into three categories. The first group are anti-hormonal and more specifically anti-oestrogen treatments, the best known of which is tamoxifen. This anti-oestrogenic treatment is effective when the breast cancer cells possess oestrogen receptors on their cell surfaces. If these receptors are not present then there is no benefit from receiving this treatment. The exception to this rule is where a small proportion of cancers which are oestrogen receptor negative display positive progesterone receptor activity. They should also receive anti-oestrogen therapies as it is felt that the negative oestrogen receptor result represents a methodological anomaly rather than the true position.

The second drug grouping of anti-cancer drugs is known as chemotherapy and is usually given intravenously. The third drug treatment is traztuzumab (Herceptin), a drug specifically designed to treat breast cancer cells that are shown to possess intrinsic genetic abnormalities with overamplification of the *HER2* gene. Cancers that possess such overamplification of the *HER2* gene tend to behave more aggressively and traztuzumab has proven efficacy in their treatment. Traztuzumab is only given when combined with chemotherapy.

Locally advanced-metastatic breast cancer

Patients who present with locally advanced-metastatic breast cancer are very unlikely to receive total cure of their cancer from any treatment or treatment combination (see Fig. 10.13). In those instances treatment is very much focused on minimizing any symptoms such as pain. In these cases radiotherapy and selected drug therapy may be used. If the cancer disseminates via the bloodstream, it can metastasize to any site within the body. The most common sites seen in clinical practice are spread to bone, liver, lungs, and brain.

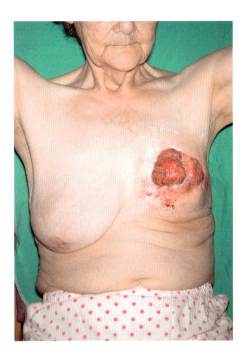

Figure 10.13 Locally invasive carcinoma.

Breast screening

Many countries including the UK offer screening to a population considered to be at high risk of developing a disease in the hope that early detection may improve outcomes for them. Breast screening in the UK offers mammography every 3 years to women aged between 47 and 73 years of age. No further investigation is performed unless the mammogram shows an abnormality or the patient reports a specific breast complaint at the time of the mammogram.

Breast screening detects a large number of asymptomatic breast cancers and the overall survival for such patients from the time of diagnosis is longer than for patients who are diagnosed following symptoms. However, this difference on its own does not prove that breast screening improves survival. If both screened patients and those with symptoms die at the same stage, all screening would have achieved would be an earlier diagnosis and awareness. This prolonged awareness of the disease could be misconstrued as a longer survival when this is not the case. In screening this is called **lead time bias**. To improve survival it has to be demonstrated that a patient has lived longer as a result of having their breast cancer found before symptoms develop than they would have lived if they had waited until the breast cancer had caused symptoms. Another form of bias that affects breast screening is that slow-growing, less aggressive tumours are more likely to be detected because the rapid doubling time of very aggressive tumours mean they are more likely to be symptomatic early. Hence if screening detects predominantly slow-growing tumours it will appear to produce a greater survival rate. This form of bias is called **length time bias**. In fact a small proportion of tumours may never have become symptomatic and patients may have been subjected to unnecessary breast surgery. However, because it is unclear which of these tumours would have developed metastatic potential, the pragmatic step is to remove all such tumours. There is no doubt that screening will save the lives of some women but the debate for health policy makers hinges on whether sufficient women benefit to justify the costs of the screening programme and a recognition of the harm some other women experience who have false-positive diagnoses or may have had unnecessary surgery for cancers that were never going to progress significantly during their lifetime.

Finals section

For revision, read the examination summary and the key points throughout the chapter and answer the questions at the end of the chapter. The good news is there are only a limited number of breast abnormalities you can be exposed to in your Finals. It is important for students to remember that examiners will be assessing your professionalism and sensitivity as well as your examination technique. Some medical schools have access to manikins that can have a variety of lumps placed inside them, and these can be used in examinations.

Key diagnostic clues

The examination of the breast is much more straightforward than that of the major systems. If you stick to your examination routine you should discover the answer. The likeliest abnormality you will encounter in the Finals is a breast lump with or without enlarged axillary nodes. It is also possible to have a patient with advanced breast cancer with hepatomegaly or ascites; or with a mastectomy with subsequent breast reconstruction.

The main clue to look for is skin dimpling, as this may hint at an underlying breast lump. If you are dealing with a breast lump the key feature is the mobility of the lump. If a lump is very mobile it is likely to be benign (in a young woman the diagnosis is likely to be a fibroadenoma). If the lump is fixed to any structures it is likely to be malignant (especially in an older woman, if it is hard with an irregular border). Even if a mobile lump proves to be an early cancer there is a greater chance of cure or control at this stage.

Some advice relating to examination

General

Use the breast examination routine given in this chapter.

The instruction

Carefully listen to what the examiner asks you to do. If you are doing an OSCE then read your instructions carefully. It is of particular importance in a breast examination that you engage with the patient, ask them if they are comfortable, explain what it is that you are going to do, and gain informed consent. Let them know that you may be speaking to the examiner throughout your examination. If you are faced with a manikin it is good practice to say to your examiners something like, 'Normally I would introduce myself to the patient and gain informed consent, and I would also ask them if they would like a chaperone present for the examination.' Even if this is not the focus of your examination it will show the examiners that you are fully conversant with these important aspects. More importantly some medical schools may allocate marks to these processes so don't forget.

General look

The patient should remove the clothes from the upper half of her body and sit on the edge of the couch or on the bed facing you. Try to ensure that your eyes are roughly at her level. Be systematic in your approach and use the routine that has been recommended. Check the hairline. Is the patient pale and appear to be wearing a wig? Are they cachexic? Is one arm larger than the other, suggesting lymphoedema? Let your wide-angled general look now become more focused for your inspection of the breasts.

Check for abnormalities in the outline or contour of the breast, particularly skin dimpling. Also check for any skin erythema. This could suggest an underlying infection. Do not be afraid to move the breast from side to side so you can see all of its surfaces including the medial, lateral, and inferior aspects. Also look carefully for any scars which may suggest previous surgery. Try not to miss the small ones which could indicate a recent biopsy procedure. Get the patient to raise her arms vertically in the air and again look for any skin dimpling.

Feel

Palpate the breast in an organized structured manner and ensure that you are using the flat of your fingers. Avoid using pinching movements and make sure that you check at intervals that your patient is comfortable. As in the routine recommended, examine the patient initially sitting up and then lying supine. **Do not forget to palpate the axillae**.

If you find any breast swelling, determine all the usual features required such as firmness, border, etc. and pay particular attention to its relationship to the overlying skin and to the deep muscles. **Always assess its mobility**.

Examination of other areas

If you suspect advanced breast cancer explain to the examiner that because you suspect a 'mitotic lesion' you would now like to proceed to examine other possible sites of spread such as the neck for lymphadenopathy, the lungs for a pleural effusion and the abdomen for any evidence of hepatomegaly. Although in the exam situation your patient will probably know their diagnosis, it is better to use a euphemism while you are still in the throes of speculation. It will also head off any awkward questions if you are completely wrong in your analysis. The examiner will usually be reassured by your reasoning and is unlikely to ask you to proceed further. If they do: **be vigilant!** as the likelihood of further signs is very high indeed.

Presentation

Try to be confident and avoid the words 'seem' or 'might'. Remember the key term to use if you find any breast abnormality is **triple assessment**. This will communicate to the examiners that you are familiar with the optimal process for making a diagnosis.

If as part of the subsequent discussion your differential diagnosis suggests a breast cancer, be sensitive to how you communicate this to your examiner in the presence of your patient. The patient deserves to be told in a prepared and sensitive way, rather than from fragments of an overheard conversation. Remember there may be OSCE stations that can investigate how you break bad news to people.

Good luck!

Questions

1 Can you remember what the abbreviation ANDI stands for and what it is?
2 What factors make an inherited form of breast cancer more likely?
3 What is involved in the triple assessment of a breast abnormality?
4 Give five causes of hyperprolactinaemia
5 What is meant by lead time bias and length time bias in breast screening?
6 What clinical features would make a breast lump more likely to be malignant?
7 In breast cancer, where are the common sites for metastasis?
8 How do you demonstrate fixity of a lump to the pectoralis major muscle and to the chest wall?
9 What are the features of a breast infection?
10 What are the three main categories of systemic treatment for breast cancer?

References and further reading

Blommers J, de Lange-De Klerke ES, Kuik BJ, et al. Evening primrose oil and fish oil for severe chronic mastalgia: a randomised, double blind controlled trial. *American Journal of Obstetrics and Gynaecology* 2002; **187**:1389–94.

Dixon M. *ABC of breast diseases*, 2nd edn. BMJ Books, London, 2003.

Hughes LE. Classification of benign breast disorders, the ANDI classification based on physiological processes within the normal breast. *British Medical Bulletin* 1991; **47**:251–7.

Levy MJ, Matharu MS, Meeran K, et al. The clinical characteristics of headache in pituitary tumours. *Brain* 2005; **128**:1921–30.

Neville EM, Freeman AH, Adiseshiah M. Clinical significance of recent inversion of the nipple: a reappraisal. *Journal of the Royal Society of Medicine* 1982; **75**:111–13.

NICE. *Familial breast cancer: the classification and care of women at risk of familial breast cancer in primary, secondary and tertiary care* (CG41), 2006. www.nice.org.uk/CG41

Santen R, and Mansell R. Benign breast disorders. *New England Journal of Medicine* 2005; **353**:275–85.

11 Neck examination

CHAPTER CONTENTS

Introduction

The neck provides support for the head and can be regarded as a large biological tunnel with important structures passing through it from the head to the rest of the

body and vice versa. As a result there are few symptoms that are specific to the neck alone. Some structures may be affected within the neck and cause symptoms that have already been discussed in the relevant chapter, for example, dysphagia in the abdominal system. The most clinically important organ in the neck is the thyroid gland and this will be discussed in detail. Another organ, the parathyroid gland, is also described. The neck normally comes under the spotlight because of a lump that has been noticed by the patient, a relative, or a friend. Therefore the emphasis of this chapter is mainly on the clinical examination of the neck.

Symptoms

The majority of neck swelling will be due to cervical lymphadenopathy of the 'glands' in the neck. As these lymph nodes are in the vanguard of the body's defence system, there are a large variety of insults that can cause them to enlarge (see Table 11.1). This can prove a challenge to your diagnostic skills, but if you adopt a systematic approach you will find that deducing the underlying cause will be readily achievable. There are other types of neck swelling which are often asymptomatic (see Table 11.4 and 'Diseases and investigations of the neck' section). All lumps can produce local and some more generalized symptoms (depending on their aetiology). If you suspect a swelling to be of thyroid origin, there are more detailed questions you should ask (which you will learn later). It is exceedingly rare for the parathyroid glands to present as a neck swelling. However, they have an important role in calcium balance and can cause distinct signs and symptoms if their function becomes disordered.

Local symptoms

Pain is an important local symptom. The majority of swellings are symptomless (unless they grow large enough to press on surrounding structures). Occasionally an organ may become painful due to infection, for example, acute lymphadenopathy secondary to tonsillitis. Other local symptoms you may encounter are discussed in the relevant chapters and include:

- hoarseness (see Chapter 5)
- stridor (*stride-or*) (see Chapter 5)
- dysphagia (see Chapter 7)
- neck pain (see Chapter 12).

Generalized symptoms

If faced with a neck swelling it is worth asking about constitutional symptoms, which could be relevant in a number of conditions. The most important symptoms to ask

Table 11.1 Some causes of cervical lymphadenopathy

Causes	Examples
Infection	
Viral	HSV, adenovirus, cytomegalovirus, measles, mumps, rubella, infectious mononucleosis, hepatitis A, B, and C, HIV
Bacterial	
Localized	Streptococcal tonsillitis/pharyngitis, mouth flora causing dental abscess, cat scratch disease
Generalized	Brucellosis, leptospirosis, syphilis, lyme disease
Fungal	Histoplasmosis, cryptococcus
Protozoal	Toxoplasmosis
Skin disease	Eczema, psoriasis (affecting the scalp)
Cancer	Any cancer of the head and neck region, metastatic spread from other carcinomas, lymphomas, leukaemias
Drugs	Carbamazepine, phenytoin, penicillin, cefalosporins
Autoimmune disease	SLE, PAN, rheumatoid arthritis
Other	Sarcoidosis

HSV, herpes simplex virus; PAN, polyarteritis nodosa; SLE, systemic lupus erythematosus.

about are weight loss, fever, and night sweats. The presence of involuntary weight loss is always a worrying sign (see Chapter 7). In the context of a neck swelling, weight loss could indicate a malignancy with lymphatic spread to nearby lymph nodes. Examples of these include thyroid cancer, bronchial cancer (see Chapter 5), and gastric cancer (Troisier's [*twa-ziers*] sign; see Chapter 7). However it could represent a solitary toxic nodule in the thyroid gland and the resultant hyperthyroidism could lead to weight loss (see 'Diseases and investigations of the neck'). The combination of weight loss, fever, and night sweats should make you think of two key conditions (both of which are treatable). These are tuberculosis and lymphoma (*lim-foe-ma*). Lymphoma is a malignant process of the haemopoietic (*he-mow-poe-i-et-ic*) system (that is, the blood-producing cells of the body including the bone marrow, liver, and spleen). There are different types of lymphoma but the most common you will hear about are Hodgkin's lymphoma and non-Hodgkin's lymphoma. They can manifest as a localized swelling of lymphoid tissue, for example, lymph node group or tonsils, or be more widespread affecting many lymph node groups, liver, spleen, and so on. In the context of lymphoma, the presence of weight loss, fever, and night sweats are classified as B symptoms and this modifies the stage of the disease (staging is a process where a disease is coded according to its severity and distribution—the stage of a disease will influence the treatment that can be offered and the ultimate prognosis). Weight loss should be more than 10% of the patient's original weight (it is sensible to use a weight from at least 6 months prior to presentation although this may be difficult to achieve practically). You will find the majority of patients cannot quantify their weight loss. Night sweats should be sufficient to drench the nightclothes and there should be an unexplained fever of >38 °C. The classical fever termed Pel–Ebstein fever (*Pieter Klaases Pel (1852–1919), Dutch physician; Wilhelm Ebstein (1836–1912), German physician*) with high swinging intermittent temperatures that recur after a few weeks is not often seen (and therefore should not be regarded as classical).

What to ask

- 'How long have you had the swelling?' (Is this acute or chronic?)

- 'Have you had a cough, sore throat, runny nose, or sinus problems?' (Is this a self-limiting viral illness or localized bacterial infection?)

- 'Have you had toothache, gum trouble or needed to go to the dentist for a recent problem?' (Again establishing if there is a local problem.)

- 'Do you have any skin rashes?' (If the scalp or neck is affected there can be localized lymph node hyperplasia, especially if there is secondary infection.)

- 'Do you have similar lumps or swellings anywhere else?' (Checking if this is not a more generalized manifestation).

- 'Have you had any night sweats? Are they sufficient to drench your night clothes or bed linen?' (This could suggest lymphoma, TB.)

- 'Have you lost any weight recently?' If yes, 'Do you know how much you have lost?' (This could again suggest TB, lymphoma, or other malignancy.)

- 'Have you been on holiday recently or travelled abroad?' If the patient answers yes, then ask details of what they did and who they were in contact with. Were they bitten, or suffered scratches or injuries? Did they have the recommended immunizations or prophylaxis? Some infections have long incubation periods so find out if they have travelled up to at least 6 months before the consultation. Some infections are endemic in certain areas; for example, brucellosis in the Mediterranean area, TB or HIV in sub-Saharan Africa. Equally, if patients are recent migrants from these areas then these infections need to be considered.

- If a simple answer is not presenting itself you may need to probe even further and ask a sexual history (see Chapter 9). Be sensitive, but you may have to enquire about sexual partners and sexual practices, and ask especially about high-risk behaviour (see Chapter 9). If positive the diagnosis can range from sexually transmitted infections to hepatitis and HIV (which can be sexually transmitted as well as through IV drug abuse).

- 'What medications are you on?' Many drugs can cause lymphadenopathy, usually due to a hypersensitivity reaction; for example, phenytoin, carbamazepine, penicillin. If you are unsure check your British National Formulary (BNF), the pharmacy, or sometimes the drug company. Don't forget about over-the-counter medications from the chemist.

Perform your review of systems because if you find a number of disparate symptoms in seemingly unrelated areas, you could be dealing with a multisystem disorder or spread from an advanced carcinoma.

Even a social history could yield dividends. Does the patient own a cat or other pets? (possible cat scratch disease). What is their occupation? (sewage workers, vets—leptospirosis). As well as smoking and alcohol, do they use recreational substances or administer IV drugs?

Significance

Most cases of cervical lymphadenopathy will be benign, self-limiting conditions especially if they are due to simple viral, upper respiratory tract infections or localized infections such as bacterial tonsillitis or dental abscesses which should respond to antibiotics. However if a swelling is present for more than 4 weeks, especially if it is still increasing in size; if it is larger than 2 cm; or there are associated features which point towards possible malignancy such as weight loss or night sweats, then this lump

Key points

- Most cases of cervical lymphadenopathy will be benign, self-limiting conditions
- Red flag signs include:
  - lack of resolution of any lump after 4 weeks
  - lump >2 cm
  - associated with constitutional symptoms such as weight loss and/or night sweats
  - any other features that would point to malignancy

needs to be referred to a specialist for further investigations. These tests could include CT scan/MRI of the relevant area or biopsy of the swelling.

Thyroid

The thyroid is a gland situated at the level of the second and third tracheal rings. It consists of two lobes connected together by a thin bridge of tissue called the isthmus (*iss-th-muss*) (see Fig. 11.1). Normally it is impalpable in most men and about 50% of women. Its function is to produce the hormones thyroxine (*thigh-rocks-in*) (T_4) and tri-iodothyronine (*try-eye-owe-dough-thigh-roe-nin*) (T_3). These hormones are responsible for regulating the metabolic processes of the body. In simple terms, if insufficient hormone is secreted the metabolic processes slow down

(in hypothyroidism) and if excessive hormone is produced these processes become overactive (in hyperthyroidism). Thyroid disorder may present clinically in one of five main ways:

- overactivity of the thyroid gland, called hyperthyroidism or thyrotoxicosis (*thigh-roe-toxic-owe-sis*)
- underactivity of the thyroid gland, called hypothyroidism or myxoedema (*mix-ee-deem-a*)
- goitre (*goy-ter*) (an enlarged thyroid gland)
- a discrete swelling or nodule in the thyroid
- eye signs in Graves' disease of the thyroid.

Note that these categories are not mutually exclusive and you can have a combination of more than one presentation, for example, a patient may have a goitre, eye signs, and hyperthyroidism in Graves' disease of the thyroid. The symptoms due to an overactive and underactive thyroid are discussed in the following sections; the other presentations are dealt with in later sections of the chapter.

Hyperthyroidism

The patient with hyperthyroidism is likely to be agitated and fidgety (which you may notice during your consultation). This behaviour could be mistakenly rationalized as understandable anxiety in the consultation or just the person's personality. The exception to this presentation is

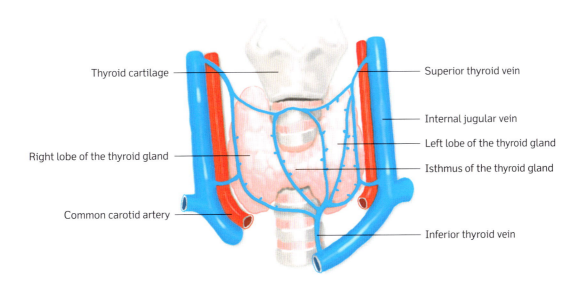

Figure 11.1 Anatomy of the thyroid.

Thyroid cartilage

Right lobe of the thyroid gland

Common carotid artery

Superior thyroid vein

Internal jugular vein

Left lobe of the thyroid gland

Isthmus of the thyroid gland

Inferior thyroid vein

the apathetic hyperthyroid patient. This patient is elderly and appears lifeless and lethargic and the condition can often be mistaken for hypothyroidism.

Questions to ask about hyperthyroidism

- 'Has there been any change in your weight?' The patient with hyperthyroidism will lose weight despite a normal or increased appetite.

- 'Has there been a change in bowel habit?' With hyperthyroidism the patient may develop diarrhoea or soft stools.

- 'Do you feel warm most of the time?' This question is an exploratory question to look for heat intolerance. If a person answers no, then clearly they do not have heat intolerance. If the answer is yes, they may still not have heat intolerance due to thyroid disorder. Supplement this question with the following one.

- 'Is increased sweating a problem?' If the answer is yes to this, then it increases the likelihood that this could be due to hyperthyroidism.

- 'Do you have palpitations?' There is an increased risk of arrhythmias with hyperthyroidism, particularly supraventricular tachycardia (SVTs) and atrial fibrillation (AF) (if the answer is yes, ask the relevant questions in Chapter 4).

- 'Do you have chest pain?' Some patients with hyperthyroidism (particularly elderly patients) may develop angina. If they have chest pain then you need to ask the relevant questions to see if their description of pain is consistent with angina. Patients with pre-existing angina may find that the frequency or severity of angina increases.

- 'Do you suffer with shortness of breath?' Patients with hyperthyroidism can develop high-output cardiac failure (if the answer is yes, prepare to ask further questions as in Chapter 4).

- 'What are your periods like?' Women with hyperthyroidism may have scanty periods (oligomenorrhoea) (*olly-go-men-no-rear*) or absent periods (amenorrhoea).

Other important questions to ask include:

- 'Are you getting snappy at people?'

- 'Do you feel anxious?'

- 'Do you have trouble falling asleep or waking up in the middle of the night?'

These are additional features of hyperthyroidism.

In addition to the above questions do not forget to take a thorough history and ask about medications (some

drugs can precipitate hyperthyroidism—see later) and a family history (some autoimmune diseases, for example, Graves' disease can be familial).

....
Tip
Always consider hyperthyroidism in any patient presenting with weight loss despite an increased appetite.
....

Hypothyroidism

The patient with hypothyroidism is likely to be lethargic and apathetic. In addition there is a slowing of mental function and poor concentration. These features can be mistaken for general apathy or diseases such as depression or dementia. They may even be dismissed simply as a function of ageing.

Questions to ask about hypothyroidism

- 'Has there been any change in your weight?' The patient with hypothyroidism will gain weight despite a poor appetite (occasionally this weight gain can be due to the retention of fluid because of cardiac failure).

- 'Has there been any change in your bowel habit?' With hypothyroidism the patient usually develops constipation.

- 'Do you feel cold most of the time?' This is an exploratory question looking for cold intolerance. If the answer is no, then it is unlikely that they have hypothyroidism. If yes then it increases the likelihood that they have it.

- 'Do you have chest pain?' Angina is common in hypothyroidism as well.

- 'Do you get short of breath?' Congestive heart failure is a complication of hypothyroidism.

- 'What are your periods like?' Women may experience very heavy menstrual bleeding (menorrhagia) (*men-owe-rage-ia*).

For a comparison of symptoms in hyperthyroidism and hypothyroidism, see Table 11.2.

Other important questions to ask include:

- 'Do you feel excessively tired?' Sometimes hypothyroidism can be mistaken for depression because of this reason.

Table 11.2 Comparison of symptoms in hyperthyroidism and hypothyroidism

System	Hyperthyroidism	Hypothyroidism
General	Agitated/listless, heat intolerance[a]	Fatigue/lethargy, sweating, cold intolerance[a]
Cardiovascular	Angina, breathlessness, palpitations	Angina, breathlessness, palpitations
Gastrointestinal	Weight loss[a], diarrhoea[a]	Weight gain[a], constipation[a]
Reproductive	Oligomenorrhoea, amenorrhoea	Menorrhagia

[a] The most discriminating symptoms for each condition.

- 'Has your skin become very dry recently?'
- 'Has your hair become dry and brittle recently?'

These are additional features of hypothyroidism.

Tip

Always consider the possibility of hypothyroidism in cases of depression or dementia (particularly in older people).

Tip

Always consider hypothyroidism in any patient with weight gain despite a poor appetite (especially in the absence of oedema).

Key points

- The combination of weight loss (despite an increased appetite), diarrhoea, and heat intolerance is highly suggestive of hyperthyroidism
- The combination of weight gain, constipation, and cold intolerance is highly suggestive of hypothyroidism

Parathyroids

The parathyroid glands are four small glands imbedded in the substance of the thyroid gland. They are involved in the regulation of calcium balance. They are rarely palpable even when they function abnormally and they usually create problems through disturbance of calcium metabolism. Like the thyroid, the parathyroids can be underactive or overactive. When overactive they produce excess parathormone (*para-thor-moan*) (PTH) and this process is called hyperparathyroidism (*high-per-para-thy-roid-ism*). Hyperparathyroidism is usually classified as primary, secondary, and tertiary. PTH causes an elevation of calcium in the blood (among other effects). With primary

and tertiary hyperparathyroidism this elevation is above the upper limit of normal for calcium and therefore causes hypercalcaemia (*high-per-cal-seem-ya*). Secondary hyperparathyroidism is the response to low plasma calcium (hypocalcaemia) and represents the body's attempt to correct this. Therefore there is no hypercalcaemia in this situation. When the glands are underactive the result is hypocalcaemia and the disease process is called hypoparathyroidism (for more details on these conditions see 'Diseases and investigations of the neck'). The symptoms and signs of symptomatic hypoparathyroidism and hyperparathyroidism are summarized in Table 11.3.

Tetany is one important sign (and should not be confused with tetanus caused by infection with *Clostridium tetani*). With tetany there is spasm of the upper and lower limb termed carpopedal spasm (the spasm of the lower limb occurs less frequently) due to hypocalcaemia or a decrease in the ionized fraction of calcium in the blood, for example, due to hyperventilation (see Case 11.1). In the upper limb there is flexion of the wrist and metacarpophalangeal (MCP) joints and hyperextension of the proximal and distal interphalangeal joints. In the lower limbs there is internal rotation of the legs and plantarflexion of the feet. Latent tetany can be demonstrated by performing two clinical tests—Trousseau's (*true-sews*) test (*Armand Trousseau (1801–1867), French physician*) and Chvostek's (*sh-vost-ex*) test (*Frantiesek Chvostek (1835–1884), Austrian surgeon*).

Trousseau's test

Trousseau's test is a test for hypocalcaemia (or a decrease in the ionized concentration of calcium, for example, following hyperventilation). It may also be positive in hypomagnesaemia and occasionally in normal people. A sphygmomanometer cuff is placed around an arm and inflated to a pressure above the systolic blood pressure of the patient. This can be maintained for a number of minutes (it is wise

Table 11.3 Comparison of symptoms in hyperparathyroidism and hypoparathyroidism

System	Hyperparathyroidism (hypercalcaemia)	Hypoparathyroidism (hypocalcaemia)
Gastrointestinal	Anorexia, nausea, vomiting, constipation	
Renal	Polyuria, polydipsia[a], nephrocalcinosis (*nef-roe-cal-sin-owe-sis*), renal stones	
Neurological	Lethargy, confusion	Paraesthesia in hands, feet, and around mouth, tetany, seizures, calcification in basal ganglia—rare cause of parkinsonism
Eyes	Metastatic calcification in conjunctiva and outer margin of the cornea (limbus)	Cataract

[a] Polydipsia = thirst.

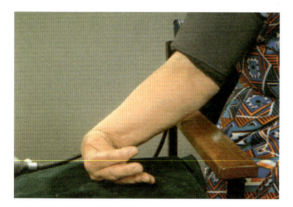

Figure 11.2 Trousseau's sign.

not to go beyond 3 minutes) and you are looking for a spasm of the hand. If this occurs, there is flexion of the MCP joints and extension of the interphalangeal joints together with opposition of the thumb. This hand posture is called main d'accoucheur (*man-da-coo-sher*) (see Fig. 11.2).

Chvostek's test

Chvostek's test involves tapping the facial nerve as it exits the stylomastoid foramen to supply the muscles of the face. Practically, this is just a few centimetres in front of the lower lobe of the ear. Feel for the ridge of bone, which runs horizontally at the level of auditory meatus of the ear; this is the zygomatic (*zy-go-mat-ick*) arch. Let your fingers drop below this ridge and about 2 cm anterior to the lobe of the ear. Now tap this area gently. A positive test is where that side of the face twitches in response. This test is felt to be less specific than Trousseau's test (in one study up to 25% of normal patients responded positively). See Fig. 11.3.

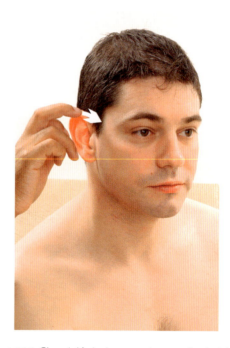

Figure 11.3 Chvostek's test: percussion over the facial nerve as it exits the stylomastoid foramen.

Key points
- Parathyroid glands secrete PTH, which has an important role in calcium regulation in the body
- Hyperparathyroidism causes hypercalcaemia in primary and tertiary hyperparathyroidism
- Hypoparathyroidism causes hypocalcaemia

CASE 11.1

Problem. A 39-year-old woman has been admitted for a partial thryoidectomy and is on her second day after the operation. The procedure took longer than anticipated but she has made a good recovery. Early on the morning of the second day she noticed pins and needles in her finger ends and around her lips, lasting about 10 minutes. She initially dismissed these symptoms but after midday they returned together with spasms of her hands and wrists. She was able to attract the attention of a nurse but shortly after this she suffered a seizure. What is happening?

Solution. An event so close to an operation should immediately make you suspicious of a surgical complication. The operation took longer than expected and this suggests that it may have been a difficult procedure with the possibility of damage to surrounding structures. The paraesthaesia of the hands and lips, together with the spasm of the hands and wrists, points to hypocalcaemia (and possibly hypomagnesaemia). Profound hypocalcaemia can also lead to seizures. During the operation it is possible to interfere with the blood supply to the parathyroid glands. This may be temporary or permanent. The glands can also be inadvertently removed, but great care is usually taken to identify and preserve them during a thyroidectomy. As the patient is symptomatic she needs treatment with calcium.

The importance of examining the neck

There are a variety of lumps that can appear in the neck. The purpose of your examination is to identify them where possible and to determine if they are benign (so you can reassure your patient) or if they herald serious disease (and therefore require further investigation and treatment).

Examination of the neck summary

1 Introduce yourself to the patient.
2 Get the patient into position.
3 Wash your hands.
4 Inspect the neck for swellings.
5 Ask the patient to stick out their tongue.*

6 Ask the patient to swallow (have a glass of water handy).*
7 Palpate the neck.
8 Auscultate the swelling.
9 Check for lymphadenopathy.
10 If you suspect a thyroid swelling, palpate the thyroid.*
11 Percuss for retrosternal extension of a goitre.*
12 Auscultate the thyroid swelling or goitre for a bruit.*
13 Check for lymphadenopathy.*
14 Assess the thyroid status.*
15 Perform any further relevant examination.
16 Wash your hands.
17 Present your findings.
* Instructions for swellings of a thyroid origin.

Examination of the neck in detail

Getting started

1 Introduce yourself to the patient

Extend your hand to shake the patient's hand and say something like, 'Hello I'm Marie Curie, a fourth-year medical student. Do you mind if I examine your neck?'

2 Get the patient into position

Unlike most examinations, the best position to examine the neck is with the patient sitting upright in a chair. The best chair to use is one with a low back so that you can palpate the neck from directly behind the patient.

3 Wash your hands

Rid your fingers of micro mingers.

4 Inspect the neck for swellings

Get your patient to elevate their chin slightly. This exposes more of the chin including the submandibular area and can accentuate any swellings in the midline. Be systematic in your inspection so that you observe all aspects of the neck. Note the position of any abnormality because you will need to examine it in more detail later.

5 Ask the patient to stick out their tongue

This request is conditional and should only be used for a discrete swelling at or near the midline of the neck. At first glance this seems a strange request but it uses a very simple principle that can identify certain types of swellings usually of thyroid origin, that is, thyroglossal (*thigh-roe-gloss-al*) cysts.

It is useful to know a little about the development of the thyroid to understand what a thyroglossal cyst is and how it behaves. The thyroid develops in the fetus as an outpouching at the base of the tongue. This descends in the neck as the thyroglossal tract ('thyro'—thyroid, 'glossal'—tongue). The thyroid matures as it descends until the isthmus comes to rest at the level of the second to fourth tracheal rings. The thyroglossal tract usually disappears when the thyroid reaches its destination, but parts of the tract may persist and may fill with fluid, producing a thyroglossal cyst. Sometimes, thyroid tissue is found in these cysts and rarely this may be the only site where functioning thyroid tissue can be found. As the thyroglossal tract is attached to the hyoid bone (and hence the base of the tongue), when the tongue is protruded the thyroglossal cyst is pulled up.

To examine, first fix your eyes on the swelling, then without shifting your gaze, say to your patient, 'Can you stick your tongue out, please?' If the lump elevates a couple of centimetres as the tongue is protruded it is likely that the swelling is a thyroglossal cyst (there are even rarer swellings that may elevate with tongue protrusion but you do not need to know these). The swelling should then return to its original position when the patient retracts their tongue.

6 Ask the patient to swallow (have a glass of water handy)

This request is designed to detect swellings of thyroid origin. The mature thyroid lies at the front of the neck in the midline and is covered by connective tissue (the pre-tracheal fascia (*fasher*)), which is attached to the trachea. Therefore when your patient swallows and the larynx elevates, the thyroid (normal or abnormal) will also elevate.

To examine, it is best to first fetch a glass or cup of water. It is remarkable how dry a person's mouth can get when they are being examined (this includes patients and students!). Say to them politely, 'Take a sip of water but don't swallow until I say.' As they take a sip of water make sure the swelling is visible and keep your eyes focused on it. Then say, 'Swallow now!', see Fig. 11.4. As your patient swallows, watch the swelling and see if it rises a few centimetres in the neck before returning to its original position. If it does, the swelling is of thyroid origin. An important

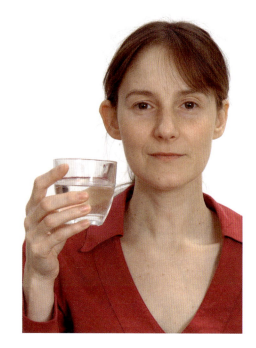

Figure 11.4 Ask the patient to swallow.

point to note is that thyroglossal cysts will also elevate with swallowing as well as tongue protrusion.

Palpation, auscultation, and percussion

7 Palpate the neck

When you palpate the neck, any swelling you identify on inspection needs to be assessed for a number of features: site, size, consistency, mobility, tenderness, margin, pulsatility, and transillumination.

- **Site**. The neck is divided anatomically into two triangles by the sternomastoid muscle (see Fig. 11.5). These are the anterior and posterior triangles. It is convention to locate any swelling found into one of these triangles. It is also important to have a working map of where the major organs are situated in the neck as this may give a valuable clue as to the identity of any lump found, for example, a midline swelling below the 'Adam's apple' could represent a thyroid nodule.

- **Size**. It is important to determine the size of any swelling. This can be done crudely with a tape measure. Baseline dimensions allow any changes in size to be monitored over time. A persistent increase in size raises the spectre of malignancy.

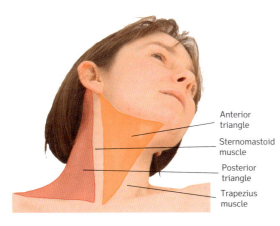

Figure 11.5 The anatomical triangles of the neck.

- Anterior triangle
- Sternomastoid muscle
- Posterior triangle
- Trapezius muscle

Table 11.4 Causes of a neck swelling

Lipoma (*lie-poe-ma*)
Epidermal cyst
Cervical lymphadenopathy
Thyroid nodule or goitre (see text)
Thyroglossal cyst (see text)
Pharyngeal pouch (see Chapter 7)
Branchial (*brank-i-al*) cyst
Cystic hygroma (*high-grow-ma*)
Cervical rib
Carotid body tumour
Salivary gland disease

- **Consistency**. Determine how soft or hard a swelling is and whether this is uniform throughout its substance. A soft swelling may represent fat- or a fluid-filled structure (cyst). A firm or rubbery swelling may indicate an enlarged organ or tissue, for example, salivary glands or lymph nodes. Hard swellings may represent malignant infiltration or calcification within its substance.

- **Mobility**. Some swellings exhibit a degree of mobility under the skin and this characteristic should be examined. Thyroid swellings will move upwards with swallowing (see step 6). If this feature is absent from a known thyroid swelling this could indicate that there is malignant infiltration of the thyroid with fixing to the surrounding structures. Lymph nodes are also mobile glands but may also become fixed if affected by malignancy or tuberculosis. When assessing mobility, hold the swelling between your thumb and index finger then try and move it back and forth in a horizontal and then a vertical plane. If it moves freely it is more likely to be benign.

- **Tenderness**. As a rule you should always check if a swelling is tender before beginning palpation. If tenderness is present this suggests an inflammatory mass such as an abscess or an organ that is inflamed secondary to infection.

- **Margin**. Assess the border of any swelling and see if it is well demarcated, for example, representing the capsule of an organ or if it is ill-defined, which could suggest infiltration by a neoplastic or inflammatory process.

- **Pulsatility**. Very few neck swellings will exhibit this property because the only major arteries in the neck are the carotid arteries. One rare swelling that exhibits this feature is a carotid body tumour (also called a chemodectoma [*key-mow-deck-toe-ma*]).

- **Transillumination**. This is a feature that can be demonstrated in fluid-filled lesions. Light from a pen torch can be directed on to one end of a swelling. If it is solid the light will be blocked. If it is a fluid-filled swelling, light will shine through it. This manifests itself as an orange glow within the swelling that diverges from the tip of the pen torch. This is best viewed in dimmed light or a blacked-out room (although this is not essential).

8 Auscultate the swelling

This aspect of the examination of a swelling is frequently forgotten. Place the diaphragm of your stethoscope over the swelling and if a bruit is present this indicates that it is either vascular in origin or it has an increased blood supply.

9 Check for lymphadenopathy

This must always be done for any neck swelling, including the thyroid. Enlarged, hard, and irregular lymph nodes may represent spread from a malignant primary. See Table 11.4 for causes of a neck swelling and Fig. 11.6 for the lymph nodes of the neck.

10 If you suspect a thyroid swelling, palpate the thyroid

If you suspect a thyroid swelling, because of its site (at or near the midline) and its elevation with swallowing, then begin palpation of the thyroid (see Fig. 11.7).

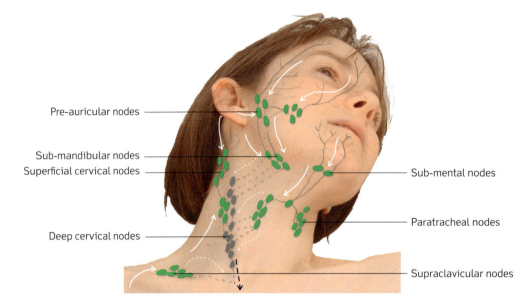

Pre-auricular nodes

Sub-mandibular nodes
Superficial cervical nodes

Deep cervical nodes

Sub-mental nodes

Paratracheal nodes

Supraclavicular nodes

Figure 11.6 Lymph node chains.

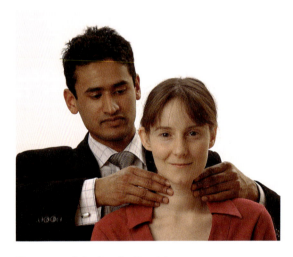

Figure 11.7 Palpating the thyroid.

Stand behind your patient and get them to depress their chin marginally to relax the strap muscles. Place your fingers on either side of the neck and map out the lobes of the thyroid. The tip of your index and middle fingers will do the work. Run your fingers around the margins of any swelling you observed earlier. Are they well demarcated or ill defined? Your analysis of a thyroid swelling or goitre should be no different from that of any other swelling. You will have already noted the site

and measured the dimensions of the swelling. Now feel the consistency of the thyroid—is it soft or firm (this suggests normal thyroid tissue) or is it 'rock hard' (this suggests thyroid cancer)? Nodules tend to be firm or hard but this does not necessarily mean malignancy (a thyroid isotope scan may be needed to determine this—see later). Check for tenderness of the thyroid as inflammation of the thyroid (thyroiditis) can occasionally cause this.

11 Percuss for retrosternal extension of a goitre

Percussion has a limited application in the neck. Occasionally a goitre may extend behind the sternum and rarely this may be its sole position (when it is called a retrosternal goitre). Percuss using the technique described in Chapter 5 (see Fig. 11.8). Begin just below the suprasternal notch and descend towards the sternal angle. Normally this area is resonant. If it is dull this suggests retrosternal extension of a goitre or a retrosternal goitre (in this context).

12 Auscultate the thyroid swelling or goitre for a bruit

See Fig. 11.9. Place the diaphragm of your stethoscope over the thyroid swelling or goitre. If a bruit is heard, this suggests overactivity of the gland (see Case 11.2) (because of the

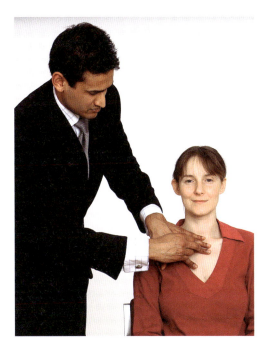

Figure 11.8 Percussion for a retrosternal extension of a goitre.

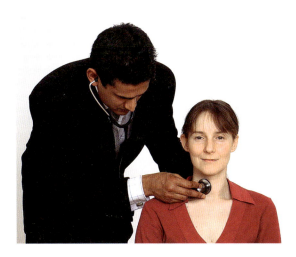

Figure 11.9 Auscultation over the thyroid gland.

requirement for an increased blood supply). If a bruit is not heard this does not rule out the possibility of hyperthyroidism.

13 Check for lymphadenopathy

Hard irregular lymph nodes in relation to a thyroid swelling could represent spread from a thyroid cancer.

CASE 11.2

Problem. You listen over a goitre but you are not sure if the bruit originates from the goitre or from the carotid artery.

  Discussion. Sometimes this distinction can prove difficult, particularly if the dimensions of the goitre are such that the diaphragm of your stethoscope overlaps the carotid artery at auscultation. It is always worth checking the aortic area to make sure that you are not hearing the radiation from the murmur of aortic stenosis. If you are still unsure remember that you should not consider this sign in isolation. If the patient has weight loss, heat intolerance, a tremor, lid-lag, and a tachycardia, the chances are that they are thyrotoxic and a bruit is consistent with their disease status. If these are absent then it is unlikely that the bruit you heard originated from the goitre.

Clinical assessment

14 Assess the thyroid status

When you find a thyroid nodule or goitre you must assess the activity of the thyroid clinically. It can only be one of three possible states:

- normal activity—euthyroid
- overactive—hyperthyroid
- underactive—hypothyroid.

  You may already have clues from your history as to what the thyroid status might be, for example:

- heat intolerance, diarrhoea, weight loss— hyperthyroid
- cold intolerance, constipation, appetite, weight gain— hypothryoid.

  Now is the time to confirm your suspicions!

- **Observe the patient**. Are they restless and fidgety?— hyperthyroid? Are they relatively relaxed?—euthyroid? Are they lethargic and disinterested?— hypothyroid?
- **Shake the patient's hand**. Are the palms sweaty?— hyperthyroid?
- **Get your patient to hold out their hands (place a piece of paper over their hand)**. Is there a tremor present?—hyperthyroid?

- **Feel the pulse**. Tachycardia—hyperthyroid? Brady-cardia—hypothyroid? Pulse rate 60–80 beats/min—euthyroid? Atrial fibrillation—associated with both hypo- and hyperthryoidism.

- **Check the eyes for lid-lag and lid retraction**. The phenomenon of lid-lag is associated with Graves' disease and is not strictly a test of thyroid status. Nevertheless it should be performed as part of your thyroid routine. Normally when the eyes follow an object that descends from above, both the globe of the eye and the eyelids move down in unison. With hyperthyroidism, the movement of the eyelids is delayed and lags behind that of the globe. To test, provide a target by holding your index finger or the tip of a pen above the head of your patient about 0.5 m in front of their face. Your patient should be able to see the target comfortably without straining their eyes or tilting their head upwards. Say to your patient, 'Keep your head still and follow my finger/this pen with your eyes only!' Now slowly move the target vertically downwards until the patient is staring down at it without straining or tilting their head. While doing this, focus on their eyes and eyelids and note if they move downwards in unison or if there is a brief delay before the eyelids follow the globe of the eye.

Lid retraction is where the upper eyelid retracts backward exposing an arc of white sclera above the cornea. In normal people the sclera is not visible except with fear, anxiety, or anger (the wide-eyed stare). The muscle controlling elevation of the eyelid (levator palpabrae superioris) is under sympathetic control. Any condition that increases circulating adrenaline or noradrenaline will cause this muscle to contract. In the context of thyroid disease these hormones are increased in hyperthyroidism. Note that this is a non-specific sign that can be seen in other conditions including fear, anxiety, or anger for the reasons just discussed. To examine, simply look for a crescent of white sclera above the apex of the cornea.

See Cases 11.3, 11.4, and 11.5 for case studies in thyroid status.

....

Tip

If you notice a crescent of white sclera below the bottom of the cornea (with the eye looking forwards naturally), this is not lid retraction. This is exophthalmos (*ex-op-thal-moss*). The cause of exophthalmos is not related to thyroid status but is autoimmune mediated (see later).

....

CASE 11.3

Problem. A 78-year-old woman is sent to the hospital's assessment unit by her GP. She has complained of abdominal pain and poor appetite over the last 3 days and has not opened her bowels for 5 days. The GP suspects constipation but would like to exclude an acute abdomen. The GP has also referred her to the psychiatrist because over the last 2 months she has become more withdrawn. She has lost interest in her hobbies and her usually immaculate house is in a state. The GP feels she is depressed and requires urgent treatment. The specialist trainee (ST4) takes one look at the letter, has a quick glance at the patient, and diagnoses hypothyroidism. Is the trainee right?

   Discussion. On this occasion yes! The GP's assessment has been good and their response has been appropriate. Profound constipation can mimic bowel obstruction with vomiting, decreased appetite, and colicky abdominal pain and therefore a surgical opinion may be necessary to exclude obstruction. However, clearly there is more going on than just an abdominal problem. The loss of interest in everyday activities could be due to depression or even a dementia (although the

time course is rapid and so this would have to be an atypical variant). The ST4's powers of deduction could become the stuff of legend after this end-of-the-bed diagnosis. However, it is based on sound medical thinking and a little bit of luck. The trainee has remembered that hypothyroidism has neuropsychiatric features that can mimic depression. Patients slow down and lose interest in life. In addition they reasoned that constipation is also a manifestation of hypothyroidism. A quick glance at the patient may have revealed coarse, thinning hair, an apathetic appearance, and perhaps erythema ab igne (a brown reticular pattern on the skin of the inner thigh or abdomen where the patient has huddled close to a heat supply to keep warm). Despite the suggestive nature of this evidence the ST4 still needed a modicum of luck as this could still have been a case of depression and they have yet to take a full history or examine the patient. The message here is that hypothyroidism is an insidious condition that can be easily missed. The key to making the diagnosis is to be constantly aware of its possibility because it is a condition that can be readily treated.

CASE 11.4

Problem. You see a 48-year-old woman who is referred to the gastroenterology clinic with chronic diarrhoea spanning 2 months. She opens her bowels between four and six times on some days and passes loose motions with no blood or mucus. During this time she has lost half a stone in weight. The GP has sent two stool samples for culture but no pathogens have been seen. You examine her and notice she looks anxious, with a tremor, and has eyes that seem to stare. She has a sinus tachycardia of 110 beats/min and abdominal examination including a rectal was unremarkable. What is the cause of her diarrhoea and weight loss?

Discussion. This is a classic case of hyperthyroidism. However, it is only obvious when all the facts are presented in this fashion. In the real world of busy clinicians it is easy for any doctor to focus on the obvious problem, for example, GP refers because of diarrhoea. The same error can be compounded by the hospital specialist, who may not see beyond their own area of expertise. Pausing to consider other possibilities may sometimes reap dividends. In this case the diarrhoea was chronic and no infective agent had been found. There was nothing in the stools to suggest an active colitic process from the history given. Clues to a cause outside the gastrointestinal tract could be recognized from the outset. The anxiety, tremor, and staring eyes do suggest thyrotoxicosis (and possibly Graves' disease). The sinus tachycardia also adds further weight. Other features to look for include heat intolerance, a goitre, and a fuller assessment of the patient's thyroid status.

CASE 11.5

Problem. You are on a GP attachment and your GP sees a 52-year-old man who has come for a follow-up visit. He presented a week ago with a sore throat and a flu-like illness. The GP suspected tonsillitis and prescribed analgesia and antibiotics. However, his throat still feels sore and he feels 'edgy' and 'lousy'. You examine his mouth and pharynx, which are normal. As you feel his neck for lymph glands you become aware that he is tender over his thyroid gland. You also notice he has a slight tremor and sweaty palms and you check his pulse and blood pressure, which are 92 beats/min and 130/50 respectively.

Discussion. This is a case of subacute viral thyroiditis. It usually begins with a viral illness. The pain in the thyroid can often be mistaken for a 'sore throat'. In some cases thyrotoxicosis can ensue which is self-limiting and this explains his continuing ill-health (he has a tremor, sweaty palms, and a tachycardia). Treatment will be further analgesia for his pain and a beta-blocker to counteract the symptoms of thyrotoxicosis. He will need further review to decide when to stop his treatment.

- **Examine the reflexes**. The sign to demonstrate here is the slow-relaxing reflex. This should only be attempted if you suspect hypothyroidism. Classically it is taught that the ankle jerk should be elicited, but those of you who are sharp eyed may notice (given the opportunity) that this can be observed at other sites, for example, biceps and triceps. The reflex is elicited in exactly the same way as you would in a neurological examination. You may notice a brief, brisk contraction followed by a more prolonged relaxation phase. In absolute terms, the whole reflex action is over in just over a second so concentration is crucial.

Tip

You must examine many normal reflexes before you can appreciate the duration of the contraction and relaxation phases and hence when the latter is delayed.

Tip

In working life, no one diagnoses hypothyroidism from slow-relaxing reflexes alone. It is a supplementary sign: one to elicit to delight your friends and colleagues when you already know the diagnosis.

Table 11.5 A contrast of signs associated with hyperthyroidism, hypothyroidism, and Graves' disease

Hyperthyroidism	Hypothyroidism	Graves' disease
Palmar erythema	Dry skin	Pretibial myxoedema
Spider naevi	Alopecia	Thyroid acropachy (*a-crow-patchy*)
Gynaecomastia	Erythema ab igne (*erry-theme-a-ab- ig-ney*)	
Proximal myopathy	Xanthelasma	
Hyper-reflexia	Hypercarotenaemia[a] (*high-per-carrot-en- ee-mia*)	
Osteoporosis	Carpal tunnel syndrome, cerebellar ataxia, myopathy, pleural effusion, pericardial effusion, ascites	

[a] Hypercarotenaemia is the finding of large amounts of β-carotene in the blood. In the context of hypothyroidism, there is the decreased conversion of β-carotene to retinol (vitamin A) in the liver leading to a large concentration in the blood. Deposition in the skin can lead to a yellow/orange pigmentation.

During your evaluation of thyroid status if you suspect a particular state, for example, hypothyroidism, then only examine relevant features from the list above, for example, hypothyroidism—bradycardia, AF, slow-relaxing reflexes, and so on. Once your examination is complete you should confirm the thyroid status of the patient by taking blood for thyroid function tests (see 'Diseases and investigations of the neck').

15 Perform any further relevant examination

Other signs associated with hyper- and hypothyroidism are contrasted in Table 11.5. Although many of these signs are associated with hyper- and hypothyroidism, they are not reliable indicators of thyroid status and therefore do not feature in the routine above. These signs do not have to be present for the respective diagnoses to be tenable.

16 Wash your hands

Cot grubby paws cause infected sores.

17 Present your findings

If the diagnosis is straightforward, mention this up front and support it with findings from your examination. If you are unsure of the diagnosis, describe your findings and give a reasonable differential diagnosis. For example,

'This young woman has Graves' disease of the thyroid. She has exophthalmos and a small, diffusely enlarged goitre. The goitre moves freely on swallowing and there is no retrosternal extension and no lymphadenopathy or bruits audible over the gland. On further examination she also has pretibial myxoedema. She is clinically euthyroid with a pulse rate that is 82 beats per minute and regular and there is no evidence of a tremor, sweating, or lid-lag.'

Or another example:

'This man has bilateral cervical lymphadenopathy. The nodes are rubbery, firm, and mobile, with some mild tenderness on palpation. In the absence of a history, the differential diagnosis is wide, including viral infections such as infectious mononucleosis (glandular fever), bacterial infections such as brucellosis, multisystem disorder such as systemic lupus erythmatosus, and neoplastic disease such as lymphoma.'

Tip

Never forget to mention the patient's clinical thyroid status when presenting a thyroid case.

Diseases and investigations of the neck

Earlier in this chapter, I have mentioned various medical conditions and investigations. In this section I now describe them. In general these descriptions are brief though certain selected topics are discussed in more detail.

Cat scratch disease

This is caused by the bacterium *Bartonella hensalae*, a Gram-negative bacillus. It is caught from a bite or scratch from a cat. It causes localized lymphadenopathy but occasionally can cause fever, malaise, and headache. More serious disease can be experienced in those who are immunosuppressed. It tends to be self-limiting but can be treated with antibiotics in the case of more serious disease.

Histoplasmosis

This is due to the inhalation of the spores of the fungus *Histoplasma capsulatum*. These spores are widespread in the environment and their growth seems to be enhanced by bird and bat droppings. Humans tend to be exposed to large quantities of the fungus during demolition of old houses, or caving. The disease is rare and it tends to be immunosuppressed patients who succumb to the disease. Mild case may have flu-like symptoms and sometimes lymphadenopathy, but in more severe infections it can disseminate throughout the body. It can behave like TB with granulomas formed in affected organs.

Cryptococcus

This is another fungus that is widespread in the environment. Two species, *Cryptococcus neoformans* and *Cryptococcus gatti*, are responsible for infections in humans. Infection occurs through inhaling the spores but in most cases the individual is asymptomatic or only develops a mild flu-like illness. As with histoplasmosis, people who are immunosuppressed are most at risk, especially patients with HIV. One of the most dangerous manifestations is cryptococcal meningitis. If this occurs the patient will need treatment with intravenous antifungal agents.

Toxoplasmosis

This is caused by the protozoon *Toxoplasma gondii*. It affects birds and mammals, and humans can be infected if they eat raw or undercooked meat, or unpasteurized dairy products. Cats are the primary host and excrete toxoplasma in their faeces, so humans (especially children) with poor hygiene can ingest it unwittingly. Most people are asymptomatic but occasionally they may exhibit flu-like symptoms and associated lymphadenopathy. It is only dangerous to people who are immunosuppressed. In these people it can affect the eyes and cause a retinitis and blindness or an encephalitis associated with seizures. Rarely a woman in the early stages of pregnancy can acquire the disease and transmit it to the fetus to cause congenital toxoplasmosis, where the baby may suffer blindness and brain damage.

Brucellosis

This is caused by *Brucella* spp. which are Gram-negative bacilli and cause infections in animals. They can be found globally but the areas of high risk include the Mediterranean region and the Middle East. Humans are infected if they ingest raw or uncooked meat or unpasteurized dairy products. Brucellosis causes a high fever, which tends to rise and fall intermittently (it can be called undulating fever). Patients can have headaches, muscle and joint pains, and lymphadenopathy. Untreated it can become chronic with intermittent relapses and granulomas can form in various organs. Treatment is with tetracyclines, aminoglycosides, or rifampicin, often in combination.

Lipoma

This is a benign fatty tumour due to the growth of adipose tissue. It is a mobile subcutaneous mass. It exhibits fluctuance although it is not cystic in nature. It does not transilluminate.

Epidermal cyst

This used to be called a sebaceous cyst. These cysts occur anywhere where there are hair follicles. They can be small or grow to several centimetres. Keratin rather than sebum is produced within them, hence the term sebaceous cyst is a misnomer. They are soft/firm, mobile, painless, and entirely benign.

Cervical lymphadenopathy

This is the most common cause of a neck swelling. There are over 300 lymph nodes in the neck. These drain areas such as the face, scalp, nose, mouth, larynx, and pharynx and can be enlarged by a variety of disease including infections, skin disease, multisystem disorders, and malignancy.

Branchial cyst

This cyst develops from the remnants of the second bran-chial clefts. The branchial clefts are four grooves seen on either side of the neck during the development of the fetus. The second, third, and fourth clefts usually disappear while the first cleft persists as the external auditory meatus. This cyst may present in late adolescence or adulthood and can be found in the upper neck over the sternomastoid muscle. The cyst is fluctuant and may transilluminate. It can be tender if it becomes infected.

Cystic hygroma

This is also called a cavernous lymphangioma. This is a con-genital lesion due to the abnormal development of the lym-phatic system. The cyst develops from primitive lymph sacs found in the neck between the subclavian and jugular veins in the embryo. The cyst is usually found in the lower third of the neck in the posterior triangle and sometimes enlarges upwards towards the ear (other areas can be affected includ-ing the tongue, chest, and axilla). It also transilluminates.

Cervical rib

Occasionally people may have a seventh cervical rib. It may be attached to the first rib or the sternum or may have no distal attachment at all. The swelling is hard, pain-less, and immobile. Cervical ribs can also be fibrous bands rather than bone. These bands often cause more complica-tions than their bony counterpart. Vascular complications include narrowing of the subclavian artery, aneurysm for-mation, thrombus formation, embolization, and ischaemia. Neurological complications include compression of the first thoracic nerve or brachial plexus lesions.

Carotid body tumour

This is also called a chemodectoma. This is a slow-growing tumour arising from the chemoreceptor cells in the carotid body at the carotid bifurcation. It is slowly growing, pain-less, and exhibits pulsatility. It is mobile in the horizontal plane but not the vertical. As a highly vascular tumour it will also have a bruit on auscultation. Finally this is one swelling that should not be biopsied.

Salivary gland disease

There are three main salivary glands: the parotid, the sub-mandibular, and the sublingual glands. The most relevant gland for the neck is the submandibular gland. A number of diseases can cause the glands to enlarge. Acute infec-tion with bacteria can lead to a swollen, extremely tender gland. A stone can often be felt within the duct of the gland and pus can sometimes be expressed into the mouth. Viral infection with a paramyxovirus (*para-mix-owe-virus*) causes mumps, which leads to enlarged glands, particu-larly the parotids. The gland is not as tender as in bacter-ial infections. Sjögren's syndrome is the combination of dry eyes and dry mouth in conjunction with a connective tissue disorder such as systemic sclerosis. The salivary glands are often painlessly enlarged in this condition. The salivary glands can also be affected by tumours. Tumours are rare and the majority of them are benign. There are many pathological forms but all tend to be firm and mobile. The malignant tumours tend to be hard and can become fixed to surrounding tissues. They spread via the blood and lymphatics and some can infiltrate along their own nerve supply.

Control of thyroid hormone production

The thyroid produces two hormones, T_4 and T_3. They are produced by modification of the amino acid tyrosine, a process that includes the incorporation of iodine extracted from the diet. Once T_4 and T_3 are manufactured they are stored within the thyroid gland for release at a later date. Once released into the bloodstream the hormones are protein bound (and in this form are inactive). Only a small proportion of hormone is free and it is this proportion that is biologically active. The thyroid gland is under the control of the anterior pituitary gland and is stimulated to function by the pituitary peptide thyrotropin (*thigh-row-trow-pin*), also known as thyroid stimulating hormone (TSH). In turn the pituitary is under the control of the hypothalamus via thyrotropin-releasing hormone (TRH). The whole process is finely tuned by a negative feedback mechanism that ensures that just the right quantity of T_3 and T_4 are produced to maintain biological processes at their optimum rate. Essentially if the T_3 and T_4 levels are too low this is 'sensed' by the anterior pituitary, which will increase the production of TSH to drive further production of T_3 and T_4. Conversely if the levels of T_3 and T_4 are too high, the production of TSH is reduced to allow the level of T_3 and T_4 to normalize (see Fig. 11.10).

Goitre

This term means the enlargement of the thyroid gland. Goitres can be classified in the following way:

- diffuse
- simple
- iodine deficiency
- due to Graves' disease
- due to Hashimoto's (*hash-ee-mow-toes*) thyroiditis
- due to subacute viral thyroiditis
- multinodular goitre.

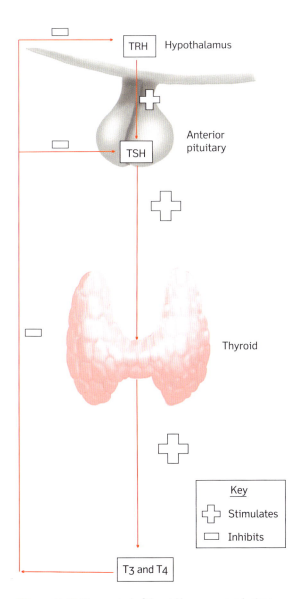

TRH   Hypothalamus

Anterior pituitary

TSH

Thyroid

Key

✛ Stimulates

▭ Inhibits

T3 and T4

Figure 11.10 The control of thyroid hormone production.

Diffuse goitre

Diffuse goitre is a goitre where there is enlargement of both lobes of the thyroid, and tends to be symmetrical. A simple goitre is a type of diffuse goitre where there is no disturbance of thyroid function (sometimes called a non-toxic goitre). A small, simple goitre may sometimes be found in some women at puberty or during pregnancy. Iodine deficiency is a common cause of a diffuse goitre worldwide. Iodine is an important cofactor in thyroid hormone synthesis and is normally found in the diet. In regions where iodine is poor in the diet this form of goitre is common, hence the term endemic goitre is also used. In the past Derbyshire in the UK was one such area, where goitres were common enough to lead to the term 'Derbyshire neck'. In the early stages the goitre is small and diffuse but later it can become large and multinodular. In some cases the patient may sometimes become hypothyroid. This has led to the introduction of programmes to introduce iodine supplementation in salt or flour which has been successful in treating this problem in some areas of the world.

Subacute viral thryoiditis

This is also called Dequervain's (*de-qwe-veins*) thyroiditis (*Fritz De Quervain (1868–1940), Swiss surgeon*). This is due to a viral infection and tends to affect females more than males. Usually flu-like symptoms are experienced, for example, headache and muscle aches and pains, and sometimes swallowing may be painful because of inflammation of the thyroid gland (this may lead to confusion with pharyngitis or tonsillitis). Patients may exhibit transient thyrotoxicosis, as stored thyroid hormone is released into the bloodstream. Note that because there is no glandular overactivity this is not hyperthyroidism. If the disease is mild no treatment is required. The patient may require analgesia for neck discomfort. If thyrotoxicosis is problematical, then treatment with a beta-blocker should suffice until symptoms settle. Occasionally the patient may go on to experience hypothyroidism, which usually lasts between 3 and 6 months.

Hashimoto's thyroiditis

Hashimoto's thyroiditis (*Hakaru Hashimoto (1881–1934), Japanese surgeon*) is also called chronic lymphocytic thyroiditis. It affects females more than males. It is an autoimmune disorder due to antibodies that react to the cells of the thyroid gland. Antibodies called thyroid microsomal antibodies are produced by lymphocytes, which infiltrate the thyroid gland and destroy thyroid cells. The condition follows a relapsing and remitting course. Early in the disease patients develop a small goitre. Occasionally some patients develop thyrotoxicosis lasting weeks or months, which may resemble Graves' disease. This is sometimes called hashitoxicosis. This phase is usually short lived as the thyroid gland is progressively destroyed. Later titres of thyroid microsomal antibodies become low or undetectable. Eventually the burden of destruction leads to hypothyroidism. Treatment is essentially symptom control. If the gland is painful analgesia can be used. If the goitre is large or there is a worry about malignancy, surgery may be contemplated. When hypothyroidism supervenes then treatment is with T_4.

Graves' disease

Graves' disease (*Robert Graves (1797–1853), Irish physician*), is an autoimmune condition affecting the thyroid. Antibodies are produced that stimulate the thyroid cells leading to their overactivity and subsequent thyrotoxicosis. It is more common in females than males. It causes a diffuse painless goitre. See Figs 11.11 and 11.12. Other features peculiar to Graves' disease include ophthalmopathy, pretibial myxoedema, and thyroid acropachy.

- **Ophthalmopathy**. See Figs. 11.13 and 11.14. This can be found in up to 60% of patients with Graves' disease. In some patients the eye signs may precede the development of the thyrotoxicosis and goitre. Exophthalmos is the most recognizable sign. This is the protrusion of the eye from its orbit. This process is also called proptosis but exophthalmos is reserved for protrusion of the eye of endocrine origin. Exophthalmos occurs independently of thyroid status. It is an autoimmune phenomenon leading to the deposition of mucopolysaccharide (*mew-co-polly-sack-a-ride*), lymphocyte infiltration, and subsequent oedema behind the eye. There is also lymphocyte infiltration and eventual thickening of the retro-orbital muscles. This combination of changes leads to protrusion of the eye. This process may impair conjugate eye movement leading to diplopia (this is called ophthalmoplegia [*op-thal-mow-plea-jah*]). Chronically there is thickening and fibrosis of the retro-orbital muscles further compounding ophthalmoplegia. Further features may develop including peri-orbital oedema, conjunctival oedema, and oedema of the cornea (chemosis) (*key-mow-sis*). In severe cases the eye is at risk of blindness because of raised intraocular pressure on the optic nerve. This is called malignant exophthalmos and is an emergency. Treatment is with high-dose steroids and occasionally surgery to decompress the orbit.
- **Pretibial myxoedema**. See Fig. 11.15. This is an uncommon condition that occurs in 1–5% of patients with

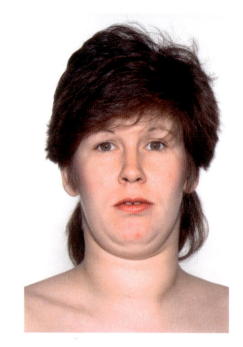

Figure 11.11 Diffuse goitre of Graves' disease.

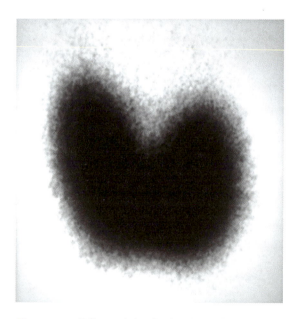

Figure 11.12 Diffuse uptake of radioactive iodine in thyroid uptake scan in Graves' disease.

Graves' disease. It is a coarse, plaque-like thickening of the skin usually over the shin (hence pretibial) but can occur elsewhere. It can be purple/blue, orange, or brown and is due to the deposition of mucopolysaccharides in the subcutaneous layer of the skin. Why a small

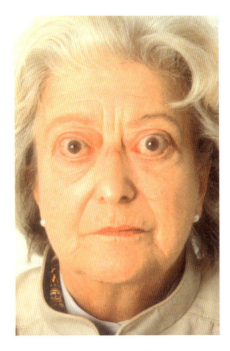

Figure 11.13 Exophthalmos due to Graves' disease.

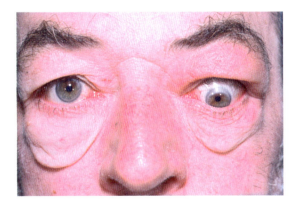

Figure 11.14 Exophthalmoplegia.

(a)   (b)

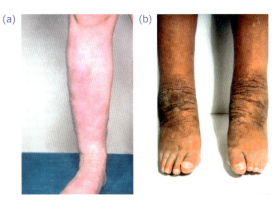

Figure 11.15 Pretibial myxoedema.

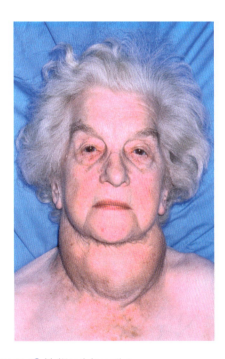

Figure 11.16 Multinodular goitre.

proportion of people with Graves' disease develop this problem is unknown.

- **Thyroid acropachy**. This is an even rarer manifestation of Graves' disease, which affects the fingers (and toes) and resembles clubbing.

Thyroid nodule

A nodule is simply a lump in the thyroid. It may be a solitary nodule or be one of a number of nodules in a multinodular goitre. A nodule is palpable if it exceeds 1 cm in diameter.

Multinodular goitre

See Figs. 11.16 and 11.17. This is a goitre where one or more nodules can be felt. With the advent of high-resolution ultrasound, impalpable nodules only a few millimetres in diameter can be detected. Therefore patients who were initially felt to have a solitary nodule can be reclassified as having a multinodular goitre. Multinodular goitres are more common in areas of iodine deficiency and affect women more than men. Nodules tend to develop in long-standing goitres and can evolve from a simple, non-toxic goitre. If nodules contain functioning thyroid tissue they can

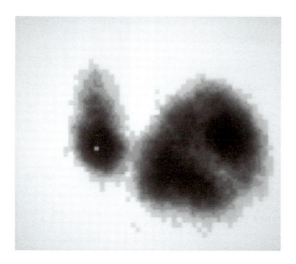

Figure 11.17 Patchy uptake in a thyroid uptake scan in multinodular goitre.

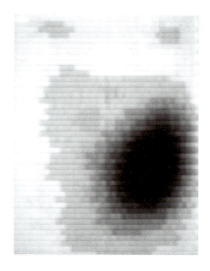

Figure 11.18 Uptake in a solitary thyroid nodule.

eventually secrete excess thyroid hormones leading to thyrotoxicosis. Patients are described as having a toxic, multinodular goitre. This tends to happen in the older patient and the classical signs of thyrotoxicosis (described earlier in the chapter) may not be apparent. They usually present with complications such as heart failure or atrial fibrillation. Complications of a large goitre (of any cause) include

- dysphagia (due to compression of the oesophagus)
- recurrent pneumonia (due to the compression of a bronchus and infection distal to the narrowing)
- stridor (due to compression of the trachea)
- hoarseness (due to compression of the left recurrent laryngeal nerve)
- venous engorgement (due to the compression of the great veins in the mediastinum).

Treatment includes anti-thyroid drugs to control symptoms if the patient has thyrotoxicosis. Definitive treatment is radioiodine therapy or surgery (particularly with complications due to a large goitre).

Solitary nodule

See Fig. 11.18. The underlying nature of a solitary nodule must always be determined. A nodule can be a cyst, adenoma—a benign collection of glandular cells (of thyroid origin)—or cancer. Note that an adenoma can be non-toxic, that is, it does not produce excess thyroid hormones. Or it may become progressively more active and secrete excess T_3 or T_4, leading to thyrotoxicosis. It is then

called a toxic adenoma. This overactivity can be sufficient to suppress activity of the rest of the thyroid gland through negative feedback. There are four ways of determining the nature of a nodule: ultrasound scanning, radionuclide scanning, fine-needle aspiration, and excision biopsy.

- **Ultrasound scanning**. This has limited value diagnostically. It can determine whether the nodule is solid or cystic (if it is cystic it is more likely to be benign). Also it may detect small nodules that are impalpable, which would suggest a multinodular goitre, a feature that would make malignancy less likely.

- **Radionuclide scanning**. A radioactive isotope (either radioiodine or technetium) is injected into the bloodstream. The isotope is taken up and concentrated preferentially by the thyroid gland. Areas of high concentration of isotope reflect increased thyroid activity and are usually described as 'hot'. Areas of low activity are conversely described as cold. A useful guide is that a functioning 'hot' nodule is unlikely to be cancerous. The majority of cancers are cold nodules. Note that although the majority of cancers are cold nodules, the majority of cold nodules are **not** cancers. Only about 10% of cold nodules are due to cancer.

- **Fine-needle aspiration**. This is the best technique for identifying a thyroid nodule. A fine needle is inserted into the thyroid and a sliver of tissue is removed for histological examination. In expert hands a diagnosis can be made on most occasions. Sometimes not enough tissue is obtained or the cell morphology cannot lead to a precise diagnosis. In cases of doubt either the aspiration can be repeated or the patient can be referred for surgery.

- **Excision biopsy**. Very occasionally, in cases of doubt, surgery is warranted. The nodule is removed along with surrounding thyroid tissue (usually a hemithyroidectomy), to provide both a diagnosis and sometimes a cure (as the nodule is removed).

Thyrotoxicosis

Thyrotoxicosis is the clinical syndrome that occurs due to an excess of free-circulating thyroid hormones T_3 or T_4. The term 'hyperthyroidism' should strictly be reserved for those cases where there is overactivity of the thyroid gland although 'hyperthyroidism' and 'thyrotoxicosis' are often used interchangeably. Cases of thyrotoxicosis that are not due to hyperthyroidism are listed under 'Other' in Table 11.6. Hyperthyroidism is termed primary when the main source driving the glandular overactivity is the thyroid gland itself. Secondary hyperthyroidism is where the source driving the overactivity is remote from the thyroid, for example, excess TSH production by the pituitary gland. In old textbooks you may see the term tertiary hyperthyroidism. This used to describe hyperthyroidism due to a hypothalamic cause. However, currently, hypothalamic causes are regarded as a secondary cause too.

See Table 11.6 for causes of thyrotoxicosis.

Table 11.6 Causes of thyrotoxicosis

Primary hyperthyroidism
Graves' disease
Toxic multinodular goitre
Toxic adenoma
Hashitoxicosis[a]
Drug induced[a]
Secondary hyperthyroidism
Thyrotropin-secreting tumour of the pituitary[a]
Other tumours
Other
Subacute thyroiditis[a]
Thyroxine ingestion (thyrotoxicosis factitia)[a]

[a] Very rare cause.

Drug-induced thyrotoxicosis

Drug-induced thyrotoxicosis may be due to excessive ingestion of T_4 or iodine-containing drugs.

- **Excessive ingestion of T_4**. Some people may take excess T_4 for a number of reasons. Overprescription by doctors rarely occurs because thyroid function tests are routinely checked and doses amended accordingly. Some patients may take excess T_4 because it gives them a high. Others may take it as part of an abnormal illness behaviour while pretending that they have not taken any (this is called thyrotoxicosis factitia (*fack-tisha*)). This usually occurs in a person with a clinical background, such as a nurse. This can be detected by the pattern of thyroid function tests, with a raised T_4, a normal T_3, and a low or undetectable TSH.

- **Iodine-containing drugs**. These drugs include amiodarone, some cough preparations, and intravenous contrast media and they can induce thyrotoxicosis in susceptible individuals (this is called the Jod–Basedow (*jod-bas-eh-dough*) phenomenon) (*Karl Adolph Von Basedow (1799–1854), German physician; Jod = iodine in German*).

TSH-secreting tumour

A tumour of the pituitary may rarely secrete TSH and drive the production of excess thyroid hormone. The key to the diagnosis of this condition is the finding of elevated T_3 and T_4 levels with a high or normal level of TSH (normally TSH would be undetectable because of negative feedback). The tumour can be demonstrated on MRI or CT scan and surgery is usually required.

Other tumours causing thyrotoxicosis

Rarely a tumour of the ovary may contain thyroid-like tissue that secretes excess T_4 or T_3. In old-fashioned textbooks this is called struma ovarii (*strew-ma-oh-vary-eye*). Thyroid isotope scans will show no uptake in the thyroid but increased uptake in the ovary. Also tumours of the testis, ovary, or bronchus can rarely secrete a peptide that behaves like TSH and stimulates the thyroid to produce excess thyroid hormone.

Hypothyroidism

See Fig. 11.19. Hypothyroidism comprises the clinical signs and symptoms caused by the decreased production of thyroid hormones due to an underactive thyroid

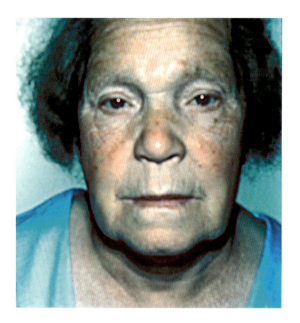

Figure 11.19 Myxoedema.

Table 11.7 Causes of hypothyroidism

Hashimoto's thyroiditis
Idiopathic/spontaneous atrophy
Previous treatment with radioiodine or thyroidectomy
Anti-thyroid drugs
Drugs
Iodine deficiency

gland (the symptoms and signs of hypothyroidism have already been described). See Table 11.7 for causes of hypothyroidism. Hashimoto's thyroiditis has already been described.

Idiopathic atrophic hypothyroidism

This is due to lymphocytic infiltration of the thyroid gland because of an unknown autoimmune trigger. Hashimoto's thyroiditis and idiopathic atrophic hypothyroidism are sometimes grouped together under the umbrella term 'lymphocytic thyroiditis' to emphasize their common autoimmune pathogenesis. Unlike Hashimoto's thyroiditis there is no goitre in this condition. It is more common in women than in men.

Previous treatment for thyrotoxicosis

If the treatment is excessive or too long in duration, then hypothyroidism may occur. It is difficult to prescribe a precise dose for radioactive iodine and hypothyroidism is a recognized complication of this treatment. Ten per cent of patients in their first year will become permanently hypothyroid. After 20 years approximately 80% of patients will develop hypothyroidism. Therefore patients undergoing this treatment require regular follow-up. If hypothyroidism does develop, treatment is with T_4 replacement. Surgical treatment with thyroidectomy can lead to hypothyroidism in 20% of cases.

Thyroid function tests

Thyroid function tests are assays for the thyroid hormones T_4 and T_3 as well as TSH levels. Different laboratories vary in what they test for and their reference ranges, but the majority now detect levels of free T_3 and T_4 (and TSH) that are independent of protein binding. Older assays used to detect total levels of T_4 and T_3 that are dependent on plasma protein concentrations. This led to problems of interpretation if the patient's plasma protein concentration varied for any clinical reason, for example, the normal increased protein concentration during pregnancy would lead to an increased total T_4 level suggesting hyperthyroidism or the decrease in plasma protein concentration in nephrotic syndrome would lead to a decrease total T_4 level suggesting hypothyroidism. In both cases, there is no true derangement of thyroid function. Some laboratories only provide T_4 and TSH levels to keep costs down and only offer T_3 in situations where it is felt the patient is clinically thyrotoxic but with a normal T_4 level (possible T_3 toxicosis). Interpreting thyroid function tests is easy if you understand the negative feedback mechanism described earlier in the control of the thyroid (Table 11.8).

Control of calcium metabolism

Most of the body's calcium is contained in the bony skeleton. Less than 1% is found in extracellular fluid. About 50% of this is bound to albumin and the rest circulates in plasma in the ionized form. The calcium in bone and in the extracellular fluid are in dynamic equilibrium and small concentrations can be mobilized from the skeleton or replaced (a process that is under hormonal control). The principle hormones involved include PTH and vitamin D. PTH is a peptide hormone secreted from the parathyroid glands and elevates plasma calcium by increasing bone resorption, increasing the intestinal absorption of calcium

Table 11.8 Key to interpreting thyroid function tests

Hyperthyroidism

$T_3\uparrow$, $T_4\uparrow$, TSH$\downarrow$

Hypothyroidism

$T_3\downarrow$, $T_4\downarrow$, TSH$\uparrow$

Rarer causes

T_3 toxicosis

$T_3\uparrow$, $T_4\rightarrow$, TSH$\downarrow$

Thyrotropin-secreting pituitary tumour

$T_3\uparrow$, $T_4\uparrow$, TSH$\uparrow$ (or $\rightarrow$)

Thyrotoxicosis factitia

$T_3\rightarrow$, $T_4\uparrow$, TSH$\downarrow$

$\uparrow$, above laboratory reference level; $\downarrow$, below laboratory reference level; $\rightarrow$, normal range

Table 11.9 Other causes of hypercalcaemia

Multiple myeloma

Malignancy

  Secondary to bony metastasis

  Secondary to parathormone-like hormone secreted from tumour

Sarcoidosis

Vitamin D toxicity (usually drug related)

Hyperthryoidism

Immobilization in Paget's disease of bone[a]

[a] *Sir James Paget (1814–1899), UK surgeon.*

with the aid of vitamin D and increasing the renal tubular reabsorption of calcium. Vitamin D is produced in the skin from sunlight. It is metabolized in the liver and kidney to its active metabolite 1,25 hydroxycholecalciferol (*hide-rocks-i-coal-ee-cal-siffer-ol*) (sometimes called calcitriol (*cal-si-try-ol*)). It increases intestinal uptake of calcium. A third hormone, calcitonin (*cal-si-toe-nin*), is produced in the parafollicular C cells of the thyroid. It decreases bone resorption and decreases renal reabsorption of calcium but it is thought to play little role in the physiological control of calcium.

Primary hyperparathyroidism

This is usually due to a parathyroid adenoma secreting excess PTH. Rarely it may be due to hyperplasia of the glands (overactivity of the glands), multiple adenomas, or a functioning carcinoma. Most commonly the patient is asymptomatic with a mild rise in plasma calcium. If the glandular activity is great enough the calcium rise can be sufficient to cause symptoms. The calcium level at which symptoms occur will vary among individuals. This is because many of the symptoms of hypercalcaemia are insidious—for example, constipation, confusion, polyuria, and polydipsia—and they may go unrecognized by the patient early in the disease. Primary hyperparathyroidism can be diagnosed by finding normal or elevated levels of

PTH in the presence of hypercalcaemia (normally PTH is low in the presence of hypercalcaemia because of negative feedback).

Secondary hyperparathyroidism

This is the response of the parathyroid glands to chronic hypocalcaemia. The most common cause is chronic renal failure (other causes include malabsorption and osteomalacia (*os-tea-owe-mal-ay-sha*)). The parathyroid glands increase their activity producing more PTH in an attempt to try to normalize the plasma calcium.

Tertiary hyperparathyroidism

This describes those cases of primary hyperparathyroidism where the parathyroid glands become autonomous and no longer respond to the normal feedback mechanisms. In these situations the plasma calcium levels can be very high.

Other causes of hypercalcaemia

See Table 11.9.

Hypoparathyroidism

This is an uncommon condition leading to decreased secretion of PTH and hypocalcaemia. The most common cause is after thyroidectomy and can be due to disturbance of the blood supply to the parathyroid glands or accidental removal of the glands. Hypocalcaemia can be transient or permanent. Idiopathic hypoparathyroidism is associated with other autoimmune disorders. Antibodies against the parathyroid gland have been demonstrated but their role in the causation of the disease is not clear. Clinical features include hypocalcaemia, cataracts, calcification of the basal ganglia, cutaneous thrush, short stature, and short fourth and fifth metacarpals.

Pseudohypoparathyroidism

This condition is rare and is due to the resistance of the target tissues to PTH. It shares many of the features of hypoparathyroidism including hypocalcaemia.

Pseudopseudohypoparathyroidism

This describes the condition where the patient has the external features of pseudohypoparathyroidism such as short stature, ectopic calcification, and short fourth and fifth metacarpals but does not have any biochemical abnormality such as hypocalcaemia. (Thankfully there is no condition called pseudopseudopseudohypoparathyroidism.)

Other causes of hypocalcaemia

See Table 11.10.

Finals

The emphasis of this section is on the short cases as this format usually causes the most uncertainty. Objective Structured Clinical Examinations (OSCEs) usually have more straightforward and standardized instructions (see 'OSCE examples'). Despite the different formats the clinical

Table 11.10 Other causes of hypocalcaemia

Malabsorption
Chronic renal failure
Osteomalacia or rickets
Acute pancreatitis

approach remains the same. For revision read the examination summary and the key points throughout the chapter and do the questions at the end of the chapter. See Tables 11.11 and 11.12 for day-to-day and Finals cases, respectively.

Some advice relating to examination problems

The instruction

The examiner may say, 'Look at the patient, what is the diagnosis?' This will usually be a spot diagnosis, for example, exopthalmos and goitre = Graves' disease of the thyroid. A variant of this instruction could be, 'Look at the patient's neck, what do you notice?' This could still be a spot diagnosis but it may also be a request to find a sign that could be the prelude to an examination in a different system, for example, Corrigan's sign (see Chapter 4), requiring a cardiovascular examination looking particularly for aortic incompetence. If the instruction is 'examine the neck' only, this suggests a thorough examination of the neck and in this circumstance a thyroid diagnosis will be high on the list of probabilities, so be prepared to execute your full thyroid routine. See Case 11.6.

General look

Continue your overall observations and look at the general demeanour of the patient.

- Are they listless and fidgety?—hyperthyroidism?
- Are they apathetic and lethargic?—hypothyroidism?
- Do they look cachexic?—malignancy?

Table 11.11 Day-to-day cases

Hyperthyroidism
Hypothyroidism
Multinodular goitre
Cervical lymphadenopathy

Table 11.12 Finals cases

Day-to-day cases
Thyroid nodule
Metastatic lymphadenopathy

CASE 11.6

Problem. You are asked to examine the neck and you do not know where to start.

Solution. Keep calm and have a strategy worked out. The most common diagnosis will be thyroid related, so it is worth glancing in three key areas:

- the eyes, looking for exophthalmos and lid retraction
- the neck in the midline, looking for a goitre or nodule
- the surrounding environment, looking for a glass of water.

If none of these features are present, then think laterally and look for abnormal pulsations in the neck, that is, raised jugular venous pressure or Corrigan's sign or look for swellings in other areas such as the supraclavicular fossa.

Inspection

You should have done this already, especially if you adopt the solution in the problem above. Get your patient to lift their chin slightly as this may make a swelling more pronounced.

Protrusion of tongue

If the swelling is at or near the midline, get the patient to protrude their tongue and observe if the swelling elevates.

Swallowing

If you suspect a thyroid swelling, get the patient to swallow and observe if it elevates.

Palpate the neck

Get the patient to flex their neck slightly to relax the sternomastoid muscles. Any swelling should be assessed for site, size, consistency, tenderness, temperature, mobility, pulsatility, and transillumination and auscultated.

Thyroid swelling

Palpate from behind the patient using the pulps of your fingers.

- Do not forget to percuss for retrosternal extension of a goitre
- Do not forget to auscultate
- Do not forget to check for lymphadenopathy.

Check thyroid status

This can be:

- hyperthyroid—irritability, tremor, sweaty, tachycardia, lid retraction, and lid-lag
- hypothyroid—apathetic, bradycardia, and slow-relaxing reflexes (check ankle jerks)
- euthyroid—relatively relaxed and normal pulse rate (on average 70–90 beats/min).

Look for other signs

Other signs include the following:

- hyperthyroid—palmar erythema, spider naevi, gynaecomastia, proximal myopathy, and hyperreflexia
- hypothyroid—dry skin, alopecia, erythema ab igne, xanthelasma, hypercarotenaemia, carpal tunnel syndrome, cerebellar ataxia, myopathy, pleural effusion, pericardial effusion, and ascites
- Graves' disease—pretibial myxoedema, thyroid acropachy, and exophthalmos.

You should be able to observe the majority of these signs with the minimum of fuss. Try not to get bogged down attempting to find every single sign that might be present. Some signs require a thorough routine all of their own, for example, proximal myopathy or ascites, and so should not be looked for unless requested or unless you have picked up on a further clue, for example, distended abdomen.

Case 11.7 suggests some follow-up questions you might ask of a patient depending on your findings.

OSCE examples

History-taking scenario

You are an FY2 working in primary care. A 32-year-old woman presents with suspected thyroid dysfunction. Please take a history and present your diagnosis. You have 10 minutes.

CASE 11.7

Problem. In a case of thyroid disease your examiners follow up by instructing you to ask some relevant questions.

Solution. This one is simple. The examiners are just testing your depth of knowledge of thyroid disease.

- If your case is a goitre, do not forget to ask about dysphagia, stridor, breathlessness, and hoarse voice. You could also ask about the possibility of previous investigations requiring contrast media, whether the patient is on medications such as amiodarone, or whether there has been any recent flu-like illness, which could cause a goitre.
- If your case is hyperthyroidism ask about heat intolerance, increased appetite, weight loss, and diarrhoea (see 'History-taking scenario').
- If your case is hypothyroidism ask about cold intolerance, decreased appetite, weight gain, and constipation (see 'History-taking scenario').

Remember:

- Introduce yourself to the patient.
- Ask the patient whether she has noticed any unintentional or unexplained weight gain or loss.
- Ask about changes to bowel habit, and elicit what these changes are.
- Ask whether the patient prefers warm or cool environments, and assess whether she is appropriately dressed for the weather.
- Ask the patient if she feels particularly irritable, fidgety or nervous; or whether she feels lethargic, has trouble concentrating, or has a low mood.
- Ask about changes to her menstrual cycle.
- Ask about palpitations, weakness, and skin changes.
- Ask if she has noticed a lump in her neck. If so, ask about a change in her voice. Also ask if she has noticed any problems with her eyes.
- Ask if there is a family history of thyroid dysfunction, and about any medications.
- Remember: hypothyroidism usually presents with a slowing down of physiological functions, so weight gain, constipation, menorrhagia, problems concentrating, lethargy and low mood point to this. Hyperthyroidism usually presents with weight loss, intolerance to heat, feeling more irritable or anxious, and scanty periods.

- Thank your patient.
- Explain that you would like to perform a thyroid examination afterwards if dysfunction is indicated by the history and you would like to perform thyroid function tests (TFTs) if indicated by the history.

Examination station

You are an FY2 working in primary care. A 59-year-old man presents complaining of having a lump in his neck. Examine him and then present your findings. You have 10 minutes.
Remember:

- Introduce yourself and gain consent; explain that you will be performing an examination of the patient's neck.
- Note whether the patient has a hoarse voice when he speaks.
- Wash your hands/use alcohol gel provided.
- Inspect the patient as a whole first. Could he have thyroid disease? Is he under/overweight? Appropriately dressed for the weather? Is he fidgety or lethargic?
- Inspect the neck without touching first, looking from the front and sides.
- Think about how you would describe the lump: its site, shape, size, colour, the skin surrounding it, its border—is it irregular or smooth?
- Ask the patient to push out his tongue. If the lump is in the midline and elevates this is a thyroglossal cyst.
- Ask the patient to swallow and look to see what happens to the lump. Is it fixed or mobile?
- Explain to the patient that you would like to feel the lump from behind. Palpate the lump, noting its temperature, texture and mobility.
- Ask if it is painful or tender, feel for pulsatility and transilluminate if appropriate to ascertain whether it is cystic or solid.
- Palpate the lymph nodes in a systematic manner, assessing the anatomical triangles of the neck, and submental, submandibular, preauricular, postauricular, and occipital nodes. Do any of them feel enlarged, painful, or hot?
- Thank your patient and wash your hands/use alcohol gel provided.
- Present your findings in a concise manner, and offer your differential diagnoses. Key differentials may be a cyst (dermoid, thyroglossal), thyroid goitre (midline), carotid aneurysm (pulsatile), lymphoma, etc.

Good luck!

Questions

1   Name three possible complications of a large goitre.

2   In what condition would you find tetany?

3   Why does a thyroglossal cyst elevate on protrusion of the tongue?

4   Which neck swelling exhibits pulsatility?

5   What 10 features should you examine for in any neck swelling?

6   If a thyroid swelling does not elevate with swallowing, give one important reason for this.

7   What cardiovascular features can you find with hypothyroidism?

8   Name four symptoms of hyperthyroidism.

9   Name four symptoms of hypothyroidism.

10   Which swellings may transilluminate in the neck?

References and further reading

Hall R, Evered DC. *A colour atlas of endocrinology*, 3rd edn. Wolfe, London, 1989.

Holt RIG, Hanley NA. *Essential endocrinology*, 6th edn. Wiley-Blackwell, Oxford, 2012.

Vanderpump MPJ, Tunbridge M. *Thyroid disease, the facts*, 4th edn. Oxford University Press, Oxford, 2008.

12 Joints

Introduction

Joints (and connective tissue) come under the field of rheumatology. The most common rheumatological conditions are osteoarthritis and rheumatoid arthritis. Osteoarthritis is usually ascribed to wear and tear or ageing (but this is incomplete and an oversimplification). Rheumatoid arthritis is a multisystem disorder that may affect many organs as well as joints. In 60–70% of cases an autoantibody called rheumatoid factor can be isolated and such cases are termed seropositive (for rheumatoid factor). How this factor is generated is still not fully understood. In contrast there is a family of conditions called the seronegative spondyloarthritides (*spon-dee-low-arth-ritty-deez*). These are a range of diseases with similar or overlapping presentations and are unified by the absence of the rheumatoid factor. These include ankylosing spondylitis (*ank-ee-low-zing-spon-dee-light-iss*), Reiter's (*writers*) syndrome, and psoriatic (*sore-ee-attic*) arthropathy.

In the following section the bulk of the history-taking will focus on symptoms from the groups above but less common groups of diseases such as the crystal arthropathies, for example, gout and pseudogout and the vasculitides (*vas-cue-litty-deez*), for example, systemic lupus erythematosus (*systemic-loo-pus-erith-mat-owe-suss*) (SLE) and temporal arteritis will be touched upon. You will also learn not to restrict your thoughts to joints alone but to the possible systemic complications that a disease may produce or to medical disease, which may have an impact on the joints.

Symptoms

The most common presentation of joint disease is pain. As with pain elsewhere there are a number of key questions you need to ask.

Joint pain

- **'Where do you feel the pain?' (site)** This is a crucial question. People can be vague about where they experience pain. Do not be satisfied with a vague waft of the hand. Get them to be specific and make them demonstrate exactly where it is. If the pain is localized to a joint it is likely that you are dealing with an arthropathy (an all-embracing term meaning an abnormality of a joint; arthralgia (*arth-ral-jah*) is a term you may also see which means pain in a joint and arthritis means inflammation in a joint). If the pain is more diffuse then it could be due to a chronic pain syndrome, for example, fibromyalgia (*fie-bro-my-al-jah*); another possibility is polymyalgia rheumatica (*polly-my-al-jah-room-attic-a*) (see 'Diseases and investigations of the joints' for both of these).
- **'Are there other joints affected?'** Always ask this. Patients may be so consumed by the pain of the offending joint that they neglect to tell you about the less troublesome joints. If one joint is affected this is called a monoarthritis (see Case 12.1), if two to four joints are affected it is called an oligoarthritis

(sometimes pauci-arthritis (*paw-si-arth-right-iss*)), and if more than four joints are affected it is called a polyarthritis. The causes of joint pain are usually different for a monoarthritis compared with a polyarthritis with some overlap in an oligoarthritis (*olly-go-arth-right-iss*) (see Table 12.1). When faced with a single hot joint, the most important diagnosis you must consider is a septic arthritis. This is an acute infection within the joint, usually due to *Staphylococcus aureus* (*staff-ee-low-cock-us-aw-ree-us*). If it is not recognized quickly, the joint can be destroyed irreparably. It is important that a single hot joint is aspirated and any fluid analysed for possible infection.

- **'How long have you had the pain?' (duration)** Acute joint pain (arthralgia) may be fleeting, for example, following a viral infection where joints may ache transiently for several hours. During such an episode there is usually no inflammation of the joints. Some systemic infections may cause arthralgias that last longer and some may cause a reactive arthritis, for example, brucellosis (*brew-sell-owe-sis*). Crystal arthropathies can cause exquisite pain in a joint for several weeks although they can be as short lived as a couple of days. Diseases such as rheumatoid arthritis or osteoarthritis may cause

CASE 12.1

Problem. A 28-year-old man presents with a painful big toe. The day before he played football and missed his evening meal. He remembered stubbing his toe during the match, but could not remember which one. Afterwards he retired to the bar where he celebrated his team's victory with copious amounts of beer. He is on no medication and has never been in hospital before. On examination, his right big toe is swollen, red, and very tender. The rest of the examination is unremarkable. What is the diagnosis?

Discussion. This patient has an inflammatory monoarthritis affecting the first metatarsophalangeal (MTP) joint. It is possible that he suffered trauma to his big toe. However, he has performed heavy exercise on an empty stomach, which he filled preferentially with alcohol! All these factors can predispose to acute gout. Furthermore acute gout is extremely painful and classically affects the first MTP joint. The diagnosis can be confirmed by joint aspiration although it is technically difficult (and painful) with a small joint.

chronic pain. Sufferers may be plagued with pain for years. The natural history of chronic pain may include episodes of more severe pain, which may represent a 'flare up' of disease. Other processes such as trauma, infection, or other rheumatological disease, for example, gout can also lead to an exacerbation of pain. Therefore you must be prepared to consider other conditions and fully evaluate your patient before finally accepting that you face a disease flare.

- **'Does the pain go anywhere?' (radiation)** This question is of limited diagnostic value with the exception of radicular pain (*rad-ick-you-lar*) (see Chapter 6) due to root or nerve entrapment, for example, sciatica. This question may also reveal that the pain is not truly joint pain but pain that just happens to span a joint. So pay special attention to how the pain is described, particularly if it seems ill defined and seems to radiate to the whole of a limb (which would favour a chronic pain syndrome). Another trap for the unwary is referred pain. In this circumstance, pain is experienced remote from its site of origin, for example, the pain caused by arthritis in a lumbar vertebra may be experienced over the hip. Diagnosing referred pain is not easy and requires the doctor to have an index of suspicion. Consider this possibility if after examination and a radiograph a joint appears normal. You may get more joy examining a joint that is more proximal.

- **'How severe is the pain?' (severity)** This question will establish how much of a problem the pain is and how it affects the patient's life. Ask the patient to score their pain out of 10, with 10 being the worst pain they have ever experienced. You will, however, have to make a judgement about the patient's personality as the same pain can be experienced differently by different individuals. A stoical individual may play down excruciating pain and conversely those with low pain tolerance may complain bitterly of the most exquisite agony. This judgement will come with experience.

- **'Is there anything that makes the pain better or worse?' (relieving or aggravating factors)** In most cases inflamed arthritic joints will be more painful with usage or stress on the joint, for example, weightbearing. There may be a history of trauma, which may aggravate pre-existing arthritis or even cause a haemarthrosis (*he-mar-throw-sis*) (blood within a joint). Ankylosing spondylitis is unusual in that back pain is worse when resting. It tends to be worse at night and eases when the patient moves during the day (unlike mechanical back pain). Most sufferers will have tried painkillers to ease their pain, usually with varying degrees of success. As a rule,

a good response to non-steroidal anti-inflammatory drugs (NSAIDs) suggests an underlying inflammatory arthritis (but remember osteoarthritis may also respond to these medications).

Table 12.1 reflects the likelihood of a diagnosis related to the number of joints affected. It remains possible that an unusual presentation of a disease may occur, for example, rheumatoid arthritis presenting initially with a monoarthritis or gout as a polyarthritis.

Stiffness

Stiffness is a subjective symptom. Many people will have experienced some joint stiffness after unaccustomed exercise or trauma to a joint or muscle. In rheumatological conditions stiffness is not transient but a persistent feature. In an inflammatory arthritis, for example, rheumatoid arthritis, stiffness is usually more pronounced when a joint is first

---

Key points

- Joint pain is the most common presentation of joint disease.
- Ask especially about the site of pain and the number of joints affected.
- Determine whether the patient has a monoarthritis, an oligoarthritis, or a polyarthritis.
- Try to ascertain whether the arthritis is inflammatory or non-inflammatory in nature.
- Always ask if painkillers have been taken (including over-the-counter remedies).

Table 12.1 Causes of a monoarthritis and polyarthritis

Monoarthritis
Septic arthritis
Crystal arthritis, for example, gout
Seronegative spondyloarthritides
Polyarthritis
Rheumatoid arthritis
Osteoarthritis
Seronegative spondlyoarthritides, for example, ankylosing spondylitis

used, for example, in the morning (morning stiffness). This stiffness is prolonged and can last more than an hour (note that morning stiffness for longer than 30 minutes is more suggestive of an underlying (inflammatory) arthritis). Ask, 'Is/are your joints stiff?' If the answer is yes, probe further.

- 'How long are they stiff for?'
- 'At what time of the day is your joint stiffness worse?'
- 'Is the stiffness related to activity or rest?'

With degenerative or mechanical arthritis, stiffness and pain tend to be worse following prolonged activity. This tends to be experienced towards the end of the day. In one particular condition, polymyalgia rheumatica (see 'Diseases and investigations of the joints'), pain and stiffness are prominent symptoms. This condition affects the proximal muscles preferentially, that is, shoulder and pelvic girdle and can be so disabling that a patient has difficulty rising from a chair or combing their hair. If you suspect this condition ask the following.

- 'Do you have difficulty combing your hair?'
- 'Do you have difficulty reaching for objects on high shelves?'
- 'Do you have difficulty rising from a chair?'
- 'Do you have difficulty climbing stairs?'

Also consider asking questions about temporal arteritis (see Case 12.6 and Chapter 6), as polymyalgia rheumatica and temporal arteritis may coexist.

Swelling

Ask if there has been swelling of the affected joint. Swelling may be due to soft tissue swelling, for example, synovitis (*sign-owe-vie-tiss*) (inflammation of the joint

lining), new bone formation due to osteophytes (*os-tea-owe-fights*), or the accumulation of fluid within a joint (effusion). Swelling may also occur around tendons (tenosynovitis) (*tea-no-sign-owe-vie-tiss*) and tendon sheaths may develop nodules. It is important to verify that swelling exists during your examination because some people will claim their joints are massively swollen even when no swelling is apparent. As joint swelling is a dynamic process it is possible that the swelling has subsided before presenting to you. This could represent a spontaneous remission or could be as a result of therapy, for example, NSAIDs or steroids. If this is the case it is worth keeping an open mind and reviewing at a later date. The concept of 'subclinical synovitis' is increasingly popular; that is, inflammation that is present and sufficient to cause symptoms, but not apparent on examination. This is important because it may still result in joint damage. The increasing use of imaging techniques, for example, ultrasound and MRI, have demonstrated this and show that clinical examination can be misleading.

Extra-articular features

Some rheumatological conditions, for example, rheumatoid arthritis, can affect other organs as well as joints. Multisystem disorders, for example, SLE, may affect joints as well as other organs. When you perform your review of systems you will detect many of these symptoms (if they exist). Generalized symptoms such as anorexia, weight loss, night sweats, and fever are common. Fatigue is an extra-articular feature that patients complain about commonly. Table 12.2 shows the more 'organ-specific' features that should be looked for.

Raynaud's phenomenon

What is it?

Raynaud's (*ray-nose*) phenomenon (*Maurice Raynaud (1834–1881), French physician*) is a common condition in which there is abnormal spasm of the arteries of the hands or feet in response to the cold. It is common,

---

Key points

- Prolonged joint stiffness lasting longer than 1 hour suggests an inflammatory arthropathy.
- Stiffness when a joint is first used (that is, morning stiffness) suggests an inflammatory arthropathy, for example, rheumatoid arthritis.
- Stiffness following prolonged activity suggests a 'degenerative'/mechanical arthropathy, for example, osteoarthritis.
- The stiffness associated with ankylosing spondylitis improves with exercise and worsens with rest.
- Stiffness and pain in the distribution of the proximal muscles should make you think of polymyalgia rheumatica.

Key points

- Swelling must be objectively verified.
- Joint swelling may be due to soft tissue growth: for example, synovial thickening, bony overgrowth, osteophytes, or fluid, for example, effusion.
- Arthritis may occur in the absence of clinical signs, that is, subclinical synovitis, but may still result in joint damage.

Table 12.2 Extra-articular features of other medical disease

Diarrhoea

Inflammatory bowel disease

Reactive arthritis

Rash

Psoriasis

SLE
  Malar flush
  Photosensitivity rash
  Livido reticularis (*live-ee-dough-re-tick-you-lar-iss*)

Behçet's syndrome (see 'Diseases and investigations of the joints')

Vasculitis

Raynaud's phenomenon

Systemic sclerosis/scleroderma (limited/diffuse)

SLE

Primary Raynaud's

Mouth

Ulcers
  SLE
  Reiter's syndrome
  Behçet's syndrome

Dry mouth
  Sjögren's syndrome[a] (see 'Diseases and investigations of the joints')
  Rheumatoid arthritis
  SLE
  Systemic sclerosis

Eyes

Scleritis/episcleritis
  Rheumatoid arthritis
Scleromalacia perforans (*s-clear-owe-mal-ay-sha-per-fur-anz*)
  Rheumatoid arthritis

Iritis (*eye-right-iss*) and uveitis (*you-vee-eye-tiss*)
  Ankylosing spondylitis

Other seronegative spondyloarthropathies, for example, reactive arthritis

Loss of vision
  temporal arteritis

Respiratory

Pleural effusion
  Rheumatoid arthritis
  SLE
  Other vasculitides

Fibrosing alveolitis
  Rheumatoid arthritis
  Vasculitis and other connective tissue disease

Cardiovascular

Pericarditis
  Rheumatoid arthritis
  SLE
  Other vasculitides

Pericardial effusion
  Rheumatoid arthritis
  SLE
  Vasculitis

Thromboembolic disease
  Anti-phospholipid (*anti-foss-foe-lip-id*) syndrome

Neuropsychiatric

Psychosis
  SLE

Stroke
  SLE
  Temporal arteritis
  Other vasculitides

Epilepsy
  SLE

Depression
  Most causes

Carpal tunnel syndrome
  Rheumatoid arthritis
  Severe osteoarthritis

Genitourinary

Urethritis (*you-reeth-right-iss*)
  Reiter's syndrome

Cervicitis (*serve-i-site-iss*)
  Reiter's syndrome

Obstetric

Recurrent miscarriages
  SLE and anti-phospholipid syndrome

SLE, systemic lupus erythematosus.
[a] *Hennik Samuel Conrad Sjögren (1899–1986), Swedish ophthalmologist.*

with the highest incidence occurring in young females. It affects the hands more than the feet and is usually bilateral. It is important to consider a cervical rib as a possible cause of unilateral Raynaud's phenomenon. Classically the hands change colour three times, from normal to white to blue and finally red. The white colour occurs due to spasm of the arteries, resulting in decreased blood in the peripheral vessels of the hands. The poor blood flow causes cyanosis and the bluish discoloration. The hands ultimately turn red as vasoactive metabolites build up in the vessels causing dilatation of the arteries. During the three stages the hands become increasingly painful and numb. In severe cases of Raynaud's phenomenon ulceration of the hands can occur. For causes of Raynaud's phenomenon, see Table 12.3.

Questions to ask about Raynaud's phenomenon

- 'Do your hands become painful in cold weather?'
- 'Do your hands change colour in the cold and what colour do they change to?' Try to elicit whether there is a triphasic colour change, that is, from white to blue and then red. The white represents the pallor of the hand as the vessels go into spasm restricting its blood supply. The blue represents peripheral cyanosis as the sluggish blood flow returns. The red phase represents a circulatory overcompensation (reactive hyperaemia (*high-per-ee-mia*) as blood surges back into the hand). This phase is also painful.

- 'How long have you had this problem?'
- 'What precautions do you take to prevent this happening?' In severe Raynaud's, people may wear gloves indoors. This question may enable you to gauge the severity of the patient's condition.
- 'Are you taking any medication?'
- 'What is your occupation?' Are they a builder or someone who works with vibrating tools? (This can cause Raynaud's phenomenon.)

If you think the patient has CREST (an acronym for major symptoms), that is, **c**alcinosis (*cal-sin-owe-sis*), **R**aynaud's phenomenon, **o**esophageal dysmotility, **s**clerodactyly, and **t**elangiectasia) or systemic sclerosis, ask the following.

- Do you have any chest or breathing problems? (associated pulmonary fibrosis.)
- Do you have any swallowing difficulties? (oesophageal dysmotility problems.)

Drug history

A drug history is always important. Take the opportunity to check if analgesia or anti-inflammatory drugs have been used and how effective they have been (do not forget to ask about over-the-counter medications and alternative or herbal remedies). Also anticipate possible side effects from medication, for example, NSAIDs—indigestion, oedema, gastrointestinal haemorrhage, renal dysfunction, and so on. Some medications can contribute to an arthropathy,

Table 12.3 Causes of Raynaud's phenomenon

Idiopathic	Known as Raynaud's disease
Connective tissue disorders	Systemic sclerosis/CREST syndrome, systemic lupus erythmatosus, polymyositis, rheumatoid arthritis, and Sjögren's (*show-grens*) syndrome (see 'Diseases and investigations of the joints')
Cervical rib, cervical spondylosis	
Increased plasma viscosity	Waldenstrom's macroglobulinaemia (*wal-den-stroms-macro-glob-you-lin- eem-ia*)* and cryoglobulinaemia (*cry-owe-glob-you-lin-eemia*)
Drugs	β-Blockers and ergot
Vibrating tools	Pneumatic drills
Endocrine	Hypothyroidism and diabetes mellitus

*Jan Gösta Waldenstrom (1906–1996), Swedish physician.

for example, diuretics can precipitate an attack of gout by decreasing the renal excretion of uric acid. An arthropathy may also be the result of a severe allergic response to any drug. This will be in the context of a severe illness affecting multiple organs including the skin. Do not forget to ask about illicit drugs, for example, intravenous heroin. With the prevalence of intravenous drug abuse increasing in this country, there has been a corresponding rise in unusual infections such as tuberculosis, hepatitis B and C, and HIV, all of which can cause arthritis.

Genitourinary history

Where appropriate, take a sexual history (see Chapter 9). This is important because reactive arthritis caused by chlamydia infection is becoming increasingly common. Also, a urethritis or cervicitis are potential symptoms of Reiter's syndrome.

Family history

Some rheumatological conditions are familial including:

- osteoarthritis
- rheumatoid arthritis
- ankylosing spondylitis (and other seronegative arthritides).

A family history of skin psoriasis is important because its presence may be indicative of psoriatic arthropathy.

Impact of illness

During your enquiries it is useful to find out what the impact of illness is on the patient's life (handicap) and their ability to function (disability). This can be done while taking a 'social history'. As you explore the patient's occupation and domestic situation, find out how the disease is affecting their life. This will also guide your treatment of the patient. If you are unable to cure their disease then appropriate aids may transform their lives, for example, a 'bathing chair' may enable a patient to have a bath safely. Also enquire about the patient's occupation, their ability to work, and the time they have taken off work—this is being increasingly used as an outcome measure in rheumatology.

Key points

- Any organ in the body can be affected by a range of rheumatological conditions
- Never forget a drug history
- Also ask about illicit drug use as intravenous drug abusers are at particular risk of infections including hepatitis, tuberculosis, and HIV
- Always assess the impact of arthritis on the patient's life

CASE 12.2

Problem. A 40-year-old Afro-Caribbean woman who has been hypertensive for several years presents with aching muscles and a rash over her arms, legs, and face. She takes bendroflumethiazide (*bend-roe-flu-meth-I-a-zide*) 2.5 mg once daily to control her blood pressure. Her mother, whom she has recently visited in the Caribbean, suffers from osteoarthritis. She has had one child who is fit and well, but four pregnancies in total. Five years ago she was treated with warfarin (*war-fa-rin*) for a deep-vein thrombosis (DVT). On examination, she is obese, but well. There is no evidence of arthritis affecting the large joints, but her left wrist joint is swollen and tender. The rash is erythematous and there are plaques affecting her cheeks, but not her nose. Elsewhere it is urticarial (*err-tick-ariel*) in nature. She has patchy hair loss. What is going on?

Discussion. This case highlights the need to be on your guard. Any one symptom could easily be explained away in isolation, for example, aching muscles and a rash could simply be a viral infection. However, if you stand back

and draw the disparate threads together you will find a unifying diagnosis. In this case the diagnosis is SLE. As you become more familiar with conditions such as SLE you will have more chance of spotting them so long as you remain alert. Typically SLE affects women, particularly of Afro-Caribbean origin, and it is characterized by a 'butterfly' rash on the face. However, any type of rash is possible. Alopecia (*allo-pea-sha*) (the loss of hair) is also a feature. Myalgia (*my-al-jah*) (muscle pain) is common and most small joints can be affected. Patients with SLE can suffer abnormalities of coagulation and there is often a history of DVT. Miscarriages are also more frequent than in the general population. The patient may have long-standing essential hypertension with a degree of renal impairment, but another possibility is lupus nephritis causing hypertension. Further blood tests may add weight to the diagnosis. In this case the anti-nuclear antibodies were positive (see 'Diseases and investigations of the joints').

The importance of examining the joints

Rheumatological problems directly affect the joints, muscles, and bones, but perhaps more importantly they affect function. Many have manifestations in other systems, for example, rheumatoid arthritis can affect the cardiorespiratory system. Similarly many general medical conditions like diabetes mellitus and acromegaly can affect the joints. For this reason it is important to look closely at a patient's joints when performing a general examination.

Examination of the joints summary

1 Introduce yourself to the patient and ask for permission to examine.

2 Ask the patient to get on to the bed (if not already there). You may need to get help!

3 Wash your hands

4 Expose the relevant joint adequately.

5 While doing steps 1–4, have a 'general look'. Is there any discomfort? Are there any aids or adaptations visible?

6 Before examining any joint, ask if it is painful.

7 With all joints, think 'Look! Feel! Move!'

8 Examine the hands and feet.

9 Examine the shoulder joint.

10 Examine the hip joint.

11 Examine the knee joint.

12 Examine the spine.

13 The GALS assessment.

14 Wash your hands.

15 Present your findings.

Examination of the joints in detail

Getting started

1 Introduce yourself to the patient and ask for permission to examine

Put out your hand to shake the patient's hand (do not squeeze too hard!). Say something like, 'Hello I'm Abraham Colles, a third-year student. Do you mind if I examine your xxxx?' (where xxxx is any joint under consideration).

2 Ask the patient to get on to the bed (if not already there). You may need to get help!

Usually this will be no problem, but if the patient is unable to get on to the bed on their own, offer your assistance if you have had moving and handling training. If not, get help from a nurse or healthcare assistant.

3 Wash your hands

Rinse away that MRSA.

4 Expose the relevant joint adequately

Make sure you can see not only the joint, but the major muscle groups around the joint and the joint proximal and distal to the one you are examining. It is probably best that you demonstrate the whole limb if examining a joint affecting an arm or leg, and the patient should strip to their underclothes if you are going to examine the spine. In this way you may appreciate any muscle wasting as a result of disuse or perhaps some subtle neurological lesion that may be contributing to a joint disorder, deformity, or swelling. Remember keyhole surgery may be desirable but keyhole examinations are not!

5 While doing steps 1–4, have a 'general look'. Is there any discomfort? Are there any aids or adaptations visible?

As soon as you meet your patient you should be assessing their general demeanour. Do they look in discomfort? Are they unwell? Note the patient's posture and ability to move. Also glance around the immediate environment and see if you can see any walking aids, for example, walking stick, Zimmer frame, or adaptations such as foam-handled cutlery to aid grip in an arthritic hand.

6 Before examining any joint, ask if it is painful

It is essential that you do not inflict any unnecessary pain with a thoughtless grab of a painful joint. This is not only undesirable and unprofessional, but you may also lose the cooperation of your patient (and fail an exam!)

Key point
- Always check if a joint is painful before examining it!

7 With all joints, think 'Look! Feel! Move!'

Remember this mantra before you examine any joint and in most cases you will perform an adequate examination (particularly if you have a mental blank).

1 **Look**. When looking at the joint(s) in question, identify any evidence of inflammation, such as redness and swelling and any obvious deformity. An old Latin summary of the signs of inflammation is

- *rubor*—redness
- *tumor*—swelling
- *calor*—heat
- *dolor*—pain
- *functio laxio*—lack of function.

2 **Feel**. When feeling the joint(s) use your fingertips to identify any evidence of inflammation, such as heat. Similarly, you will be able to locate any source of pain or swelling. Bimanual palpation of a joint is the most sensitive method of palpation. Can you feel the joint line clearly? If so, inflammation is unlikely. Synovitis is usually felt as a boggy swelling (like feeling a grape) and is usually tender. Bony swelling is usually hard and non-tender. Feel along the tendons while moving the joint—you should be able to palpate any tendon sheath swelling or tenosynovitis, which may cause crepitus (*crep-it-us*) (see later).

3 **Move**. Ask the patient to move the relevant limb in all planes (active movement) and compare that with passive movement (you move the limb for the patient). A restricted range of movement may be due to pain, muscle weakness, mechanical problems, effusion, or inflammation.

Hands and feet

8 Examine the hands and feet

As the hands are the most important functionally these will be concentrated on exclusively (although many aspects of hand examination are relevant to the foot). You should first be aware of the anatomy of the hand (see Fig. 12.1). The hand examination is straightforward (see Fig. 12.2).

Expose the forearms and elbows. Ask the patient if they can do this for you. Gently help them if they cannot. This will give you an idea of the degree of function they have. Now crouch down next to the patient. You should

have a systematic order in which you examine hands. The author tends to use the following routine:

- nails
- skin
- bones and joints
- muscles
- elbows

> ### Key points
> - The classical features of inflammation are redness, pain, heat, swelling, and loss of function
> - Remember 'Look! Feel! Move!'

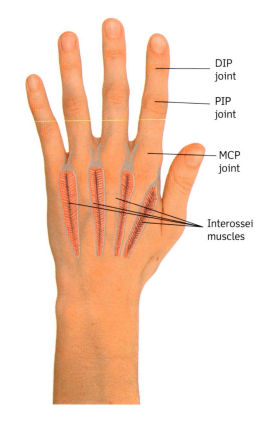

Figure 12.1 The hand showing the interossei and metacarpophalangeal, proximal interphalangeal, and distal interphalangeal joints. DIP, distal interphalangeal; PIP, proximal interphalangeal; MCP, metacarpophalangeal.

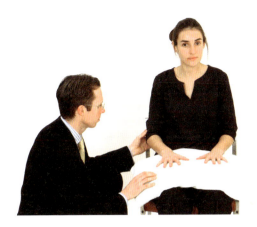

Figure 12.2 Correct position for examining the hands.

- function
- neurological examination
- vascular examination.

Nails

Examine the nails very carefully. Look for signs shown in Table 12.4. See Fig. 12.3.

Skin

Look at the skin carefully. Do not restrict your gaze to the hands but also look at the arms and face. Look for steroid-induced purpura associated with the treatment of rheumatoid arthritis; the skin will also be papery thin (also check for a 'moon face' and 'buffalo hump' suggesting steroid-induced Cushing's syndrome (see Chapter 13). Also look for the signs shown in Table 12.5. See Fig. 12.4. Look for linear scars suggesting previous surgery such as decompression of the carpal tunnel or tendon sheaths or joint replacement.

Bones and joints

Inform the patient that you are now going to concentrate on the bones and joints in the hands. Say, 'I am now going to look at the bones and joints in your hands. I am going to gently squeeze over the joints, tell me if they hurt.' You should look, feel, then move the bones and joints. Are there any bony deformities, such as Heberden's (*hebberdens*) nodes (*William Heberden Sr (1710–1801), English physician*) to suggest osteoarthritis? Osteophytes (small bony outgrowths around the joint margin) develop in osteoarthritis; when found at the distal interphalangeal (DIP) joints, they are called Heberden's nodes; those found at the proximal interphalangeal PIP joints are called Bouchard's (*boo-shards*) nodes (*Charles Joseph Bouchard (1837–1915), French physician*). Look and feel for joint swelling—is there any synovitis (boggy soft tissue swelling around the joint)? Carefully palpate along the digits. If the metacarpophalangeal (MCP) joints look swollen, ask the patient to clench their fist. Normally, you will see the knuckles clearly defined. If synovitis is present there will be generalized swelling around the knuckles obscuring their definition. Remember that swollen joints may be painful. Joints may become dislocated (displacement of the ends of bones forming a joint so that they do not touch) and subluxed (partial dislocation, so that there is some contact with the ends of bones within the joint). These changes occur typically in rheumatoid arthritis. See Table 12.6 for some signs of joint disease. The hand changes in rheumatoid arthritis are characteristic and should be learned as they are common (see Fig. 12.5 and Table 12.7). Remember to expose and look at the elbows for any rheumatoid nodules. They are also found over many of the extensor tendons and along the ulna border of the forearm. Ask the patient to both flex and extend the wrist joints. Again joint swelling or pain will restrict this movement. It is also worth considering the patterns of symptoms and signs. The existence of a symmetrical MCP synovitis may indicate rheumatoid arthritis, whereas DIP and large joint involvement suggest a seronegative spondyloarthritides such as psoriasis.

Muscles

The muscles can be normal or wasted. You should concentrate on the pattern of wasting:

- **disuse atrophy**—generalized wasting of the muscles of the hand
- **ulnar nerve lesion**—wasting of the hypothenar eminence and dorsal and palmar interossei (*inter-ross-ee-eye*) (intrinsic muscles of the hands) with sparing of the thenar eminence
- **median nerve lesion**—wasting of the thenar eminence.

Generalized wasting of the small muscles of the hand is common in chronic arthritides affecting the hands. Specific wasting relating to a mononeuropathy is less

Table 12.4 Comparing nail signs with their associated diseases

Sign	Description	Disease suggestive of
Pitting and splitting	Multiple tiny nail depressions	Psoriatic arthropathy
Onycholysis (*on-ee-coal-lie-sis*)	Separation of the nail plate	Psoriatic arthropathy
Hyperkeratosis (*high-per-kerra-toe-sis*)	Exuberant nail growth	Psoriatic arthropathy
Longitudinal ridging	Small ridges along the nail length	Rheumatoid arthritis
Nailfold infarcts	Tiny black streaks	Vasculitis
Nailfold capillaries	Tiny blood vessels in nailfold	Scleroderma/SLE
Periungual (*perry-un-gwal*) erythema	Redness of the nails	Connective tissue disease
Gottran's papules	Scaling pink/purple papules over knuckles	Dermatomyositis
Sclerodactyly (*s-clear-owe-dack-tilly*)	Skin tightening	Scleroderma
Raynaud's phenomenon	White fingers in the cold, changing to blue and then red on warming	Systemic sclerosis, scleroderma/SLE[a], and primary Raynaud's

[a] SLE, systemic lupus erythmatosus.

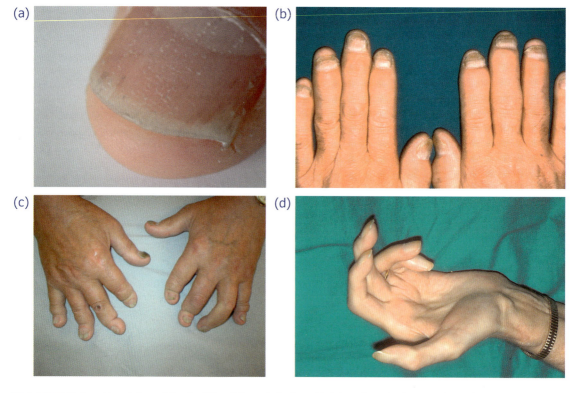

Figure 12.3 Nail and hand signs: (a) nail pitting; (b) onycholysis and joint swelling due to psoriatric arthropathy; (c) onycholysis and arthritis mutilans; (d) sclerodactyly.

Table 12.5 Comparing skin signs with their associated diseases

Signs	Disease suggestive of
Psoriatic plaques on extensor surfaces	Psoriatic arthropathy
Telangiectasia	Systemic sclerosis
Tophi (*toe-fie*)	Chronic tophaceous gout
Rheumatoid nodules (elbows)	Rheumatoid arthritis
Palmar erythema	Rheumatoid arthritis
Tight, thick, shiny skin	Systemic sclerosis
Papery thin skin with purpura	Steroid treatment—likely to be rheumatoid arthritis
Atrophy of the pulp of the finger	Systemic sclerosis
Calcinosis	Systemic sclerosis
Scleroderma facies (*fay-seize*) (beaked nose, small mouth, and telangiectasia)	Scleroderma

(a) (b)

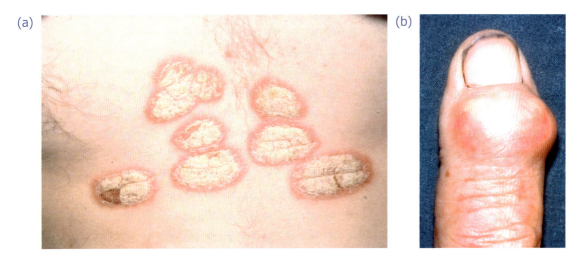

Figure 12.4 (a) Psoriatic plaques; (b) gouty tophus.

common. However, carpal tunnel syndrome secondary to rheumatoid arthritis is the cause of a median nerve palsy (see Chapter 6). The affected muscles will demonstrate a reduction in power and there will be sensory loss in the distribution of the nerve.

Elbows

An essential part of the examination of the hands is to look at the elbows. Ask the patient if you can look at their elbows (show them how you want them to be positioned—see Fig. 12.6). Look carefully at the elbow joint and also along the ulnar border of the forearm. Gently run your fingers over these areas. You should be looking and feeling for rheumatoid nodules and gouty tophi. Note that the presence of rheumatoid nodules in a patient with rheumatoid arthritis increases the chance of them being seropositive for rheumatoid factor (over 80%) (see Fig. 12.7). Ask the patient to place their hands back on the pillow, but this time with palms facing upwards. Quickly re-examine the hands from this angle. Look for palmar erythema, Dupuytren's contracture, any muscle wasting in the palms, and any scars of previous surgery.

Table 12.6 Some signs of joint disease

Sign	Disease suggestive of
Heberden's nodes	Osteoarthritis
Bouchard's nodes	Osteoarthritis
Synovitis	Often associated with rheumatoid arthritis
Subluxation	Rheumatoid arthritis

Key points

- Always inspect for nail changes
- Observe the skin for thinness, purpura, and rashes
- Note any deformities of the hand. Are they symmetrical and characteristic of rheumatoid arthritis?
- Look for the pattern of muscle wasting. Disuse? Carpal tunnel syndrome?
- Never forget to inspect the elbows especially for rheumatoid nodules or plaques of psoriasis
- Never forget to check function

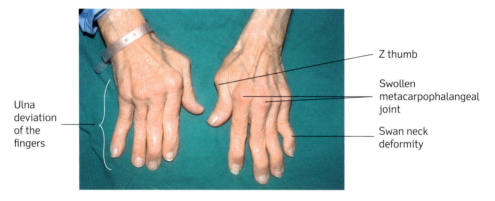

Figure 12.5 Rheumatoid hands.

Function

It is extremely important to assess function. The author assesses gross function by asking the patient to perform five specific tasks.

- Undo and redo a button.
- Remove a pen top and demonstrate how they would write a letter.
- Unscrew the top of a small container or medicine bottle (it is useful to carry one with you into an examination, see Fig. 12.8).
- Demonstrate how they comb the back of their hair (this also assesses external rotation of the shoulder).
- Pick different-sized coins up from a table, see Fig. 12.8.

Remember that these functions will be limited by pain or deformity secondary to the arthritis so ask, 'Is pain stopping you from doing that task?' as it may not always be obvious.

Neurological examination

Any examination of the hands should include a neurological assessment. This is covered in Chapter 6.

Vascular examination

Also palpate the ulnar and radial pulses (see Chapter 4).

Shoulders

9 Examine the shoulder joint

The primary function of the shoulder is the placement of the hand. It is a mobile joint, but as a consequence is less stable. Stability is provided by the rotator cuff, a collection of muscles and tendons that surround the shoulder joint. The muscles involved are supraspinatus (*soup-ra-spin-ay-tus*), infraspinatus (*in-fra-spin-ay-tus*), subscapularis (*subs-cap-you-lar-iss*), and teres (*terrys*) minor. Ask the patient to remove their clothing above the waist. This will provide you with an ideal opportunity to observe the shoulders (you may instantly see which shoulder is affected).

1 **Look**. Look at the shoulders from all angles, comparing each side with the other. Look for areas of skin discoloration, swelling, and muscle wasting. Swelling may represent an effusion or, if overlying the clavicle,

Table 12.7 The hand changes of rheumatoid arthritis

Changes	Explanation
Swelling of the MCP and PIP joints	Synovial thickening/synovitis
Swan neck deformity	Hyperextension of PIP joints with fixed flexion of MCP and DIP joints
Boutonnière (*boot-on- knee-air*) deformity	Fixed flexion deformity of PIP joint with extension contracture of DIP and PIP joints
Z deformity of the thumb	Subluxation at the base of the thumb
Palmar erythema	
Triggering of the finger	Flexor tendon nodule interrupting smooth movement of tendon in tendon sheath
Ulnar deviation of the fingers	Subluxation at the MCP joints
Rheumatoid nodules	Fibrinoid material surrounded by inflammatory cells

DIP, distal interphalangeal; MCP, metacarpophalangeal; PIP, proximal interphalangeal.

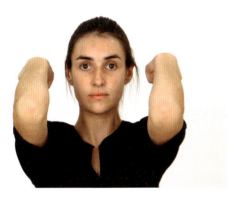

Figure 12.6 Correct exposure of elbows.

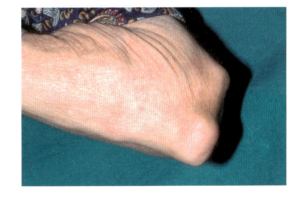

Figure 12.7 Rheumatoid nodule at the elbow.

a previous fracture. Muscle wasting affecting the deltoids will result in a flattened shoulder. This could be secondary to a neuropathy. Supraspinatus and infraspinatus (the muscles running from the scapula to the shoulder joint) will waste in chronic tendonitis or acute tear. Ask the patient to flex their biceps (ideally against resistance) looking for a ruptured biceps tendon. You will see a tightly contracted mass of biceps muscle either sitting high in the arm or distally near the elbow. See Fig. 12.9. Now ask the patient to push against a wall. This will reveal any winging of the scapula. Any pathology affecting the long thoracic nerve or the muscle it supplies (serratus (*sir-rate-us*) anterior)

will cause the scapula to 'wing' or rotate so that it becomes a prominent bulge through the muscles of the back.

2 **Feel**. Gently palpate the shoulder and feel for swelling or crepitus. Crepitus is a grating, crunchy sensation you feel when a joint moves while your fingers are applied to it (it can sometimes be heard). It indicates degenerative changes within the joint. Swelling may be due to effusions, bursitis, dislocation, or old fractures and crepitus may be due to degenerative changes within the glenohumeral (*glean-owe-humour-al*) or acromioclavicular (*a-crow-me-owe-cla-vick-you-lar*) joints. Palpate over the dorsal spine and the interscapular

(a)

(b)

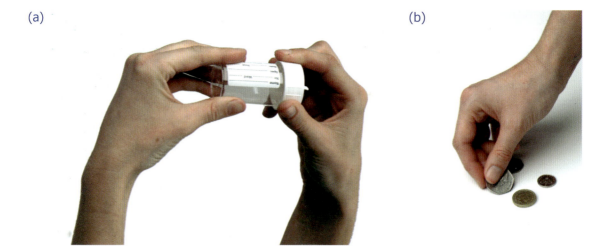

Figure 12.8 Testing hand function.

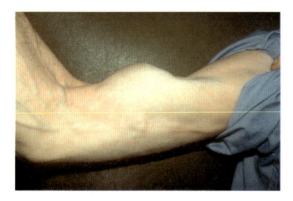

Figure 12.9 Ruptured long head of biceps tendon.

area. These areas are called trigger points and pain here may be suggestive of fibromyalgia (a benign, functional condition, giving rise to various aches and pains in muscles). There are many definitions for fibromyalgia, which include specific numbers of tender points throughout the skeleton. Remember tenderness in the interscapular area could equally be related to muscle spasm from a problem related to the thoracic spine. Check the supraclavicular fossa for any evidence of lymphadenopathy and sternoclavicular joints for evidence of arthropathy.

3 **Move**. See Fig. 12.10. Assess both the active and passive movements of the shoulder joint and try to quantify them in terms of degrees of movement. When testing shoulder movement it is important to make sure you are not simply getting scapula movement contributing to movements of the shoulder. So observe the scapula during your assessment. Assess

- abduction
- adduction
- flexion
- extension
- internal rotation (with the elbow flexed at 90°)
- external rotation (with the elbow flexed at 90°).

Any limitation of movement is significant and may reflect underlying pathology affecting the glenohumeral joint. Other causes of impaired movement are capsular or subacromial bursitis, subacromial (*sub-a-crow-me-al*) impingement, rotator cuff tear, and tendonitis. Usually abduction is affected first. There may be signs of inflammation or an effusion. Limitation of active movement **only** suggests pathology of the muscles and tendons around the shoulder joint (the rotator cuff). Active movement is often painful. Limitation of active **and** passive movement suggests pathology of the shoulder (glenohumeral) joint itself. Limitation of movement may be due to pain or be 'mechanical' (bony or joint capsule) or inflammation. There are exceptions to any rule and capsulitis (*cap-sue-light-iss*) is one of these. With capsulitis, there is loss of passive as well as active movement yet the glenohumeral joint is normal. Perform a brief examination of the acromioclavicular joint. Look

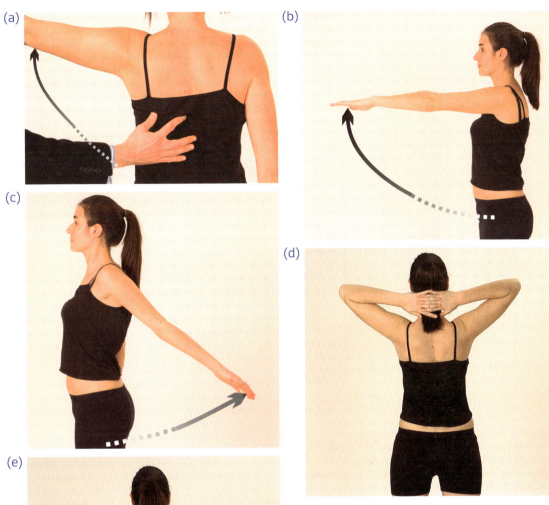

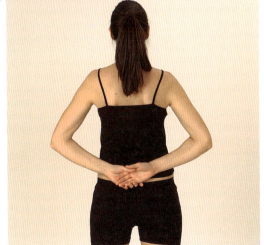

Figure 12.10 Assessing shoulder movements: (a) abduction, (b) flexion, (c) extension, (d) external rotation, (e) internal rotation.

and feel the joint: undertake the scarf test—ask the patient to touch their opposite shoulder with the tip of their index finger. Observe the movement and note any tenderness. Other signs include mid-arc pain, which suggests rotator cuff tendonitis and subacromial impingement. Loss of external rotation suggests capsulitis.

Hips

10 Examine the hip joint

The hip is a ball and socket joint and has a major role in weightbearing. Disorders of the hip will present with pain and a limp. Examine the following:

- observe the gait
- measure leg length
- hip flexion
- hip abduction
- hip adduction
- internal rotation
- external rotation.

1 **Look**. Look as your patient walks into a clinic or on the ward. Do they have an antalgic gait? This is a limp secondary to pain in any part of the leg. With hip disease the patient will lean towards the affected side to minimize movement of the hip on walking. A Trendelenburg (*trend-ellen-burg*) gait (*Friedrich Trendelenburg (1844–1924), German surgeon*) is usually due to chronic hip disease. Here the patient will lean away from the affected hip. The pelvis on the unaffected side drops when they stand on the affected leg

> ### Key points
> - The shoulder is a mobile joint and is relatively unstable; hence it is prone to dislocation and subluxation
> - A major contribution to the stability of the shoulder is by the rotator cuff muscles
> - Movements at the shoulder joint include abduction, adduction, flexion, extension, and internal and external rotation

(in fact, you should ask the patient to stand on one leg then the other to emphasize this—this is called Trendelenburg's sign).

....
Tip
Do not forget to look for neurological causes for an abnormal gait.
....

Now measure the leg length from the anterior iliac spines (the bony protuberance over the upper pelvis) to the medial malleolus (*mal-lee-owe-lus*) (over the ankle joint) of the same side. This is called the **true leg length** because it simply measures the femur plus tibia/fibula (a difference of 1 cm between right and left legs is normal). But the patient could have identical true leg lengths and still look as though one leg is shorter than the other! This is usually due to problems with the pelvis or hip joint (or spine, for example, scoliosis) and for this reason you should also measure the **apparent leg length**. The apparent leg length is from the umbilicus to the ipsilateral medial malleolus and takes into consideration the pelvis and hip joint (a difference of >2 cm is significant). Any tilting of the pelvis, for example, from curvature of the spine, will produce unequal apparent leg length despite the true leg length being equal.

2 **Feel**. Feel around the hip joint for any area of local tenderness. Feel over the greater trochanter (*trow-canter*) (this can easily be seen and felt when the patient is on their side, it is the bony protuberance on the lateral aspect of the upper thigh and is an important site of muscle insertions). The most common problem here is trochanteric bursitis (painful inflammation of the bursa overlying the greater trochanter).

3 **Move**. You can test all the movements of the hip (except hip extension) while the patient is supine. Start with passive movements and follow this order.

    (1) **Hip flexion**. See Fig. 12.11. Flex the hip with knee bent. It should reach 120°.

    (2) **Hip abduction**. See Fig. 12.12. Keep the legs straight and stabilize the pelvis with your left hand by placing it over the anterior iliac spine. Draw the right leg towards you (or left leg away from you) using your right hand to support the calf muscles. Once the pelvis starts to deviate (you will feel it start to abduct in line with the leg), this is

the point of maximum hip abduction. It is usually about 45°.

(3) **Hip adduction**. See Fig. 12.13. You can keep your hands in the same position as for abduction, but this time move the right leg away from you across the midline (or left leg towards you). Again, keep the leg straight and pelvis still. The normal angle of adduction is about 30°.

(4) **Internal and external rotation of the hip**. See Figs. 12.14 and 12.15. This is one of the earliest and most reliable signs of hip disease. Flex the knee to 90° and rotate the foot laterally, thereby turning the hip inwards. Similarly with external rotation, rotate the foot medially. You should be able to achieve 45° of both internal and external rotation.

(5) **Extension of the hip**. Ask the patient to turn over so that they are prone; keeping the leg straight extend the hip. After performing the passive movement for each action get the patient to repeat the movement actively and note any pain or limitations of movement.

Knees

11 Examine the knee joint

The knee joint is a modified hinge joint. Its stability depends on internal structures (cruciate [*crew-she-ate*] ligaments and menisci [*many-sky*]) and external structures (collateral ligaments and surrounding muscles) (see Fig 12.16). The menisci are crescent-shaped pieces of cartilage found in the medial and lateral aspect of the knee joint. They are relatively unstable and susceptible to injury. Both the seronegative spondyloarthritides (such as psoriatic arthropathy and ankylosing spondylitis) and rheumatoid arthritis commonly affect the knee.

Key points
- Always examine the gait of a patient with hip problems
- Movements at the hip joint include abduction, adduction, flexion, extension, and internal and external rotation
- Difficulty with internal rotation of the hip is one of the earliest signs of hip disease

Observation of the knee

Remove clothing covering the patient's lower limbs, but remember to cover the patient's groin to protect their modesty. Now look at the legs. There are certain features to look out for:

- genu varum (*jen-oo vair-um*)
- genu valgum (*jen-oo val-gum*)

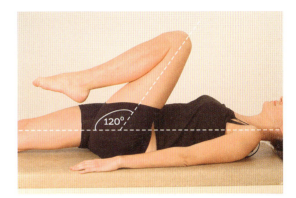

Figure 12.11 Hip flexion.

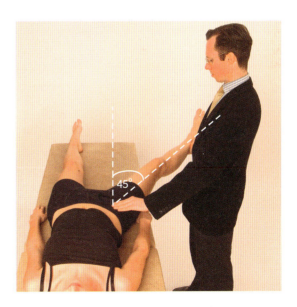

Figure 12.12 Hip abduction (ensure the pelvis is stabilized).

- genu recurvatum (*jen-oo re-curve-ate-tum*)
- muscle wasting.

Genu varum

See Fig. 12.17. This is medial displacement of the tibia on the femur causing an outward bowing of the leg. Such 'bowing' of the legs can be due to rickets, injury, or

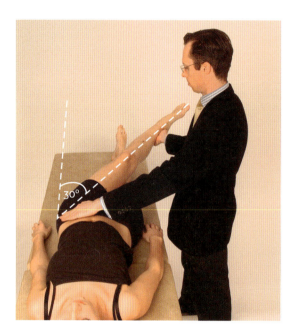

Figure 12.13 Hip adduction.

infection. Sometimes an abnormality of the epiphyseal (*epi-fizzy-al*) growth plate or of the medial aspect of the knee may also cause genu varum.

Genu valgum

See Fig. 12.18. This is lateral displacement of the tibia on the femur. Again this may be due to injury, infection, or abnormalities of either the epiphyseal growth plate or of the lateral compartment of the knee. It is seen more commonly in inflammatory joint disease such as rheumatoid arthritis.

Genu recurvatum

See Fig. 12.19. This is hyperextension of the knee beyond 10°. This may be associated with hypermobility syndromes. For example, Ehlers–Danlos (*err-luz-dan-loss*) syndrome or pseudoxanthoma elasticum (*sue-dough-zan-though-ma-elastic-um*). Benign hypermobility syndrome is the most common cause where lax ligaments due to abnormal collagen synthesis permit excessive movements at joints (in lay terms, being 'double-jointed').

Muscle wasting

Look at the quadriceps muscle bulk. Any chronic painful knee condition will cause it to waste. You will need to examine many quadriceps muscles before you can appreciate subtle loss of muscle bulk. To monitor the rate of muscle wasting or recovery, it may be necessary to measure the circumference of the quadriceps (see Fig 12.20). Do this at 10 cm above the superior pole of the patella.

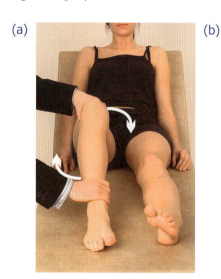
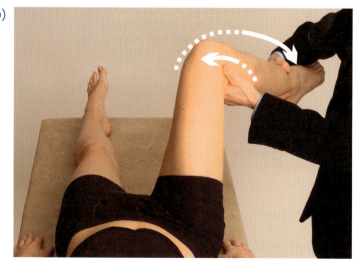

Figure 12.14 Internal rotation of the hip. (a) Start position; (b) end position.

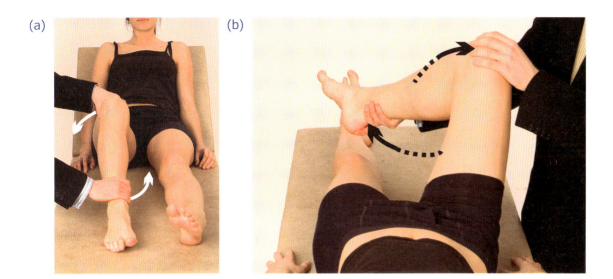

Figure 12.15 External rotation of the hip. (a) Start position; (b) end position.

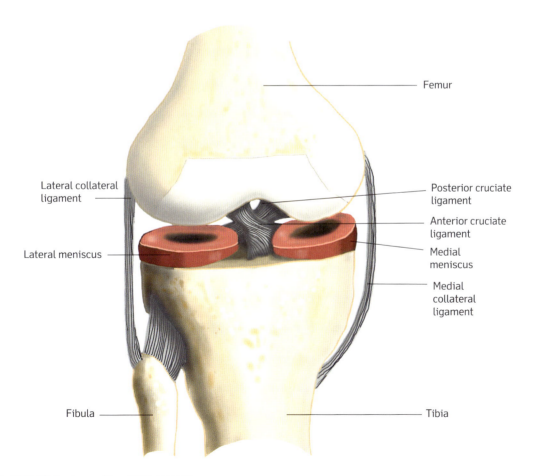

Femur

Lateral collateral ligament

Posterior cruciate ligament

Anterior cruciate ligament

Lateral meniscus

Medial meniscus

Medial collateral ligament

Fibula

Tibia

Figure 12.16 Anatomy of the right knee joint.

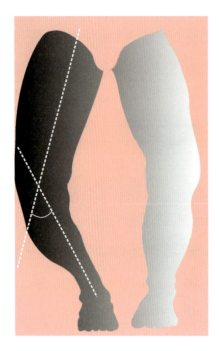

Figure 12.17 Genu varum.

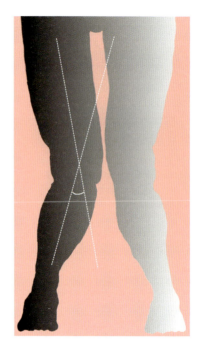

Figure 12.18 Genu valgum.

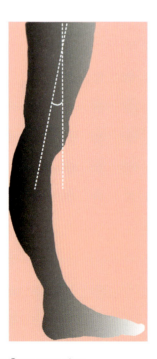

Figure 12.19 Genu recurvatum.

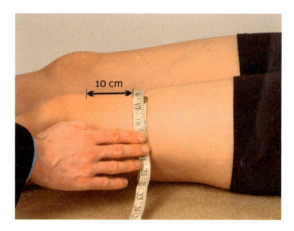

10 cm

Figure 12.20 Circumferential measurement of the quadriceps muscle.

Examination of swelling

There are many causes of a swollen knee. Often in a young fit person it is secondary to trauma causing a haemarthrosis. However, there are several inflammatory conditions that may cause it (see Table 12.8). The swelling can be due to fluid, bony growth, or synovial thickening. Swellings secondary to fluid are either generalized (an effusion) or localized (a bursa). There are a few clinical tests for effusions. For each test, start with the patient sitting on a couch or bed with their knees extended and exposed. First, inspect the knee for either an obvious suprapatellar pouch effusion or loss of the normal contours of the parapatellar gutters. Then perform the following more specific tests.

Bulge test

See Fig. 12.21. This is a test for small effusions. Stroke the fluid around the knee with the palm of your right hand from the medial joint line proximally into the suprapatellar pouch. Now place your left hand across the medial aspect of the joint margin with the thumb resting on the patella. This will prevent any fluid passing back down the medial side of the knee. You can now stroke the fluid from the suprapatellar pouch back down the other (lateral) side of the knee using the dorsum of the right hand running down the lateral joint line. A bulge of fluid at the medial patella gutter confirms a small effusion.

Patellar tap

See Fig. 12.22. This is a test for larger effusions. With the knees extended, place your left hand on the suprapatellar

Table 12.8 Causes of a swollen knee

Septic arthritis
Rheumatoid arthritis
Osteoarthritis
Pseudogout
Gout

pouch (to contain the effusion within the pouch) and gently milk any fluid towards the patella, making sure you maintain downward pressure on the thigh (see Fig. 12.22). Now place your right hand on the patella and tap it. If fluid is present you will feel the patella descend before tapping against the underlying bone. Compare this with yourself (assuming you have no effusion). There should be no downward displacement of the patella or 'tapping' sensation. Note that if the effusion is very tense these tests will be less accurate. If the swelling looks localized, then consider a bursitis. Check its position and see if it correlates anatomically with a bursa. With any localized swelling define the consistency, dimensions, tenderness, presence of pulsation, reducibility, and transillumination (if a swelling transilluminates, it will glow when you shine the light from a pen torch through it—indicating the presence of fluid).

Ruptured Baker's cyst

A Baker's cyst (*William Morrant Baker (1839–1896), English surgeon*) is a swelling of clinical importance. It lies in the popliteal fossa (at the back of the knee) and if it ruptures precipitates sudden calf pain. The knee swelling may reduce and the calf may become swollen with pitting oedema. The most important differential diagnosis is that of a DVT as both produce similar signs (calf swelling, oedema, pain, and often redness). Patients presenting in this way should be investigated with an ultrasound scan of the veins of the leg (to check their patency) or a venogram (contrast is injected into the veins of the foot to see if there is good flow back up the leg. If the flow is blocked this suggests a clot in the vein). Ultrasound is particularly useful because it can also be used to confirm any fluid in

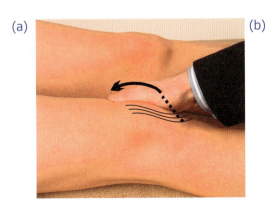
(a)
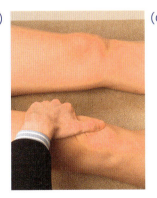
(b)
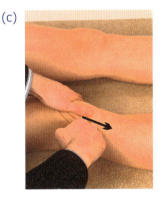
(c)

Figure 12.21 The bulge test: (a) stroking fluid proximally into the suprapatellar pouch; (b) holding the fluid in the suprapatellar pouch; (c) stroking fluid distally from the suprapatellar pouch.

the knee joint, any remnants of the Baker's cyst, or any evidence of soft tissue oedema.

Examination for stability

The knee depends on a number of structures for its stability. This includes the cruciate ligaments, the collateral ligaments, the capsule of the knee, and the menisci. You should test for the stability of the collateral ligaments and the cruciate ligaments.

There are two collateral ligaments, the medial and lateral collateral ligaments. These ligaments run vertically on either side of the knee and prevent any medial (varus) or lateral (valgus) movement. To test the collateral ligaments, the knee should be flexed at about 20°. Hold the ankle with one hand and support the thigh with the other. To stress the lateral collateral ligament, apply a valgus (lateral) force to the joint. If you are examining the right leg, do this by pushing the ankle medially (away from your body) with your right hand and simultaneously pulling the inner aspect of the knee laterally with your right hand. To stress the medial collateral ligament, apply a varus (medial) stress to the knee, pull the ankle laterally (towards **your body**) with your right hand while simultaneously pushing the outer aspect of the knee medially with your left hand. Check the joint line between the tibia and femur for any separation. Any weakness or tear of the collateral ligaments will become apparent as a lateral (or medial) movement associated with a widening of the joint line on the opposite side of the knee. See Figs. 12.23 and 12.24.

There are two cruciate ligaments, the anterior and posterior cruciate ligaments. The anterior cruciate ligament runs from the anterior aspect of the femur to the posterior

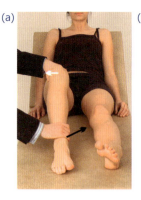
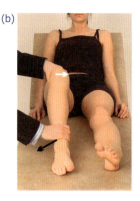

Figure 12.23 Assessment of the collateral ligaments. (a) Stressing the medial collateral ligament: the white arrow represents the force generated by the left hand to stabilize the knee (to prevent its movement). The right hand attempts to move the ankle medially. (b) Stressing the lateral collateral ligament.

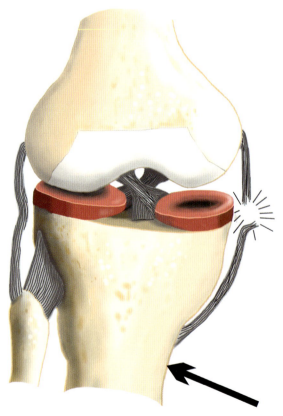

Figure 12.24 Collateral tear showing angulation and separation. Any lateral movement of the tibia will cause undue displacement and angulation.

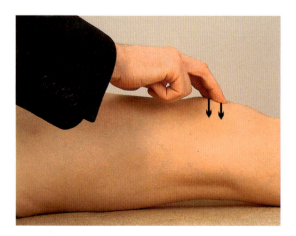

Figure 12.22 The patellar tap.

aspect of the tibia. Similarly, the posterior cruciate ligament runs from the posterior aspect of the femur to the
anterior aspect of the tibia. They prevent any anterior or
posterior movement of the femur on the tibia. The anterior
cruciate prevents the tibia slipping forward in a horizontal
plane from the femur (and is essential for climbing down
a flight of stairs). The posterior cruciate prevents the tibia
slipping backwards on the femur.

Anterior cruciate assessment

Lachman's (*lack-mans*) test is used. The knee should be
flexed at about 30°. Hold the femur securely by placing
your left hand at the back of the thigh. Now hold the tibia
with your right hand over the back of the calf muscles. Try
to pull the tibia forwards on the femur. An intact anterior
cruciate ligament will prevent any anterior movement. Any
movement greater than 5 mm anteriorly is suspicious.

Anterior cruciate assessment

The anterior drawer test is used; it is similar to the Lachman's test, but the knee is flexed at 90°, see Fig. 12.25.
The hip should not be in internal or external rotation as
this prevents the anterior cruciate being assessed. For this
reason it is inferior to the Lachman's test. If the tibia is
internally rotated inadvertently it tightens the posterior

cruciate. If there is now any anterior movement this will be
due to a posterior cruciate tear.

Posterior cruciate assessment

The posterior drawer test is used. The knee should be
flexed at 90°. If there is a posterior cruciate tear, there
will be posterior subluxation of the tibia on the femur
leading to the loss of convexity of the upper tibia compared with the normal one. See Fig. 12.26. Performing
an anterior drawer test will correct this (the posterior
drawer sign). As mentioned above you can also perform
an anterior drawer test while the tibia is in internal rotation to assess the posterior cruciate.

Range of movement

In testing the range of movement of the knees, there are
several steps that you should consider:

- prone-lying test
- active hyperextension of the knee
- quadriceps lag
- passive extension of the knee
- active flexion of the knee
- passive flexion of the knee.

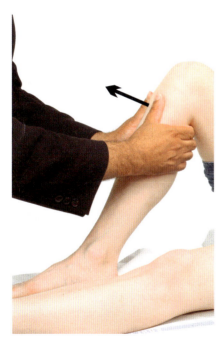

Figure 12.25 The anterior drawer test: stressing the
anterior cruciate ligament.

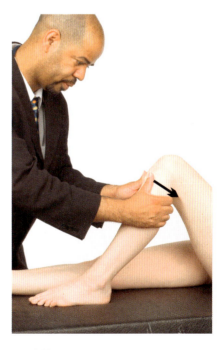

Figure 12.26 The posterior drawer test: stressing the
posterior cruciate ligament.

Prone-lying test

A flexion deformity of the knee could be missed on simple observation. The prone-lying test is a good way of demonstrating a flexion deformity. Ask your patient to lie prone on the bed or couch with their feet over the edge. The knees should extend naturally as the anterior aspect of the leg comes to rest on the examination surface. If there is a flexion deformity, the affected leg will remain elevated above the couch from the knee down. Chronic hamstring tightness, occurring in sportsmen and sportswomen, will produce a flexion deformity. The resistance to extension will be gradual on passive examination. A locked knee will produce a sudden painful resistance to extension and it represents the presence of intra-articular debris, for example, from meniscal tears. This requires orthopaedic attention.

Active hyperextension of the knee

When the patient is in the supine position, ask them to lift their heels off the couch while keeping their knees touching it. This is active hyperextension of the knee. Normal individuals should be able to hyperextend the knee joint to no more than 10° above the horizontal (see Fig. 12.27). Hyperextension beyond this is called genu recurvatum. See Fig. 12.19.

Quadriceps lag

Now ask the patient to lift the lower limb off the couch with the knee extended. This will reveal any quadriceps lag, due to weakness. Essentially it takes a little longer for the leg to be raised because it is weaker than the other leg.

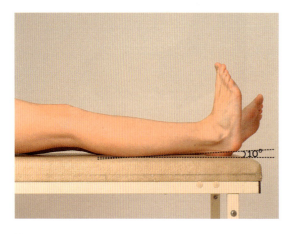

Figure 12.27 Normal hyperextension of the knee.

Passive extension, active flexion, and passive flexion of the knee

Ask the patient to (actively) flex the knee. Compare both sides. Now passively extend the knee and compare it with the other side. Repeat the knee flexion as a passive movement. The range of movements should be full, equal, and painless (see Case 12.3).

Key points

- Note any deformity of the knee joint (the prone-lying test may unmask a subtle fixed-flexion deformity)
- Always check the integrity of the knee ligaments with a painful knee
- If the knee is swollen perform the bulge test or the patella tap
- During active extension of the knee look out for quadriceps lag, which suggests weakness of that muscle group
- A ruptured Baker's cyst can mimic a DVT

CASE 12.3

Problem. A 32-year-old man injured his knee while playing football. It had swollen up to the size of a balloon but he did not seek medical help. After a 'few days in bed' the swelling had gone down and he went back to work as an accountant. He has presented to the hospital emergency department because he has found on occasions his knee has 'seized up' and that he is unable to extend his knee. One episode was so painful he had fallen to the floor. What is the problem and what should be done?

Discussion. Ideally you should get a clearer account of the mechanism of injury, for example, a direct blow to the knee or a twisting injury, to enable you to predict the possible consequences. However, an important complication has ensued. He has developed a locked knee. This is an orthopaedic emergency because if he is not treated promptly he could damage his joint further. He will need arthroscopy to inspect the joint as it is likely that he has damaged a meniscus and a fragment or flap may be impeding the extension of the knee. As part of his examination you should also check the integrity of his ligaments to see if there is any joint instability.

Spine

12 Examine the spine

Back pain is one of the most common causes of absence from work in the UK. Because the spine has many important functions (scaffold for the limbs, protection for the spinal cord, and a vibration damper), the slightest disorder will affect function dramatically. Patients with back problems usually present to their GP; however, those with acute severe back pain often attend the emergency department. There are several important causes of back pain. Most commonly it results from injury (trauma) through actions such as lifting heavy objects incorrectly or twisting suddenly (see Case 12.4), but occasionally a patient with back pain will be found to have a more sinister cause. Warning signs for possible serious spinal pathology include

- fever and unexplained weight loss
- bladder or bowel dysfunction
- history of carcinoma
- ill health or presence of other medical illness
- progressive neurological deficit
- disturbed gait or saddle anaesthesia
- age of onset <20 years or >55 years
- steroid use
- HIV infection.

Causes of back pain are shown in Table 12.9. For the purposes of examination, the spine can be divided into three segments: the neck (cervical spine), the upper back (thoracic spine), and the lower spine (lumbar spine). You should ask the patient to remain standing if you are going to examine the whole of the spine. If you are examining the neck, the patient may sit down.

Table 12.9 Causes of back pain

Trauma
Tumour
Inflammation
Infection
Mechanical/degenerative

Cervical spine

1 **Look**. Watch the patient as they walk into the room and study how they are holding their neck. Ask the patient to sit down if you are examining only the neck. Look at the neck from the front (anteriorly) and from the sides (laterally). When looking at the neck anteriorly, observe whether the neck is held straight or if it is twisted (torticollis) (*taut-ee-coll-iss*). Torticollis in an adult is often due to trauma (injury), chronic scarring of the cervical spine, or disorders of the cervical discs. In infants it can be caused by tumour of the sternocleidomastoid muscle. When observing the neck laterally, look for the normal curvature of the neck (convex forward—lordosis [*lord-owe-sis*]). It becomes exaggerated in ankylosing spondylitis to compensate for the abnormal backward curvature (kyphosis [*kye-foe-sis*]) of the thoracic spine that occurs in this disorder. See Fig. 12.28.

2 **Feel**. Palpate the neck to identify areas of local tenderness, which could represent inflammation or injury. Feel for enlarged lymph nodes. It is easiest to palpate from behind the patient, but remember to tell them exactly what you are about to do, as it is alarming to be grasped by the neck from behind!

3 **Move**. The neck has several basic movements (flexion, extension, lateral flexion, and rotation) that should be assessed (see Fig. 12.29). You should give clear explanations of the exact movement that you would like. It is

(a) 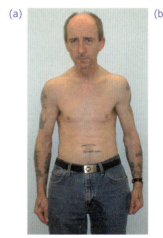 (b)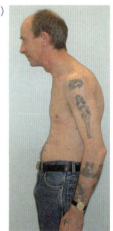

Figure 12.28 Ankylosing spondylitis. The disease is not apparent when viewed from the front, but the typical question-mark posture is readily apparent when viewed from the side.

preferable to show the patient the desired movement yourself. For example, if you ask your patient to place their left ear on their shoulder, they may do so by simply lifting up their left shoulder to touch their ear! This demonstrates good shoulder movement but defeats the purpose of the examination, that is, lateral flexion of the neck.

There are a couple of supplementary tests that should be considered when examining the neck.

- **Lhermitte's (*ler-meets*) sign (the barber's chair sign)**. (*Jacques Jean Lhermitte (1877–1959), French neurologist/psychiatrist.*) Flexion of the neck produces paraesthesia in the arms and sometimes legs due to nerve irritation. This occurs in multiple sclerosis.
- **Reverse Lhermitte's sign**. This occurs when parasthaesia occurs in the arms on neck extension. It is due to cervical myelopathy (see 'Diseases and investigations of the joints').

Thoracic spine

1 **Look**. Observe the spine from the back (posteriorly) and the sides (laterally). The normal thoracic spine curves backwards slightly (kyphosis) (see Fig. 12.30) and the vertebrae should be aligned vertically on top of one another. Any curvature in the lateral plane is abnormal and is called a scoliosis (*scoe-lee-owe-sis*) (see Fig. 12.31). The normal thoracic kyphosis can increase gradually in chronic disorders such as ankylosing spondylitis, osteoporosis, or degenerative disc disease. It can occur acutely due to infection or fracture of the vertebrae. An angular kyphosis called a gibbus (*gib-bus*) may result. A

small degree of lateral curvature is acceptable but more pronounced scoliosis can be due to

- leg length inequality
- postural (only occurs when the patient is sitting down)
- neurological disease (syringomyelia or neurofibromatosis)
- congenital (absent or fused vertebral discs)
- infected vertebral discs
- tumour (primary or metastatic) affecting the vertebrae.

However, commonly no cause is found and the cause is said to be idiopathic.

2 **Feel**. Gently feel along the spine and percuss individual vertebrae to locate areas of tenderness. A painful vertebra is significant and should alert you to the possibility of a collapsed vertebra (Case 12.4), infection of the intervertebral disc, or a tumour affecting the spine.

3 **Move**. Measure the distance from the first thoracic disc (D1) to the last (D12) (see Fig. 12.32) (D = dorsal, synonymous with thoracic) and ask the patient to bend over (anterior flexion); the distance between these two points should increase by at least 3 cm. Ask the patient to run one hand down the side of their leg. This is lateral flexion and should achieve about 15° from the midline on either side. Next, assess rotation by holding the patient's pelvis (or asking them to sit down) and ask them to twist to look over one then the other shoulder. Remember that flexion, extension, and lateral flexion of the thoracic spine are closely linked with that of the lumbar spine and can be difficult to separate. Measuring the anterior flexion of the thoracic spine is demonstrated in Fig 12.32.

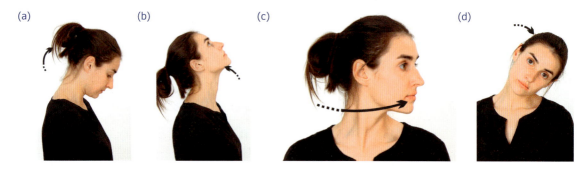

(a)　　　(b)　　　(c)　　　(d)

Figure 12.29 Neck movements: (a) flexion, (b) extension, (c) rotation, and (d) lateral flexion.

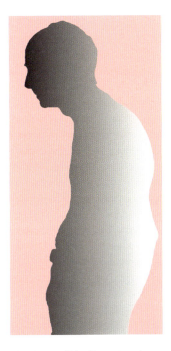

Figure 12.30 Kyphosis of the thoracic spine.

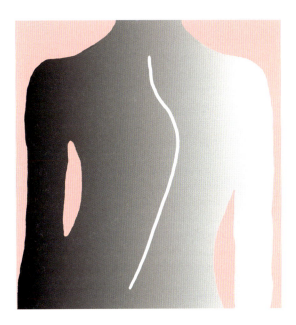

Figure 12.31 Scoliosis of the thoracic spine.

Lumbar spine

1 **Look**. Observe the lumbar spine both laterally and posteriorly. The lumbar spine has a lordosis. Determine whether the lordosis is exaggerated or lost. Is there a coexistent scoliosis? See Table 12.10 and Fig. 12.33.

2 **Feel**. Gently feel along the vertebrae for areas of focal tenderness and percuss each one in turn.

3 **Move**. Movement of the lumbar spine is closely linked with that of the thoracic spine and it is difficult to isolate movements to one particular segment of the spine. In fact, there are specific tests for measuring flexion of the lumbar spine as there are for measuring flexion of the thoracic spine. Schober's (*show-burrs*) test is the best of these. When the patient is standing, identify the posterior superior iliac spines or the dimples of Venus, that is, L5 (see Fig. 12.34) and mentally draw a line from one to the other. From the midpoint of this line measure 10 cm upwards and mark this point with a pen. Ask the patient to bend forwards to touch their toes and re-measure the distance from the pen mark back to the midpoint between the posterior superior iliac spines. The distance should be at least 15 cm. A reduction in flexion is often seen in ankylosing spondylitis. Normally the length of the lumbar spine should increase when

Key points

- The spine provides a scaffold for the limbs and organs, is a shock absorber, and protects the spinal cord
- The spine is conveniently divided into the cervical, thoracic, and lumbar regions
- Normally the cervical spine has a lordosis, the thoracic spine a kyphosis, and the lumbar spine a lordosis; look out for loss or exaggeration of these curvatures
- Palpate and percuss each vertebra (and paraspinal area) and look for tenderness
- Perform Schober's test to quantify flexion of the lumbar spine

bending forward. Also assess lateral flexion and rotation to see if they are full and equal.

13 The GALS assessment

The overall integrity of the musculoskeletal system can be screened very quickly. Indeed, most of the examination can be done without touching the patient, by simply asking the patient to follow your movements (it is easier to show someone what you mean than to describe it to them). The main signs of rheumatic disease are swelling and deformity, plus pain and difficulty

CASE 12.4

Problem. A 72-year-old male smoker is admitted with severe back pain. This occurred after he tried lifting a heavy bag of compost while leaning forward in an awkward position. He took solpadol, which gave some temporary relief but the pain is as strong as ever. On examination, he has a kyphosis and is tender around D10–D12. The pain is severe enough to restrict any movement of the spine. A radiograph reveals generalized osteopenia of the spine and wedge fractures of D9–D12. How should he be managed?

Discussion. Clearly he has sustained fractures of several vertebrae resulting from his attempt to lift a heavy weight with a poor technique. Osteoporosis is prevalent in old age and leads to fragile bone architecture, which can predispose to fractures (even with trivial forces). It is a disease that affects women predominantly (one in three women over 50 years) but what is not widely appreciated

is that it can affect men too (one in 12 men over 50 years). Despite this, your patient is a 'young fit' older person (assumed, as he is still gardening) and therefore you need to consider other pathological causes of osteoporosis. Check that he is not on steroids and he needs screening for thyrotoxicosis, malabsorption, liver disease, myeloma, and other malignancies including prostate cancer with prostate specific antigen. He will need regular analgesia until his pain settles and treating in the acute setting with the intravenous bisphosphonate (*buy-foss-phone-ate*) pamidronate (*pam-id-roe-nate*) (which also has a good analgesic effect). If no secondary causes of osteoporosis are found he should continue with oral biphosphonate treatment to protect his spine, have a dual energy X-ray absorphometry (DEXA) bone scan to monitor the density of bone and be advised to stop smoking as this is a risk factor for osteoporosis.

(a) 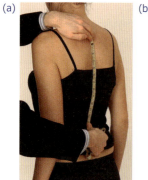 (b)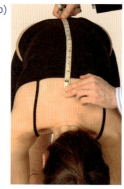

Figure 12.32 Measuring anterior flexion of the thoracic spine.

Table 12.10 Causes of a loss of lordosis and exaggerated lordosis

Loss of lordosis
Degenerative disc disease

Exaggerated lordosis
Spondylolisthesis[a]
Fixed flexion deformity of the hips
Pregnancy
Obesity

[a] Spondylolisthesis (*spon-dee-loll-iss-thesis*) is the forward movement of a vertebra on the one below it (and tends to occur in the lumbar spine).

with movements. Consequently, the minimum screening examination involves

- looking for any swelling or deformity and for any abnormal position or posture of the limbs or individual joints
- observing the patient move and looking for any difficulty or restriction of movement.

The order in which the system is examined is not important and depends on the situation (outpatients, ward, and so on) and the patient. Essentially four components

must be assessed and can easily be remembered using the acronym GALS (**g**ait, **a**rms, **l**egs, **s**pine). This is a rapid and efficient way of assessing the integrity of the musculoskeletal system. It is **not** a diagnostic examination. It is a screening procedure to indicate which aspects of your examination require more detailed assessment. As the patient performs a movement, enquire if it is painful. If abnormalities are noted, examine these in more detail as described earlier. Once you become familiar with all aspects of the rheumatological examination you will be able to perform the GALS screen quickly and efficiently.

Gait

This can be done as the patient walks towards you in any clinical setting. Look for a normal symmetrical gait. Disorders of the musculoskeletal system can lead to a variety of gait abnormalities including loss of symmetry, stiffness, and pain on walking. Some patients need walking aids, others need help with transfers. You should observe how easily they manage to sit and get up from a chair. Look at their knees (varus, valgus, flexion deformity?), look at their feet (pronation, valgus deformity, toe posture?), and look for unsteadiness—especially when turning. Make a note of their posture—look for normal spinal curvatures (cervical lordosis, thoracic kyphosis, and lumbar lordosis).

Arms

Hand

Ask the patient to perform the prayer sign (see Fig. 12.35). It tests wrist extension (and when reversed, flexion), MCP and PIP joint extension, and flexor tendon and soft tissue stretch. Ask the patient to make a fist—are they able to cover their nails? Assess the 'pinch' and 'power' grips (see Fig. 12.36). With the patient's hand extended, look for 'squaring' of the hand, for carpometacarpal (CMC) osteoarthritis, and osteophytes at DIP joints (Heberden's nodes) or PIP joints (Bouchard's nodes). Perform a lateral squeeze by gently and progressively squeezing across MCP joints, noting any tenderness that may be found in an inflammatory arthritis. Examine for synovial swelling (synovitis) and look for loss of joint contours. Feel for soft tissue swelling obscuring the normal joint outline and for synovitis at the PIP joints. Remember synovial thickening has a similar consistency to a grape! Tendon sheaths are lined with synovium; feel for thickening and crepitus in rheumatoid arthritis and 'triggering' due to a nodule (rheumatoid arthritis or SLE).

Elbow

The elbow extends to at least 180°, but not usually beyond 190°. It flexes to allow the fingers to touch the shoulder easily. Test the proximal radioulnar joint with the elbow tucked in. Ask the patient to turn their hand palm down (pronation), then palm up (supination).

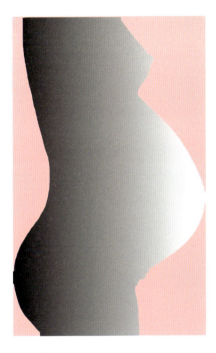

Figure 12.33 Exaggerated lordosis due to pregnancy.

(a)

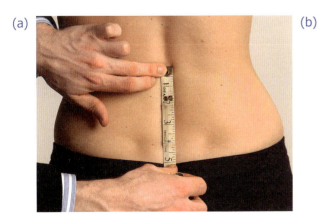

(b)

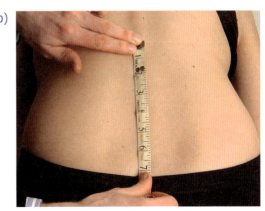

Figure 12.34 Schober's test: (a) standing, (b) touching toes.

Shoulder

Check shoulder abduction and elevation, noting the transition from glenohumeral movement to scapulothoracic movement. Internal rotation is a functionally important movement for dressing. Also assess external rotation; it is especially restricted in lesions of the shoulder capsule.

Spine

You cannot examine the spine with the patient fully dressed because you will need to see and feel the anatomy.

Cervical region

The patient may sit or stand for this. The levator scapulae (*le-vay-tor-scap-you-lee*) is often tender to gentle squeeze in cervical spine problems and also in fibromyalgia. The neck becomes stiffer with age so loss of movement does not always indicate disease (lateral flexion is more sensitive for detecting symptomatic lesions).

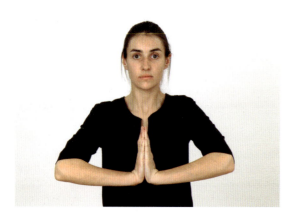

Figure 12.35 The prayer sign.

(a)   (b)

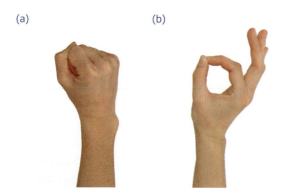

Figure 12.36 (a) Fist; (b) pinch.

Dorsal region

Ask the patient to sit (to eliminate rotation at the pelvis and legs) and then rotate their torso.

Lumbar region

With the patient standing ask them to touch their toes noting separation of the lumbar spinal processes. If the patient complains of back pain or if movement is restricted, further assessment is warranted and more so if there is leg pain or paraesthesiae.

Legs

Hip

With the patient supine, check hip flexion.

Knee

Abnormal swelling may be due to fluid, bony, or soft tissue swelling—look for loss of the normal contours and test for effusions.

Foot and ankle

Inspect the sole for calluses, look for abnormal separation of the toes, then gently squeeze the metatarsal heads. Examine for asymmetry or abnormal posture. Pain or observed abnormalities require further assessment.

Wash your hands

14 Wash your hands

Don't bug your patients.

Presentation of findings

15 Present your findings

Now start your presentation. If your findings point to a diagnosis, then be confident and mention this up front, for example,

> 'The diagnosis is rheumatoid arthritis because there is a symmetrical deforming inflammatory arthropathy with evidence of swan neck and boutonnière deformity of the fingers. There is a Z deformity of the thumb and palmar erythema. There is wasting of the small muscles of the hands and ulnar deviation of the fingers. The distal interphalangeal joints are spared and there are nodules at the elbows. This is consistent with rheumatoid arthritis and the presence of nodules increases the likelihood of the patient being

seropositive for rheumatoid factor. I would now like to go on and examine the chest for any signs of pleural effusion, the skin for steroid-induced changes, and the eyes for scleritis.'

Cases 12.5 and 12.6 illustrate some clinical scenarios.

Diseases and investigations of the joints

In the earlier parts of this chapter, various medical conditions have been mentioned. In this section they are now described. In general these descriptions are brief though certain selected topics are discussed in more detail.

Ehlers–Danlos syndrome

See Fig. 12.37. Ehlers–Danlos syndrome (*Edvard Lauritz Ehlers (1863–1937), Danish dermatologist; Henri Alexandre Danlos (1844–1912), French dermatologist*) is a disease of connective tissue of which there are different subtypes. The main characteristic of this condition is hypermobile joints ('double-jointedness'). The skin tends to be thin but elastic. It also exhibits poor healing producing typical 'fish-mouth' scars and pseudotumours (calcified haematomas). Patients may have kyphoscoliosis or genu recurvatum and are prone to spontaneous

pneumothorax, gastrointestinal haemorrhage, dissecting aneurysm, ruptured aortic aneurysm, and aortic and mitral incompetence.

Pseudoxanthoma elasticum

See Fig. 12.38. This is an inherited disorder of elastin with different subtypes. The hallmark feature is the appearance of the skin, which resembles a 'plucked chicken'. The skin of the flexures—axillae, neck, antecubital fossa, and groins—tends to be loose. The patient has hypermobile joints and may exhibit genu recurvatum. Complications include gastrointestinal haemorrhage, ischaemic heart disease, and aortic and mitral incompetence.

Fibromyalgia

This is one of the chronic pain syndromes. The pain tends to be ill defined and not limited to the joints and the pain is sometimes described as 'all over the body'. There is no identifiable pathology connected with this syndrome yet there may be multiple tender spots all over the body. It tends to occur in patients who exhibit psychiatric symptoms such as poor sleep, lassitude, and irritability, and conditions such as tension headaches, irritable bowel syndrome, and chronic fatigue syndrome. This does not mean

---

CASE 12.5

Problem. A 54-year-old woman is referred to clinic with neck pain. She also has pain in her shoulders, wrists, and hands, which she has had for 2 years and 'nobody has done a thing about it.' She is unable to sleep at night and her appetite is poor. She says she has swelling of all her joints and she is stiff all over every day. She suffers with headaches and has irritable bowel syndrome, which has flared up recently. She works as a secretary and is having a stressful time at the moment. On examination the pain is not limited to any specific joint and there are several points over her neck, trapezius muscle, shoulders, and back that are tender to the touch. Although she says her joints are swollen, they are normal with no signs of inflammation. She has a full range of movement of all her joints. What is the diagnosis?

Discussion. This case seems difficult at first sight and it is easy to be overwhelmed by the amount of pain and the patient's multiple symptoms. Some clues are apparent, however. The pain is diffuse and not confined to a

joint and despite the patient complaining bitterly of joint swelling there is no objective evidence for this. The pattern of symptoms is not consistent with inflammation, that is, inflamed joints are not stiff all the time and the patient has a full range of movement. With the diffuse nature of the pain and multiple tender spots the diagnosis is likely to be fibromyalgia. This is an ill-defined condition with no discernible pathology (see 'Diseases and investigations of the joints') and tends to be linked with disorders such as tension headache, irritable bowel syndrome, and chronic fatigue syndrome. These conditions tend to get worse at times of stress and it is notable that the patient is under pressure at work. It is said that such people should not be overinvestigated because this will reinforce the idea that something serious is wrong. This is a sensible approach, although in practice a beleaguered GP may well refer to a number of specialists over time as symptoms recur and an insistent patient pleads for something to be done.

that this condition is 'all in the mind'. It does, however, mean that plenty of reassurance is required that there is no life-threatening illness going on and that the treatment (including physiotherapy, graded exercise, improving sleep disturbance, and addressing psychological issues/depression/anxiety) will be different from standard rheumatological regimens.

Gout

Gout is one of the 'crystal arthropathies' and is due to deposits of monosodium urate monohydrate into joints and tendons. It affects men more than women and commonly causes a monoarthritis or oligoarthritis, but polyarthritis resembling rheumatoid arthritis can occur. It produces a hot painful joint (classically the first MTP joint of the big toe). Uric acid is a breakdown product of the purine (*pure-een*) bases guanine (*gwar-neen*) and adenosine (*add-den-owe-seen* or *adder-no-seen*) in DNA and RNA. Increased serum levels of uric acid (hyperuricaemia) (*high-per-you-reek-ee-mia*) may be due to increased production of uric acid or decreased excretion by the kidney. Although hyperuricaemia is a prerequisite for gout not everybody with high uric acid will develop gout. Gout may be recurrent and can become chronic. In chronic gout a large deposition of uric acid crystals may

---

CASE 12.6

Problem. A 72-year-old woman gives a 3-week history of progressive pain and stiffness in her shoulders and hips. It has gradually worsened so that she cannot get out of a chair easily and is unable to climb stairs, forcing her to sleep downstairs. She also has difficulty combing her hair and her scalp feels sore when she attempts this. Getting food out of the top cupboards in the kitchen has been impossible. She has also had drenching night sweats and has lost a stone in weight. Examination revealed very little. There was no joint inflammation and she had good power in all her limbs although movements were limited by pain. There were no rashes but she was tender over her right temporal artery. What is the diagnosis?

Discussion. The history suggests a proximal muscle problem and possibly a myopathy. However, the patient's power is preserved and movements are limited by pain only. Other important clues are the tender temporal artery and the soreness when she combs her hair. The diagnosis is polymyalgia rheumatica and it is likely that she has temporal arteritis. Systemic features such as nights sweats and weight loss can accompany temporal arteritis. Even so, it is worthwhile excluding other possible causes, for example, polymyositis, underlying malignancy, and even an atypical presentation of rheumatoid arthritis. Further investigations should include a temporal artery biopsy, creatine kinase (CK) enzyme, rheumatoid factor, and a possible search for malignancy. Treatment with steroids rapidly improved her symptoms.

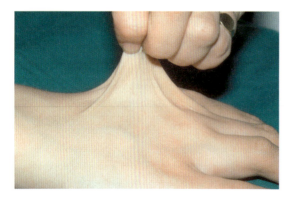

Figure 12.37 Ehlers–Danlos syndrome. The skin is elastic and distensible.

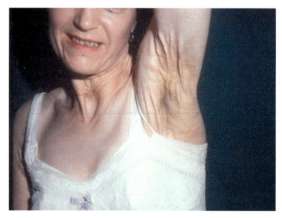

Figure 12.38 Pseudoxanthoma elasticum.

lead to tophi (a cheesy-looking exudate). These tophi can be found in joints, tendon sheaths, and the helix of the ear (see Figs 12.39 and 12.40). The diagnosis of gout is made by joint aspiration and demonstrating the characteristic crystals (needle-shaped, negatively bire-fringent (*bye-re-fringe-gent*) crystals on polarizing light microscopy).

Pseudogout

This is another cause of a 'crystal arthropathy' due to the deposition of calcium pyrophosphate (*pie-roe-foss-fate*) crystals. As the name suggests pseudogout can mimic gout clinically with the production of one or more hot painful joints. The pain tends to linger longer than in classical gout (may last for weeks). The diagnosis, like that for gout, is made on joint aspiration and finding positively birefringent crystals of calcium pyrophosphate on polarizing light microscopy. Deposition of calcium pyrophosphate in cartilage is called chondrocalcinosis (*con-dro-cal-sin-owe-sis*) and can be seen as fine white lines on the articular surface of the affected cartilage on radio. Many metabolic diseases can cause this appearance, for example, myxoedema, hyperparathyroidism, and Wilson's disease. However it is important to note that chondrocalcinosis is often asymptomatic and is therefore distinct from pseudogout.

Septic arthritis

This is due to active infection of a joint by microorganisms. Usually the infection is bacterial but viral (and in immunocompromised patients fungal) infections can occur. The most common bacterial agent in adults is *Staphylococcus aureus*. This form of arthritis leads to a hot, painful joint,

which the patient is reluctant to move. This presentation always warrants a joint aspiration for diagnostic purposes. If this diagnosis is missed irreparable damage may occur. So do not miss it!

Psoriatic arthropathy

Psoriasis is a skin disease with plaques that have a red base with a silvery scaly surface and are found on the extensor surfaces especially over the elbows (see Fig. 12.4), scalp, in the navel and behind the ears. Some 15–20% of patients with psoriasis develop arthritis (in a small number of cases the arthritis may predate the psoriasis). Why joint disease develops in some people and not in others is unclear. Five main patterns of joint disease are seen:

- distal joint disease affecting predominantly the DIP joints of the hands and feet
- mono- or oligoarthropathy
- a symmetrical polyarthropathy resembling rheumatoid arthritis
- arthritis mutilans (*mute-till-anz*)—a rare, severe destructive arthritis leading to gross deformity
- sacro-iliitis (*say-crow-eye-lee-eye-tiss*).

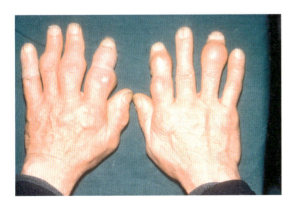

Figure 12.39 Chronic tophaceous gout.

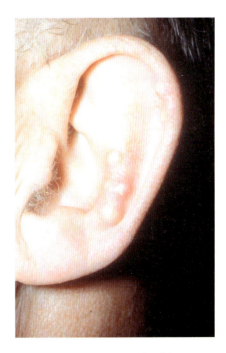

Figure 12.40 Gouty tophi at the helix of the ear.

There may be overlap between many of the groups above. Psoriatic arthropathy is usually associated with nail changes including nail pitting and splitting; onycholysis (separation of the nail plate); and hyperkeratosis (exuberant overgrowth of keratin of the nail).

Reiter's syndrome (reactive arthritis)

Classically Reiter's syndrome (*Hans Conrad Julius Reiter (1881–1969), German physician*) has been described as a triad of signs: arthritis, genital tract inflammation, and conjunctivitis. This syndrome is triggered by a specific infective episode. When first described it was thought to be a sequelae of sexually transmitted disease, for example, chlamydia but now it is also recognized following a diarrhoeal illness. It affects men more than women and predominantly affects young adults. It is classified as one of the seronegative spondyloarthritides and shares many clinical features although the arthritis tends to affect the lower limbs. A characteristic desquamating rash affecting the palms and soles of the hands and feet called keratoderma blenorrhagica (*ke-rat-owe-derma-blen-owe-ra-jicka*) may occasionally be seen. Other features include iritis and painless ulceration of the mouth. Treatment is symptomatic and directed at the underlying cause.

Behçet's syndrome

Behçet's (*beh-shays*) syndrome (*Hulusi Behçet (1889–1948), Turkish dermatologist*) is a multisystem disorder that is usually classified with the seronegative spondyloarthritides. It most commonly presents as a monoarthritis or an oligoarthritis. It is associated with mouth and genital ulceration, skin rash, sterile pustules, iridocyclitis of the eyes, and thromboembolic disease.

Seronegative spondyloarthritides

This is a collection of conditions with similar clinical presentations, which share the absence of the rheumatoid factor. Common features include

- inflammation of the sacroiliac joints (sacroiliitis)
- an asymmetrical peripheral arthritis
- an enthesopathy (*en-thee-sop-pathy*) (inflammation at the site of tendon insertion)
- an iritis or anterior uveitis.

Ankylosing spondylitis

This is one of the seronegative spondyloarthritides. It is more common in men and is associated with HLA B27. It has a predilection for the spine. Initially it starts as local sacroiliitis and it can progress to affect the whole spine. Calcification of the interspinous ligaments occurs and in advanced cases there is fusion of the spine (a process called ankylosis). On a radiograph this looks like a bamboo cane and is sometimes referred to as a bamboo spine. A compensatory cervical lordosis is required to enable the patient to look forward. When viewed from the side the patient looks like a question mark (hence they are described as having a question-mark posture). See Fig. 12.28. Remember to perform Schober's test. They also have poor chest expansion and rely on 'diaphragmatic' respiration. Measure chest expansion using a tape measure and record the circumference of the chest on expiration at the nipple line. This should increase by 4 cm on inspiration but is substantially reduced in ankylosing spondylitis. Other features include iritis, aortitis and aortic incompetence, conduction defects of the heart, and apical fibrosis of the lungs.

Systemic sclerosis

This is a disorder that is recognized by its characteristic skin appearance (tight, hard, and waxy). This may be limited (called CREST) or diffuse (termed scleroderma). Other organs may be affected and the term systemic sclerosis is used (although many people use the term systemic sclerosis and scleroderma synonymously). It affects females more than males and there is a strong association with Raynaud's phenomenon. Other features include reflux oesophagitis and stricture, oesophageal dysmotility, small bowel hypomobility, and bacterial overgrowth leading to malabsorption, lung fibrosis, and renal failure. There is also another variant called limited cutaneous systemic sclerosis (formerly called CREST syndrome; it is worth remembering its earlier name because, as mentioned previously, this is an acronym for its major symptoms).

Polymyalgia rheumatica

This is a condition in which the disease process is poorly understood. There is an overlap with temporal arteritis, but a vasculitic process cannot explain those cases of polymyalgia rheumatica that occur in isolation. It affects females more than males and tends to affect patients over the age of 50 years and those of white European origin. It causes pain and stiffness (**not weakness**) of the proximal muscle groups (shoulder and pelvic girdle muscles). The stiffness is worse in the morning and lasts for hours. Patients experience difficulty getting out of a chair and climbing stairs and they also experience difficulty combing their hair and reaching for objects over their heads. Other features include non-specific symptoms of anorexia, weight loss, night sweats, and fatigue. There are usually raised inflammatory markers, that is, erythrocyte sedimentation rate (ESR) or plasma viscosity. It is essentially a clinical diagnosis and responds rapidly to steroid treatment. Polymyalgia rheumatica may need prolonged treatment over a number of years as it has a tendency to relapse off steroids.

Rheumatoid arthritis

This is a multisystem inflammatory disorder that affects synovial joints and is characterized in some cases by the presence of rheumatoid factor. It affects females slightly more than males. Its most common presentation is a symmetrical polyarthritis that develops over weeks or months, although more acute presentations occur. There is morning stiffness for longer than 1 hour. The synovial lining of a joint becomes inflamed, which if untreated will lead to erosion of cartilage and bone (typically periarticular osteoporosis and erosion). Later on in the disease process deformities of the joints may develop. There may be non-specific features such as fever, sweats, anorexia and weight loss, and fatigue. There may be vasculitic features such as nail fold infarcts, digital gangrene, ulcers, scleritis or episcleritis, peripheral neuropathy, and mononeuritis multiplex. Other organs may be involved:

- lungs—pleural effusion, lung fibrosis, rheumatoid nodules, bronchiolitis (*bron-key-owe-light-iss*), and Caplan's (*cap-lanz*) syndrome (rheumatoid nodules and pneumoconiosis) in miners
- heart—pericarditis and endocarditis—aortic incompetence and myocarditis
- neurological—carpal tunnel syndrome, cervical myopathy, peripheral neuropathy, and mononeuritis multiplex
- keratoconjunctivitis sicca (*ker-rat-owe-con-junk-ti-vie-tiss-sicker*) syndrome or Sjögren's syndrome
- spleen—Felty's syndrome—enlarged spleen and hypersplenism leading to anaemia (occasionally pancytopenia) (*pan-site-owe-pee-nia*)
- anaemia—drug-related anaemia—gastrointestinal loss due to NSAIDS, bone marrow suppression due to gold or penicillamine (*penny-sill-am-mean*), the anaemia of

chronic disorders, dietary, for example, folate deficiency, or an association with pernicious anaemia (vitamin B_{12} deficiency).

Diagnostic criteria have been drawn up by the American Rheumatism Association and the American College of Rheumatology. Seven criteria have been identified:

1 morning stiffness of greater than 1 hour
2 arthritis of the hand joints
3 arthritis of at least three types of joints (PIP, MCP, wrist, elbow, knee, ankle, and MTP)
4 symmetrical arthritis
5 rheumatoid nodules present
6 rheumatoid factor present
7 joint erosions on radiographs of wrists and hands.

Four of the seven criteria must be present to establish the diagnosis of rheumatoid arthritis. Criteria 1–4 must be present for at least 6 weeks.

Vasculitis

The systemic vasculitides are a collection of disorders caused by inflammation and fibrinoid necrosis of blood vessels. This inflammatory process can be primary, that is, the underlying cause is not known or secondary to another disease, for example, rheumatoid arthritis. Primary vasculitis can be classified according to the size of blood vessel affected, that is,

- large vessel—for example, temporal arteritis
- medium vessel—for example, polyarteritis nodosa
- small vessel—for example, GPA.

Some conditions are more common at certain ages, for example, Kawasaki (*cower-sack-ee*) disease (*Tomisaku Kawasaki (1925–), Japanese paediatrician*)—childhood and temporal arteritis—old age. Other conditions have a predilection for certain organs, for example, temporal arteritis—temporal arteries and Churg–Strauss syndrome (*Jacob Churg (1910–), Polish-born American pathologist; Lotte Strauss (1913–1985), American pathologist*)—lungs. Most diseases can be diagnosed by biopsy of an affected organ and treatment is often steroids with or without steroid sparing agent.

Osteoarthritis

This is a chronic joint disorder resulting in progressive damage to cartilage and subchondral bone. It used to be regarded only as a degenerative disorder because it affected older people. However, other factors may play a role including genetic factors (composition of cartilage) or mechanical stress—for example, obesity, repetitive high-impact activity, or trauma with disordered repair (increasing evidence is supporting the role of inflammation in the genesis of osteoarthritis). Symptoms include pain that is worse with activity but settles on resting, stiffness after a period of inactivity, and in more advanced cases deformity of the joint. Pathologically there is a gradual thinning of articular cartilage leading to a decrease in the joint space. Later as cartilage destruction is complete (or near complete), underlying bony surfaces may become eroded and sclerose in an attempt at repair. The bone response may be sufficient to produce bony outgrowths at the joint margins called osteophytes. In the hands these osteophytes produce hard swellings at the DIP joints (Heberden's nodes) and at the PIP joints (Bouchard's nodes). If the hands demonstrate these nodes the patient is described as having nodal osteoarthritis (more common in females). Often there is a 'square hand' deformity due to subluxation of the base of the first metacarpal. If more than three joints are affected the condition is known as generalized osteoarthritis.

Systemic lupus erythmatosus

SLE is a multisystem disorder of unknown cause where antibodies are directed against constituents of biological cells including the nucleus and surface antigens. Practically any organ in the body can be affected although certain patterns of disease are seen, for example, skin only (cutaneous lupus). It affects females more than males and it is more common in black people (not Africans). Other features include

- **skin**—malar rash in classical 'butterfly distribution', photosensitivity rash, discoid rash called discoid lupus erythematosus, which can be found in isolation, vasculitic rash, livido reticularis, alopecia (hair loss), and Raynaud's phenomenon
- **mouth**—ulcers
- **cardiovascular**—pericarditis, endocarditis, and myocarditis
- **lungs**—pleurisy, pleural effusion, and pulmonary fibrosis
- **neurological**—psychosis, epilepsy, dementia, strokes, and peripheral neuropathy
- **gut**—chronic active hepatitis and splenomegaly
- **rheumatological**—arthralgia and arthritis
- **gynaecological**—amenorrhoea and recurrent abortions

- **haematological**—anaemia of chronic disease, haemolytic anaemia, hypersplenism, and anti-phospholipid syndrome leading to recurrent thromboses (see Case 12.2).

Keratoconjunctivitis sicca syndrome

This affects the eyes and is due to the decrease or lack of production of tears leading to 'dry eyes'. The lack of lubrication results in gritty eyes that can become easily inflamed and infected. It is often found in association with a 'dry mouth' called xerostomia (*zero-stow-mia*), which is another unpleasant condition that can lead to poor dental hygiene and subsequent tooth and gum disease.

Sjögren's syndrome

This can be primary (keratoconjunctivitis sicca and xerostomia on their own) or secondary in association with a connective tissue disease, for example, systemic sclerosis, SLE, or rheumatoid disease.

Inflammatory markers

C-reactive protein (CRP), plasma viscosity, and ESR are markers of inflammation. They will be elevated regardless of the cause of inflammation and so are non-specific. They provide a guide to the degree of inflammation and can be used to monitor progress with treatment.

Rheumatoid factor

Rheumatoid factor is an autoantibody and its production may be a way for the immune system to aggregate immune complexes so they can be removed more easily by the spleen and other immune organs. Most assays detect an IgM antibody that is directed against the constant region (Fc) portion of IgG. Enzyme-linked immunosorbent assay (ELISA) testing is capable of detecting other classes of rheumatoid factors (IgG, IgA) but these are not widely used clinically. The latex test is reported in a titre with most laboratories considering >1:40 as positive. The nephelometry test is usually reported in international units (IU) and the normal range is dependent on the specific laboratory (usually <20 IU). Rheumatoid factor is not a sensitive or specific test for rheumatoid arthritis. There are a variety of clinical conditions that can be positive for the rheumatoid factor (therefore limiting its specificity). In fact it can be present in up to 10% of the normal population. It is most useful as a prognostic indicator because those who are rheumatoid factor positive typically have a more aggressive disease. It is positive in up to 60% of cases with early disease and 75% with established disease. It is also useful in confirming a clinical impression that a polyarthritis that looks like rheumatoid arthritis is even more likely to be so. It is also used to follow patients with Sjögren's disease to predict the development of lymphoma.

Anti-nuclear antibodies

There are many anti-nuclear antibodies. These are antibodies found in the serum, which are directed against certain components of the nucleus of a cell. Different anti-nuclear antibodies are positive in certain conditions, however they are not entirely specific and so cannot be thought of as a powerful diagnostic tool. They can be divided into anti-nuclear antibodies and extractable nuclear antigens. See Table 12.11. Other important markers include anti-neutrophil cytoplasmic antibody (ANCA). C-ANCA is positive in 90% of patients with active generalized GPA, but is frequently seen in polyarteritis nodosa, idiopathic necrotizing, and crescentic glomerulonephritis. P-ANCA is a useful marker for vasculitis-associated

crescentic glomerulonephritis, but is present in other systemic necrotizing vasculitic disorders including polyarteritis nodosa and Churg–Strauss syndrome and it is present in <10% of SLE patients. It is commonly seen in ulcerative colitis.

Bone scan

A bone scan, involving the intravenous injection of radioisotopes, is useful for detecting malignant deposits in the bone. Patients may present with bone pain and weight loss. Inflammation can also be detected on bone scans and although a bone scan is not useful for diagnosing one rheumatological disorder from another, it can give information about patterns of inflammation, which may be helpful diagnostically. Note that DEXA bone scans use X-ray beams to measure the density of bone and should not be confused with an isotope bone scan.

Joint aspiration and injection

Most joints can be punctured to either remove fluid (for therapeutic or diagnostic purposes) or to inject drugs. For

Table 12.11 Anti-nuclear antibodies and their possible associations

Anti-nuclear antibody	Disease suggestive of
Double-stranded DNA (dsDNA)	SLE
Single-stranded DNA (ssDNA)	Drug-induced SLE
Anti-histone	Drug-induced SLE
Anti-centromere	CREST syndrome
Anti-nucleolus	Systemic sclerosis
Anti-speckled	Systemic sclerosis
Extractable nuclear antigens	
Smooth muscle (Sm)	SLE
Anti-Ro (SSA)	Sjögren's, SLE, and neonatal lupus
Anti-La (SSB)	Sjögren's, SLE, and neonatal lupus
Anti-Scl 70	Systemic sclerosis
Ribonucleoprotein (RNP)	Mixed connective tissue disease and SLE
Anti-Jo-1	Polymyositis and fibrosing alveolitis

DNA, deoxyribonucleic acid; SLE, systemic lupus erythematosus.

Table 12.12 Diagnostic features of joint aspirates

	Normal	OA	RA	Septic	Gout	Pseudogout
Appearance	Clear, thick	Clear, thick	Yellow, thin	Pus, thick	Clear, thin	Clear, thin
WBC count	+	+	++	++++	++	++
Crystals	None	None	None	None	Present	Present
Culture	Sterile	Sterile	Sterile	Positive	Sterile	Sterile

OA, osteoarthritis; RA, rheumatoid arthritis; WBC, white blood cell.

example, an inflamed knee joint due to rheumatoid arthritis can be punctured to

- remove fluid that is causing a painful effusion
- inject steroids and local anaesthetic to suppress inflammation
- exclude another cause, for example, gout, pseudogout, infection, or haemarthrosis.

Alternatively, a patient presenting with a swollen knee, who is not known to suffer from arthritis, may have the knee joint aspirated as a diagnostic procedure. The most important differential diagnosis here is septic arthritis. Certain conditions can be diagnosed after examination of the joint fluid. Consequently, fluid removed from a joint should be sent to the microbiology department for microscopy, culture, and sensitivity and to the biochemistry department for examination under polarized light. See Table 12.12. Checking the white blood cell count of the aspirate is not performed routinely nowadays. Gout can be diagnosed and differentiated from pseudogout by the examination of joint fluid under polarized light.

Table 12.13 Day-to-day cases

Rheumatoid arthritis
Osteoarthritis
Gout

Table 12.14 Finals cases

Day-to-day cases
Psoriatic arthropathy
Chronic tophaceous gout
Ankylosing spondylitis
Systemic lupus erythematosus
Raynaud's phenomenon

Arthroscopy

Arthroscopy entails the direct examination of the joint. A flexible telescope (arthroscope) is introduced into the joint under local anaesthetic. The arthroscope has a small diameter and many joints can be investigated using this technique. Once in the joint, an examination of the structures can be undertaken and the nature and extent of inflammation assessed. In addition fluid can be removed for diagnostic and therapeutic purposes and drugs can be administered. Occasionally minor surgical procedures can also be performed.

Finals section

The emphasis of this section is on the short cases as this format usually causes the most uncertainty. The objective

structured clinical examinations (OSCEs) usually have more straightforward and standardized instructions. Despite the different formats the clinical approach remains the same. For revision read the examination summary and the key points throughout the chapter and do the questions at the end of the chapter. See Tables 12.13 and 12.14 for day-to-day and Finals cases, respectively.

Key diagnostic clues

Unlike other systems there is no key diagnostic clue. When dealing with the joints, it is most important to determine if there is a true arthritis or synovitis as the causes are different to joints that are not inflamed. Palpation is the key here. A swollen joint that feels boggy suggests synovitis. If it feels hot to the touch this suggests that the inflammatory process is active.

Some advice relating to examination problems

Rheumatology cases are great for examiners! There is a wide variety of rheumatological conditions to choose from and patients are often well despite their illness. Patients can be used for both long cases and short 'spot' cases. In the spot case cardinal features of rheumatological conditions should prompt a diagnosis, for example, the butterfly rash of SLE. When faced with a spot case be prepared to answer supplementary questions on the disease you have identified (see Chapter 13).

The instruction

The examiner may ask you 'Look at this patient. What is the diagnosis?' (or some variant). This would suggest a spot diagnosis (see Chapter 13). The more likely instruction would be 'Examine this patient's hands.' See Case 12.7.

General look

Before you plunge into your examination of the hand, sneak a peek at the face and the rest of the body. A patient with a plethoric, round face with purpura on the arms may be cushingoid as a result of steroid treatment for rheumatoid arthritis.

Position the hand

If there is obvious deformity, ask the patient if their hands are painful. If a pillow is handy get them to rest their palms

---

CASE 12.7

Problem. You are unsure when asked to examine the hands whether to check the joints or to perform a neurological examination.

Solution. Do not panic, your observation is the key. Quickly look at the hands and determine if there are any abnormalities. Thankfully most joint disease will be immediately obvious. Look for swelling or deformities. If these are spotted you are home free (but do not relax too much as there is still work to be done). If there are no obvious abnormalities visible **then** it is sensible to begin a neurological examination.

---

on them. If there is no pillow hold the hands very carefully so as not to cause discomfort.

Look

Always start with the nails otherwise the signs could be missed. Look for pitting, onycholysis, and hyperkeratosis (psoriasis) or splinter haemorrhages and nail fold infarcts (vasculitis). Turn the hands over. Is there any palmar erythema? (rheumatoid arthritis?). Also look for any deformity and any obvious pattern, for example, do the fingers deviate to the ulnar side? (rheumatoid arthritis). Is there any swan neck or boutonnière deformity of any fingers? Are the deformities symmetrical, that is, affecting both hands in a similar fashion? (probably rheumatoid arthritis). If asymmetrical this is more likely to be a seronegative spondarthritides or gout (in chronic tophaceous gout look for cheesy-looking material exuding from a joint). Now scan the arms quickly for purpura (steroid treatment?), skin plaques of psoriasis, or rheumatoid nodules.

Feel

Now observe all the DIP joints and note any swelling. Do they feel soft and boggy (synovitis?) or hard? (Heberden's nodes). Do the same for the PIP joints (Bouchard's nodes) and the MCP joints. Check the wrist for any deformity and synovitis before running your hand down the ulna border of the forearm to the elbow. You may palpate rheumatoid nodules that were not apparent on inspection. A fluctuant swelling at the elbow suggests olecronon bursitis (gout? rheumatoid arthritis?). Double check and make sure there are no occult plaques of psoriasis on the extensor surface of the elbow.

Move

You need to perform a quick check of function. Get your patient to undo and do up buttons, hold a pen, and so on.

Remember!

You could be shown rheumatoid feet! Do not panic, simply follow the steps for the examination of the hand and the signs are similar.

Supplementary clues

With joint disease of the hands you will usually have an idea what condition you are dealing with early on (you hope). So to add the finishing touches to the examination you can demonstrate extra relevant findings (but see Case 12.8); for example, with rheumatoid arthritis pull

CASE 12.8

Problem. You have finished your examination of rheumatoid hands but you are unsure whether to progress to a neurological examination.

Solution. You realize that a neurological deficit is possible with rheumatoid arthritis but to embark on a 'neuro' examination will be time consuming. Worse still, if you hesitate your examiners may (wrongly) assume that you are clueless. The author's approach is to say up front that they have concluded their examination but ordinarily would perform a neurological examination because they are aware that rheumatoid arthritis can cause neurological deficits. Also be alive to any clues such as wasting of the thenar eminence, which could suggest a carpal tunnel syndrome. If this is the case the author would modify their statement and say 'I would normally go on to perform a neurological examination particularly as I have noticed marked wasting of the thenar eminence which raises the possibility of carpal tunnel syndrome.' In this way the examiners will give you due credit for your knowledge and will usually let you know if they expect you to proceed with a neurological examination.

down the lower eyelid and inspect for scleritis or episcleritis or with chronic tophaceous gout inspect the pinna of the ear for deposition of gouty tophus. It is important to note that these manoeuvres are not essential but demonstrate that you have a good working knowledge of the disease you are suspecting, including any extra-articular manifestations.

Presentation

Try to be confident—avoid the words 'seems' or 'might'!

OSCE examples

History-taking station

You are an FY1 in the emergency department. A 34-year-old woman has presented with an acutely swollen left knee. Please take a history from the patient and present your findings to the examiner. You should then discuss differential diagnoses and further management.

Remember:

- Introduce yourself to the patient.
- Take a pain history (remember SOCRATES; see Chapter 4).
- Ascertain if there is a decreased range of movement of the left knee.
- Ask specifically about fever and feeling unwell over the past 2 days (if this is positive this raises the possibility of a septic arthritis).
- Past medical history—this lady has poorly controlled asthma and is on regular courses of steroids.
- Check drug history, social history, and family history; ask specifically for rheumatoid arthritis or gout.
- 'Any injuries lately?'—i.e. a possible source of infection (this patient had an infected blister the previous week).
- Ask if there are any other swollen joints.
- Thank your patient.
- Give a succinct presentation to the examiner.
- Differentials are septic arthritis/gout/pseudogout/rheumatoid arthritis.
- Most important investigation: urgent joint aspiration—send for microscopy, culture and sensitivities and radiography of left knee.
- Other tests include: FBC, U&E, CXR, urinalysis, blood cultures.

Examination station

Perform a GALS examination on this 17-year-old man who presents with low back pain. Perform the Schober's test. There is no need to take a history.

Remember:

- Introduce yourself to the patient and gain consent to examine.
- Wash your hands/use alcohol gel provided.
- First, ask the screening questions—'Are you in any pain at the moment?' 'Can you walk up stairs?' 'Do you have problems with moving your hands, for example doing your buttons up on your shirt?'
- Perform a thorough GALS examination, adopting the 'look, feel, move' formula, telling the examiner what you are assessing for at each stage.
- Continuously compare the left and right side of the body looking for symmetry.
- Schober's test: make a mark on the lumbar spine at the level of the posterior iliac spine. Measure out a line from

5 cm below to 10 cm above the mark. Ask the patient to bend forward as far as they can. If the line does not lengthen by at least 5 cm there is reduced lumbar flexion (e.g. in ankylosing spondylitis).

- Thank your patient and wash your hands/use alcohol gel.

Good luck!

Questions

1 Name three nail changes in psoriatic arthropathy.
2 Which structures are responsible for the stability of the knee?
3 What is carpal tunnel syndrome?
4 What do the terms kyphosis, scoliosis, and lordosis mean?
5 Name three possible respiratory complications associated with rheumatoid arthritis.
6 What are the causes of a knee effusion?
7 How do you perform a patella tap?
8 What are the five main features of limited systemic sclerosis (CREST syndrome)?
9 If faced with a single 'hot' joint, what is the most important diagnosis to consider?
10 In chronic tophaceous gout, where might you find deposition of tophi?

References and further reading

Adebajo A. *ABC of rheumatology*, 4th edn. BMJ Publishing/Wiley-Blackwell, Oxford, 2010.

Bellamy N. *Colour atlas of clinical rheumatology*. Kluwer, Lancaster, 1985.

Boyle AC. *Colour atlas of rheumatology*. Wolfe, London, 1986.

Doherty M, Dacre J, Dieppe P, Snaith ML. The 'GALS' locomotor screen. *Annals of Rheumatological Disease* 1992; **51**:1165–9.

Doherty M, Doherty J. *Clinical examination in rheumatology*. Wolfe, London, 1992.

Gross JM, Fetto J, Rosen E. *Musculoskeletal examination*, 2nd edn. Blackwell Science, Oxford, 2002.

13 Spot diagnosis

Introduction

A spot diagnosis is not the diagnosis of acne. Spot cases are an assortment of different diseases with visible signs that can lead to an instant diagnosis. Any system, for example, the endocrine, dermatological, or neurological, can be used and the only factor they have in common is the instruction 'Look at this patient! What is the diagnosis?' (or a variant of this). The spot diagnosis requires a different skill from the ones you have been learning so far. It requires the instant recognition of clinical signs (in contrast to the usual methodical approach). The key to the spot diagnosis is experience. Once you have seen the clinical signs again and again, you will be able to process the information quickly and make that snap diagnosis. It is as simple as that. The only difficulty with some spot cases is that subtle signs can be easily overlooked. However if you can develop a 'trigger' for these conditions, that is, some clue that will prompt your recall, then you will not miss them.

The spot case scenario can be unnerving for any student because rather than plunging into a comfortable, well-rehearsed routine, they are literally put 'on the spot'. The situation is made even more nerve-wracking because

any system can be affected and where do you start looking? The aim of this chapter is to acquaint you with the more common spot cases that you will encounter as a student and to give you some system of approach to spot diagnosis.

The importance of spot diagnosis

Although the spot case is now less frequently used in exam settings it can still be used in ward teachings. The spot technique is valuable because it can provide a shortcut to a diagnosis, for example, while taking a history, you notice the staring eyes of a patient with exophthalmos. You then make the connection with their weight loss and diarrhoea, that is, they have Grave's disease of the thyroid and are thyrotoxic. Everyone is impressed by the clinician who stands at the end of the bed and plucks the diagnosis out of the air without touching the patient. As you gain in experience the 'general look' that you are cultivating with all systems can become your passport to a crucial diagnosis. This skill is essential in today's busy clinical environment especially as you climb the career ladder. Your exposure time to patients can be extremely limited if you are in general practice, or doing a busy clinic and even on ward rounds in hospitals. Therefore the ability to make a spot diagnosis is an essential part of any doctor's arsenal and why it is being taught here. However, here are some notes of caution about using the spot technique in clinical practice.

- First impressions can be misleading, for example, the telangiectasia you thought were spider naevi from a distance could be due to other disease on closer inspection, for example, systemic sclerosis (see Case 7.7 and Fig. 13.13).
- Your diagnosis could be accurate but the disease could have no connection with the patient's symptoms.
- Your diagnosis could be accurate and relevant but the patient could have other pathology in other systems. This is called comorbidity and it is especially important in older people.

The approach to the spot case

The spot case tests your ability to notice signs and formulate a diagnosis. Sometimes in your finals this is all that is required. More often, however, the spot case will be the basis for further examination or questions. This could be an opportunity for you to demonstrate your knowledge of the case. So if you can, seize the initiative. The instruction is all-important in the spot case. It may be specific, for example, 'Look at this patient's leg'. The focused case is usually straightforward as you do not have to hunt very far to find the lesion. The only problem you face is not recognizing the sign (if this is the case do not freeze, describe what you see and try and come to a sensible conclusion; if necessary give a differential diagnosis). The more general commands, 'What is the diagnosis?' or 'Look at this patient: what is the diagnosis?' are more difficult. As the range of possible cases is so wide, you have to be more systematic in your inspection. Even then some cases can still be strikingly obvious at first glance.

Start by getting an overall impression of the patient. This first glance may be sufficient for you to reach a diagnosis. If this is the case, spend a few more seconds gathering extra clues that might strengthen the diagnosis before reporting back to the examiners (do not spend too much time or you might appear clueless). If the diagnosis is not immediately obvious, pay attention to the patient's demeanour and mood. Do they seem apathetic and expressionless? (Parkinson's disease? myxoedema?). Are they listless and agitated? (thyrotoxicosis?). Do they

have a hunched posture? (which might suggest Parkinson's disease or vertebral fractures due to osteoporosis (Cushing's syndrome?), Paget's (*pah-jets*) disease, or acromegaly). Also check skin colour. Do they appear pigmented (the most common causes are racial or tanning) but in an examination setting this may be more relevant (Addison's disease? haemochromatosis (*he-ma-crow-ma-toe-sis*)?). Does the skin appear yellow (jaundice?). After a brief global assessment if answers are still not forthcoming, it is time to inspect your patient in more systematic detail. The author prefers a 'top-down' approach because I find the majority of information about a person is packed into the head and face. First check the shape of the head. Is the forehead enlarged? (Paget's disease?). Is there unusual balding (myotonia dystrophica) or hair loss (alopecia)? (systemic lupus erythmatosus (SLE)? myxoedema?). Assess the shape of the face. Is it round and moon-shaped? (Cushing's syndrome?). Check for symmetry of the face. Is there drooping of one side of the face? (facial nerve palsy?).

Now assess the eyelids and check for symmetry. Is there drooping of one of the lids? Is it a complete ptosis (third nerve palsy?) or a partial ptosis? (Horner's syndrome?). Look at the eyes and again compare both sides. Do they have a staring quality? (exophthalmos?). Or is there evidence of yellow sclerae? (jaundice?). Check the nose. Is it enlarged and bulbous? (acromegaly?). Or is it pinched and 'beak' like? (systemic sclerosis?). Inspect the lips. Are they thin and drawn with radial furrows surrounding them? (systemic sclerosis?). Or are there multiple red 'spots' that could suggest telangiectasia (hereditary haemorrhagic telangiectasia (HHT)?) or speckled pigmentation? (Peutz–Jehgers (*perts-yay-ga*) syndrome?) (*Johannes Laurentius Augustinus Peutz (1886–1957), Dutch physician; Harold Joseph Jeghers (1904–1990), American physician*). At this point it is worth scanning the rest of the face for other areas of discolouration. There may be telangiectasia on the cheeks (spider naevi?) or a 'butterfly rash' (SLE?).

Now leave the face and study the neck underneath. Is there a diffuse swelling in the midline? (goitre?). Or is there a more discrete lump? (multinodular goitre or thyroid adenoma?). Trace along the edge of the neck until you reach the clavicles on each side and check for lumps there too (malignant lymph nodes? On the left side, Virchow's [*ver-coughs*] node?). Finally study the limbs. If they are exposed, check to see if there are any telangiectasia (spider naevi?) or purpura (Cushing's syndrome?). Is there deformity of the limbs? (Paget's disease?). Are they held in an unusual posture (for example, flexion at the elbow and internal rotation of the arm due to hemiplegia)?

This list may seem daunting but as you see more signs and gain in experience, you will find that you process information rapidly and automatically. Do not try to remember all the conditions that have been mentioned so far. In fact there are many more conditions that could have been added. The aim has been to give you a systematic approach to the spot case, a blueprint for seeking out abnormalities (especially those that are subtle and easily missed). You do not need to stick with the sequence described. You could do it in reverse order or some other personal preference. The important thing is that your adopted routine does not miss anything.

In the next section a number of diseases that are commonly used as spot cases have been chosen. The list is not comprehensive and it is likely that you will face a condition that is not on the list. Here cases that you will have to diagnose from a general look at the patient (rather than a more focused study of part of the body) have been concentrated on. For each case a specific feature (or features) that **triggers** the author's recall of that condition (much as large animal and trunk triggers the image of an elephant) has been picked.

Below the triggers, other features of the disease that can prompt you to search for further confirmatory signs or to ask relevant questions have been summarized. If you can, take charge and be bold in your finals. Tell your examiners what you are suspecting and why and tell them you would like to check (or ask questions) to determine if other features of the condition are present. If they give you permission, go for it. If not, they may have questions about the case they may test you on instead.

....

Tip
For conditions that are not described try and work out the features that can act as triggers for you.
....

Tip
Be prepared to ask simple questions on the causes, investigation, treatment, and complications of the disease you have spotted.
....

Spot cases

Paget's disease

What is it?

It is a disorder of bone of unknown cause, leading to a lack of coordination between bone formation and bone lysis

(destruction). The result is bone that may be enlarged but soft with poor tensile strength.

Trigger features

- Shape of the head—enlargement of the forehead.
- Elderly patient.

The person is usually elderly and their forehead may be enlarged (called frontal bossing). This can give the face a triangular outline (with the base of the triangle being formed at the top of the head and the point by the chin (see Fig. 13.1). The presence of a hearing aid will reinforce the diagnosis because deafness may be caused by Paget's disease affecting the ossicles (the tiny bones of the middle ear that normally conduct sounds to the inner ear).

Other features

- Bowing of the long bones—the humerus, tibia, and femur may bend under the weight of the body (see Fig. 13.2).
- Pathological fractures—bones may fracture due to relatively minor stresses.
- Kyphosis—the spine may curve due to vertebral fractures.
- Optic atrophy—the second nerve can be trapped by expanding bone leading to atrophy.
- High-output cardiac failure—the affected bone is very vascular early in the disease and sufficient blood can be shunted into the bone to force the heart to work harder to compensate.

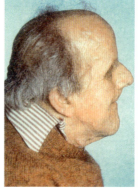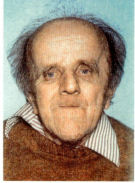

Figure 13.1 Paget's disease: note the frontal bossing of the forehead, giving the head a typical triangular shape.

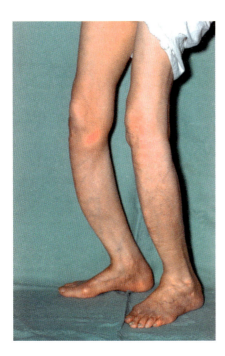

Figure 13.2 Paget's disease: bowing of the tibia bilaterally.

- Spinal cord compression—this can occur either due to vertebral fracture or more rarely due to brainstem invagination (*in-vaj-in-ay-shun*) (called platybasia [*plat-ee-base-ia*]). Normally, the weight of the skull and its contents are balanced by an upward force, produced by the cervical vertebrae. If Paget's disease affects the base of the skull, this upward force can push the softened base and the brainstem upwards, with disastrous consequences.

....

Tip

Deafness is prevalent in older people and therefore Paget's disease is not necessarily the cause of hearing impairment.

....

Parkinson's disease

What is it?

It is a chronic neurological disorder due to depletion of dopamine in the basal ganglia.

Trigger features

- An apathetic, mask-like face
- Usually an elderly person

- Flexed posture
- Pill-rolling tremor.

Examinations are stressful situations for patients as well as students. So if someone appears to be staring blankly without expression you should be suspicious about Parkinson's disease. The patient tends to be elderly, although younger people are afflicted (for example, Michael J. Fox, the actor) and they may have a hunched posture. If you see a pill-rolling tremor, breathe a sigh of relief as this helps clinch the diagnosis. This has not been put in as the most important trigger because the tremor is not always produced to order in the examination setting. People have been known to stare for ages in the hope of seeing the tiniest flicker and have been disappointed.

If you are certain you are dealing with Parkinson's disease, seize the initiative and tell your examiners,

'The patient has a mask-like, expressionless face and I suspect they have Parkinson's disease. I would like to assess their tone, with your permission.' Most examiners will allow this. Introduce yourself to the patient and ask if you can examine their arms. Then test for cogwheel or lead-pipe rigidity (see Chapter 6).

Other features

- Slow movements (bradykinesia)
- Rigidity (these first two features together with the tremor are the hallmarks of Parkinson's disease)
- Greasy skin (seborrhoea)
- Excessive drooling (sialorrhoea)
- Tiny spidery writing (micrographia)
- Shuffling gait
- Prone to falling
- Postural hypotension.

....

Tip

If you see a tremor, observe the hand closely. Pay particular attention to the thumb and make sure it is pill-rolling in nature because there are other forms of tremor that have been mistaken for a parkinsonian tremor.

....

Tip

Note the response from the patient when you ask for permission to examine them. If their voice is quiet and lacks volume this is dysphonia, another feature of Parkinson's disease.

....

Exophthalmos

See Figs. 13.3 and 13.4.

What is it?

This is the protrusion of the eyes from the orbit due to retro-orbital infiltration and oedema and the most common cause is autoimmune thyroid disease. Sometimes you may hear the term proptosis used. Both terms mean the same thing with the exception that exophthalmos is usually reserved for proptosis of thyroid origin. Twenty-five per cent of patients with Grave's disease have exophthalmos. Exophthalmos is unrelated to thyroid status (that is, hyperthyroid, euthyroid, or hypothyroid; see Chapter 11) and may precede the development of Grave's disease.

Trigger feature

● Staring eyes.

   This spot case is easily missed. The patient (usually a woman) seems to be staring at you (sometimes to the point of rudeness), but then staring can be normal human behaviour. You have to remind yourself that you are in an examination and this may be your only clue. If you make the connection between staring eyes and exophthalmos you are on your way. Look carefully at the eyes, especially around the iris. If you can clearly see white sclera under the bottom margin of the iris (and also possibly the top margin), it is likely that the patient has exophthalmos.

Exophthalmos tends to be assymetrical. Some people advocate you look over the top of the patient's head from behind, while they are seated. From this position you can see how far the eye is protruding from the orbit. Although this visually confirms that the eye is protruding, it does not add any further useful information.

Other features

● Corneal ulceration—as the eye protrudes further from the orbit, the cornea becomes exposed and dry (as it loses the lubricating properties of blinking). It then becomes prone to ulceration and infection.

● Chemosis—as the eye protrudes the venous and lympatic drainage can be obstructed leading to oedema of the conjunctiva and periorbital oedema. In advanced cases the conjunctiva can become very red and swollen.

● Malignant exophthalmos—the pressure in the orbit becomes so great that it compresses the optic nerve or its blood supply, threatening sight. Note that this is not dependent on the degree of exophthalmos.

● Ophthalmoplegia—this is where eye movements are affected leading to diplopia. This occurs because of infiltration and oedema of the ocular muscles. In long-standing cases there may be fibrosis of the muscles leading to further impairment of movement (see Fig. 11.14).

● Goitre—this is usually a smooth diffusely enlarged goitre (this may be the subject of a spot case—see later).

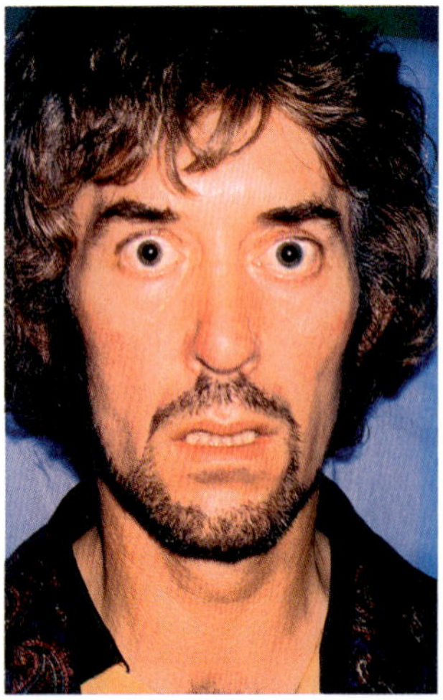

Figure 13.3 Exophthalmos due to Grave's disease.

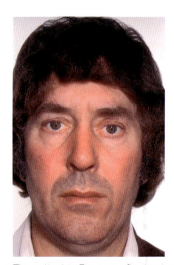

Figure 13.4 The patient in Fig. 13.3, after treatment.

Goitre

See Fig. 11.16.

What is it?

This is the enlargement of the thyroid gland.

Trigger features

- Swelling at the front of the neck.
- (A glass of water nearby.)

This can be easy to miss. However, if you stick to your systematic review, which includes the neck, you should pick this up (especially if your patient is a woman). If you see a goitre, quickly check for exophthalmos. Then say to your examiners,

'I have noticed a midline swelling in the neck, which is smooth and symmetrical. There is no exophthalmos. The likeliest cause is a goitre. I would like to confirm that it moves with swallowing and check the patient's thyroid status.'

If your examiners permit it, get a glass of water (one may be conveniently handy and is a further clue to a thyroid case) and observe if the swelling rises with swallowing. If it does, this confirms that it is of thyroid origin. Also check for lymph nodes around the neck. Then go on to check the thyroid status (see Chapter 11 and 'Thyrotoxicosis' and 'Myxoedema' in this chapter).

....

Tip

If you get a case with a discrete nodule or lump in the midline, get the patient to stick out their tongue to exclude a thyroglossal cyst (see Chapter 11) even if you see a glass of water present. Then go on to get the patient to swallow some water to determine if the swelling is a thyroid nodule. You will still need to check for lymph nodes and to assess the thyroid status as before.

....

Other features

- Dyspnoea (due to compression or deviation of the trachea)
- Cough
- Stridor (inspiratory noise due to obstruction of the trachea)

- Dysphagia (compression of the oesophagus from large goitre)
- Hoarse voice (due to left recurrent laryngeal nerve compression)
- Horner's syndrome (due to compression of the sympathetic nerves in the neck).

Thyrotoxicosis

What is it?

This is a condition due to the excess secretion of thyroid hormones.

Trigger features

- Patient looks anxious, listless, and fidgety
- Fine postural tremor.

This is another tricky spot case because there is sometimes very little to go on. Sometimes your examiners may give you some supplementary information to guide you. Your only physical clue may be that your patient (usually a woman) seems listless and agitated. If possible, watch her hands and see if you can glimpse a fine tremor when she moves them. In some cases thyrotoxicosis will be combined with Grave's disease and exophthalmos and a goitre may be additional clues. Tell your examiner,

'This young woman looks restless and fidgety and this suggests thyrotoxicosis. There is no obvious exophthalmos or a goitre but I would like to check this patient's thyroid status fully.'

If you are on the right lines your wish is likely to be granted. If you are wrong (some people can become anxious when they are on show for an examination), the examiners should give you credit for your thinking and will gently steer you in the right direction. Now check the thyroid status (see Chapter 11).

1 Observe the outstretched arms for a postural tremor.
2 Check for sweaty palms.
3 Check the pulse for a tachycardia.
4 Check the pulse for atrial fibrillation.
5 Look for lid retraction.
6 Look for lid-lag.

Other features

- Fatigue
- Heat intolerance

- Increased appetite
- Weight loss (despite increased appetite)
- Diarrhoea
- Angina
- Tachycardia
- Atrial fibrillation
- Heart failure
- Spider naevi
- Palmar erythema
- Osteoporosis
- Mild hypercalcaemia
- Proximal myopathy
- Amenorrhea (absent periods) in women.

Myxoedema

See Figs 13.5 and 13.6.

What is it?

This is a coarse thickening of the skin and subcutaneous tissues due to the deposition of mucopolysaccharides, which occurs in association with an underactive thyroid (sometimes myxoedema is used synonymously with hypothyroidism **but** hypothyroidism can occur without myxoedema).

Trigger features

- Apathetic expression
- Coarse thickened facial features
- Thinning of the hair.

Myxoedema is a condition that is easily missed. The patient is usually elderly (and female). Sometimes the skin has a yellowish tinge due to hypercarotenaemia (see Case 7.8). Also check to see if the patient has exophthalmos or a goitre. Occasionally patients with Grave's disease develop spontaneous hypothyroidism. More commonly it is the result of treatment for thyrotoxicosis with radioactive iodine or thyroidectomy (look carefully for a scar in the collar region of the lower neck—surgeons try to make them as invisible as possible). If you think you are dealing with myxoedema say to your examiners,

'This patient has an apathetic expression and has coarse thickened features and thinning hair. This suggests that the patient has myxoedema and with your permission I would like to check her pulse and her reflexes.'

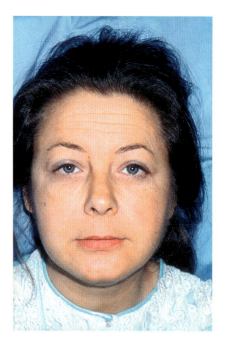

Figure 13.5 Myxoedema.

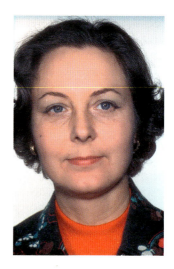

Figure 13.6 The same patient as in Fig. 13.5, after treatment.

If permission is granted, introduce yourself to the patient and ask if you can examine her briefly. Listen to her voice when she responds. Is it hoarse and croaky? This is another feature of hypothyroidism. Check to see if the patient has a bradycardia and then assess her ankle reflexes (you are looking for a slow-relaxing phase to the reflex).

Tip

If the patient is not in an optimum position for testing the ankle reflexes it is okay to check the biceps or triceps for the same slow-relaxing phenomenon.

Other features

- Fatigue
- Cold intolerance
- Weight gain
- Carpal tunnel syndrome
- Angina
- Pericardial effusion
- Cerebellar ataxia
- Depression
- Menorrhagia in women.

Acromegaly

See Fig. 13.7.

What is it?

Acromegaly ('acro'—extremities, 'megalos'—big) is a condition that causes enlargement of the bones, soft tissues, and organs of the body. It is due to the excess secretion of growth hormone from a pituitary tumour. The critical feature is that the epiphyses (the growing ends of bones) are fused. If they are not then giantism occurs as the bones can grow without restriction.

Trigger feature

- A large head with large coarse features.

The patient with acromegaly is fairly unmistakable. They have a large head with prominent supraorbital ridges, a large bulbous nose, and thick lips. They have a prominent lower jaw (prognathism) which can make the lower teeth protrude beyond the upper ones. The teeth may also become widely separated although this will not be obvious until you speak to the patient.

Other features

- Enlarged hands (see Fig. 13.8) and feet—hands have a 'doughy' feel because of increased thickness of the soft tissues
- Increased hat size and increased glove and shoe size
- Greasy skin (seborrhoea)
- Kyphosis
- Osteoarthritis
- Hepatomegaly, splenomegaly, and renal enlargement
- Cardiomyopathy
- Hypertension
- Diabetes
- Carpal tunnel syndrome (see Chapter 6)
- Proximal myopathy (see Chapter 6)
- Also features due to pituitary tumour

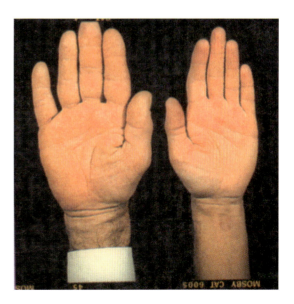

Figure 13.8 Acromegalic hand next to a normal hand for comparison.

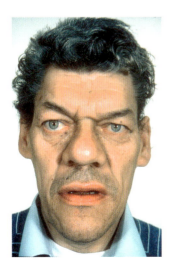

Figure 13.7 Acromegalic facies.

- Headache
- Bitemporal hemianopia (see Fig. 6.9).

Cushing's syndrome

See Figs. 13.9 and 13.10.

What is it?

Cushing's syndrome (*Harvey Cushing (1869–1939), American neurosurgeon*) is a collection of physical signs and symptoms caused by a chronic excess of cortisol.

Causes

- Long-term steroid treatment—the most common cause.
- Pituitary tumour causing adrenocorticotropic hormone (ACTH) secretion—this hyperstimulates the adrenals (hyperplasia) to secrete excess cortisol (this is called Cushing's disease).
- Ectopic ACTH production—this is secreted by tumours, for example, bronchial carcinoma; in some cases the development of the cancer is so rapid that the full features of Cushing's syndrome are not seen.
- Adrenal tumours—adenomas and carcinomas.

Trigger features

- Fat, round face (moon face)
- Central obesity
- Purpura.

If you see a patient with a fat, round face do not dismiss this as simple obesity (especially in an examination setting). The distribution of fat is different in Cushing's syndrome. It tends to accumulate centrally around the neck and trunk (on the neck it causes a 'buffalo hump' and the obese abdomen develops purple stretch marks called striae (see Fig. 7.19). The limbs become thin and wasted, leading to what has been called a 'lemon-on-a-stick appearance'. Scan the face and exposed limbs for any sign of bruising. If you see purpura it makes the diagnosis of Cushing's syndrome more likely (it occurs because of fragile dermal blood vessels and thinning of connective tissue that normally supports them).

Other features

- Thin skin
- Osteoporosis
- Hypertension
- Diabetes
- Proximal myopathy
- Depression
- Psychosis
- Amenorrhoea in women.

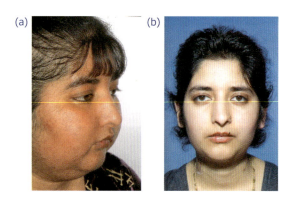

(a)   (b)

Figure 13.9 Cushing's syndrome: (a) cushingoid facies before treatment; (b) cushingoid facies after treatment.

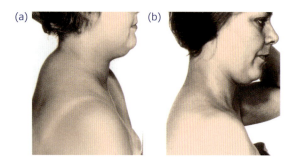

(a)   (b)

Figure 13.10 Cushing's syndrome: (a) buffalo hump of Cushing's syndrome; (b) the same patient after treatment.

Addison's disease

See Figs. 13.11 and 13.12.

What is it?

Addison's disease (*Thomas Addison (1793–1860), English physician*) is a disorder due to lack of the hormones cortisol and aldosterone because of damage or destruction of the adrenal cortex.

Causes

- Autoimmune
- Tuberculosis involving the adrenals

(a)
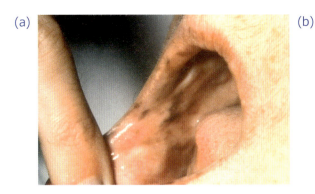

(b)
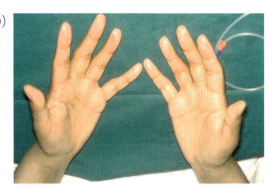

Figure 13.11 Addison's disease: (a) pigmentation of the buccal mucosa; (b) pigmentation of the palmar creases.

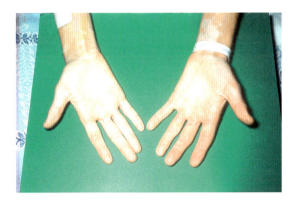

Figure 13.12 Vitiligo in a patient with Addison's disease.

- Septicaemia (meningococcal sepsis with adrenal involvement is known as Waterhouse–Friderichson (*water-house-frid-er-rick-son*) syndrome) (*Rupert Waterhouse (1873–1958), English physician; Carl Friderichson (1886–1979), Danish paediatrician*)
- Bilateral adrenalectomy (*a-dren-a-leck-tummy*) (used to be performed for malignant diseases and Cushing's syndrome)
- Secondary causes of adrenal underactivity occur and include long-term steroid therapy and pituitary or hypothalamic disorders that lead to a decrease in ACTH production.

Trigger feature

- Generalized brown pigmentation of the skin (and recent scars).

This is obviously a non-specific trigger that has other causes. It also highlights what an insidious condition Addison's disease is. Most of its signs and symptoms are non-specific and you need a very high index of suspicion

to detect it. If you meet someone who is inappropriately brown and unwell, this disease **must** cross your mind. The pigmentation is due to the lack of adrenocortical hormones, which normally provide feedback to the pituitary. In the absence of these hormones the pituitary secretes even more ACTH and a by-product of this hypersecretion is the stimulation of melanocytes leading to pigmentation.

Other causes of brown pigmentation

- Haemochromatosis (sometimes slate grey)
- Nelson's syndrome (this occurs following bilateral adrenalectomy where the lack of adrenocortical hormones produces a hypersecretion of ACTH as before)
- Ectopic ACTH production (usually from hormone-secreting cancers, for example, small cell tumours of the bronchus).

If you see a pigmented individual, you have to be more flexible in your approach. Tell your examiners,

'I have noticed generalized brown pigmentation of the patient. If they have not been to a hot country for a holiday or been on a sun-bed, then the possible causes include Addison's disease, Nelson's disease, ectopic ACTH production, and haemochromatosis. With your permission I would like to examine the patient further and ask some questions.'

If this is allowed, introduce yourself to the patient and ask to examine their hands. Look at the palmar creases and see if they are pigmented. Look at the elbows and search for any scars. Note whether these are pigmented too (only recent scars that have formed when Addison's disease has been active will be pigmented). Ask the patient to open their mouths and examine the buccal cavity with a pen torch. Are there areas of pigmentation here too? Other possible areas of pigmentation include the nipples and areas of friction such as the elbows and knees. If pigmentation is present in these areas then this suggests Addison's disease. If you have time, ask if the patient has had both their adrenals removed (this would suggest Nelson's syndrome). Ask about other symptoms of Addison's disease (see 'Other features', next).

Other features

- Anorexia
- Weight loss
- Vomiting
- Fatigue
- Diarrhoea or constipation
- Hypotension
- Postural hypotension
- Hypoglycaemia.

Systemic sclerosis

See Fig. 13.13.

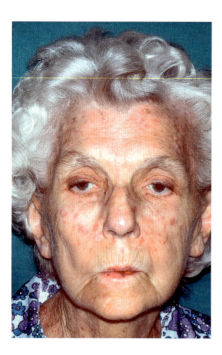

Figure 13.13 Facies of systemic sclerosis. Note the thin-drawn mouth with radial furrows (pseudorhagades) and telangiectasia.

What is it?

It is a generalized disease of connective tissue that leads to the proliferation of collagen and fibrosis of skin, subcutaneous tissue, small blood vessels, and organs. Its cause is unknown.

Trigger features

- 'Beak'-shaped nose
- Thin-drawn mouth
- Radial furrows around the mouth (pseudorhagades) (*sue-dough-rag-aids*)
- Telangiectasia.

The patient (usually a woman) has an unmistakable appearance. Despite this, each sign on its own can be overlooked unless you are wary. I find the area around the nose and the mouth very helpful in the recognition of this disorder. Once you have twigged the diagnosis, you have an opportunity to demonstrate your knowledge. Tell your examiners that you suspect systemic sclerosis; explain why and say that you would like to examine the hands for evidence of sclerodactyly (*s-clear-owe-dack-tilly*) (atrophy of the fingertips), the changes of Raynaud's phenomenon, and calcinosis.

Other features

- Shiny, waxy-looking skin
- Sausage-shaped fingers (early changes of Raynaud's phenomenon)
- Dysphagia
- Lung fibrosis
- Renal failure
- Pericardial effusion
- Cardiomyopathy.

Facial nerve palsy

See Fig. 6.31.

What is it?

This is a lesion of the facial nerve, which can be due to an upper or a lower motor neuron cause.

Trigger feature

- Facial asymmetry with drooping of one side of the face (occasionally people can have bilateral facial nerve palsy, which can be difficult to spot but you should not encounter this in an undergraduate examination).

This is one case that should be easy to spot. However, there is plenty of work to be done. You need to demonstrate whether the facial nerve palsy is an upper motor neuron (UMN) or a lower motor neuron (LMN) lesion. Tell your examiners,

'I can see drooping of the left side of the face, which indicates a facial nerve palsy. I would like to determine whether it is an upper or lower motor lesion and look for clues to its aetiology *(ee-tea-ollow-jee* [cause]).'

Introduce yourself to the patient and assess the facial nerve in detail. Get your patient to blow out their cheeks, show their teeth, screw their eyes up tight, and raise their eyebrows. If they are unable to screw their eyes up tight or raise their eyebrows this is a LMN lesion (see Chapter 6). Having demonstrated a LMN lesion, quickly check for any potential causes. Look at the cheeks in the parotid area for signs of a swelling (parotid tumour) or a scar of a previous operation. With a pen torch, look around the ear and the external auditory meatus for signs of herpetic vesicles (Ramsay–Hunt syndrome). Very rarely a cerebellopontine tumour can cause a LMN lesion. So ask the patient if they have trouble with their hearing (cranial nerve VIII, cochlear) or have been falling (cranial nerve VIII, vestibular). If you have time, check for nystagmus (see Chapter 6). If you demonstrate a UMN lesion, the most common cause is a stroke. Immediately look at the position of the limbs. Is one arm internally rotated with flexion at the elbow and is the corresponding leg internally rotated with the knee in extension and with plantarflexion of the foot? This is the classical position for hemiplegia.

Horner's syndrome

See Fig. 13.14.

What is it?

This is a collection of three physical signs:

- partial ptosis of an eyelid (partial droop of the lid)
- small pupil (miosis)
- absence of sweating (anhydrosis) *(an-high-drow-sis)*.

Enophthalmos is mentioned in some books (the eye sinks back into the socket), but it is unclear whether this is a true phenomenon or an illusion caused by the ptosis itself (see 'Trigger feature' and Case 5.16).

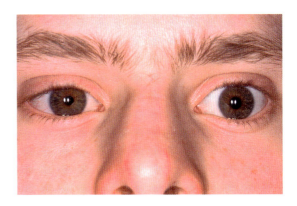

Figure 13.14 Horner's syndrome. There is a partial ptosis as the right eyelid encroaches on the iris along with miosis of the right pupil.

Trigger feature

- Slight droop of an eyelid.

Horner's syndrome is another sign that is very easy to miss. Even its most obvious marker, partial ptosis, can be hard to spot for the unwary. So when inspecting the eyes, spend time checking for symmetry between them. If you do suspect a Horner's syndrome you need to move in closer to confirm your findings. Let your examiners know what you are doing, say,

'I have noticed a partial ptosis of the right eyelid and I am suspecting a Horner's syndrome. With your permission I would like to examine the pupil for miosis.'

Introduce yourself to the patient and see if the relevant pupil is constricted when compared with the other. If it is, then it is likely you are dealing with Horner's syndrome. You can check for anhydrosis crudely by running your index finger down one side of the forehead and then the other. Normal skin sweats slightly and has a soapy feel as you run your finger down it. If there is absence of sweating, the skin is dry, and your finger will glide smoothly without resistance. Demonstrating enophthalmos is not necessary. It is now believed that this is an illusion due to depression of the palpabral fissure.

Tip

Further examination is important because in elderly people a partial ptosis may be a consequence of ageing. This is because the levator muscle can become weak or become detached from the lid.

Tip

In an examination setting there may not be time to do this, but if there is very little difference between the pupils because of bright ambient light take your patient to somewhere gloomy (and explain why, lest they become suspicious of your intentions). In a darker environment, the normal pupil will dilate appropriately and make any differences between the two pupils more obvious.

Tip

To confuse the issue, miosis may be a normal consequence of ageing, plus elderly people may be on eyedrops, for example, for glaucoma, which can constrict (some can dilate) the pupil, so it may be worth asking if they have eye problems and if they are on eye drops.

Hereditary haemorrhagic telangiectasia

See Fig. 13.15.

What is it?

HHT is an inherited condition (autosomal dominant) whereby patients develop telangiectasia in the skin and mucous membranes. These vessels are weak and may lead to bleeding.

Trigger feature

- Red blebs on the face, particularly around the lips.

There are a number of conditions that may cause telangiectasia of the face including systemic sclerosis (see 'Systemic sclerosis' section) and chronic liver disease (spider naevi). However, HHT causes lesions around the lips, buccal mucosa, and tongue. Therefore if you see telangiectasia especially around the lips (and there is no evidence of systemic sclerosis or jaundice), say to the examiners,

'I have noticed lesions reminiscent of telangiectasia on the face and around the lips. I would like to demonstrate that they are telangiectasia and I would like to inspect the buccal mucosa and tongue because I am suspecting hereditary haemorrhagic telangiectasia.'

If allowed, blanch a lesion and see if it refills. Then ask the patient to open their mouth and inspect with a torch. Make sure that you inspect the underside of the tongue. If lesions are present in the mouth the diagnosis is HHT.

Other features

- Iron deficiency anaemia
- Gastrointestinal haemorrhage
- Haemoptysis
- Epistaxis (nose bleed).

Peutz–Jehgers syndrome

See Fig. 13.16.

What is it?

This is an inherited disorder (autosomal dominant), leading to a combination of pigmentation of the skin and mucous membrane and polyposis of the intestines.

(a) 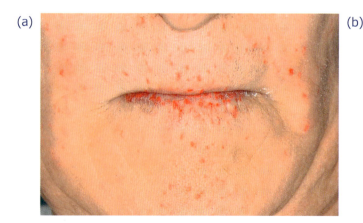 (b)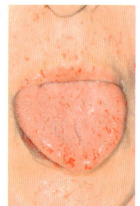

Figure 13.15 Hereditary haemorrhagic telangiectasia: (a) telangectasia around the lips; (b) telangectasia on the tongue.

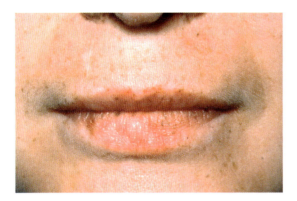

Figure 13.16 The perioral pigmentation of Peutz–Jehgers syndrome.

Trigger feature

- Brown freckly pigmentation around the lips.

This sign is easy to miss, but if you do home in on this sign then the diagnosis is straightforward. You just need to keep this in mind when you do your systematic scan of the face. Pigmentation can also be found on the hands and feet.

Other features

- Polyps in the bowel (histologically they are hamartomas)
- Iron deficiency anaemia
- Gastrointestinal haemorrhage
- Rarely malignant change.

Jaundice

See Fig. 13.17.

What is it?

Jaundice is the yellow discoloration of the skin and sclerae due to the deposition of the bile pigment bilirubin (see Chapter 7).

Trigger features

- Yellow sclerae
- Yellow skin.

Jaundice can be easy or difficult to spot depending on the underlying cause. A full-blown obstructive jaundice may jump out at you whereas someone with mild Gilbert's

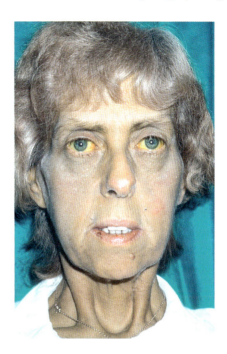

Figure 13.17 Jaundice: this patient looks cachexic, which suggests a malignant cause for her jaundice.

syndrome may not be readily noticeable from the end of the bed (it would be unfair for examiners to try to get you to spot the latter without getting you to examine the face closer). If you notice yellow skin, check for scratch marks, which suggest itching (pruritis) and see if you notice any telangiectasia, which could be spider naevi and might indicate chronic liver disease. Often a spot case of jaundice will be a prelude to a full examination of the gastrointestinal tract. Tell your examiners that you have noticed yellow skin and sclerae and you suspect jaundice. You would like to confirm this and perform a fuller examination of the abdomen to determine a cause and to look in particular for signs of chronic liver disease.

Other features

These depend on the cause of jaundice. Usually this is chronic liver disease and so you should be familiar with the signs (see Chapter 7).

References and further reading

Ryder REJ, Mir MA, Freeman EA. *An aid to MRCP PACES*, 4th edn. Wiley-Blackwell, Oxford, 2012.

14 Examination of the child

Introduction

The clinical examination of children is not just a cut-down version of that carried out in adults but a complete adaptation. Paediatric examinations need to be tailored to the individual child and the techniques employed will depend on their age, understanding, and level of coop-eration. Examination of the infant or very young child will be mostly observational and opportunistic, such as observing walking or breathing and listening to the heart while the child is quiet. The ability to engage the child is a skill that will develop through practice and experience, but can be enhanced by involving a parent, using a play therapist, and carrying out the examination in a child-friendly environment. It should also be remembered that young children when confronted with a strange situation and an unknown adult may become intimidated and overwhelmed. Recognizing this, it can be helpful to place yourself at the child's level and make the examination playful and relaxed.

Children are in general healthy and robust. The identification of the normal in a child is as important as the abnormal, such as distinguishing an innocent heart murmur from a pathological one. Never underestimate the relief that parents feel when they are reassured that their child is healthy. As children grow physically, mentally, and emotionally throughout their childhood the examiner should take every opportunity to assess adequate growth and development. You should also consider health promotion, child safety, parenting skills, and child protection issues in each consultation and discuss appropriately. Finally, a good experience with the medical profession in childhood will be remembered, and will allow a good relationship to develop and continue into adulthood.

The assessment of the child is a huge topic and hence this chapter is not comprehensive. We have, however, tried to provide a structure to enable students to use their developing skills fruitfully in examining a wide range of children. There is also some emphasis on the extremes of childhood (i.e. the newborn and the adolescent) with some discussion on topics unique to these areas. Good luck!

Terminology

- **Neonate**: baby up to 28 days of age.
- **Infants**: babies are considered to be infants up to the age of 1 year (from the Latin *infans*, *in*=not and *fans*=speak).
- **Preschool child**: a child under 5 years of age; this can be further divided into younger (1–3 years) and older (3–4 years) preschool child.
- **School-age child**: child age 5–16 years can be divided into younger (5–10 years) and older (11–16 years).
- **Adolescent**: child from puberty.
- **Parent**: parent or main caregiver (e.g. foster carer).

History

In paediatrics the history is one of the most important aspects of your assessment. When it is done well the correct diagnosis can sometimes be ascertained from the history alone. History-taking is an art that needs to be practiced and an invaluable skill in any chosen speciality. Taking a successful history from a parent or carer can be challenging but also very rewarding. The best place to learn how to take a history is on the wards, in clinics, and in the emergency department. Take every opportunity to practice the skills learnt from this chapter, as medicine is best learnt from the bedside. Excellent communication skills are required when taking a history regarding a child. It is important that you are a perceptive and receptive listener. It is vital that the parental and child's concerns are listened to sympathetically. Always begin with open questions as this will inevitably reveal far more information. For example, 'Tell me what is worrying you about your child.'

Tip

Always listen to the concerns of the parent or carer. If they are worried you should be too.

History-taking in the paediatric setting has many similarities to that of adult medicine and some of the basic principles which you will have already learnt will be applicable. The major difference is that the information obtained is from a third party, normally the parent or carer. The information provided to you may be modified by the parents' perceptions and fears. You should also involve the child as much as possible. From around 4 years old, the child may be able to contribute but still try to involve them if they are younger. Always use an interpreter if there is a language barrier. Avoid using family or friends to maintain confidentiality.

When taking the past medical history take a detailed history of any previous illnesses or accidents. Recurrent attendances may be a flag for possible child abuse, or a more significant disease; for example, repeated fractures could be non-accidental or be the product of an underlying bone disease.

Additional aspects of a paediatric history to cover can be easily remembered by the mnemonic 'BINDS':

- **B**irth, pregnancy and neonatal
- **I**mmunization
- **N**utrition and growth
- **D**evelopment
- **S**ocial

Birth, pregnancy, and neonatal

This should include a detailed birth history including the birth weight, the mode of delivery, and any complications during the pregnancy and neonatal period.

Immunizations

Check that the child is up to date with their immunizations as per the UK immunization schedule (Table 14.1) This information may be documented in the personal child health record which is also referred to as the 'red book' (Fig. 14.1).

Nutrition and growth

Take a good dietary history; a 24 hour recall is sometimes asked for on the first visit to a paediatric outpatient clinic. If an infant is taking formula feeds ask how many bottles and how much milk is being given per feed. In a breastfed baby ask how long the baby feeds normally and how often. Establish if the child has been growing well; this information will be in the 'red book'.

Development

Ask specifically about any concerns raised by the parents, nursery, or school. Do the parents feel that their

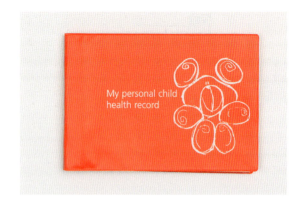

Figure 14.1 The personal child health record ('red book').

development is on a par with their elder siblings or peers? Ask about specific developmental milestones which are covered later in this chapter.

Social and family history

The child's social background is an essential component, so draw a detailed family tree (Fig. 14.2). This may highlight hereditary conditions or social difficulties.

- Ask who is in the family and who lives at home.
- Ask about consanguinity (genetic relationship between parents, commonly first cousins) as this will increase the risk of genetic disorders.
- Ask about the parents occupations as this will provide insight into the family's socio-economic status. Identify if they have pets as this may be relevant in cases such as asthma.
- Always consider the possibility of abuse and the welfare of the child should always be at the forefront of your mind.
- Ask about the health of the other children at home and determine if they have any special needs.

The commonest acute presentations of infants and toddlers are infections as their developing immune system are introduced to new pathogens; respiratory and gastrointestinal infections make up the bulk of these. Accidents are also common in mobile children. This age group have the largest numbers of emergency attendances and admissions to medical services. Pyrexia, cough, and vomiting are common presenting symptoms and it is important to take a good history in order to ascertain the underlying diagnosis. Pyrexia is probably the most anxiety-provoking symptom. Most children will have a non-specific viral illness, but it is important to elicit aspects of the history that may suggest a more significant problem, particularly meningitis. Associated

Table 14.1 UK immunization schedule

Age	Vaccine
2 months	DTaP/IPV/Hib (diptheria, tetanus, pertussis (whooping cough), polio, Hib) PCV (pneumococcal)
3 months	DTaP/IPV/Hib Men C (meningococcal)
4 months	DTaP/IPV/Hib Men C PCV
12–13 months	Hib/Men C PCV MMR (measles, mumps, and rubella)
3 years and 4 months to 5 years	DTaP/IPV/Hib MMR
Girls age 12–13 years	HPV (human papillomavirus)
13–18 years	Td/IPV (tetanus/diphtheria/polio)

(a)

(b)

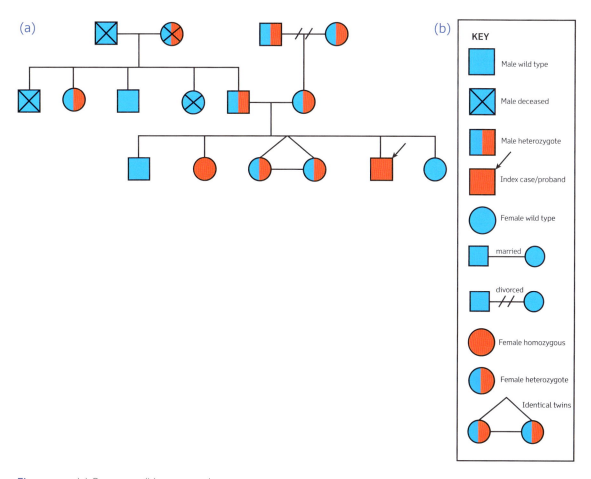

KEY

▪	Male wild type
⊠	Male deceased
◧	Male heterozygote
▪	Index case/proband
●	Female wild type
▪—●	married
▪—//—●	divorced
●	Female homozygous
◖	Female heterozygote
△	Identical twins

Figure 14.2 (a) Genogram; (b) genogram key.

symptoms such as rash, coryza (runny nose), wheeze and respiratory distress, bowel and urinary changes are important to ask about. Events leading up to development of a cough may be relevant, for example, a child who has inhaled a foreign body. It is important to think about possible diagnoses in order to frame the history-taking process. Examples of common symptoms can be seen in Table 14.2.

Newborn history/background

A neonate is defined as an infant less than 28 days of age and it is therefore clear that a history will have to be gathered from a number of other sources. Maternal and infant records should be quickly reviewed before examining the newborn. Maternal age, parity, antenatal scans, fetal growth, details of any antenatal tests including triple test, amniocentesis, serological tests for infection (HIV, hepatitis B&C, rubella, syphilis) and any obstetric or medical illness

during pregnancy should be sought from maternal records and will provide useful clues. History of any maternal drug use, maternal medications, social history, and child protection concerns will have implications on the health and well-being of the infant. Perinatal events like onset of labour, presence of fetal distress, risk factors for sepsis (maternal pyrexia during labour, prolonged rupture of membranes), nature of delivery, condition at birth, and need for resuscitation should be checked from infant records. Check with the midwife looking after the baby if she/he has any concerns about the baby.

Adolescent history

The adolescent patient is often poorly served by health services. This is especially evident at the time of transition to adult services during the latter phase of adolescence. Adolescents will complete growth and puberty, acquire a

Table 14.2 Common symptoms

Main symptom	Additional symptom(s)	Possible diagnoses
Pyrexia	Cough and coryza	Viral upper respiratory tract infection
Pyrexia	Cough ± difficulty in breathing	Lower respiratory tract infection, e.g. pneumonia
Cough	Stridor	Croup, foreign body, bronchiolitis
Cough	Wheeze	Bronchiolitis, asthma
Vomiting	Diarrhoea	Gastroenteritis, allergy
Effortless vomiting	Infant	Reflux, gastroenteritis
Vomiting	Pyrexia	Urinary tract infection, sepsis, meningitis

Key points

- The additional components of a paediatric history include:
  - **B**irth
  - **I**mmunizations
  - **N**utrition and growth
  - **D**evelopment/school
  - **S**ocial and family history
- If there is a language barrier, avoid using a family member or friend to interpret, to maintain confidentiality
- Make sure that the child's immunizations are up to date
- The child's personal health record (the 'red book') contains a wealth of valuable information
- Cough, pyrexia, and vomiting are common presenting symptoms

new body shape and develop their sexual and personal identity. Children at the start of puberty are still largely dependent on their parents who are responsible for their health, financial, and personal needs. However, by the end of adolescence individuals become almost entirely responsible for their own well-being, with increasing independence from their parents.

The basic structure of a medical history remains unchanged when assessing an adolescent patient. However, some modifications are needed, such as the addition of pubertal assessment (if indicated) and an altered focus in the social history. Importantly the direction of questioning during the history-taking should be towards the adolescent themselves, rather than their parent/s or carer/s, thus acknowledging the adolescent's emerging adult status and independence. Provide the patient with time to explain their concerns and also listen to them. It is important to both gain trust and show respect for their evolving maturity.

The presence of parents/carers and friends can both augment and hinder the history-taking process. Support from a caring and non-judgemental companion will be of benefit for the adolescent. However, certain questions may become embarrassing for some adolescents in the presence of certain company (e.g. discussing acne or bowel habits in front of a partner, or sexual history in front of a parent), and the history-taker should take this into consideration.

Tips

- If necessary, companions should be politely asked to leave the room before any sensitive questions are asked.
- Raise this possibility as routine practice at the start of the consultation to prepare all parties to avoid embarrassing the adolescent or raising unnecessary suspicion among the parents.
- Alternatively, taking the patient for examination in a separate room after history-taking is another strategy to allow more sensitive questions to be asked in private without the need to ask the companion to leave during the consultation.

Developmental history/pubertal assessment

During assessment of growth and development in the history the adolescents' pubertal status should be established and in females the presence of menarche and pattern of menses should be ascertained. Ask at what age the first signs of puberty have been seen. If puberty has started check that progression through puberty is occurring appropriately. Some adolescents may not know they are in puberty, especially boys, and it can be useful to enquire about greasy skin or hair, body odour, or changes in mood.

Family and social history

Family history in the adolescent, as with history-taking in the younger child, should include a family tree. Other relationships may become important such as any partners or offspring.

In taking a social history it is important to assess risk taking behaviour in an adolescent such as smoking and experimenting with recreational drugs. These issues should be sensitively enquired about alongside an individual's alcohol consumption and sexual activities. This is also an opportunity for health promotion and issues such as safe sex practice to avoid sexually transmitted infections, contraception, and smoking cessation can be discussed.

....

Tips

Often the best way to ask about these without sounding too judgemental is to ask 'How much alcohol do you drink in a month?' or 'Which drugs have you tried' rather than the more accusatory 'Do you smoke/drink alcohol/take drugs?'

....

Establishing the patients' current circumstances regarding schooling, higher education, or career aspirations as well as situation at home and hobbies can be most useful in painting a picture of their current life and future plans. An interest in these issues will again help strengthen the sense of trust and respect that the patient feels towards the examiner.

Eating disorders are most common in adolescence and young adulthood. Dietary habits should be discussed during an adolescent history-taking, especially if issues such as eating disorders are suspected.

At the end of the history you can check if the adolescent or their parent has any issues not yet addressed which they wish to raise with you.

Special considerations when examining a child

Examination skills are taught throughout the medical school curriculum and are vital to becoming a proficient doctor. The methodology of examining adults has been covered in depth within the other chapters of this book. Many of the principles already learnt will be applicable to children. However, this knowledge and skill will need to be adapted to enable the successful examination of a child or adolescent.

Within this section we hope to highlight the differences between the paediatric and adult examination. We endeavour to improve your confidence in working with children because although they are a challenge they are fun to work with! See Case 14.1.

The key considerations are:

- Children are less cooperative and one needs to be opportunistic. Playful diversions are effective!

- Children present with very different pathology. Observation skills are the most important tool of examination—rushing to formally examine a young child can lead to upset and results in a suboptimal exam.

- Be aware of the developmental capability and age of the child. For example, a child who has stranger anxiety (develops from 6 months of age) will not respond well to being taken out of a parent's/carer's arms to be put on an examination couch.

- Build a rapport with the child and gain their trust; make the examination into a game and use age appropriate

CASE 14.1

Problem. I am very wary of examining children as I am worried about upsetting a child or even causing pain.

Discussion. This is a very normal worry that all students have. Children will often be frightened of strangers and it can be very daunting to be faced with a crying child. It provokes concern not only for you, but more importantly for the parent(s). This is where good communication skills are vital. Talk calmly to the child and parents explaining what you are going to do. It is unlikely that you will hurt the child by doing a normal examination but ensure that the child is out of danger when carrying out your examination. Also remember to talk to the child, and if old enough enquire whether they have pain anywhere. Examine the child at their level even if this means being on your knees. There is nothing scarier than a person looming over you. Be opportunistic in your approach; for example, in between crying episodes you may be able to listen to the child's chest with a stethoscope. Most importantly, develop your observation skills. For example, a young child who is vigorous, alert, and combative is unlikely to be very unwell. Despite all your best efforts the child may still become upset. If you have tried to distract and comfort the child then it may be worthwhile to consider deferring the examination till the child is more settled.

toys. Once the child is less wary you may be able to touch the child, for example, placing the stethoscope.

It is helpful to think about children in four different age categories; infant (0–1 years), preschool (1–4 years), school age (5–10 years), and adolescents.

Infants

Make funny noises and smile a lot to distract the child. Sometimes it is helpful to use a pacifier such as the child's dummy or a clean little finger (get the parents' permission before doing this). Ensure that the child is close to the parent from the age of 6 months as this is when stranger anxiety manifests.

Preschool

Examine the child on the parent's lap as much as possible (Fig. 14.3). Demonstrate what you are about to do on a doll or their favourite toy or on the child's parent. Allow the child to hold your stethoscope so that they can become familiar with it.

School age

A more adult style examination is suitable, but always talk through the examination and ensure they know what you intend to do. Try and make it 'fun' and not too intimidating. With adolescents respect their modesty, offer to perform the examination without their parent, and always use a chaperone.

Adolescents

See 'Adolescent examination'.

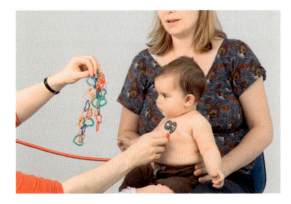

Figure 14.3 Child being examined on the parent's lap, while being distracted with a toy.

Key points

- Try to establish a rapport with the child by making the consultation fun and non-threatening
- Involve the child during the history-taking process
- Good communication skills are the key to eliciting a detailed history and obtaining the correct diagnosis
- Adapt your examination approach to the developmental stage of the child
- Concentrate on developing your observational skills.
- If the child becomes upset despite your best efforts then withdraw graciously

In summary, the key to examining children successfully is to develop your observation skills and to be opportunistic. Children will often be frightened of strangers. Preparation is essential. The only way to learn the skills of a good paediatrician is by practicing on the wards and in clinics.

Examination of the child summary

1. Get your equipment ready.
2. Introduce yourself to the child and parent and ask permission to examine.
3. Wash your hands.
4. Position the child and make them comfortable.
5. General inspection of the child.
6. Examine the hands.
7. Inspect the head, face, and neck.
8. Inspect the skin.
9. Examine the cardiovascular system.
10. Examine the respiratory system.
11. Examine the abdominal system.
12. Examine the genitourinary system.
13. Examine the musculoskeletal system.
14. Examine the nervous system.
15. Assess development of the child.
16. Assess hearing and vision.
17. Assess ear, nose, and throat.

18 Thank the child and parent.

19 Wash your hands.

Examination of the child in detail

Getting started

1 Get your equipment ready

Make sure that you have everything you need for your examination. This will be age dependent. Common to all ages are the following:

- Stethoscope
- Measuring tape
- Age-specific growth charts
- Pen torch or other light source

It is also advantageous to have an ophthalmoscope but these should be available on the ward or clinic. When examining an adolescent boy you may need access to Prader's orchidometer (see 'Adolescent examination').

··

Tip

It is not necessary to buy a specific paediatric stethoscope. In an older child an adult stethoscope is fine. For a younger child there should be appropriate stethoscopes available on the ward where you are based.

··

2 Introduce yourself to the child and parent and ask permission to examine

Say something like 'I am Ernst Moro, a fourth-year medical student. Is it all right if I examine xxxx?'

3 Wash your hands

Clean mitts for the little mites.

4 Position the child and make them comfortable

Where and how you do this will depend on the child's age, as discussed before (see 'Special considerations when examining a child').

5 General inspection of the child

Take a minute to stand at the end of the bed and look at the child and the space around them. In an OSCE examination this will allow you time to remain calm and collected in the heat of the moment. A lot of information can be obtained from inspecting the bed space. For example, if a child has asthma they may be connected to a saturation monitor or have an aerochamber (a small volumatic device designed for children to improve the delivery of drugs to the lungs; see Chapter 5) present by the bedside. See Table 14.3.

One of the most important skills to learn is the ability to identify well versus unwell children. A drowsy child, or one who is irritable, is likely to be unwell. Paradoxically a child who is uncomplaining during an examination (in some cases) could also be brewing a serious illness. Recognizing a sick child early can alter the outcome significantly and improves with experience. Look specifically for pallor, jaundice, or cyanosis (see Chapters 4, 7, and 5 respectively for the significance of these). Is there a rash? If so, check to see if it is blanching or non-blanching. A non-blanching rash raises the suspicion of meningococcal septicaemia (see Fig. 14.6). Also request some basic observations such as temperature, pulse, blood pressure, respiratory rate, and oxygen saturations. Some of the normal values will vary with the child's age as demonstrated in Table 14.4.

Table 14.3 Things to look for in a general inspection

Does the child look well or unwell?
Lethargic/irritable/alert?
Signs of pain/discomfort?
Signs of dehydration?
Child's demeanour/cleanliness
Scars

Key points
- Always assess the child's general appearance
- Does the child look unwell? Drowsiness, irritability and not complaining when being examined (in some cases) may be worrying features
- Always check for pallor or cyanosis
- Are there any rashes? If so, are they blanching or non-blanching?
- Always review the vital signs

Table 14.4 Normal values in children

Age	Heart rate (beats/min)	Respiratory rate (respirations/min)	Systolic blood pressure (mmHg)
<1	110–160	30–40	70–90
2–5	95–150	25–35	80–95
5–12	80–120	20–25	90–110
>12	60–100	15–20	100–120

Table 14.5 Causes of clubbing in children

Respiratory
Cystic fibrosis
Tuberculosis
Cardiovascular
Congenital heart disease with right-to-left shunt
Infective endocarditis
Gastrointestinal
Inflammatory bowel disease
Coeliac disease
Autoimmune hepatitis
Other
Thyrotoxicosis
Idiopathic

Detailed examination

6 Examine the hands

The hands can provide a lot of clues towards a diagnosis. Look for signs of clubbing. The most common causes in children are listed in Table 14.5. Look for a single transverse palmar crease which is a sign associated with a number of syndromes including trisomy 21 (Down's syndrome). Note, however, that this sign is not pathognomonic for trisomy 21 and may be present in normal children. Look for signs of anaemia and endocarditis such as splinter haemorrhages and Janeway lesions.

7 Inspect the head, face, and neck

Start by looking at the child's face and determine whether there are any dysmorphic features (see the 'Newborn examination' section). For neonates and young infants palpate the anterior fontanelle assessing whether it is sunken or bulging (see Table 14.14 and 'Newborn examination' section, also see Case 14.2). Look for any asymmetry of the skull and measure the head circumference. Children may have abnormal moulding of the head predominantly due to outside pressure on the skull in response to their sleeping positions as babies. Sometimes there may be premature fusion of one or more of the cranial sutures which causes an abnormality in the head shape referred to as craniosynostosis (*cray-knee-owe-sin-os-toe-sis*).

Look for any signs of jaundice, cyanosis, or anaemia as you would for an adult. Remember that the causes of jaundice will be different in children compared to adults (see Table 14.6). Examine the neck feeling for lymph nodes. Children often have small palpable lymph nodes in the anterior and posterior triangle which are associated with conditions such as acute tonsillitis. If the lymph node is large then this may be a cause for concern (Table 14.7).

8 Inspect the skin

Have a more focused look at the colour of the skin: confirm pallor, jaundice, or cyanosis if you spotted this on inspection. Does the child have a rash? Children can have a variety of rashes. It is useful if you can recognize rashes such as chickenpox and measles (see Figs. 14.4 and 14.5).

The first thing to establish is whether the rash is blanching or non-blanching. Parents are taught to perform the 'glass test' which involves pressing a glass over the rash and determining whether it disappears with pressure (Fig. 14.6). There are several causes of a non-blanching rash (Table 14.8). Any non-blanching rash must be taken seriously as it can herald meningococcal meningitis/septicaemia.

Tip

Always assess the child's rash in the context of the child's physical state. Do they look well or unwell?

CASE 14.2

Problem. I am unsure of what to look and feel for when examining an infant's fontanelle and sutures.

Discussion. This is a part of the paediatric examination that is very specific to infants and young children. The anterior fontanelle is usually closed by 18 months and the posterior one by 6 months. Place your hand on the infant's head just at the forehead and move it back, maintaining contact with the scalp. A sunken fontanelle will feel as if there is a 'dip' on top of the scalp. The child may also have features of dehydration (see Table 14.14). A bulging fontanelle will feel like a tense 'bump' on the scalp. The child may be unwell with pyrexia and lethargy and meningitis should be considered. When examining all infants feeling the fontanelle is important. Take all the opportunities you can to feel a normal fontanelle as this will increase your chances of recognizing an abnormal one. It is also important to feel the sutures between the skull bones. It is normal for an infant to have a small gap of 1–2 mm, but a large gap (>5 mm) between the skull bones and large fontanelles may mean that a child has hydrocephalus (a build-up of cerebrospinal fluid around the brain causing the skull bones to separate). Overriding sutures may be normal in a newborn baby and the skull bones will separate over a few days. In an older infant if there is no gap between the skull bones and a ridge is felt, craniosynostosis should be considered.

Look for any abnormal shaped marks or suspicious bruises such as those on the ear or over the spine as these may be features of physical abuse (Fig. 14.7). See Case 14.3.

9 Examine the cardiovascular system

Most children have healthy hearts and a normal cardiovascular system. When examining the cardiovascular system in children you are usually looking for signs of congenital heart disease and more rarely acquired disease (e.g. heart failure).

Dysmorphia

Inspect the child's face for dysmorphic (*dis-more-fick*) features, as cardiac conditions are sometimes associated with syndromes; examples are listed in Table 14.9. Dysmorphic features are an unusual configuration of the normal structures of the face that give an unusual and sometimes characteristic appearance.

Key points

- Commence any examination by inspecting the child from the end of the bed
- Make sure you learn how to recognize the unwell child
- With bruising/injury in unusual places, of an unusual shape or of a recurrent nature, you may have to consider child abuse

Nutritional status

Comment on the nutritional status of the child and ask to plot their growth parameters on a growth chart—a child who is clammy, tachypnoeic, pale, and/or failing to thrive may be in heart failure.

Cyanosis

The presence or absence of cyanosis will help to determine the type of congenital heart defect (see Table 14.10). If the defect allows a right-to-left shunt then the blood flow will bypass the lungs preventing oxygenation (and hence cyanosis).

Examine the pulses

In infants, feel for the brachial pulse. In older children feel the radial pulse. Examine left and right pulses simultaneously to determine if there is any delay which would be suggestive of coarctation of the aorta. Assess the rate, character, and rhythm of the pulse.

Blood pressure

Measure the child's blood pressure using an appropriately sized cuff. Any paediatric ward or clinic should have a range of cuff sizes available. Choose a cuff that covers about two-thirds of the upper arm.

Capillary refill time

Assess the child's capillary refill time by pressing on the sternum for 5 seconds with a finger or thumb, and noting the time needed for the colour to return once the pressure is released. The normal capillary refill time is 2 seconds or less.

Jugular venous pressure

You will be accustomed to looking at the jugular venous pressure (JVP) in adults, but this is rarely done in children.

Carotid pulse character

Check the carotid pulse.

Table 14.6 Causes of unconjugated and conjugated hyperbilirubinaemia in children and infants with jaundice

Unconjugated hyperbilirubinaemia	Conjugated hyperbilirubinaemia
Breast milk jaundice	Chromosomal (e.g. trisomy 21)
Physiological	Endocrine (e.g. hypothyroidism)

Haemolytic disease:
    Rhesus incompatibility
    ABO incompatibility
    Glucose-6-phosphate dehydrogenase deficiency
    Haemoglobinopathy (e.g. sickle cell/thalassaemia)
    Sepsis
    Microangiopathy (e.g. haemolytic-uraemic syndrome)
	Infections:
	    Bacterial, e.g. septicaemia/UTI
	    Viral, e.g. hepatitis A, hepatitis B, cytomegalovirus
	    Parasitic, e.g. malaria

Drugs	Drugs
Polycythaemia (raised red cell count)	Metabolic e.g. galactosaemia
Endocrine e.g. hypothyroidism	Genetic (e.g. cystic fibrosis, Alagille syndrome)
Genetic (e.g. cystic fibrosis)	Parental nutrition
Hereditary: Gilbert disease	

Table 14.7 Worrying features of enlarged lymph nodes

Rapid and progressive enlargement of the node(s)
Fixed to underlying tissues
Larger than 3 cm
Ulceration of the skin
Onset in the neonatal period
Inflammatory mass >3 cm present for >6 weeks despite treatment

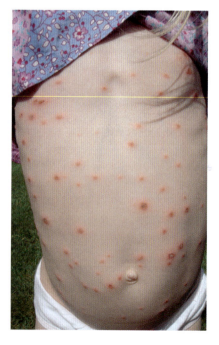

Figure 14.4 Chickenpox.

Examine the chest

Look for any scars which may suggest previous cardiac surgery. Feel for the apex beat, noting the position and character of the impulse. In children this is normally in the fourth intercostal space, midclavicular line. Ascertain whether there is dextrocardia. Feel for heaves over the sternum (an indicator of pulmonary hypertension) and thrills over the praecordium.

Auscultation

- Listen in all four areas (aortic, pulmonary, mitral, and tricuspid).

- Comment on whether both first and second heart sounds are present and whether a murmur is audible. If present comment on whether it is systolic or

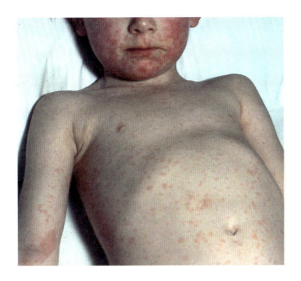

Figure 14.5 Measles.

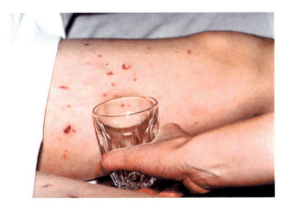

Figure 14.6 Child with a non-blanching rash—the 'glass test' demonstrated.

Table 14.8 Causes of a non-blanching rash in children

Infection: meningococcal disease, other bacterial sepsis, viral illness

Trauma/mechanical/idiopathic thrombocytopenic purpura

Henoch–Schönlein purpura

Acute leukaemia

Haemolytic-uraemic syndrome

(a)   (b)

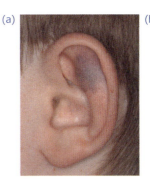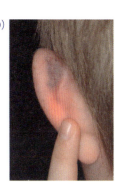

Figure 14.7 (a) and (b) A bruised pinna due to child abuse. Reproduced from Welbury R, Duggal M, Hosey MT, *Paediatric Dentistry*, 4th edn, 2012, with permission from Oxford University Press.

CASE 14.3

Problem: I am very worried that when examining a child I will make a mistake in describing a bruise as suspicious when in fact it is not or vice versa.

Discussion: This is a worry for even the most experienced paediatrician, so you are in good company. Indeed, it is a very contentious issue. It has been shown that there is no characteristic way a bruise evolves so it is not possible to say that a particular colour of bruise is more likely to make it suspicious or accidental. One of the most important clues particularly in an infant or young child is whether there is a definite plausible cause for the bruise—this can be elicited from the history. If this is not the case then suspicions may be raised. Think about the location of the bruise—is it in an unusual place such as on the ear or on non-bony areas? (see 'Paediatric diseases and investigations' section and Fig. 14.28) Also think about the developmental age of the child. For example, a 2-month-old baby is not mobile and is thus unlikely to have sustained a bruise from falling. The most important thing to remember is to report your findings to a senior member of the medical team and do not confront parents as this will definitely get you into trouble!

diastolic, the site of maximal intensity, whether it radiates; attempt murmur-enhancing moves and then comment on the grade of the murmur (see cardiovascular system examination for adults in Chapter 4).

- Murmurs are relatively common in children but the majority are innocent murmurs. For a murmur to be

Table 14.9 Syndromes in congenital heart disease

Common syndromes	Cardiac condition
Trisomy 21 (Down's syndrome)	AVSD, VSD
Trisomy 13 (Patau's syndrome)	VSD, double outlet right ventricle
Trisomy 18 (Edward's syndrome)	VSD, double outlet right ventricle
Turner's syndrome	Coarctation of the aorta
DiGeorge syndrome	Tetralogy of Fallot
	Familial VSD
	Interrupted aortic arch
	Conotruncal anomalies
	Common arterial trunk
William's syndrome	Aortic stenosis
	Pulmonary artery stenosis
Noonan syndrome	Hypertrophic cardiomyopathy
	Pulmonary valve stenosis

AVSD, arterioventricular septal defect; VSD, ventricular septal defect.

Table 14.10 Cyanotic and non-cyanotic heart conditions

Cyanotic heart conditions	Non-cyanotic heart conditions
Tetralogy of Fallot	Ventricular septal defect
Transposition of the great arteries	Atrial septal defect
	Patent ductus arteriosus
	Pulmonary stenosis
	Coarctation of the aorta
	Aortic stenosis

Table 14.11 Congenital cardiac abnormalities and their associated murmurs

Cardiac condition	Associated murmur
Ventricular septal defect	Harsh pansystolic murmur at the lower left sternal border
Atrial septal defect	Systolic murmur at the upper left sternal edge with fixed splitting of the second heart sound
Pulmonary stenosis	Ejection systolic murmur in the pulmonary area
Aortic stenosis	Ejection systolic murmur in the aortic area
Persistent ductus arteriosus	Continuous or systolic murmur at the left infraclavicular area. Also radiates to back between scapulae

classified as innocent it must have the following characteristics (remember the 5 Ss); **s**oft, **s**ystolic, **s**hort (never pansystolic), a**s**ymptomatic, heard at the left **s**ternal edge. Innocent murmurs have a musical quality; they do not radiate and vary with the child's posture and position. Innocent murmurs have no clinical significance and the heart is structurally normal. Some of the other types of murmurs associated with structural abnormalities are detailed in Table 14.11.

- Auscultate posteriorly to detect any murmurs which may radiate to the back (e.g. persistent ductus arteriosus).

- Listen to the lung bases for signs of pulmonary oedema and feel for hepatomegaly. Note that peripheral oedema is rarely seen in children with heart failure.

- To complete the examination it is necessary to feel the femoral pulses because if the femoral pulses are weak or absent this may suggest coarctation of the aorta. For a school-age child and in an examination setting always ask before proceeding as this part of the examination may be considered inappropriate.

Tip

Heaves are felt for in the same way as in adults. You will usually need to apply a little less pressure and use only the heel of your hand in a small child.

Table 14.12 Signs of respiratory distress in children

Sign	Comments
Subcostal recession	Indrawing under the costal margin
Intercostal recession	Indrawing between the ribs
Tracheal tug	Inward and downward pull of trachea
Grunting	An expiratory sound made by infants as they exhale against a closed glottis. This provides increased PEEP and keeps their lower airways open
Nasal flare	The nasal alae are seen to flare indicting that there is increased work of breathing
Head bobbing	Use of scaleni and sternocleidomastoid muscles to assist ventilation

PEEP, positive end-expiratory pressure.

10 Examine the respiratory system

The factors contributing to respiratory distress in children are diverse and different from those in adults. The rib cage is cartilaginous, thus making it more compliant, which is why children can show marked signs of respiratory distress (see Table 14.12 and Case 14.4). The ribs are also perpendicular to the spinal column and so there is less of the 'bucket handle' motion of the ribs during respiration; in addition, the intercostal muscles and accessory muscles of ventilation are immature.

When tasked with examining a baby or toddler it is hard to complete all the elements of the respiratory exam. Below is a suggested approach to the younger, less compliant child.

- **Observation**. Comment on any dysmorphic features, supplementary oxygen, cyanosis, abnormal breathing noises (grunting/stridor/wheeze), clubbing, respiratory rate, signs of respiratory distress (see Table 14.12), chest expansion, nutritional status, anaemia, and any scars.
- **Auscultation** (do this early before they cry!). Listen in the same areas as you would for an adult.

CASE 14.4

Problem: I find it difficult when performing a respiratory exam on a young child to describe different types of recession.

Discussion: Recession is a clinical sign of respiratory distress which occurs as increasingly negative intrathoracic pressures cause indrawing of part of the chest. This is different to adults due to the compliant nature of a young child's chest. Usually children under 2 years have a 'softer' rib cage and so when negative pressure is exerted you can see the whole chest move! In sternal recession you can see whole or part of the sternum being 'sucked' in; it is a sign of significant respiratory distress. Subcostal recession is indrawing under the rib cage (under the costal margin). Adults and older children will use their accessory muscles and may demonstrate intercostal recession (indrawing between the ribs), their rib cages are more 'bony' and less 'flexible'.

- **Palpation**.
  - Palpate the apex beat—dextrocardia and primary ciliary dyskinesia are associated with the condition Kartagener's (see 'Kartagener's syndrome' in 'Paediatric diseases and investigations' section).
  - Palpate the trachea.
- **Percussion**. This is not always done in very small children as it is often not very helpful and can distress the child.
- **Examine the liver**. The liver is pushed down with hyperexpanded lungs.
- **ENT examination**. Always do last as it causes the most distress.

In older children the more conventional adult approach can be used but with some important emphases:

- Inspect the child's chest for any chest wall abnormalities such as pectus excavatum and pectus carinatum (Fig. 14.8), barrel chest, or Harrison's sulcus (see Table 14.13 and Case 14.4).
- Look for signs of eczema as children with asthma often have other atopies such as eczema/hay fever.
- Tactile vocal resonance is infrequently performed in children of all ages.

- Percussion of the chest is of little value in infants.
- Peak flow measurements are only of use in a child of approximately 5 years or older (some younger children may grasp the technique so it may be worth a try).

....

Tip
Always talk through your examination with the child and warn them before doing any uncomfortable procedure such as feeling for the trachea.

....

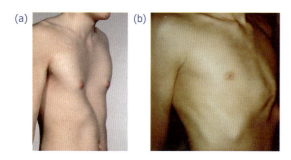

Figure 14.8 Chest abnormalities: (a) pectus excavatum; (b) pectus carinatum.

Cases 14.5 and 14.6 explore some of the difficulties you might have in examining the respiratory system of a child.

11 Examine the abdominal system

The examination of the abdomen is similar to that of an adult with some important emphases:

- Do they have a nasogastric tube, intravenous cannula, or gastrostomy in situ?
- Nutritional status—plot the child's growth on a growth chart. If there are major concerns regarding malnutrition it is advisable to measure the child's mid upper arm circumference (MUAC). This should be at least 14 cm in children aged between 6 months and 5 years.
- Look for signs of peripheral oedema as this may be a feature of nephrotic syndrome (see 'Paediatric disease and investigations' section).
- Inspect the child's buttocks; if they are wasted, this may be a feature of coeliac disease (see 'Paediatric disease and investigations' section).
- Look for any signs of dehydration. The indicators of dehydration are listed in Table 14.14.
- Observe the abdomen for any scars of previous operations.

Table 14.13 Chest wall deformities

Name	Type	Comments
Pectus excavatum	Congenital	Commonest congenital chest wall deformity A depression in the lower anterior chest due to abnormal growth of lower ribs and sternum. Usually noticed at birth but can worsen in adolescence. Usually asymptomatic. May be related to Marfan's syndrome
Pectus carinatum	Congenital	Second commonest congenital chest wall deformity A protrusion of the chest wall. Usually asymptomatic and presents in adolescence
Harrison sulci	Acquired	A fixed groove under the rib cage at the insertion of the diaphragm. Children who have severe asthma especially when their rib cage is at its most compliant (<2 yrs) may develop Harrison sulcis. It is thought to be due to longstanding strain on the diaphragm due to increased work of breathing leading to a fixed deformity. It may also be present in rickets: a lack of mineralized calcium in bones causes the diaphragm to pull the softened bone inward
Barrel shaped	Acquired	An increased anterior-posterior diameter is seen which looks 'barrel' shaped. This suggests air trapping caused by chronic lung disease such as asthma or cystic fibrosis

CASE 14.5

Problem. When I am doing respiratory examination on children I find it difficult to know when to diagnose a child with bronchiolitis or a bacterial pneumonia.

Discussion. This can be difficult, particularly in an infant, as both can present with pyrexia and on examination tachypnoea and crepitations may be present. A child with pneumonia will have focal signs including localized crackles and reduced air entry over the affected area and a high-grade temperature. A child with bronchiolitis will have wheeze and crackles throughout the chest and typically has a low-grade temperature (<38 °C).

- Check for abdominal distension. The causes of abdominal distension are the 5 Fs; **f**at, **f**latus, **f**luid, **f**aeces, or **f**etus (always possible after puberty). Constipation is one of the most common causes of abdominal distension in children.

- Before palpating, stop and establish whether the child is in any discomfort. If they have pain ask them where it hurts and examine this area last and cautiously.

- For palpation of the abdomen you ideally want the child lying on their back and flat, but this may not be possible. Often it is necessary to feel the abdomen with the child lying across the parent's lap. Start by examining lightly in the nine areas that you are accustomed to in adults. Then, if there is no discomfort, progress to deeper palpation. You are assessing for any signs of guarding, rebound tenderness or percussion tenderness which are signs of peritonitis. Then palpate and auscultate for a liver and spleen.

Tip
When palpating the abdomen get down to the child's level to avoid exerting too much pressure on the abdomen.

- In newborns and infants it is normal to be able to feel a liver edge 1 cm below the costal margin.

- It is important to start palpation as low down as possible in the right iliac fossa to avoid missing substantial organomegaly.

CASE 14.6

Problem. I am confident at hearing wheeze in a child on auscultation. However, I am not sure when to diagnose asthma or when it should be diagnosed as viral-induced wheeze.

Discussion. It is important to consider the history in detail. Usually a child is not considered to have asthma until they are at least 1 year old, as when a child is less than 1 year old they are likely to have episodes of wheeze only related to colds and less likely to respond to management with bronchodilators. A younger preschool child may have a triggering factor of a viral upper respiratory tract infection (i.e. a cold) which would make you consider viral wheeze. Some of these children will grow out of these types of symptoms. If a child has recurrent and interval symptoms (e.g. cough at night), a personal or family history of atopy, and triggers other than colds such as exercise, exposure to pets, damp, and pollen, then asthma is a more likely diagnosis. These children will be more likely to respond to bronchodilators. Further information can be obtained from the British Thoracic Society guidelines on asthma.

Table 14.14 Signs of dehydration in children

Mild (5%)	Moderate (5–10%)	Severe (>10%)
Dry mouth and lips	Dry mouth and lips	Dry mouth and lips
Normal urine output	Reduced urine output	No urine output >12 h
Alert	Lethargic	Decreased GCS
Fontanelle normal	Fontanelle sunken	Fontanelle very sunken
Skin turgor normal	Skin turgor reduced	Skin turgor very reduced
Pulse normal	Tachycardia	Tachycardia
Normotensive	Normotensive	Hypotensive
Capillary refill <2 seconds	Capillary refill 2–3 seconds	Capillary refill >3 seconds

- Palpate for the kidneys using the balloting technique previously learnt. If the kidneys are palpable then they are likely to be enlarged. Loin tenderness might indicate underlying pyelonephritis and needs further evaluation with urinalysis.

- Finally, check the groin for any hernias—older children can find this embarrassing so always ask before proceeding or if in an exam check with the examiner first.

- To complete your examination you would normally want to perform a rectal examination. However, rectal examinations are rarely performed in children and should *only* be done by an experienced paediatrician or surgeon. The examination should include external inspection of the anus to look for any fissures or dilatation which may be a feature of constipation or sexual abuse.

- On completion of the abdominal system examination, inspect the child's urine and stool.

11 *Examine the genitourinary system*

In preschool children check boys for undescended testes, hydrocoeles, and hernias. In girls inspect the external genitalia if they complain of urinary symptoms because they may have vulvovaginitis (inflammation or infection of the vulva and vagina). This can be caused by inadequate hygiene in prepubertal girls.

Urinary tract infections (UTIs) are common in children and if untreated are associated with renal scarring in young children. The symptoms in infants and young children are often non-specific, making a diagnosis difficult. Any child presenting with a fever should have their urine tested. All children under the age of 6 months with a proven UTI will need some form of imaging. This will normally be an abdominal ultrasound scan 6 weeks after the infection has been treated; however, further investigations may be required. In older children, if the UTI is caused by an atypical organism or is recurrent, then other investigations such as a DMSA (dimercaptosuccinic acid) or MCUG (micturating cystourethrogram) scan may be warranted.

12 *Examine the musculoskeletal system*

The best approach to assessing the musculoskeletal system in children is to use pGALS (Table 14.15). pGALS

Table 14.15 A brief summary of the pGALS assessment tool

	Manoeuvres	Assessment
Gait	Observe the child standing and then watch them walk Get the child to walk on their heels and tiptoes	Look at their posture and habitus, look at their skin, and look for any deformity Look at the foot posture and the child's feet and ankles
Arms	Observe the child's hands held out in front and then get them to turn them over and make a fist Touch the tips of each of the fingers Squeeze the MCP joints Assess the hands pressed together, palm to palm and back to back Reach up and touch the sky and look at the ceiling Put the hands behind their head Ask the child to open their mouth wide and try to put 3 of their fingers in their mouth	Look for any muscle wasting to the hands, forearm, or upper arm Look for any swelling over the joints Assess the range of movement of the wrists, elbow, and shoulder joints Assess for any pain on movement Look for any restriction in manual dexterity
Legs	Feel for any effusions in the knee Active movement of the knees Passive movement of the hips	Look for any muscle wasting to the thigh or calves Look for any swelling over the joints Assess the range of movement of the knees and hips Assess for any pain on movement
Spine	Try to get the child to touch their shoulder with their ear Ask the child to bend down and touch their toes	Range of movement of the neck Range of movement of the thoracolumbar spine Assess for any signs of a scoliosis

stands for paediatric gait, arms, legs and spine; it is a screening tool designed for school-age children, based on the adult version. If an abnormality is detected further evaluation of that joint is required. The full version can be accessed from the arthritis research campaign website **http://www.arthritisresearchuk.org/**. At an undergraduate level this tool should be sufficient in any examination setting. The sequence of pGALS is essentially the same as that in adults but with some additional assessments for the feet, ankles, wrists, neck, and temporomandibular joints.

Tips

- Young children have difficulty localizing or describing pain.
- Rather than vocalizing pain, children may present with a change in behaviour, decreased sleeping, or a regression in their attainment of developmental milestones.

13 Examine the nervous system

It may seem a daunting task to examine a toddler's or infant's neurology as they will not be able to comprehend or respond to the usual commands. It is within this system that your observation skills will be crucial. The components of paediatric neurological examination are the same as in the adult (tone, power, reflexes, sensation, coordination, and cranial nerves) but cannot be done in the same manner in younger children because of their variable cooperation. Your approach to assessing a 10-year-old's neurology will be quite different to that for a 1-year-old, which is why this section has been divided into two parts following the assessment of conscious level.

Assess the child's conscious level

As in adults, it is important to carry out a rapid neurological assessment in an unwell child. This is part of the ABCDE approach and should be done formally to avoid unhelpful terms such as 'comatosed' or 'unrousable' which will be interpreted differently by different clinicians.

The AVPU scale is an easy and quick method of assessing consciousness.

- A–**A**lert
- V–Responds to **V**oice
- P–Responds to **P**ain
- U–**U**nresponsive to all stimuli

Explain to the parent/child what you are going to do. If the child is awake they are A (Alert). If the child is not awake, check for responsiveness to voice by talking to them. V (Responds to **V**oice) can be documented if they open their eyes, move, cry, speak (or behave appropriately if non-verbal—e.g. cry, babble). Response to a painful stimulus should be assessed if there is no response to voice. Pain should be produced by pressing firmly on the supraorbital notch (beneath medial end of eyebrow) with your thumb (see Table 14.16). Finally if there is no response at all the child is U (Unresponsive) and appropriate emergency steps need to be taken to manage the child.

The Glasgow Coma Scale (GCS) is more detailed and takes a little longer than the AVPU. It may be done after a first assessment with the AVPU scale. GCS was initially devised as a scale for head injuries. A total score should be given with the component subscores to give an indication of the level of consciousness (see Case 3.12 in Chapter 3). For children under the age of 5 there is a modified scale (see Table 14.16). For those over 5 the adult score can be used.

- Pain should be produced by pressing firmly on the supraorbital notch (beneath medial end of eyebrow) with your thumb, except for M4, which is tested by pressing hard on the flat nail surface with the barrel of a pencil.
- If signs are asymmetrical, score the best response.
- If in doubt repeat after 5 minutes and ask for help.
- Score as usual in the presence of sedative drugs.

Plot over time on an appropriate chart to assess changes in GCS

Examination of the baby or preschool child

Take time to observe the child while dressed and playing. This should provide a basic understanding of whether the child has any significant neurological abnormality. Developmental skills will provide important neurological clues. Visual inspection is the most useful part of the examination so avoid upsetting the child by doing procedures that will yield less information (e.g. examining reflexes on a crying child). Muscle wasting, gait, and coordination can be assessed by watching a child play.

Pay particular attention to the following:

Overall size and proportions of the child

Does the child's head seem disproportionately large compared to the body, which may represent hydrocephalus?

Table 14.16 Child's Glasgow Coma Scale

	>5 years	<5 years
Eye opening		
E4	Spontaneous	
E3	To voice	
E2	To pain	
E1	None	
C	Eyes closed (by swelling or bandage)	
Verbal		
V5	Orientated (in person or place or address)	Alert, babbles, coos, words or sentences to usual ability (normal)
V4	Confused	Less than usual ability, irritable cry
V3	Inappropriate words	Cries to pain
V2	Incomprehensible sounds	Moans to pain
V1	No response to pain	
T	Intubated	
Motor		
M6	Obeys commands	Normal spontaneous movements
M5	Localizes to supraorbital pain (>9 months of age) or withdraws to touch	
M4	Withdraws from nailbed pain	
M3	Flexion to supraorbital pain (decorticate)	
M2	Extension to supraorbital pain (decerebrate)	
M1	No response to supraorbital pain (flaccid)	

Measure the head circumference and plot the value on a growth chart.

Dysmorphic features

Does the child have a syndrome which is associated with neurodisability? Is there any drooping of the mouth or an expressionless face, which may be a feature of a myopathy (e.g. myotonic dystrophy)?

Head

Note the head shape, cranial sutures, fontanelle, and head circumference. If the child has had raised intracranial pressure in the past then they may have a ventricular reservoir or ventriculoperitoneal shunt.

Eyes

Observe the child's eye movements. If there are roving movements then the child may be blind. Is there nystagmus or a squint?

Movement

Is there evidence of marked wasting of any of the limbs? Is the child using one hand more than the other? Developing hand preference below the age of 18 months is a feature of cerebral palsy. If there is scissoring of the legs then this may be a feature of a spastic diplegia. Is the child able to walk or run? In addition, observe the child's coordination.

Limbs and spine

Next, undress the baby to the nappy and inspect the child's limbs for signs of deformity and muscle bulk. Look at the child's back to assess for any signs of spina bifida (abnormal tufts of hair, pits or swellings) or corrective surgery. See Case 14.7.

Tone

- Tone can be assessed by picking up a child; this is easier and more useful in an infant who has less 'stranger

CASE 14.7

Problem: What are the clinical features of spina bifida?

Discussion: Spina bifida is an example of a lower motor neurone lesion. Like spastic cerebral palsy, power will be decreased. Unlike cerebral palsy, tone will be decreased and reflexes will also be diminished or absent and there is no clonus. There may also be bladder and bowel disturbance. It is important to look for signs of hydrocephalus as this can be associated with spina bifida.

awareness'. If the child feels as if they are 'slipping through your hands' this may be an indication of poor tone.

- Scissoring of the legs is a sign that there is spasticity at the hip abductors (tested by abducting the hips) and toe pointing indicates spasticity at the plantar flexors (tested by dorsiflexing the foot).
- Head control and tone can be assessed when a child is lying prone—can they lift their head off the couch?
- Head and trunk control can be assessed by putting the child in a sitting position.
- A younger infant can be pulled into a sitting position and an older infant may be able to sit with or without support.
- Assessment of the older infant or toddler on a parent/carer's lap is appropriate, and provided the child is settled and relaxed it should be possible to move the limbs to assess limb tone which may be reduced or increased.
- It is important to attempt to assess for clonus. This is done in the same manner as an adult but with a gentler stretching force. Changes in tone may indicate cerebral palsy (see Case 14.8).

Power

- Formal power testing will not be possible in the younger age group.
- Observation of gross motor skills will provide signs of whether power is affected. In the younger infant vigorous kicking and antigravity movements are likely to indicate normal power.
- Putting the child in a standing position and assessing lower limb power can be helpful. In the older infant and toddler, sitting, crawling, and walking can be observed.
- Note any asymmetrical movement, for example, a child with a unilateral cerebral palsy (hemiplegia).

Table 14.17 Result of increase tone or contracture at various joints (and bulbar muscles)

Joint	Result
Ankle	Plantar flexion Varus/valgus deformity of foot
Knee	Flexion
Hip	Flexion Limited adduction Internal rotation
Wrist	Flexion Pronation
Elbow	Flexion
Shoulder	Adduction
Bulbar muscles	Dysphagia Drooling—inability to swallow secretions Possible unsafe swallow

CASE 14.8

Problem: I find it difficult to understand what clinical features to look for in a child with cerebral palsy.

Discussion: Cerebral palsy is an umbrella term for a non-progressive insult to the developing brain (80% antenatal, 10% perinatal and 10% postnatal) resulting in motor problems. It is an upper motor neuron lesion; There will be evidence of reduced power, increased tone, and brisk reflexes. In a child with early motor delay it is important to think of cerebral palsy. An infant may initially be very hypotonic and then develop hypertonia and spasticity. Clonus may be elicited. If hypertonia is present it is important to assess if a joint can be actively or passively placed in a normal position, if this is not possible the child may have a fixed deformity (Table 14.17). Cerebral palsy is usually spastic (unilateral or bilateral); older terminology includes hemiplegia, diplegia, and quadriplegia (see Table 14.18). Cerebral palsy may also be ataxic (7%), dyskinetic (4%), or mixed (4%).

Table 14.18 Cerebral palsy terminology

Affected side	Old terms	New terms
One side— right or left	Hemiplegia	Unilateral
Both sides	Diplegia	Bilateral A description of pattern can also be given, e.g. lower limbs affected > upper limbs
	Quadriplegia	Bilateral A description of pattern can also be given, e.g. lower limbs affected equally to upper limbs

Sensation and proprioception examination

- Formal examination of sensation and proprioception is also not possible in a preschool child.

- Some idea as to whether sensation is intact can be obtained from the history and observing how a child responds to light touch, for example, tickling.

- In an older child sensory examination can be done more formally but it is important not to cause pain. If a painful procedure (e.g. venepuncture) is required as part of the investigation of a child, the response to this can add to the assessment.

Reflexes

- The same principles for eliciting reflexes in adults can be applied provided the child is relaxed.

- Putting 1–2 fingers on the tendon (particularly for upper limbs) and tapping your own fingers with the tendon hammer will limit any pain felt by the child and should elicit the reflex.

- An extensor plantar response will be present until approximately 8 months of age.

- Also assess the primitive reflexes as outlined under the newborn check.

- Protective reflexes (Table 14.19) develop as primitive reflexes are disappearing.

Table 14.19 Protective reflexes

Age	Reflex	Description
4–5 months	Downwards parachute	When held above floor and quickly lowered as if falling upright, child will extend and abduct both legs
6–7 months	Sidewards protective	If child sitting and is tipped off balance will put arm out to other side to counterbalance
8–9 months	Forwards protective	If child falls forwards will extend arms forwards
9–10 months	Backwards protective	If child pushed backwards in sitting position both arms extend to prevent falling

- If primitive reflexes persist this may indicate emerging neurological disorder such as cerebral palsy and may prevent protective reflex development.

Coordination

- Coordination can be examined by assessing and observing fine motor skills, for example, when playing with toys or drawing.

- There may be evidence of tremor or ataxia. In a child older than 2 years, finger–nose and heel–shin manoeuvres can be tried.

- A 3-year-old should be able to stand on one leg momentarily.

Tip

Neurological examination in the infant and young preschool child is mainly based on observation.

Cranial nerve examination

- Assessment of cranial nerves II–IV and VI is also primarily based on observation.

- Look for any asymmetry of the face which provides gross information about cranial nerve involvement (predominantly VII).

- Try to get the baby to follow a toy. Cranial nerve VII again can be assessed by observing the child when they smile or cry as a facial palsy may become apparent.

- Cranial nerve VIII will need to be assessed more formally, as explained in step 14.

- Cranial nerves IX, X, and XII can be assessed by observing the child's suck and swallow.

- Sometimes a toddler may stick out their tongue on command, enabling you to assess cranial nerve XII.

Examination of the preschool and school-age child

In this age group you can attempt to perform a similar examination to that in an adult. The key is to make the examination fun and to reward the child with plenty of praise and encouragement. The basic principles of assessing tone, power, coordination, reflexes, and sensation in adults still apply to children. Revise this by referring to the relevant chapters in this book. Also examine for signs of meningitis in the same way by assessing for photophobia and looking for Kernig's sign, etc. (see Case 14.9 and Fig. 6.82).

CASE 14.9

Problem: How can I examine a baby for meningitis?

Discussion: It is important to realize that it is often hard to recognize a neurological disorder in very young children and babies as they do not present in the classical way. For instance, a 4-month-old baby with meningitis is unable to tell you that they have a headache or photophobia and you won't be able to assess for Kernig's sign. Therefore you have to rely on your clinical acumen and listen to what the parents are saying. If the parent is telling you that their child is irritable, hard to console, and prefers to be left alone rather than being cuddled then this is a sign of meningeal irritation and the child could easily have meningitis. Often clinically the only signs are that the child has a high-pitched cry, is irritable, and may have increased tone. If such signs and symptoms are present, especially with a fever, then a full septic screen including a lumbar puncture is necessary.

There are differences from the adult investigation, and some useful tips are as follows:

- At the beginning of the examination examine the back and observe the child's gait. When asking the child to do certain manoeuvres, ensure that the task is age appropriate.

- When assessing the gait assess for stiffness as this may suggest an upper motor neuron lesion. If the child has a broad-based gait this may imply cerebellar pathology. A waddling gait may indicate a form of muscular dystrophy such as Duchenne's muscular dystrophy (DMD).

- If your examination is suggestive of DMD then ask the child to lie on his back on the floor and then ask him to attempt to stand up. A child with DMD will roll onto his front, assume the prayer position, and then walk up his legs with his hands due to a proximal weakness. This is referred to as Gower's sign (Fig. 14.9).

- Some of the commands for assessing power are often quite difficult for children to understand, so it is necessary to adapt them so that they are more familiar and child-friendly. For example when assessing the child's power in C5 (shoulder abduction) and C6–8 (shoulder adduction) ask the child to 'flap like a chicken'. If necessary show them what you want them to do.

Cerebellar examination

Assess for signs of cerebellar pathology as it is common for CNS tumours to manifest with cerebellar signs. Use the techniques you would use for adults. The signs of a

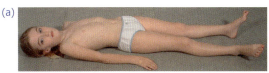
(a)

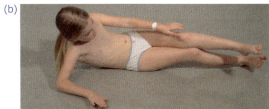
(b)

(c) 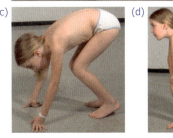   (d)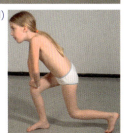

Figure 14.9 Gower's sign.

cerebellar lesion are easily remembered using the mnemonic 'DANISH':

- **D**ysdiadochokinesia
- **A**taxia
- **N**ystagmus
- **I**ntention tremor
- **S**taccato or slurred speech
- **H**ypotonia

Cranial nerve examination

Cranial nerve examination is time consuming. It should be done in full if clinically indicated. The examination needs to be adapted according to age and development of the child. See Table 14.20.

Tip

When performing fundoscopy ask the child to look at a picture in front of them and then ask them about it. Turn the room lights off if the child will let you.

14 Assess development of the child

Child development is a dynamic process. Organized neurological progression and interaction with the

Table 14.20 Summary of cranial nerve examination

Cranial nerve	Function	How to assess
Olfactory (I)	Sense of smell	Ask if they have had any change in their sense of smell or taste
Optic nerve (II)	Visual acuity, visual fields, colour vision, pupillary light and accommodation reflex (sensory part)	Check visual acuity using a Snellen chart, assess visual fields, colour vision using Ishiara plates, pupillary light and accommodation reflexes and fundoscopy
Oculomotor nerve (III)	Eye movements and pupillary light and accommodation reflex (motor part)	Inspect for ptosis and a squint. Check for nystagmus and ask about diplopia
Trochlear nerve (IV)	Eye movements	Inspect for ptosis and a squint. Check for nystagmus and ask about diplopia
Trigeminal nerve (V)	Facial sensation, muscles of mastication, and corneal reflex (sensory part) (rarely performed in children)	Test facial sensation over all 3 sensory divisions. Ask the child to grit their teeth and feel the masseters
Abducens nerve (VI)	Eye movements	Inspect for ptosis and a squint. Check for nystagmus and ask about diplopia
Facial nerve (VII)	Facial muscles, taste to anterior 2/3 of the tongue and corneal reflex (motor part)[a]	Ask the child to screw their eyes tight, blow out their cheeks and show their teeth
Vestibulocochlear nerve (VIII)	Hearing and balance	Weber's and Rinné's tests
Glossopharyngeal nerve (IX)	Sensation of palate and pharynx and gag reflex (sensory part)[a]	Get the child to open their mouth and say 'aaah'
Vagus nerve (X)	Palatal and pharyngeal muscles and the gag reflex (motor part)[a]	Get the child to open their mouth and say 'aaah'
Accessory nerve (XI)	Sternomastoid and trapezius muscles	Ask the child to shrug their shoulders and then ask them to stop you pressing down. Then get the patient to turn their head to the right and then left, each time ask them to stop you pushing their head back into the middle
Hypoglossal nerve (XII)	Motor supply of the tongue	Ask the child to open their mouth and look at their tongue for any wasting or fasciculations. Then ask them to put their tongue out and wiggle it from side to side

[a] Note that the gag reflex and corneal reflex are very rarely performed in children and should not be conducted unless specifically asked to do so.

surrounding environment enable a child to become independent over a relatively short space of time; an immobile non-verbal infant will develop into a walking communicating child.

Any insult to the developing brain (ante-, peri-, or postnatal) can result in significant developmental and neurological consequences. Other causes of developmental delay may be genetic or congenital (Table 14.21).

Developmental delay may be global, affecting all domains of development, or may be isolated to one or two specific modalities: for example, autism affects language and communication skills. There is an array of

Table 14.21 Causes of global developmental delay

Antenatal	Antepartum haemorrhage
	Maternal infection (e.g. influenza)
	Congenital infection
	Drugs: prescription and recreational
	Alcohol exposure
Perinatal	Hypoxic insult (e.g. birth asphyxia)
	Infection (e.g. group B streptococcus)
Postnatal	Prematurity complications (e.g. intraventricular haemorrhage)
	Infection (e.g. meningitis)
	Metabolic (e.g. hypoglycaemia; hyperbilirubinaemia)
Genetic	Chromosomal (e.g. trisomy 21, fragile X)
	Duchenne muscular dystrophy
	Phenylketonuria

confusing terminology in this area; significant global delay in the preschool child will almost invariably result in a child who has a **learning disability**. A developmentally normal child may have a **learning difficulty** that is not picked up until the child is at school. Learning disability is defined as an IQ of less than 70; the child will have other difficulties such as social and self-help skills. The onset of disability will be before 18 years of age. Learning difficulty relates to a child's specific educational difficulties such as dyslexia, where IQ is intact. Learning disability and difficulty are not the same but the terms are often used interchangeably; this should be avoided especially when discussing children with their parents. See Case 14.10.

Families of learning-disabled children are likely to have had many hospital visits. Take the time to read the notes of such children so that you are au fait with the child and their condition. There is nothing more upsetting or annoying to a family than having to repeat lots of sensitive information. This has to be balanced with getting the relevant information from the family about the current episode. Seek advice from parents and do not assume you know all the answers; they know their children better than you do. If a parent feels that the child is in pain ask them why they believe this—for example, changes in behaviour, eating habits, bowel habits. Try to tread carefully so as not to cause offence or distress. If in doubt ask a senior colleague.

CASE 14.10

Problem: When seeing children with developmental delay and learning disabilities I am not sure what the best way is to approach them and their families.

Discussion: This can be very challenging. The most important thing is not to assume the child is unable to contribute to the consultation. With an older child you can address the child directly in the same way you would in any other consultation. It may be that their response will be limited; however, it is better to do this than to undermine any ability that the child may have. One big mistake that can be made is in assuming a child in a wheelchair is learning disabled as well as physically disabled. If the child is finding it difficult to respond or is not able to respond, seek permission from the child to ask the parent or carer.

Key points

- Learning disability and learning difficulty are **not** the same
- Learning disability will have impact on IQ whereas a learning difficulty will not
- A learning-disabled child will have the onset of disability before 18 years of age

Students often struggle with developmental examination assessment as there is no equivalent examination in adults. Although assessment of development is often challenging because of the varying cooperation of a young child, it is also rewarding and enjoyable, especially when you succeed in gaining valuable information! The assessment can be divided into four main categories:

Posture and movement

Posture of a child is more important in a young infant and gross (big) movements become more relevant as they get older and begin to harness these skills. Impairment in movement skills may be a sign of a developmental problem such as cerebral palsy.

Fine motor, vision, and manipulation

Fine motor skills include movement and use of the hands. To develop these skills children will need to have adequate vision so it is important to think about these two components together.

Hearing and communication

In order to acquire verbal communication skills there is a recognized ordered process from non-verbal to verbal. Hearing needs to be intact for children to be able to do this in a normal fashion. However, children who have significant hearing impairment can still learn to communicate. Depending on the level of impairment, this can still include some verbal communication.

Social behaviour and play

Development in this area is often subtle to begin with and will start with soft signs of carer recognition and regard and then play skills and social behaviour will become more obvious. It is sometimes forgotten that impairment in this area can be very debilitating.

....
Tip

When reporting back your findings to an examiner divide the areas of development into the four described earlier to ensure a systematic approach. Always give an age range (e.g. 9–12 months) as parents/carers do not like hearing that their child is likely to be 9 months old when in fact they are 12 months!
....

Table 14.22 shows a detailed outline of preschool development. It is helpful to divide developmental milestones into 3 monthly time periods. There are developmental 'red flags' that should raise concern when assessing development in a child (see Table 14.23). In a child with early motor delay it is important to think about cerebral palsy. Combining a developmental examination and a neurological examination will assist in making a diagnosis. Beyond the age of 5 years, normal development is more abstract because children are in the process of becoming adolescents and young adults and mature at different rates. There will be huge variety in skills attainment when compared to younger children; for example, one developmentally normal child may be able to swim where another struggles despite equivalent motor development in both children. Learning and cognitive ability is monitored in school using tests and other educational achievements.

The actual assessment of development should be done in a room with plenty of space and suitable toys—but not too many, as this can be distracting. For the younger child a play mat will be useful. A parent or carer should be present to support the child. A successful assessment hinges on you gaining the child's trust. With a preschool child, particularly above the age of 2 years, it will be easier to engage the child's cooperation as you may be able to use

verbal communication and stimulate their interest in certain activities, for example, building bricks, drawing.

There are formal developmental screening tests such as Denver II, which is widely used and requires training. It is a useful surveillance tool to monitor children at risk for development delays or where there is a suspicion of delay. It contains 125 items which are divided into four areas: gross motor, fine motor/adaptive, personal/social, and language skills. A line is drawn at the child's chronological age and skills that cross the line are tested. It is easy to use and understand and to obtain the test and training materials see the further reading and reference section at the end of the chapter. There are other tests of development (e.g. schedule of growing skills, Griffiths, and Baileys) but these are often more time consuming and are beyond the scope of undergraduate teaching (see also 'References and further reading'). See Case 14.11 for some tips on putting developmental theory into practice.

....
Tip

When assessing fine motor manipulation don't use a very small object as the child may choke. You can use 'hundreds and thousands' if available (with parental permission) or use the end of a pen/pencil with an interesting top such as a small toy or ball. Initially see if they use a palmar grasp to take the pen; then cover the pen shaft and see if they will use a pincer grasp for the toy.
....
Tip

Gross motor skills in an infant can be observed in a '360° manoeuvre' by initially placing the child on their back (you may already find them in this position) and then pulling them up to sit, then placing in a standing position, then putting them on their front, and lastly placing them on their back again. During this manoeuvre you can also put the infant in ventral suspension to assess tone and head control (see Fig. 14.23).
....

15 Assess hearing and vision

Hearing and visual milestones have been outlined in Table 14.21. Part of neurological and developmental history and examination includes some assessment of vision and hearing. This may be obtained from information from a parent or carer but will also include personal observation.

Vision

The most common visual disorder in children is a squint (medical term is strabismus [*stra-biz-mus*]). This can affect

Table 14.22 Developmental milestones in the preschool child

Age (months)	Posture and movement	Fine motor and vision	Hearing, language, and communication	Social behaviour and play
3	Head control when pulled to sit When held in standing bends knees When prone lifts head and chest wall in midline	Brings hands together in midline; reaches out to grasp Hand regard Fixes and follows through 180° and also up and down Defensive blink	Turns head/eyes to sound Settles to sound of recognizable voice Shows enjoyment when spoken to Coos	Looks intently at carer Excited prior to feeds Takes pleasure in routines such as bathtime
6	Sits supported with good head control When put in standing position bounces up and down When prone lifts head and chest wall up and supports on arms Rolls back to front (5–6 months; front to back (6–7 mths)	Uses palmar grasp to grasp objects Transfers objects Interested in toys and objects at 30-cm range using both eyes together	Turns to recognizable voice or sound at ear level Vocalizes vowel sounds eg. a-a, goo Laughs when happy, screams when annoyed	Enjoys physical play Starting to become anxious of strangers Puts hand on bottle/breast when fed Starting to wean
9	Sits unsupported and able to correct position Pulls to stand Rolls or crawls to move	Enjoys exploring and manipulating toys Uses index finger to point at objects Object permanence	Turns to quiet noise Babbles ma-ma, da-da Responds to name Understands no and yes	Stranger awareness Plays peek-a-boo Attempts to take spoon while feeding
12	Crawls Cruises on furniture May walk alone	Mature pincer grasp Puts objects in container Points to objects in the distance Recognizes familiar faces	Knows familiar tunes Imitates adult voices	Waves bye-bye Demonstrates use of object (e.g. hairbrush) Helps with dressing
15	May walk alone Crawls upstairs	Interested in books Scribbles Uses both hands	Says up to 6 words Understands simple instructions	Explores environment Looks to carer for support
18	Walks well Starting to run Walks upstairs holding hand	Turns several pages of book Builds tower of three cubes	6–20 recognizable words Listens Obeys instructions (e.g. 'put coat on') Points to body parts	No sense of danger Plays alone well but needs adult reassurance

(continued)

Table 14.22 (*continued*)

Age (months)	Posture and movement	Fine motor and vision	Hearing, language, and communication	Social behaviour and play
24	Runs Walks up stairs, holding rail, two feet to a step	Holds pencil using thumb and first two fingers Turns pages of book singly Stacks 6–7 cubes	50+ words and short sentences Refers to self by name Asks questions (e.g. names of objects)	Plays alongside other children Tantrums Feeds self well with spoon Attempts to verbalize toilet needs
30	Jumps with two feet off step Throws ball	Recognizes photos of self Hand preference Does inset puzzles	200+ words Short sentences 2–3 words Knows full name	Pretend play, e.g. tea parties/puts dolls to bed Toilet trained
36	Walks up stairs alternate feet Climbs Rides tricycle Throws a ball overhand and catches Kicks ball well	Threads beads Matches colours Cuts with toy scissors	More structured sentences Knows several nursery rhymes Counts 1–10	Imaginative play Fewer tantrums Fondness for siblings Likes helping adults with household jobs
48	Stands on one foot 3–5 seconds Rides tricycle well	Copies cross and letter Builds three steps with cubes Matches and names colours	Grammar correct Knows full name and address	Understands the idea of past, present, and future More independent; knows own mind
60	Hops Walks on narrow line Skips	Throw and catches ball well Draws pictures Colours in pictures neatly	Enjoys jokes Uses newly learnt words correctly	Dresses and undresses alone Uses knife and fork well

Table 14.23 Some red flags in developmental assessment

Parent/carer concern

Regression (i.e. skills that a child gained initially but has now lost)

Motor skills not attained (e.g. poor head control at 4 months; not sitting by 9 months; hand preference before age of 18 months; not walking by 18 months)

Discordant development (i.e. development in one area does not match that in another)

Family history of developmental problems

up to 7% of children and is higher in those with a learning disability. Therefore it is important to be able to examine for a squint. Note that in babies up to 3 months of age an intermittent squint can sometimes be seen as their vision develops and is normal. Students often find squint examination tricky. However, if the exam is performed in a logical organized manner then it will become easier with time.

Squint: what is it?

This is where the eyes fail to work as a functioning pair and their visual axes no longer intersect on the target of gaze. When this occurs the child will either experience diplopia or blurred vision. In young children if this is not corrected the brain will learn to suppress the image from the affected

CASE 14.11

Problem. I have a good theoretical understanding of neurological and development examination in young children. However, I am finding it difficult to put it all into practice.

Discussion. Development assessment is not easy particularly in infants who are developing stranger awareness. Observation is the key and must start from the first time you see the child. Look around the child and see if there any other clues, such as hearing aids, walking aids, glasses, adapted prams, or wheelchairs. You may be able to talk to a parent/carer while watching the child playing. Getting down to the child's eye level also helps. Do not try to examine the child immediately as this will inevitably make them upset. Try to engage a child with an interesting toy; you can involve the parent in this. To begin with, it is better to encourage skills that you think the child will be able to do. Making a child perform something that they cannot do will immediately make the child upset and defensive. Once a developmental assessment is going well, ascertain what skill a child is unable to do. The developmental age for that particularly domain will be between that and the previous skill they were able to do. It is vitally important to continually praise the child as this will encourage them to cooperative further. You may have to ask a parent or carer to help with parts of the assessment and also check with them whether the child is able to do the tasks at home or school, because not all children perform well in front of an audience.

eye and will become irreversible. This is known colloquially as a lazy eye or medically as amblyopia (*am-bli-owe-pia*).

Causes

- Due to refractive errors of the eye (concomitant). This is the commonest cause in childhood.
- Paralysis of the muscles of the eye (known as incomitant). These are rare in children and may be secondary to a cranial nerve palsy, raised intracranial pressure or a feature of a benign syndrome such as Brown's or Duane's.

How to examine

1 **Inspection**. Check for any obvious eye abnormalities or asymmetry. Look for any dysmorphic features. Children with trisomy 21 or those with epicanthic folds and a low

broad nasal bridge can give the impression of a squint (called a pseudosquint). If a squint is obvious on your initial observation this is known as a manifest squint or heterotropia (*het-er-owe-troe-pia*). If the affected eye is turned medially towards the nose this is known as a convergent squint or esotropia (*ee-so-tr-owe-pia*). If the eye is turned laterally away from the nose it is known as a divergent squint (exotropia). More rarely the eye can turn upwards (hypertropia) or downwards (hypotropia).

2 **Corneal light reflection**. If you suspect a squint but are not too sure, observing the corneal light reflection may give an additional clue. Using a torch, shine the light centrally onto the nasal bridge and ask the child to look at the light. The light reflection should be seen approximately in the middle of each pupil. If there is any asymmetry a squint is likely to be present.

3 **Cover test**. The cover test is a more dynamic way of demonstrating or uncovering a squint. It can be performed in one of two ways:

- the unilateral cover test (cover/uncover test); testing for a manifest squint
- the alternating cover test.

- **Unilateral cover test (cover/uncover test)**. This is used to test for a manifest squint. It is performed by asking the child to fix on an object/picture. For a successful assessment this needs to be a suitably interesting picture and can usually be performed on a child from the age of 2. When the good eye is covered with an occluder or a hand (allow at least 5 seconds) the affected eye takes up fixation of an object (so long as there is no paralysis of the ocular muscles, i.e. an incomitant squint). This demonstrates a manifest squint. If the eye moves out laterally to take up fixation this is a convergent squint and if the eye moves in medially this is a divergent squint, that is, the eye moves in the opposite direction to the squint. This should be repeated a minimum of three times for certainty. Conversely if the affected eye is covered by an occluder, the other eye will not move as it is the dominant eye and will already be focused on the target.

- **Alternating cover test (cross-cover test)**. This is used to test for a latent squint. It is performed similarly but with the occluder used in a different way. If no manifest squint is demonstrated either on inspection, light reflection, or the unilateral cover test, the eyes will initially appear symmetrical. The occluder covers one eye briefly for 1–2 seconds before it is quickly moved to the other eye (before binocular fixation can occur). This rapid movement causes one eye to dissociate functionally from the other and the covered eye will move to its rest or 'squint' position. When the occluder is removed, the eye resumes fixation. If there is a discernible movement of the eye to take up fixation, you have demonstrated a latent squint or heterophoria (*het-er-owe-for-i-a*). In this circumstance if the eye moves out laterally to fix the target it is termed esophoria (*ee-so-for-i-a*) and if it turns in medially it is called exophoria. If no compensatory movement occurs during the testing then no latent squint has been demonstrated. This does not mean that the child does not have a squint as their squint may be intermittent and only becomes noticeable when the child tires. When this occurs this is known as decompensation. Thus a latent squint may decompensate into an intermittent squint which can in turn decompensate further into a manifest squint. Children with squints should be seen in the first instance by an orthoptist who if necessary will refer to an ophthalmologist to complete a full ocular assessment.

Other visual tests

- **Eye movements**. In a young child try and get them to follow a light or a toy with their eyes (as in the cranial nerve examination).

- **Acuity**. This can be formally examined in an older child with a LogMAR chart and in a younger child with pictures. Test each eye separately.

- **Fundoscopy**. Check whether there is a red reflex present and if possible carry out fundoscopy. This can be exceptionally difficult in the young child.

Hearing

Hearing surveillance is initially tested in the newborn period (see 'Newborn examination'). Conductive hearing loss secondary to 'glue ear' (otitis media with effusion, OME) is very

Table 14.24 Risk factors for sensorineural hearing loss

Prematurity/low birth weight
Family history
Ear and craniofacial abnormalities
Congenital infections (e.g. CMV, toxoplasmosis, rubella)
Ototoxic medication (e.g. gentamicin)
Genetic syndromes (e.g. trisomy 21)
Childhood infection (e.g. meningitis, mumps, measles)

CMV, cytomegalovirus

common; up to 50% of school-age children will have one episode. Ongoing OME can affect learning, language, and behaviour. Some children will need grommets. Sensorineural hearing loss (SNHL) occurs in 1–2 children per 1000. See Table 14.24 for risk factors for sensorineural hearing loss.

If concerns arise in later infancy and childhood this is usually first noticed by parents. A full examination should be done if parents have concerns about hearing, particularly looking for ear or facial abnormalities. A formal hearing assessment should also be done. Previously a distraction test was done for every child at 8 months but this was not a very accurate test so is no longer part of routine child surveillance. Hearing milestones are outlined in Table 14.22.

16 Assess ear, nose, and throat

Always leave the ENT examination until the last as it is the least well tolerated. It is important to do the ENT examination well as it may provide the clue as to why the child has a high fever and may prevent further and sometimes painful procedures being required. Be clear with your instructions to parents in terms of the correct position to hold the child, as they will need to do the restraining. Figure 14.10 demonstrates the correct positioning. Then, using the auroscope, examine the ear canal and tympanic membrane looking for signs of an otitis media or foreign body or wax. Repeat this on the other side. Next position the child so they are on the parent's lap facing towards you. Get the parent to place one arm around the child's body and one arm over their head (see Fig. 14.11). Gently using a tongue depressor prise the child's mouth open and examine the dentition and the oropharynx. Pay close attention to the child's tonsils looking for pus or exudate.

> ## Key points
>
> - There are two types of squint, concomitant (non-paralytic) and incomitant (paralytic)
> - Concomitant squints are the most common and are usually due to a refractive error
> - Concomitant squints may be convergent (affected eye turns inward: esotropia) or divergent (affected eye turns outwards: exotropia). Incomitant squints are rare in children and may be secondary to a cranial nerve palsy, raised intracranial pressure, or a feature of a benign syndrome
> - Remember 'tropias' are manifest squints and 'phorias' are latent squints

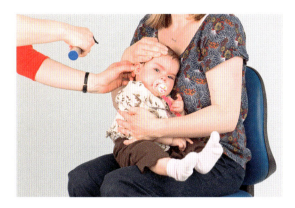

Figure 14.10 Examination of the ear.

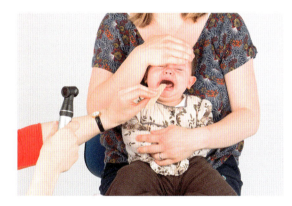

Figure 14.11 Examination of the oropharynx.

17 Thank the child and parent

This is sometimes forgotten when you are trying to make sense of your findings.

18 Wash your hands

This is easily forgotten too.

Newborn examination

The neonatal examination, or newborn check as it is called, might be the first contact that the parents and the baby have with a doctor and is very useful for allaying parental anxiety. It also provides an excellent opportunity for the early identification of congenital abnormality. The newborn check is usually carried out in the hospital by a trained health professional before the baby is discharged home. This is followed by another check at 6–8 weeks, usually at the GP's surgery. It is important to document

Key points

- Apply a systematic approach to your examination
- Build up a rapport with the child first as this will gain their trust
- Never forget the role of the parents in supporting the examination for young children
- Leave uncomfortable parts of the examination until the end
- At the end of every system examination plot the child on an appropriate growth chart
- Wash your hands before and after every examination
- Clinical skills are developed at the bedside, so get practising

the details of the newborn check in the baby's notes as well as in the child health record, including the details of follow-up if needed.

Aims of the neonatal examination

1 To assess well-being and general health:
   - Feeding
   - Meconium
   - Urine
   - Weight/head circumference

2 To provide an opportunity to talk to parents:
   - Allay anxiety
   - Address concerns if any

3 To detect obvious congenital anomalies

Some of the conditions that might not be detected during the newborn check include:

- **Congenital heart diseases**. There are certain congenital heart diseases that are dependent on a patent ductus arteriosus, for example, hypoplastic left heart, pulmonary atresia to provide systemic or pulmonary circulation. The ductus arteriosus normally closes within a few days after birth and these conditions become apparent after the closure of the ductus arteriosus. Coarctation of aorta can also present within a few days after birth.

- **Inborn errors of metabolism**. These will usually present later (time needed for the metabolites to accumulate).

The parents need to be aware of this and should be asked to seek medical advice if they are concerned about their child.

In an ideal setting, the newborn examination is performed in the presence of both parents. It is important to introduce yourself and explicitly state the purpose of the newborn examination. It is important to maintain hand hygiene precautions before examining a child.

The newborn examination is quite different from examining an adult or even an older child because the examination has to be tailored to each individual baby and their moods. It might be appropriate to start with listening to the heart first if the baby is quiet and to leave uncomfortable procedures (hips, eyes) to the last as they might upset the baby. You will have to explain to the parents what you are going to do and sometimes the examination will have to be carried out at different times depending on whether the baby is quiet or not. If you are in doubt about a finding, always seek a second opinion from your senior as some findings may not be clear cut.

Tips

- Ensure that the baby is warm.
- Make sure your hands are warm and clean.
- Offer feeds if the baby is upset.

Begin by introducing yourself and then check if the parents have any particular anxieties about the baby. A general chat about how the baby is feeding and the adequacy of feeding is useful before examination. Check with the parents if it is the ideal time for examination. Meconium is the dark green coloured stools that are normally passed by newborn babies. Babies generally pass meconium within the first 24 hours and most of them pass urine within the first 24–48 hours. Delayed passage of meconium could be associated with intestinal abnormalities like Hirschsprung's (*Her-sh-prungs*) disease or meconium ileus. Delayed micturition, or a poor urine stream especially in a male infant, can be associated with urinary obstruction, for example due to the presence of posterior urethral valves.

Newborn babies sleep between 16–18 hours a day and some parents might be anxious about this.

Get your equipment ready

- Stethoscope
- Ophthalmoscope
- Measuring tape
- Specific growth charts
- Light source
- Gloves

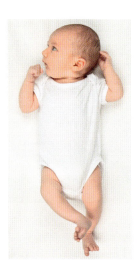

Figure 14.12 A normal neonate.

Examination of newborn

Begin the examination by observing the infant, looking especially at their general tone and activity. A normal newborn infant when awake has increased flexural tone with all four limbs flexed and moving symmetrically (Fig. 14.12). Excessive floppiness in an infant usually suggests underlying disease which can be either systemic (e.g. infection, hypoglycaemia) or neuromuscular problems. The next step is to undress the baby fully but always ensure that the baby is warm (use blankets to keep the baby warm). Dirty nappies are almost inevitable and changing nappies is perhaps an essential skill to be learnt by neonatal trainees!

Record the baby's weight and head circumference on an appropriate growth chart (sex, gestation, etc.) This is vitally important to enable the early identification of growth retardation (see Table 14.25). Babies whose weight is less than the 10th centile are termed 'small for gestational age' (SGA) and might be growth retarded. Large for gestational age (LGA) babies have birth weights greater than the 90th centile and might have associated maternal diabetes (see Table 14.26).

Measuring head circumference

Measure head circumference by using a flexible tape measure. Use the occipitofrontal circumference and ensure that the most prominent points in the skull are included. Ideally, head circumference should be measured three times and the maximum measurement obtained should be used as the baby's head circumference (Fig. 14.13). Head

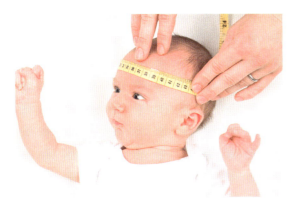

Figure 14.13 Measuring head circumference.

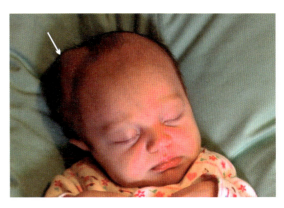

Figure 14.14 Cephalhaematoma.

Table 14.25 Causes of growth disturbance

| **Intrauterine growth retardation (IUGR)** |
| Utero-placental insufficiency |
| Maternal smoking |
| Congenital infections |
| Chromosomal disorders |
| **Large for gestational age (LGA)** |
| Infant of diabetic mother |
| Constitutional |
| Beckwith–Weidemann and other syndromes |

Table 14.26 Causes of an abnormal head circumference

| **Microcephaly** |
| Congenital infections |
| Chromosomal disorders |
| Fetal alcohol syndrome |
| Familial microcephaly |
| **Macrocephaly** |
| Hydrocephalus |
| Hydranencephaly |
| Subdural hematomas |

circumference less than 3 SD from the mean is defined as microcephaly (2nd centile) and macrocephaly is defined as head circumference greater than the 91st centile (see Table 14.26).

The examination of the head should include feeling for the anterior fontanelle, which is a membranous portion of the skull over the frontal region above the forehead and normally measures about 4 × 4 cm. A wide-opened anterior fontanelle is associated with some chromosomal abnormalities like trisomy 21, or hydrocephalus. Caput succedaneum (*ca-put sucks-a-dane-ee-um*) is a common finding in the newborn and is the result of oedema and swelling of the subcutaneous tissue during the trauma of delivery. This spontaneously resolves within a few days and needs no treatment. Cephalhaematoma (*ke-fal-he-ma-toe-ma*) is a subperiosteal hematoma of the scalp and is a fluctuant swelling that is bounded by the sutures and takes a few weeks to disappear (Fig. 14.14). Look for any evidence of birth injuries, as instrumental delivery can be associated with scalp and facial bruising.

Skin

Look for the colour of skin, particularly for pallor or jaundice. Jaundice is seen in about 60% of term infants and is due to the immaturity of the liver. This usually resolves within the first week. Jaundice occurring in newborns before the first day or persisting for more than 14 days needs further evaluation to rule out underlying causes. There are numerous rashes that are seen in a newborn, most of which are physiological and disappear without any treatment (see Table 14.27 and Fig. 14.15).

Table 14.27 Common skin conditions in neonates

Condition	Distribution	Colour	Action
Erythema toxicum	Trunk/limbs	Red	Reassurance
Mongolian spot	Back/sacrum	Blue	None
Stork bite	Face	Red	Reassurance
Port wine stain	Face	Red/ blue	*r/o associated conditions such as Sturge–Weber syndrome
Milia	Nose	Yellow	Reassurance
Pustule	Anywhere	Yellow	Antibiotics

*r/o = rule out

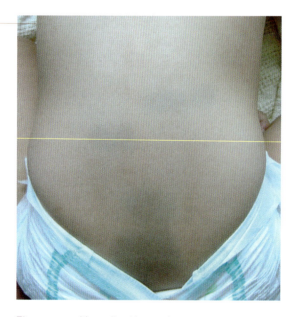

Figure 14.15 Mongolian blue spot.

Face

Examine the face for any obvious bruising or any marks. It is important to examine the baby's facial features; if they look abnormal don't forget to check both parents, in case these are inherited. Some of the commonly seen dysmorphic features are listed in Table 14.28 in conjunction with trisomy 21 (Down's syndrome). See also Case 14.14.

Table 14.28 Common dysmorphic features of trisomy 21 (Down's syndrome)

Flat occiput (brachycephaly)
Low-set ears
Upslanting/downslanting eyes
Epicanthic fold
Hypertelorism (wide nasal bridge)
Depressed nose
Small jaw (micrognathia)
Protuberant tongue
Talipes
Loose skin behind the neck
Single palmar crease
Overriding digits
Clinodactyly (see text)
Hypotonia
Sandal gap (wide gap between the great toe and 2nd toe)

Look for any birthmarks (naevi/hemangioma) on the face. The presence of a port wine stain, especially if limited to one-half of the face will need evaluation to rule out Sturge–Weber syndrome. This is associated with intracerebral hemangiomas which can result in seizures.

Eyes

It is very difficult to examine eyes as newborn infants are naturally photophobic. Examine them in subdued lighting, as babies will tend to open their eyes in this setting. NB. Do not force open the eyelids as this is uncomfortable for the neonate and can disrupt the examination.

Tip
Gentle rocking of the head is helpful in opening the eyes of the newborn infant.

Inspect the eyes for any asymmetry. Upslanting or downslanting eyes are significant in the presence of other

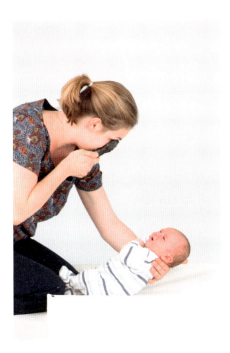

Figure 14.16 Examining for the red reflex.

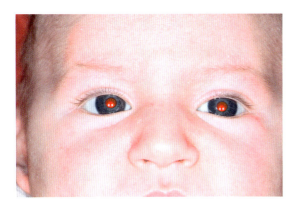

Figure 14.17 Red reflex.

dysmorphic features and can provide clues to a diagnosis. Examination of the red reflex is vital to rule out congenital cataracts or tumours and is done by shining the light on the eyes and looking for the presence of a red glow (this is similar to the 'satanic red eye' effect you see in uncorrected photographs of people's faces; see Figs. 14.16 and 14.17; also see Case 14.12).

Mouth

Look for an abnormally small jaw (micrognathia) (*my-crow-g-nath-ia*). Open the mouth of the baby using your fingers, especially the little finger just to open the lips and

gums. Avoid using a tongue depressor as it can cause trauma. In a crying baby, it is easy to examine the mouth and palate. Look for the presence of an abnormally large tongue (hypothyroidism) or a protuberant tongue (Down's syndrome). Natal teeth are uncommon but can cause difficulty with feeding. If they are loose, they need to be removed as there is a risk of aspiration.

Palate

Examination of the palate is vital to identify cleft palate (Fig. 14.18). It is important to both **look** and **feel** for the defect as it is difficult to diagnose a submucosal cleft palate by inspection alone.

Ears

Check the ears for the presence of any preauricular pits, skin tags. Low-set ears are a common dysmorphic characteristic which in the presence of other features might indicate an underlying syndrome.

Neck

Inspect the neck for any sinus, swelling, or deformity. Common neck swellings include cystic hygroma, branchial cyst, or sternomastoid tumour.

Respiratory examination

Count the respiratory rate (see Table 14.29) and look for the signs of excessive work of breathing in a newborn which

(a) 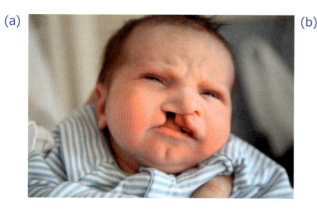 (b)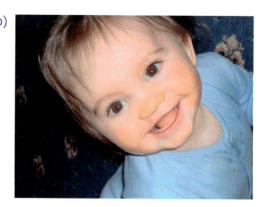

Figure 14.18 Cleft palate: (a) before surgery; (b) after surgery.

Table 14.29 Normal values of vital signs in the newborn

Heart rate	120–160 /min
Respiratory rate	40–60 /min
Blood pressure	70/40 mmHg

includes tachypnoea, nasal flaring, the presence of sub-costal or intercostal retractions, and grunting. The presence of any of these signs indicates the need for urgent evaluation and intervention in that particular individual.

Cardiovascular examination

Auscultate the chest for heart sounds and murmurs. Murmurs are very common in the neonatal period due to the cardiopulmonary adaptive changes. The examination of femoral pulses is an important aspect of cardiovascular examination. Use your thumbs to appreciate the volume of both femoral pulses simultaneously. Unequal or absent femoral pulses indicate possible coarctation of the aorta and the neonate needs further evaluation with an echocardiography, especially if unwell. Routine use of pulse oximetry in identifying abnormal postductal saturations (lower limb) has been increasingly used to detect congenital heart diseases that would have been difficult to pick up on routine examinations. Blood pressure measurements are not routinely done in newborns but should be performed if there is a suspicion of congenital heart disease or if they are unwell.

Abdominal examination

Examine the abdomen for the presence of any mass, swelling, or organomegaly. The liver, spleen, and kidneys can sometimes be palpable in newborns. Inspect the umbilical cord for any discharge, redness, or induration around the site. Umbilical granuloma are common and they indicate excessive granulation tissue at the umbilicus after the remnant of the cord has fallen off. They might need treatment if they persist for weeks or if large enough to cause concern.

In boys, palpate both the testes and check if they are present in the scrotum. Abnormal swellings in the scrotum include inguinal hernia or hydrocele. See Case 14.13. Inspect the urethral opening and ensure that there is no hypospadias (where the urethral opening is located on the under surface of the penile shaft). If there is hypospadias, the neonate should be referred to the urologists as it might require surgical correction later. The parents should be advised not to circumcise the baby if this is part of their culture.

Limbs

Inspect both the upper and lower limbs for any obvious birth injuries. Check tone and movement of all the limbs and count all the digits.

Upper limbs

Check the clavicles for the presence of any fracture or discontinuity. Erb's palsy is usually due to traction injury to the brachial plexus during delivery. The neonate keeps the affected arm extended with the wrist pronated and fingers extended. If diagnosed, the neonate needs referral to a physiotherapist and usually has a good prognosis (Fig. 14.19).

Single palmar crease

Also known as a simian crease, this is associated with syndromes, particularly Down's syndrome. Clinodactyly is where there is incurving of the little finger towards the other fingers and is also associated with Down's syndrome.

CASE 14.13

Problem: When examining a newborn male I find it difficult to decide whether the testes are descended and whether I am missing other diagnoses such as a hydrocele or inguinal hernia.

Discussion: Testes should have descended in a term baby bilaterally. You may have to 'milk' them downwards as they may be retractile. If you cannot feel one or both, the baby needs to be referred to a paediatric surgeon. If a swelling is seen or felt in the scrotum this may be a hydrocele or hernia. In fact they share a similar aetiology. In fetal life the processus vaginalis (PV) should be obliterated as the testicle descends; however, if it remains and has a small diameter then fluid accumulates and cause a scrotal swelling called a hydrocele. If the persisting PV has a large diameter then abdominal contents can push through and an indirect inguinal hernia will result. Therefore during your examination you will not be able to get above the swelling. A swelling that can be transilluminated (i.e. using a pen torch as a light source on the surface of the scrotum) is more likely to be a hydrocele.

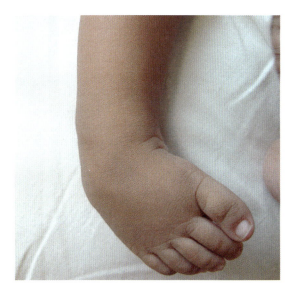

Figure 14.20 Talipes equinovarus.

Lower limbs

Look for any asymmetry of creases and the tone of both the lower limbs. Talipes is a condition where there is an incurving of the foot at the ankle (*talus* means ankle; *pes* means foot, in Latin) See Fig. 14.20. Sometimes you will see the full description, talipes equinovarus; the old lay term for this was club foot. The deformity is variable and can be postural. Identification of talipes during examination requires referral to a physiotherapist. Always rule out spinal cord abnormalities, associated hip dislocation, or neurological/neuromuscular problems in bilateral talipes.

Hip examination

Examination of the hips is an important part of the newborn check. For this, the baby needs to be lying supine on a flat surface with full exposure. Explain to the parents what the examination involves as it can be uncomfortable for the baby. The objective of the hip examination is to screen for developmental dysplasia of the hip (DDH) where there is an abnormality of the hip joint that causes dislocation (see Table 14.30 for risk factors for this condition). Examination should start by inspecting the limbs for the presence of leg length discrepancy and/or asymmetry of the skin creases. There are two components of the hip examination:

Ortolani's test (reduction)

This is to test whether the hip is already dislocated. It is usual to examine one hip at a time. Examine the

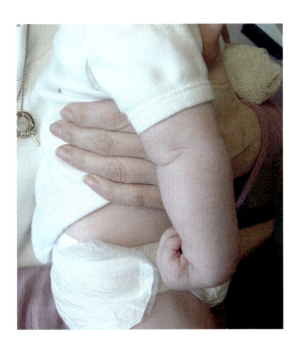

Figure 14.19 Erb's palsy.

Table 14.30 Risk factors for developmental dysplasia of hip (DDH)

Female infant
Breech presentation
Family history of DDH
Neurological/neuromuscular disorders

baby on his/her back with the knees flexed to 90°. Grasp the baby's thigh with the middle finger over the greater trochanter and the thumb on the lesser trochanter. Lift the thigh upwards, at the same time gently abducting it. This brings the femoral head from its posterior position to opposite the acetabulum. In a dislocated joint, the femoral head moves forwards, giving rise to a 'clunk' (see Fig. 14.21).

Barlow's test (dislocation)

This test is to assess if the hip is prone to dislocation. With one hand fixing the pelvis with the thumb anteriorly over the symphysis pubis, the other fingers posteriorly over the coccygeal region, the other hand grasps the baby's thigh in the same way as in the Ortolani test and the thigh is pushed gently downwards while adducting it. Dislocation is palpable as the femoral head slips over the posterior lip of the acetabulum. In a neonate with suspected DDH, a hip ultrasound is warranted and an orthopaedic opinion should be sought. Even in the absence of a clunk, the presence of 'clicky' hips might need evaluation with a hip ultrasound, especially in the presence of any of the risk factors in Table 14.30 above.

Neurological examination

Neurological examination of the newborn involves assessing the tone and posture of the infant. Normal, term, newborn babies have a flexed posture and are vigorous with their movements. Floppy babies are hypotonic and have abducted thighs adopting a 'frog's legs' posture. On ventral suspension, i.e. holding the baby with one hand under the abdomen and the other hand over the back in the prone position (see Fig. 14.22), the normal newborn will display some extensor tone in the neck. Floppy babies will show poor extensor tone in the neck and their overall floppiness makes them assume the shape of the letter C. The commonly tested neonatal reflexes include the Moro's reflex, suck reflex, and grasp reflex.

(a)
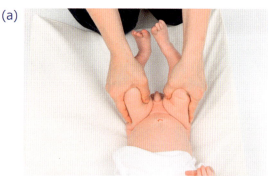

(b)
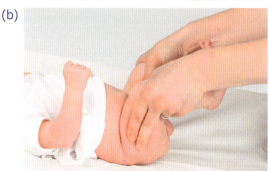

(c)
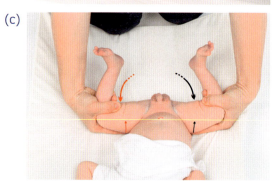

Figure 14.21 Ortolani's test: (a) starting position; (b) starting position, side view; (c) end position.

Moro reflex

This reflex is elicited by placing one hand under the infant's shoulders and the other under the head and then gently but suddenly dropping the head by several centimetres. A full response consists of a sudden abduction and extension of the arms, followed by adduction and flexion (Fig. 14.23). An asymmetrical Moro reflex suggests either a brachial nerve palsy or a birth injury. An absent Moro reflex is seen in neonates who are generally 'unwell' or in neuromuscular/neurological problems. The palmar and plantar grasp reflexes are elicited by applying pressure to

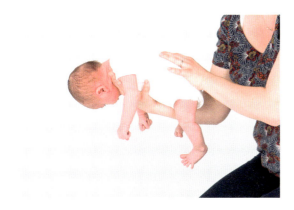

Figure 14.22 Ventral suspension.

(a)   (b)

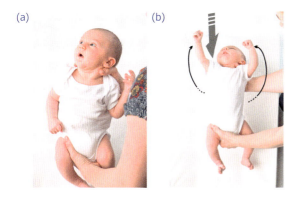

Figure 14.23 Moro reflex: (a) starting position; (b) demonstrating the abduction and extension of the arms.

the palm and sole respectively which results in flexion of fingers or toes.

Neonatal screening

All neonates undergo a universal hearing screen at birth and if it is abnormal they are offered a follow-up assessment with evoked response audiometry. The UK National Screening Committee recommend that all babies in the UK are offered screening for phenylketonuria (PKU), congenital hypothyroidism (CHT), sickle cell disorders (SCD), cystic fibrosis (CF), and medium-chain acyl-CoA dehydrogenase deficiency (MCADD). This is usually done with a heel prick sample obtained at 5–7 days of age.

Adolescent examination

As adolescents start their journey to adulthood they often become self-conscious about their bodies, so reassurance,

---

CASE 14.14

Question: I am not very confident about whether a newborn infant is dysmorphic or not. How do I go about this?

   Discussion: This is a very common challenge for juniors as there can be a wide variation in how the newborn infant looks. It is important to look at both parents as neonates can bear striking resemblance to their parents. There might be important clues from history—age of the mother (higher risk of Down's syndrome in older mothers), abnormalities in antenatal scans (increased nuchal fold thickness, presence of renal, cardiac abnormalities, and presence of growth retardation) and family history of genetic disorders. It is hard to define the clinical features soon after birth as many infants have bruised/swollen face and scalp from delivery. A useful tip is to examine the baby repeatedly after giving time for the swelling/bruises to settle down. The presence of feeding difficulties, excessive floppiness (hypotonia), and intrauterine growth retardation increases the suspicion of underlying problems. A senior review is always warranted when there is the possibility of dysmorphism. Midwives and neonatal nurses are very experienced in handling babies and are very helpful in differentiating normal features from dysmorphism.

---

empathy, and professionalism are all important in reducing embarrassment during the examination. Consent should always be obtained (at least verbally) prior to any examination. Competent adolescents should be able to express their wishes with regard to consent for examination (and treatment) and these wishes should be respected by the examiner.

A child is legally defined as a person less than 18 years of age. However, the laws with regards to consent are different for those above or below the age of 16 years of age. If a child of 16 or 17 years of age is deemed competent to make a decision then they can consent to a procedure. If a child of 16 or 17 is not deemed competent then a person with parental responsibility can make that decision for them (with the child involved as much as possible).

A child under 16 years of age is not automatically presumed to be legally competent to make decisions about their health care. However, children under 16 can be deemed competent to give valid consent if they have 'sufficient understanding and intelligence to enable him or her to understand fully what is proposed'. The Gillick competency and Fraser guidelines can be used to assess whether a child is mature enough to make and understand the implications of their own decisions.

Chaperones are always needed during examination of pubertal status. This should not be a relative or carer of the patient, but another professional (e.g. a nurse or another doctor). Chaperones may also be appropriate if exposure of the patient is needed for a thorough examination (e.g. examination of a female chest).

Growth

Midparental height (MPH)

This measurement helps to distinguish between genetic and constitutional growth disturbances. It calculates the expected height of a child based on their parent's height. A healthy child's final height will be normally distributed around the MPH and this therefore prevents unnecessary investigations. In situations where there is a large difference between parents' heights then the MPH is less reliable.

The mean difference in final adult height is 14 cm between women and men, so when calculating the MPH for a girl, subtract 14 cm from the father's height, and for a boy add 14 cm to the mother's height. The midpoint between the parent's corrected heights is the MPH, and the target range is calculated on the MPH ±8.5 cm in females and 10 cm in males, representing the 2nd and 98th centiles for MPH (Table 14.31).

Height velocity

This is the rate of growth of a child and it should be calculated at intervals of 6–12 months. It can then be plotted on a chart and if it crosses several centiles, further investigations should be carried out.

Pubertal staging

Puberty consists of a series of predictable events and its staging is vital in the clinical assessment of all children in order to establish if their development and peak height velocity is within normal limits. The staging system most commonly used is the Tanner staging (see Fig. 14.25).

Table 14.31 Calculation of the midparental height for a female

Mother's height (MH)= 156 cm
Father's height (FH)= 185 cm
MPH = (MH + FH)/2 − 7
= (156 + 185)/2 − 7
= 164 cm
Range = 164 cm ± 8.5 cm

Phases of childhood growth

Normal growth can be divided into three phases—infancy, childhood, and pubertal growth—which are regulated by slightly different mechanisms but represent a continuum. During infancy, the major regulating influence is nutritional status in addition to normal thyroid status and adequate emotional support. Linear growth is initially rapid, about 25 cm in the first 12 months of life, although the rate of growth (height velocity) decreases markedly during this phase. The childhood growth phase begins at approximately 6 months but predominates from the age of 3, and is primarily driven by growth hormone, although normal thyroid function is needed for normal growth. The height velocity during this phase can range from 4 to 8 cm/year. There is little difference between the height and weight velocity in the growth of girls and boys during this phase and both have a slowly decelerating growth until puberty.

During puberty, the adolescent growth spurt is caused by increasing levels of androgen and oestrogens produced by the gonads in males and females respectively. This is as a result of hypothalamic–pituitary–gonadal activation which in turn results in a significant increase in growth hormone secretion.

In females, the adolescent growth spurt coincides with the start of puberty and is breast development, and starts approximately 2 years earlier than in males. The peak height velocity (fastest rate of growth) reaches approximately 8 cm/year, and occurs on average at about 12 years of age. Consequently, the onset of menstruation (menarche) which follows the peak height velocity represents a time when the height velocity is falling, and only approximately 5 cm of height on average will be gained after menarche. The average age of menarche in UK females is 12.9 years. In males, the adolescent growth spurt coincides with a testicular volume of 10–12 mL and occurs when male puberty is already well established. The peak height velocity is reached at a testicular volume of 12–15 mL (approximately 14 years of age). The amplitude of peak height velocity reaches approximately 10 cm/year in males, and the average difference in adult height between males and females is 13–13.5 cm.

Decimal age and height velocity

Expression of age as a decimal makes calculations, especially of height velocity, much easier and more accurate. Every day is a fraction of a year, so each day is equal to 1/365th of a year. The table of decimals of year is found on clinical growth charts, and shows what decimal fraction of a year has elapsed each day.

To calculate the decimal age of a child seen in clinic on the 20 October 2013 and born on 12 March 2001, the decimal birthday (2001.192) is subtracted from the decimal clinic appointment (2013.800) (see Fig. 14.24):

$$1997.192 - 2009.800 = 11.608 \text{ years}$$

Height velocity is calculated by dividing the difference in height (cm) by the difference in interval (decimal years).

Bone age

The bone age is used to assess the skeletal maturity of growing children by using a radiograph of the left wrist and hand. The final adult height is only reached when the bony epiphyses fuse in the long bones of the leg and in the vertebrae. Skeletal maturity is therefore a good guide to how much growing has been done and how much remains. A delayed bone age compared to the child's chronological age means there is greater potential for growth, and the opposite is true for an advanced bone age.

Puberty

Normal pubertal development follows a set sequence of events, although the onset and duration varies considerably between individuals. In girls, the first stage of pubertal development is breast budding, and the peak height velocity occurs at B2–3 (see chart in Fig. 14.25). Menarche occurs towards the end of puberty and is accompanied by a marked deceleration in height velocity. In boys, the first stage of pubertal development is the enlargement of the testes from less than 4 mL to more than 4 mL, although the increase in growth rate occurs with testicular volumes of 6–10 mL.

In order to correctly assess the pubertal stage of development of any child (see Table 14.32), it is important to use the Tanner criteria, which can be found on clinical growth charts (see Fig. 14.25), and a Prader orchidometer

(Fig. 14.26) in boys. Assessment of pubertal staging in girls includes breast (B), pubic hair (P), and axillary hair (A) development, and in boys genital development and testicular volume (G), in addition to pubic and axillary hair. Penile length, which is measured from the base of the penis to the tip of the glans, is useful in excluding hypogonadism, particularly in obese males, as firm compression of the suprapubic fat pad often reveals the penis to be normal sized.

In females, assessment of the uterine shape, size, and endometrial echo by pelvic ultrasound can also give an indication of oestrogen effect and is a useful technique in pubertal assessment. If there is diagnostic uncertainty regarding pubertal assessment, biochemical investigation can also be carried out.

Precocious puberty and delayed puberty

Precocious puberty

This is a general term meaning early sexual development, and can either be caused by true central precocious puberty (TCPP), where normal puberty occurs because of abnormally early activation of the hypothalamus, or precocious pseudopuberty, which is caused by abnormal secretion of sex steroids and is independent of the hypothalamic–pituitary axis. TCPP is defined as occurring before the age of 8 years in girls and before 9 years in boys, in the UK. TCPP is unusual in males and is much less likely to be idiopathic in origin, so will require a thorough investigation of possible underlying causes.

Delayed puberty

This is defined as the absence of secondary sexual characteristics in females by 13 years of age or in males by 14 years of age. It can either be central or peripheral depending on the site of the problem (i.e. within the hypothalamic–pituitary axis or in the gonads respectively).

Most causes of delayed puberty are due to simple constitutional delay in growth and puberty (CDGP). Typically the child has normal childhood growth, but with a delayed puberty and growth spurt. Their bone age is, however, sufficiently delayed to result in a normal predicted final adult height, and often there is a family history of delayed puberty. It is most common in boys and can be a cause of great distress because of teasing or embarrassment at being significantly smaller and younger looking than their peers.

Although it is important to differentiate CDGP from other causes such as familial short stature or hypogonadotrophic hypogonadism, it is not usually necessary to carry out any investigations other than bone age estimations

DECIMAL YEAR CALCULATION

	1	2	3	4	5	6	7	8	9	10	11	12	13	14	15	16	17	18	19	20	21	22	23	24	25	26	27	28	29	30	31
JAN	000	003	005	008	011	014	016	019	022	025	027	030	033	036	038	041	044	047	049	052	055	058	060	063	066	068	071	074	077	079	082
FEB	085	088	090	093	096	099	101	104	107	110	112	115	118	121	123	126	129	132	134	137	140	142	145	148	151	153	156	159			
MAR	162	164	167	170	173	175	178	181	184	186	189	192	195	197	200	203	205	208	211	214	216	219	222	225	227	230	233	236	238	241	244
APR	247	249	252	255	258	260	263	266	268	271	274	277	279	282	285	288	290	293	296	299	301	304	307	310	312	315	318	321	323	326	
MAY	329	332	334	337	340	342	345	348	351	353	356	359	362	364	367	370	373	375	378	381	384	386	389	392	395	397	400	403	405	408	411
JUN	414	416	419	422	425	427	430	433	436	438	441	444	447	449	452	455	458	460	463	466	468	471	474	477	479	482	485	488	490	493	
JUL	496	499	501	504	507	510	512	515	518	521	523	526	529	532	534	537	540	542	545	548	551	553	556	559	562	564	567	570	573	575	578
AUG	581	584	586	589	592	595	597	600	603	605	608	611	614	616	619	622	625	627	630	633	636	638	641	644	647	649	652	655	658	660	663
SEPT	666	668	671	674	677	679	682	685	688	690	693	696	699	701	704	707	710	712	715	718	721	723	726	729	731	734	737	740	742	745	
OCT	748	751	753	756	759	762	764	767	770	773	775	778	781	784	786	789	792	795	797	800	803	805	808	811	814	816	819	822	825	827	830
NOV	833	836	838	841	844	847	849	852	855	858	860	863	866	868	871	874	877	879	882	885	888	890	893	896	899	901	904	907	910	912	
DEC	915	918	921	923	926	929	932	934	937	940	942	945	948	951	953	956	959	962	962	967	970	973	975	978	981	984	986	989	992	995	997

Figure 14.24 Decimal year calculator.

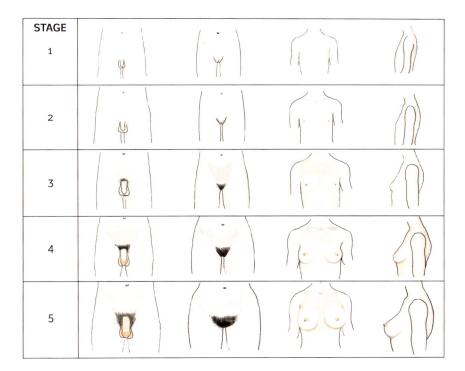

Figure 14.25 Tanner staging.

Key

Male

Genital development: (G)
Stage 1 Preadolescence—testes, scrotum, and penis about the same size as in early childhood
Stage 2 Enlargement of scrotum and testes. Skin on scrotum reddens
Stage 3 Enlargement of the penis; length initially
Stage 4 Increased size of penis with growth and breadth and development of glans. Testes and scrotum larger
Stage 5 Genitalia adult in size and shape

Pubic hair: (P)
Stage 1 No pubic hair
Stage 2 Sparse growth of long, slightly pigmented, downy hair, chiefly at base of penis
Stage 3 Considerably darker, coarse, and more curled hair spread sparsely over the junction of the pubes
Stage 4 Pubic hair is adult in type but considerably smaller with no spread to medial surface of thighs
Stage 5 Adult in quantity and type

Female

Breast development: (B)
Stage 1 Preadolescence, elevation of papilla only
Stage 2 Breast bud stage; elevation of breast and papilla as small mound
Stage 3 Further enlargement of breast and areola with no separation of their contours
Stage 4 Projection of areola and papilla to form secondary mound above breast
Stage 5 Projection of papilla only due to recession of areola

Pubic hair: (P)
Stage 1 No pubic hair
Stage 2 Sparse growth of long slightly pigmented downy hair, chiefly on the labia
Stage 3 Considerably darker, coarse, and more curled hair spread sparsely over the junction of the pubes
Stage 4 Pubic hair is adult in type but considerably smaller with no spread to medial surface of thighs
Stage 5 Adult in quantity and type

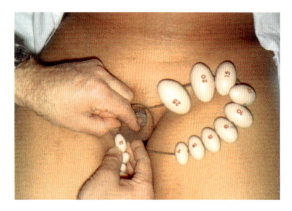

Figure 14.26 Prader orchidometer.

Table 14.32 Clinical assessment of puberty

Plot the height and weight of the adolescent
Calculate the midparental height and the target range (cm)
Calculate the height velocity using the decimal age
Assess the pubertal stage using Tanner criteria ± orchidometer
Bone age radiograph of the left wrist and hand.

and the prognosis is very positive. Occasionally in boys over 13.5 years, a short course of testosterone therapy may be offered in order to precipitate puberty. See Cases 14.15, 14.16, and 14.17 for case studies about puberty.

Paediatric diseases and investigations

Within this section we have endeavoured to give a brief account of several conditions mentioned within this chapter. The information below is simply an overview and is not a substitute for a core paediatric textbook.

Acute lymphoblastic leukaemia

One-third of all childhood cancers are leukaemia and the most common form is acute lymphoblastic leukaemia (ALL), a cancer of immature lymphocytes (lymphoblasts).

Aetiology

The causes of childhood ALL are usually unknown (though it is more common with certain genetic conditions such as Down's syndrome).

CASE 14.15

Problem: A 13-year-old girl is referred to you with delayed puberty. You notice that she is short and that her predicted height is below her midparental target range. She also has no secondary sexual characteristics. There is no family history of delayed puberty. Is this a case of simple CDGP or could there be something else going on?

Discussion: The combination of delayed puberty and short stature in a female should always prompt the examiner to consider Turner's syndrome as a diagnosis. Turner's syndrome is caused by complete or partial absence of one of the X chromosomes so that the karyotype is 45X instead of 46XX, and this occurs in 1 in 2500 live female births. These girls are always short and this may be the only clinical feature. Most girls with Turner's syndrome will also have ovarian malformation, where the ovaries consist of streaks of ovarian tissue which is unable to produce sufficient levels of oestrogen or ova. Although the uterus and external female genitalia are normal, these girls will require replacement oestrogen at puberty and are infertile. There may also be abnormalities of other internal organs such as the aorta and kidneys. Investigations include a karyotype analysis and a pelvic ultrasound scan.

CASE 14.16

Problem: When examining young girls who are obese with increased height and breast development, how do I know that they are not in true precocious puberty?

Discussion: Commonly children who are obese are tall for their age and often have an advanced bone age. However, usually the height velocity does not keep increasing. They are prone to a slightly early puberty, but their final height is not adversely affected and they become normal-sized adults (unlike in precocious puberty). In girls, breast development is the first sign of puberty but it can be difficult to detect differences between fat tissue and breast tissue in obese girls, therefore monitoring for other signs of growth and puberty may be required.

Symptoms

At presentation symptoms can include bleeding tendencies (e.g. nose bleeds/bruising) secondary to low platelet levels, increased susceptibility to infections due to abnormal white blood cell production and anaemia (causing tiredness and lethargy).

CASE 14.17

Problem: You see a 15-year-old boy in clinic who is a lot shorter than his peers; his height is below the bottom centile and he has lost some weight recently. Academically he has not been doing as well at school and he has been complaining of diarrhoea and abdominal pain. His testes are both 4 mL in volume and he has a few pubic hairs. What investigations (if any) would you want to do?

Discussion: While simple CDGP is the most common cause of delayed puberty and short stature in boys, it does not explain his weight loss, poor academic performance, and abdominal symptoms. A diagnosis of Crohn's disease was indicated by the elevation of inflammatory markers (ESR) and confirmed following an endoscopy and barium follow through.

It is important to take a full history and examination in adolescents, as successful treatment of the underlying disease may reverse the short stature and delayed puberty. Testosterone therapy is not usually required in such cases. Although growth hormone is occasionally used for chronic diseases to improve short stature, it is not a licensed indication for inflammatory bowel disease and further endocrine evaluation may be considered. Children with Crohn's disease may have decreasing height velocity before the gastrointestinal manifestations of the disease become established.

Diagnosis

This is made by finding blast cells in abnormally raised numbers in the bone marrow and often the peripheral blood.

Treatment

This is mainly with chemotherapy. Overall survival is now greater than 90% in the UK with improved chemotherapy regimens.

Atrioventricular defect

An atrioventricular defect (AVSD) is a deficiency (hole) in the atrioventricular septum of the heart.

Aetiology

This is the most commonly associated heart defect in children with Down's syndrome.

Diagnosis

The diagnosis is made by cardiac ultrasound (cardiac echo). A complete AVSD is a hole in the wall between the atria and a hole in the wall between the ventricles with one common valve between these four chambers. In a partial AVSD there is no direct intraventricular communication of the atrial defect. In AVSD pulmonary hypertension is caused by left-to-right flow across the defect.

Symptoms and treatment

Patients are likely to need treatment for heart failure (diuretics) and most AVSDs require surgical intervention within the first 6 months of life.

Autism

Autism is a lifelong condition that manifests in early childhood; it is usually recognized after the age of 2 years although signs may have been present earlier.

Aetiology

The aetiology of autism is unknown but it is likely to have a genetic basis. The MMR is not a cause of autism and the research surrounding this particular health scare was seriously flawed. There are a number of coexisting comorbidities including epileptic seizures and learning disabilities. Autism is also common in children who have tuberous sclerosis. Autism is included under an umbrella term of autistic spectrum disorders (ASD); this includes Asperger's syndrome. The prevalence of ASD is approximately 1/100.

Diagnosis and symptoms

Children are diagnosed with autism if they meet certain criteria; these include impaired social interaction, impaired social communication, and restricted interests with rigid and repetitive behaviours.

Treatment

There is no cure for autism, and it can have a profound effect on children and their families particularly as the condition is not well understood. Management includes intensive behavioural, educational, and psychological input. A lot of other 'alternative' interventions are used but there is no evidence that any of these treatments have a positive effect.

Beckwith–Wiedemann syndrome

Aetiology

This is a congenital growth disorder associated with defects in chromosome 11.

Symptoms

These include neonatal hypoglycaemia, being LGA, poor feeding, large prominent tongue and eyes, umbilical hernia or omphalocele, horizontal earlobe creases, organomegaly, hemihypertrophy, undescended testes and increased risk of certain tumours (Wilms' tumour and adrenal carcinoma).

Diagnosis

This is made clinically on phenotypic features and on genetic testing.

Treatment

There is no specific treatment for Beckwith–Wiedemann syndrome other than the management of any of its associated problems, such as for poor feeding.

Bronchiolitis

Aetiology

Bronchiolitis is caused by many viruses. The most common pathogen is the respiratory syncytial virus (RSV). Most children are aged 1–9 months.

Symptoms

The disease is characterized by coryzal symptoms, increased shortness of breath, wheeze, and cough. The main findings on examination are signs of respiratory distress, wheeze, and fine end-inspiratory crackles.

Diagnosis

Bronchiolitis is diagnosed by performing a nasopharyngeal aspirate (NPA) which looks for common viruses.

Treatment

Supportive only. Babies with low oxygen saturations will require oxygen therapy and if they are having feeding difficulties then a nasogastric tube may be required or even intravenous fluid. Some infants require a period of mechanical ventilation.

Cerebral palsy

Aetiology

Cerebral palsy is a disorder caused by a non-progressive lesion within the developing fetal or infant brain leading to difficulties in movement and posture. There are many different types and causes of cerebral palsy including spastic hemiplegia, spastic diplegia, spastic quadriplegia, dyskinetic, mixed cerebral palsy, hypotonic cerebral palsy, and monoplegia.

Diagnosis

This is made clinically and investigations can include brain imaging to assess areas affected.

Treatment

This is supportive and addresses the effects of the child's cerebral palsy on areas such as feeding, joint positioning, and associated symptoms such as seizures. The aim is to prevent complications and improve function and quality of life.

Child protection and safeguarding

It is the duty of every doctor who has contact with children to safeguard and protect their welfare (relevant UK legislation is the Children Act 2004). Safeguarding aims to ensure that children are provided safe and effective care in childhood and protected from maltreatment. You should always consider whether a child is at risk of abuse or being abused at every consultation with a child. It is beyond the scope of this chapter to detail the systematic examination of a child for a child protection medical examination. However, it is important that all students and doctors who have contact with children are aware of the basic signs of child abuse and the procedures to follow if abuse is suspected. Figure 14.27 details the potential sites of injury which should raise suspicion that injury is non-accidental.

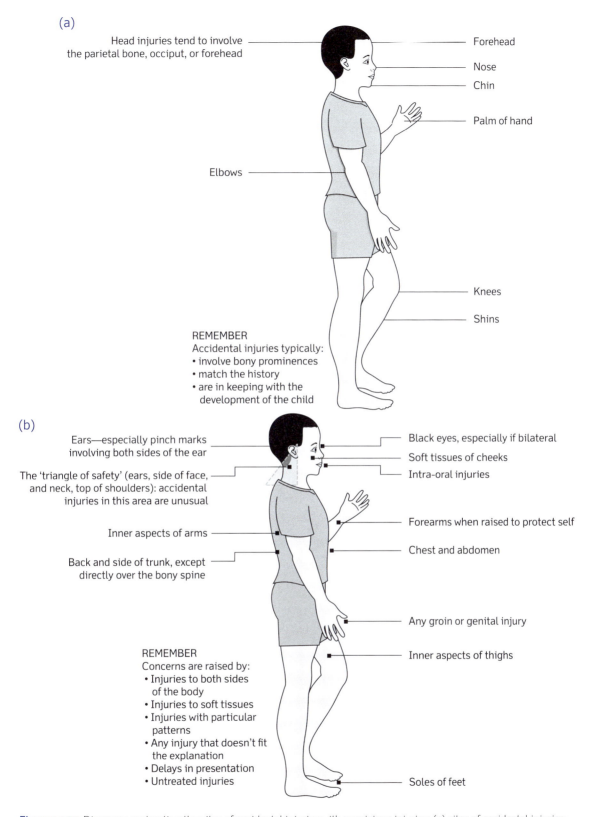

(a)

Head injuries tend to involve the parietal bone, occiput, or forehead

Forehead

Nose

Chin

Palm of hand

Elbows

Knees

Shins

REMEMBER
Accidental injuries typically:
• involve bony prominences
• match the history
• are in keeping with the development of the child

(b)

Ears—especially pinch marks involving both sides of the ear

The 'triangle of safety' (ears, side of face, and neck, top of shoulders): accidental injuries in this area are unusual

Inner aspects of arms

Back and side of trunk, except directly over the bony spine

Black eyes, especially if bilateral

Soft tissues of cheeks

Intra-oral injuries

Forearms when raised to protect self

Chest and abdomen

Any groin or genital injury

Inner aspects of thighs

REMEMBER
Concerns are raised by:
• Injuries to both sides of the body
• Injuries to soft tissues
• Injuries with particular patterns
• Any injury that doesn't fit the explanation
• Delays in presentation
• Untreated injuries

Soles of feet

Figure 14.27 Diagrams contrasting the sites of accidental injuries with suspicious injuries: (a) sites of accidental injuries; (b) sites of injuries that should cause concern.

Reproduced from Harris J, Sidebotham P, Welbury R et al. *Child protection and the dental team: an introduction to safeguarding children in dental practice.* COPDEND: Sheffield, 2006. **www.cpdt.org.uk**

The legal definition of child abuse is taken from the Children Act 1989 and states that 'The child is suffering or likely to suffer significant harm and the harm is attributable to lack of adequate parental care or control'. There are four categories of abuse which a child can be registered as being at risk of on a social services child protection plan. These are:

- physical abuse
- sexual abuse
- neglect
- emotional abuse.

Children can be subject to more than one form of abuse. Physical abuse is the same as non-accidental injury. An inconsistent or changing explanation for the injury, or an injury which is incompatible with the mechanism given or for the developmental stage of the child, should raise alarm and prompt further investigation for child abuse.

The UK National Society for the Prevention of Cruelty to Children (NSPCC) provides the following definitions of the other categories of abuse:

- **Child sexual abuse** is defined as 'abuse which involves persuading or forcing a child to take part in sexual activities, or encouraging a child to behave in sexually inappropriate ways'.
- **Emotional abuse** is defined as 'severe and persistent ill treatment which adversely affects a child's emotional health and development'.
- **Neglect** is when the 'essential needs of a child' (e.g. adequate food, water, shelter, warmth, protection, and health care provided by attentive, dependable, and kind carers) are persistently not met.

If you suspect that a child is being abused or is at risk of abuse, you have a duty to act. You should report your concerns to a senior professional (e.g. the consultant looking after the child) and if required also to social services or the police. This should be done according to local and national safeguarding guidance. Both the General Medical Council (GMC) and National Institute for Health and Care Excellence (NICE) have guidance on the appropriate management of potential child abuse (see 'References and further reading').

Coarctation of the aorta

Aetiology

This is narrowing of the aorta, usually distal to the left subclavian artery adjacent to the insertion of the arterial duct.

Symptoms

The child will often present in the neonatal period with circulatory collapse. Absent femoral pulses or radiofemoral delay are clinical signs of aortic coarctation.

Diagnosis

This is confirmed by cardiac ultrasound.

Treatment

Medication must be given intravenously (prostaglandin infusion) to keep the ductus arteriosus patent and maintain this alternative circulatory route before arranging emergency cardiac surgery to correct the coarctation.

Coeliac disease

Aetiology

Coeliac disease is an autoimmune disorder that involves a heightened immunological response to ingested gliadin in gluten (found in wheat, barley, and rye) in genetically susceptible people. Coeliac disease is associated with other autoimmune conditions.

Symptoms

The disease can present any time after weaning (peak 9 months to 3 years). The condition predominantly affects the small intestine. The symptoms include chronic or intermittent diarrhoea, failure to thrive, or faltering growth. Persistent or unexplained gastrointestinal symptoms including nausea and vomiting, recurrent abdominal pain, cramping or distension, or unexplained iron-deficiency anaemia may also be present.

Diagnosis

To screen for coeliac disease a blood test for tissue transglutaminase (tTGA) is the first-choice test alongside total IgA levels. If the tTGA result is positive then a small intestine biopsy (endoscopic duodenal or jejunal) will be required to confirm the diagnosis. The characteristic features on the biopsy include subtotal villous atrophy.

Treatment

A lifelong gluten-free diet is necessary. Affected children should be monitored as they are at increased risk of small-bowel lymphoma if the diet is not adhered to.

Congenital hypothyroidism

Aetiology

Congenital hypothyroidism (CHT) is caused by reduced or absent thyroid hormones from birth. CHT is mostly caused by anatomical defects (e.g. thyroid aplasia), with some causes due to disordered thyroxine metabolism or rarely hypothalamic–pituitary axis dysfunction.

Symptoms

If undetected and untreated it is associated with irreversible neurological damage and impaired growth.

Diagnosis

CHT is screened for on the 'heelprick' blood spot test shortly after birth as part of the newborn screen.

Treatment

For a confirmed case, treatment is with lifelong thyroxine hormone replacement therapy and regular monitoring to ensure levels remain in the normal range.

Croup/epiglottitis

Aetiology

Croup occurs from 6 months to 6 years of age. Parainfluenza viruses are the commonest cause although other viruses can also cause croup.

Symptoms

The condition is characterized by a barking cough, harsh stridor, hoarseness, coryza, and low-grade fever.

Diagnosis

Croup must be differentiated from epiglottitis which is a life-threatening condition caused by *H. influenzae*. In epiglottitis the child normally looks toxic, is drooling, and has a very high fever.

Treatment

For croup, treatment is with oral dexamethasone or nebulized budesonide. In severe cases nebulized adrenaline can be administered. If epiglottitis is suspected do not approach the child, but arrange urgent senior help including an anaesthetist and ENT surgeon for airway management as IV antibiotics will be required, but IV cannulation can cause total airway blockage secondary to the child's distress.

Cystic fibrosis

Aetiology

CF is the commonest lethal recessive disease of white Europeans. In the UK 1 person in 25 people is a carrier and 1 in 2500 white infants have CF. CF is caused by impairment in the cystic fibrosis transmembrane regulator (CFTR) function. The defect is carried on chromosome 7. There are over 1000 mutations responsible for CF, but the ΔF508 mutation is the commonest. The function of the CFTR is as a chloride-ion channel but also to inhibit the epithelial sodium channel. Therefore if the CFTR is defective there is reduced fluid production at the respiratory epithelial surface and enhanced sodium resorption.

Symptoms

As a consequence of the CFTR defect secretions are viscous and there is impaired mucociliary clearance, increasing the risk of infections. Other organs are also affected including the gut, pancreas, liver, and reproductive system. Children classically present with recurrent chest infections, bulky greasy stools, and failure to thrive.

Diagnosis

The gold standard for diagnosing CF is a sweat test. Other investigations include a sputum or cough swab, chest radiograph, and DNA for genotyping. CF is now often screened for on the Guthrie card by testing for immunoreactive trypsin which is raised in CF.

Treatment

This is based on the prevention of infection with, for example, prophylactic flucloxacillin, intense physiotherapy, optimization of nutrition, and assisting the absorption of fat with exocrine pancreatic supplements (e.g. Creon) and fat-soluble vitamins. Children with CF often require 2-week admissions for IV antibiotics. There are many new/emerging therapies which are improving survival rates.

Developmental dysplasia of the hip

Aetiology

The term 'developmental dysplasia of the hip' (DDH) refers to a spectrum of pathology, ranging from mild acetabular dysplasia with a stable hip through more severe forms of dysplasia, often associated with neonatal hip instability, to established hip dysplasia with or without later subluxation or dislocation. It affects 1–3% of newborn infants.

Symptoms

The condition may be asymptomatic in the newborn period even in the more severe cases. If missed, the condition can lead to later complications such as arthritis of the hip.

Diagnosis

All babies are screened for DDH during their routine newborn check using Ortolani and Barlow's tests to detect hip instability or dislocation of the hip. Babies who were born breech or with a family history of developmental dysplasia are screened with a routine hip ultrasound scan.

Treatment

Clinically dislocated or dislocatable hips need orthopaedic intervention in the neonate either by using a harness to hold the hips in position or operative techniques.

DiGeorge syndrome

Aetiology

This is caused by a deletion on chromosome 22.

Symptoms

Children with this condition normally have cardiac abnormalities (especially tetralogy of Fallot), abnormal facies, hypocalcaemia, thymic aplasia (causing immunodeficiency), and cleft palate.

Diagnosis

This is made on genetic testing by fluorescent in situ hybridization (FISH).

Treatment

This is tailored to the individual as a wide variety of symptoms is seen in individuals with this condition.

Duchenne's muscular dystrophy

Aetiology

DMD is one of over 20 types of muscular dystrophy. The genetic abnormality associated with DMD (X-linked recessive) causes a defect in the production of the dystrophin protein (important in muscle fibres). DMD affects only males (with very rare exceptions) and the defective protein results in gradual muscle cell breakdown and loss causing progressive muscle weakness.

Symptoms

Affected boys usually develop difficulties in walking at around 1–3 years of age. Pelvic girdle muscle weakness is prominent (making it difficult to stand from sitting on the floor) and calf pseudohypertrophy can be seen. Some individuals with DMD may have associated learning difficulties. With progression of the disease boys are often unable to walk by late childhood (8–10 years), become wheelchair dependent, and have a considerably shortened life expectancy (around 25 years).

Diagnosis

Boys affected by DMD may have a raised serum creatinine kinase (CK). Diagnosis is made by genetic testing for specific genes, and muscle biopsies in conjunction with the above clinical picture.

Treatment

Many types of treatments are now available to deal with the progressive weakness and other complications of DMD (cardiomyopathy, respiratory failure, and recurrent chest infections) and may extend life expectancy and improve quality of life.

Erb's palsy

Aetiology

Erb's palsy, also known as brachial plexus paralysis, is a condition which is mainly due to birth trauma.

Symptoms

Traumatic delivery following forceps or shoulder dystocia may cause injury to the brachial plexus resulting in a classical involvement of the upper limb involving extension of the elbow and pronation of the forearm and flexion at the wrist (waiter's tip hand). The paralysis can be partial or complete; the damage to each nerve can range from bruising to tearing.

Diagnosis

This is made from the combination of the above clinical picture and an appropriate history of trauma.

Treatment

Some babies recover on their own, but some may require physiotherapy and rarely surgical intervention.

Fetal alcohol syndrome

Aetiology

Excessive alcohol ingestion by the mother during pregnancy can lead to fetal alcohol syndrome.

Symptoms

Children with the condition have a saddle-shaped nose, maxillary hypoplasia, absent philtrum, and short thin upper lip. The condition is associated with developmental delay and cardiac defects.

Diagnosis

This is made from the combination of the above clinical picture and an appropriate history of alcohol ingestion in pregnancy.

Treatment

This is tailored to the individual as a wide variety of phenotypes is seen in individuals with this condition.

Fragile X

Aetiology

Fragile X syndrome is the most common form of inherited learning difficulties in boys. It is caused by an increased number of gene code repeats on a fragile area of the X chromosome, causing a change in the *FMR1* gene which codes for a protein needed for brain development (if defective this is produced in lower levels or not at all). Females can be affected (due to X-inactivation), but are usually less severely affected.

Symptoms

As well as developmental delay there are some characteristic physical features including long facies with a large forehead and prominent jaw. Affected individuals can have hyperextensible joints and decreased muscle tone as well as flat feet and large testes at puberty.

Diagnosis

This is made on genetic testing.

Treatment

This is supportive and tailored to the individual needs of those affected.

Haemolytic-uraemic syndrome

Aetiology and symptoms

This is a triad of acute renal failure, microangiopathic haemolytic anaemia and thrombocytopenia. It typically occurs following gastroenteritis caused by *E. coli* O157:H7. There may be multiorgan involvement.

Diagnosis

This is made clinically when the above triad is seen and can be supported by microbiological findings of an *E. coli* infection.

Treatment

Supportive, including blood product transfusion and dialysis.

Henoch–Schönlein purpura

Aetiology

Henoch–Schönlein purpura (HSP) is a form of vasculitis which is thought to be triggered by a virus. It typically occurs between the ages of 3 and 10 years.

Symptoms

It is characterized by a purpuric rash to the lower limbs and buttocks, arthralgia, periarticular oedema, abdominal pain (may be secondary to intussusception), and glomerulonephritis.

Diagnosis

This is made on the clinical picture.

Treatment

This is supportive in this self-limiting condition, including pain relief. Monitoring for renal complications is advised (regular urine dipstick testing for protein/blood). Parents are warned of the signs of potential complications of HSP and advised to seek medical attention if these occur (e.g. intussusception, testicular pain).

Hirschsprung's disease

Aetiology

This condition is associated with the absence of ganglion cells from the mesenteric and submucosal plexuses of part of the large bowel. The abnormal bowel extends from the rectum proximally to affect a variable length of bowel.

Symptoms

The condition normally presents within the neonatal period with a failure to pass meconium.

Diagnosis

This is made on rectal biopsy.

Treatment

Surgical intervention is often required to remove the aganglionic section of bowel.

Hydrocoele

Aetiology

A hydrocoele is an abnormal collection of fluid within the remnants of the PV.

Symptoms

These scrotal swellings are usually fluctuant and characteristically transilluminate with a torch held against the scrotum.

Diagnosis and treatment

Normally hydrocoeles resolve by the age of 2 years and do not require any surgical intervention unless persistent.

Hydrocephalus

Aetiology

Hydrocephalus is a disturbance of formation, flow, or absorption of cerebrospinal fluid (CSF). This leads to a rise in pressure within the central nervous system. The most common causes of congenital hydrocephalus are obstruction of the cerebral aqueduct flow, Arnold–Chiari, or Dandy–Walker malformation. In preterm infants hydrocephalus may result from a severe intraventricular haemorrhage. Hydrocephalus in older children may be acquired following a serious head injury.

Symptoms

Hydrocephalus is detected clinically by several signs and symptoms which include a bulging fontanelle or rapid increase in the head circumference while the cranial sutures are still open. Downward cast of the eyes ('sunsetting') may be apparent in any age group. Signs of raised intracranial pressure are seen in the older child when the cranial sutures are fused.

Diagnosis

Made on clinical picture and cranial imaging (e.g. cranial ultrasound or MRI).

Treatment

This is undertaken by neurosurgery and includes procedures such as ventriculoperitoneal shunt insertion.

Hypoplastic left heart

Aetiology and symptoms

This is underdevelopment of the left side of the heart which leads to cyanosis. The mitral valve is small or atretic, the left ventricle is redundant, and there is normally aortic valve atresia. The condition is often associated with coarctation of the aorta.

Diagnosis

Diagnosis is made on cardiac ultrasound scanning.

Treatment

The condition is associated with a very poor prognosis and may be considered inoperable. Palliative surgical procedures or cardiac transplant may be undertaken.

Immune-mediated thrombocytopenic purpura

Aetiology

Immune-mediated thrombocytopenic purpura (ITP) is the commonest cause of thrombocytopenia in childhood. It is caused by an immune-mediated destruction of platelets within the reticuloendothelial system. It mainly occurs between the ages of 2 and 10 years and is thought to be triggered by a virus.

Symptoms

Children affected by ITP will bruise easily and develop purpura. They may also have epistaxis and mucosal bleeding.

Diagnosis

This is made on full blood count in the absence of other causes for the haematological picture seen.

Treatment

Normally treatment is not required and parents are simply advised that their children should refrain from contact sports or similar violent activities to avoid head injury. If there is suggestion of active bleeding then a course of prednisolone may be commenced. In rare cases immunoglobulins are required. Platelet transfusions are only used if there is acute life-threatening haemorrhage, as platelets are quickly consumed.

Juvenile idiopathic arthritis

Aetiology

Juvenile idiopathic arthritis (JIA) is a type of childhood autoimmune arthritis which can occur over a short period of time or can develop into a chronic condition.

Symptoms

Initial symptoms are usually non-specific, such as decreased appetite and weight loss, a salmon pink rash, lethargy, and flu-like symptoms. Following the early signs there is development of joint swelling (often wrist/ankle/knee/hands/feet). The pain associated with these joint swellings is often worse in the morning, improving with use as the day passes. Deformities of the joints can develop over time. There are three types of JIA: polyarticular (affects five or more joints in the first 6 months of the disease), oligoarticular (affects four or fewer joints in the first 6 months of the disease), and systemic (arthritis, fever, and a classic 'salmon pink' rash).

Diagnosis

This is made clinically and by undertaking autoimmune serum tests. JIA is associated with iridocyclitis and patients with JIA require regular slit lamp examination to detect the development of this condition which can cause permanent eye damage if left untreated.

Treatment

This may include the use of steroids and other immunosuppressant drugs.

Kartagener's syndrome

Aetiology

Kartagener's syndrome is characterized by the combination of primary ciliary dyskinesia and dextrocardia. Primary ciliary dyskinesia is associated with a defect in cilia function. The lack of effective ciliary motility causes abnormal mucociliary clearance.

Symptoms

This results in recurrent or persistent respiratory infections, sinusitis, otitis media, and male infertility. Diagnosis is made from nasal brushings which are analysed under an electron microscope revealing an abnormality in the cilia.

Treatment

The management is similar to CF in that children require intense physiotherapy and recurrent antibiotics to combat recurrent infections and colonization.

Kawasaki disease

Aetiology

Kawasaki disease (KD) is an acute, self-limiting vasculitis occurring predominantly in younger children. A cause has not been identified although theories including a superantigen-mediated pathway have been proposed.

Symptoms

KD is characterized by a sudden onset of a high fever which lasts for more than 5 days and four or more of the following: polymorphic rash, bilateral non-exudative conjunctivitis, mucositis (strawberry tongue, lip cracking), cervical lymphadenopathy, and desquamation of the fingers and toes. The child is often very miserable and irritable.

Diagnosis

There is no specific test for KD, but a raised white cell count, thrombocytosis, raised ESR and CRP, and low plasma lipids are some of the features associated with the condition.

Treatment

The most serious complication is the development of coronary artery aneurysms. KD is managed with aspirin (for at least 6 weeks), immunoglobulins, and intense cardiac monitoring and follow-up.

Medium-chain acyl-CoA dehydrogenase deficiency

Aetiology

MCADD is an autosomal recessive condition due to a mutation in the *ACADM* gene causing either an absent or dysfunctional medium-chain acyl-CoA dehydrogenase (MCAD) enzyme (which is essential for breaking down fats to release energy).

Symptoms

These usually appear in infancy or childhood with hypoglycaemia (causing drowsiness and lethargy which can lead to coma, brain damage, and even death) during periods of fasting or illness.

Diagnosis

MCADD is screened for on the 'heelprick' blood spot test shortly after birth as part of the newborn screen.

Treatment

Management involves eating regularly and having sugary drinks during periods of illness to prevent hypoglycaemia.

Meconium ileus

Aetiology

In meconium ileus, low or distal intestinal obstruction results from the impaction of thick and viscous meconium in the distal small bowel.

Symptoms

There is a failure to pass meconium within 48 hours of birth, and a high risk of ileal perforation is associated with this condition.

Diagnosis

Meconium ileus is strongly associated with CF and all children with meconium ileus should be fully investigated for the condition.

Treatment

Surgical, with removal of the meconium plug.

Meningococcal septicaemia

Aetiology

Meningococcal disease can cause bacterial meningitis or septicaemia or a combination of both. It is due to infection with the gram negative bacteria meisseria meningitis (meningococcal).

Symptoms

The commonest symptoms are limb pain, pale or mottled skin, or cold hands and feet. The majority of affected children will develop a rash which in the early stages may be maculopapular and blanching. This nearly always develops into a non-blanching petechial or purpuric rash.

Diagnosis

This is made on microbiological culture and PCR detection of the bacteria.

Treatment

Meningococcal septicaemia is a medical emergency. Children with suspected meningococcal disease need intravenous antibiotics as quickly as possible. The antibiotic of choice is dependent on local policy; however, third-generation cephalosporins are the commonest therapy. If the child is seen in general practice IM benzylpenicillin can be given before sending them to the emergency department.

Nephrotic syndrome

Aetiology and symptoms

Nephrotic syndrome is a disorder of the kidneys characterized by heavy proteinuria, hypoalbuminaemia, and generalized oedema and often associated with hyperlipidaemia. In children the most common type of nephrotic syndrome is minimal change disease (MCD) (80%). Other types include focal segmental glomerulosclerosis (FSGS) and mesangiocapillary glomerulosclerosis (MCGN).

Diagnosis

This is made clinically and on renal biopsy.

Treatment

Most patients with MCD respond to systemic steroid treatment, but many develop a relapsing remitting course.

Noonan's syndrome

Aetiology

This is an autosomal dominant inherited condition.

Symptoms

The range of clinical features is vast and includes a short webbed neck, mild learning difficulties, pectus excavatum, short stature, and pulmonary stenosis or atrial septal defect.

Diagnosis

This is made clinically and can be supported by genetic testing.

Treatment

This is symptomatic and includes the treatment of any cardiac abnormalities and in some individuals the use of growth hormone to improve final height.

Patent ductus arteriosus

Aetiology

Also called persistent ductus arteriosus. This is the failure of closure following birth of the ductus arteriosus which connects the pulmonary artery to the descending aorta. It typically occurs in preterm neonates.

Symptoms

It is detected clinically by bounding femoral pulses and/or a systolic murmur at the left sternal edge.

Diagnosis

Made on cardiac ultrasound scan.

Treatment

Only required if symptomatic. Fluid restriction, indomethacin, or ibuprofen are initially tried. If these fail then surgical duct ligation may be required.

Phenylketonuria

Aetiology

Phenylketonuria (PKU) is an inherited condition (autosomal recessive) characterized by the inability to break down phenylalanine (found in many protein-containing foods such as milk and eggs as well as the sweetener aspartame). Infants with PKU lack the enzyme phenylalanine hydroxylase. Phenylalanine is involved in the production of melanin, hence those with the condition often have lighter hair/skin than unaffected siblings.

Symptoms

Untreated this condition causes phenylalanine and other harmful toxins to build up in the body resulting in damage to the central nervous system and brain damage. An odd 'musty' odour can sometimes be detected on the breath and skin due to these toxins.

Diagnosis

All babies in the UK are screened for PKU on the 'heelprick' blood spot test shortly after birth as part of the newborn screen. If this is positive then further blood and urine testing is undertaken to confirm the diagnosis.

Treatment

The treatment for such individuals is a lifelong diet extremely low in phenylalanine, particularly while still growing in childhood as well as during conception and pregnancy. The outcome is good if the diet is followed.

Posterior urethral valves

Aetiology

Posterior urethral valves (PUV) are excess flaps of tissue in the urethra that cause obstruction to the urinary flow. This congenital condition occurs only in boys and about 1 in 8000 babies.

Symptoms

The degree of urinary outflow obstruction will determine the severity of the condition. In severe obstruction, there might be dilatation of the urinary tract including the bladder and bilateral vesicoureteric reflux. Boys with PUV can present with poor urinary stream, propensity to develop UTIs, and chronic renal failure.

Diagnosis

Early detection of PUV is essential to prevent lasting renal damage and is made by MCUG.

Treatment

Treatment of the valves is surgical by endoscopic valve ablation.

Spina bifida

Aetiology

Spina bifida is a type of neural tube defect which includes a range of spinal cord malformations. Spina bifida cystica (myelomeningocele) is the most common type of spina bifida and is usually found in the lumbar region. The spine is bifid and a cyst forms. Nearly all patients with spina bifida cystica have an Arnold–Chiari malformation (downward displacement of the cerebellar tonsils through the foramen magnum).

Symptoms

A meningocele, a cystic swelling of the dura and arachnoid, protrudes through the spina bifida defect in the vertebral arch. Patients with spina bifida cystica will usually have some degree of lower limb paralysis and sensory loss, bladder and bowel dysfunction, and cognitive dysfunction. Hydrocephalus and brainstem compression can also occur.

Diagnosis

The lesions can be detected antenatally by ultrasound scan and maternal serum alpha-fetoprotein (AFP).

Treatment

Treatment is neurosurgical (usually in a specialist centre) to correct the defect and children often have sequelae which require multidisciplinary team management tailored according to the individual needs.

Sturge–Weber syndrome (encephalotrigeminal angiomatosis)

Aetiology

Sturge–Weber syndrome is a rare neurocutaneous disorder that is present at birth with angiomas involving the leptomeninges (leptomeningeal angiomas) and skin of the face. The cutaneous angioma is called a port wine stain.

Symptoms

Children with this condition will have a port wine stain, commonly on their face, at birth. Depending on the site of the lesions, which are usually in the parietal and occipital regions, there will be a variety of neurological manifestations. These include seizures, focal deficits, such as hemiparesis, headaches, and developmental disorders.

Diagnosis

This is made clinically and brain imaging is used to investigate the presence of intracerebral involvement.

Treatment

Seizure control may improve the neurological outcome. Seizures need treatment with medications and if this fails, epilepsy surgery may be considered in suitable patients. Complications include glaucoma, hemiparesis, and stroke-like episodes. The patient's quality of life depends on how well the symptoms can be prevented or treated. Regular review by ophthalmology and neurology is required.

Tetralogy of Fallot

Aetiology

This condition is defined by four anatomical abnormalities: ventricular septal defect (VSD), overriding aorta, right ventricular outflow tract obstruction (pulmonary stenosis), and right ventricular hypertrophy. It is associated with DiGeorge syndrome.

Symptoms

This is the commonest cause of congenital cyanotic heart disease. Children may present with cyanosis and signs of acute heart failure in the neonatal period and with cyanotic 'spells' where there is worsened cyanosis and syncope.

Diagnosis

Made on cardiac ultrasound scanning.

Treatment

Surgical, by closure of the VSD and widening of the pulmonary outflow tract. Children may require more than one surgical intervention.

Turner's syndrome

Aetiology

Females with Turner's syndrome have the karyotype 45X.

Symptoms

The clinical features are short stature, lymphoedema of the hands and feet in the neonate, neck webbing, cubitus valgus, wide-spaced nipples, heart defects (coarctation of the aorta), ovarian dysgenesis, normal intelligence, and horseshoe kidneys.

Diagnosis

Genetic testing confirms the presence of a single X chromosome.

Treatment

Includes the administration of growth hormone to improve final height and surgical intervention as required for any cardiac defects.

Ventricular septal defect

Aetiology

A VSD is a single or multiple holes in the ventricular septum of the heart. VSD is a common congenital heart defect which can occur alone or in combination with other heart defects.

Symptoms

Patients with a small VSD may be asymptomatic, but may have a systolic murmur audible on cardiac examination (loudest at the apex). Larger VSDs may result in signs and symptoms of heart failure (e.g. poor feeding and slow weight gain, sweating with feeds) in infants.

Diagnosis

Made by cardiac ultrasound scan.

Treatment

Patients with a small hole may often require no treatment (other than monitoring) as this may close spontaneously with time. Larger VSDs may present with heart failure secondary to left to right shunting across the defect. Larger defects may require both medical (diuretics) and surgical intervention.

Williams' syndrome

Aetiology

This syndrome is due to a microdeletion on chromosome 7 and is usually sporadic.

Symptoms

The clinical features include short stature, hypercalcaemia, supravalvular aortic stenosis, and mild to moderate learning difficulties. Characteristics also include a stellate pattern iris and 'cocktail party' speech.

Diagnosis

Made by the clinical features above and confirmed on genetic testing (FISH).

Treatment

This is supportive and focuses on ameliorating the associated abnormalities including avoidance of taking extra calcium and repair of any cardiac abnormalities.

DMSA scan

This is a type of radionuclide scan using dimercaptosuccinic acid (DMSA). It is used most commonly to identify any sign of scarring to the kidneys following a urinary tract infection.

Micturating cystourethrogram

A micturating cystourethrogram (MCUG) is an investigation which involves injecting a contrast medium into the bladder via a catheter. A series of real-time radiographs (fluoroscopy) are subsequently taken. This is the only way of demonstrating vesico-ureteric reflux.

Finals section

Key topics that feature in the exam

We appreciate that the prospect of being faced with a child in a clinical examination fills most candidates with a feeling of impending doom. Do not fear! You will now be equipped with plenty of tips which will assist you in the heat of an exam. This section will cover some of the common and key topics which you are likely to face in a paediatric clinical exam (see Table 14.33). It is beyond the scope of this book to cover all the potential topics. Please note that the format and timings for the scenarios will vary depending on which medical school you attend. See Cases 14.18–14.22 for advice relating to examination problems in paediatrics.

OSCE examples

History-taking scenario

A 9-month-old baby has been brought to the emergency department following a presumed fit. You are the FY1 doctor working in the emergency department. Take a focused history from the mother. You do not need to examine the child. Once you have completed the history explain to the mother what you think is the most likely diagnosis and how you wish to manage the child. You have 10 minutes.

The examiner will expect you to:

- Determine whether this was a febrile or an afebrile seizure.
- Ascertain the duration of the seizure.
- Was it definitely a fit or a rigor? Did the child lose consciousness? Was it partial or generalized? Was there a witness?
- Was there a postictal phase?
- Take a history with regards to other aspects of the history focusing on the past medical history, development, and family history of epilepsy and febrile seizures.
- Explanation: statistics on the frequency (3% of children aged 6 months–5 years), risk of the child developing epilepsy (1% will develop epilepsy), and the chances of the child having another febrile seizure (1 in 3). The mother may ask about the effects on the child's development (no impact). Say you will provide a leaflet if the emergency department has one.

Table 14.33 Common Finals cases

History-taking topics
Fever
Rash
Vomiting
Diarrhoea
Febrile convulsion
Asthma control
Recurrent abdominal pain/acute abdominal pain
Examinations
Respiratory: cystic fibrosis
Cardiovascular: innocent murmur
Gastrointestinal: inflammatory bowel disease
Neurological: squint assessment, cerebral palsy
Development assessment
Syndromes: trisomy 21/Turner's syndrome
Information giving/explanation
Explain to a mother the complications associated with Down's syndrome
Demonstrate how to use an inhaler/aerochamber/peak flow meter
Explain to a mother how to manage nocturnal enuresis
Plotting weight and height on a growth chart and interpreting growth charts
Infant colic
Urinary tract infection management and investigations
Immunization counselling
Explain neonatal jaundice
Counsel mother about benefits of breastfeeding

Examination scenario

You are the FY1 working in primary care. A 5-year-old girl presents to your surgery with a fever. Perform a thorough cardiovascular examination on this child and present your

CASE 14.18

Some advice relating to examination problems in paediatrics

Problem: How will I manage to complete the whole examination of the child in the allocated time?

Solution: You will never be asked to examine every system of the child in one scenario. Therefore it is important to read the question carefully to ensure that the correct system is examined. Always check what the focus of the station is, e.g. history-taking, examination of a system, or information giving.

CASE 14.19

Problem: The child refuses to cooperate or becomes distressed.

Solution: Remember that the choice of patient needs to be practical. The examiner is unlikely to bring either an unwell child or an extremely young child or baby to the examination. Therefore your subject is likely to be a relatively healthy, cooperative, and non-intimidating school-aged child! If the child is not willing to cooperate or becomes upset, do not panic. This does not mean that you have failed. Children get tired and grumpy, so don't take it personally. The important thing to remember is that a lot of information can be gathered through **observation**. You will lose marks if you try to persist with the examination and upset the child further.

CASE 14.20

Problem: The child will not perform certain milestones during a development assessment.

Solution: This is not an uncommon occurrence as children are not performing monkeys! Ask the examiner if it would be all right to ask the mother/carer some questions instead. This is always helpful when performing a development assessment. The examiner is more likely to score you highly if you use your initiative and observational skills rather than trying to examine an unhappy child and distressing them.

CASE 14.21

Problem: Will I be marked down if I do not examine the child in a systematic way?

Solution: The examiner will expect you to be opportunistic. If you are confronted with a toddler then it would be wise to auscultate the chest first before the child becomes upset. If there are areas which you have had to leave out due to lack of patient cooperation explain to the examiner what these areas were.

CASE 14.22

Problem: How do I describe dysmorphic features without upsetting the carer or child?

Solution: This is always tricky and you must be confident with your diagnosis before stating that a child looks dysmorphic. If you think that a child has trisomy 21 describe the features that you see: For example, 'On examination I note that Jack has epicanthic folds, a single palmar crease, and low-set ears, features which are consistent with a diagnosis of trisomy 21'. If you are not sure whether the child is dysmorphic do not comment on this.

findings and diagnosis to the examiner at the end. You have 10 minutes.

The examiner will expect you to:

- Demonstrate a good rapport with the child and demonstrate respect for the child's modesty.
- Perform a thorough cardiovascular examination with a systematic approach.
- Present your findings in a succinct manner.
- Demonstrate that you have heard a murmur and try to describe the murmur as soft and systolic at the left sternal edge with no radiation.
- Conclude your examination by asking to plot the child's height and weight on an appropriate growth chart (children with trisomy 21 and Turner's syndrome have a specific growth chart).
- Explain that the most likely diagnosis is an innocent murmur.
- Understand the management of an innocent murmur.

Information giving

You are the FY1 working in a paediatric clinic. An 8-year-old girl, accompanied by her mother, presents with bedwetting. Take a focused history and discuss the various management options with the family. You have 10 minutes. The examiner will expect you to:

- Determine whether this is primary or secondary nocturnal enuresis.
- Ensure that there are no contributory factors, e.g. spina bifida, urinary tract infection, or constipation.
- Take a history of the child's fluid intake.
- Include a detailed social and family history.
- Explain how common nocturnal enuresis is, preferably with statistics (nocturnal enuresis occurs in 10% of 5-year-olds, 5% of 10-year-olds).
- Explore the various management options, e.g. star charts, enuresis alarms, drug options.
- Provide a leaflet if available.

Questions

1 Name three causes of a non-blanching rash in children other than meningococcal septicaemia.
2 What are the five signs of respiratory distress in children?
3 What are the four domains of development?
4 Provide four examples of 'red flags' that could be relevant to a child with possible developmental delay.
5 How might an infant present with cerebral palsy?
6 How do you diagnose trisomy 21 and what treatment is available?
7 What is the first stage of pubertal development in girls?
8 How will you differentiate a respiratory condition from a cardiac condition in the newborn infant?
9 Which hormones are responsible for the adolescent growth spurt?
10 What are the antenatal risk factors that might indicate underlying congenital abnormalities in neonates?

References and further reading

Advanced Life Support Group (ALSG). *Advanced paediatric life support*, 5th edn. Wiley-Blackwell, Chichester, 2011.

British Paediatric Neurology Association (BPNA). *Child's Glasgow coma scale*, revised, 2001. http://www.bpna.org.uk/audit/GCS.PDF

Denver II tool. To obtain test and training materials for the Denver II tool, contact DDM, Inc. 1(800) 419–4729, Sales@denverII.com, or UK Hogrefe Ltd., 4630 Burgner House, Oxford Business Park South, OX4 2SLJ, UK, +44(0) 1865 402900, http://www.hogrefe.co.uk

Department for Education. *What is the difference between safeguarding and child protection?* http://www.education.gov.uk/popularquestions/a0064461/safeguarding-and-child-protection Accessed 11 February 2013.

Foster HE, Jandial S. pGALS—a screening examination of the musculoskeletal system in school-aged children. *Hands On. Reports on the Rheumatic Diseases;* series 5, no.15, 2008. http://www.arthritisresearchuk.org/shop/products/publications/information-for-medical-professionals/hands-on/series-5/h015-series-5.aspx

General Medical Council (GMC). *Protecting children and young people: The responsibilities of all doctors*, 2012. http://www.gmc-uk.org/guidance/ethical_guidance/13257.asp Accessed 11 February 2013

Jordan N, Tyrrell J. Management of enlarged cervical lymph nodes. *Current Pediatrics* 2004; **14**:154–159.

National Society for the Prevention of Cruelty to Children (NSPCC). *Worried about a child? Online advice.* http://www.nspcc.org.uk/help-and-advice/worried-about-a-child/online-advice/online-advice_wdh85524.html Accessed 11 February 2013.

NICE Clinical Guidance. *Urinary tract infections in children (CG54)*, August 2007.

NICE Clinical Guidance. *Feverish illness in children (CG47)*, May 2007.

NICE Clinical Guidance. *Diarrhoea and vomiting in children under 5 (CG84)*, April 2009.

NICE Clinical Guidance. *When to suspect child maltreatment (CG89)*, December 2009.

Raine J, Donaldson M, Gregory J et al. *Practical endocrinology and diabetes in children*, 2nd edn. Blackwell, Oxford, 2005.

Sheridan MD. *From birth to five years: children's developmental progress*, 3rd edn (revised and updated by Ajay Sharma and Helen Cockerill), Routledge, New York, 2008.

Wheeler R. A plea for consistency over competence in children. *BMJ* 2006; **332**:807.

15 Chest radiograph

Introduction

The chest radiograph (CXR) is one of the most commonly requested investigations. All CXRs will be reported by an experienced radiologist, at a later date. As a junior doctor, after admitting your patient, you will be expected to interpret the CXR straight away. So, it is not surprising that as a student your seniors will test you on the wards or even in examinations!

The CXR is an important investigation. It allows us to diagnose both acute and chronic pathology affecting the cardiorespiratory system. It is a non-invasive, relatively cheap, and easily performed investigation. However, ionizing radiation is potentially harmful. You should be especially aware of exposing pregnant women to X-rays. They can cause radiogenic cancers and hereditary disorders. Radiation protection regulations have been designed to prevent this. The CXR will not occur frequently in the examination setting, but once you have qualified there will be no avoiding it. It is strongly advised that you master the art of CXR interpretation. It involves recognition of certain patterns. The more you see or indeed look for these patterns, the more easily you will be able to spot them. Of course, you must also think about the clinical features associated with the CXR. Often in the examination, you will be given a short resumé to point you in the right direction. Before the various patterns of CXR pathology are discussed, you must first appreciate how a CXR is produced and be able to identify the normal structures on a CXR.

How X-rays are produced

X-rays are generated in vacuum tubes that produce a beam of radiation. This beam is then directed at the patient's chest. X-rays are absorbed to a variable degree by different body tissues depending on their density. The amount of radiation emerging from the other side of the patient is reflected in different shades of grey on a film that catches the X-rays. Black areas indicate low-density tissue (e.g. air in the lungs). White areas indicate high density (bone). Strictly speaking, an X-ray is the radiation that is produced by the machine and directed at the patient, and the radiograph is the picture that we look at. Despite this, most people (including doctors) colloquially refer to the radiograph as an X-ray.

The normal chest radiograph

See Fig. 15.1. CXRs are usually taken on full inspiration. The normal CXR is termed PA, meaning the X-rays pass through the patient from posterior (P) to anterior (A). Sometimes a patient is too unwell to leave their bed and they will have a portable CXR where the radiation beam is directed from the anterior to posterior (this is called an AP CXR).

A CXR (except in a few circumstances) should be taken on full inspiration. The direction from which the film is taken is important. As you can see from Table 15.1, the direction of projection will change the size of structures seen on the CXR. The PA CXR taken on deep

inspiration provides most information about the chest and is the gold standard. Alternative angles of projection may be used for other reasons (see Table 15.2). You must be able to identify the structures and landmarks on a normal CXR before considering any pathology. Figure 15.2 is a schematic diagram of the important features seen on a normal CXR.

Tip

If possible, CXRs should be taken in the radiology department where a good quality PA film can be produced. This maximizes the chance of getting useful diagnostic information.

Table 15.1 Differences between PA and AP films

	PA	**AP**
Heart	Not magnified	Magnified
Scapula	Rotated away from the lungs	Superimposed on the lungs
Clavicles	Cross lungs about 5 cm below apices	Projected above lung apices

Table 15.2 Different angles of projections and their indications

Angle	The indication
PA	Gold standard
AP	Unwell, bedbound, or immobile patient
Lateral	To localize opacities or masses
Expiration	To identify a small pneumothorax or bronchial obstruction
Lateral decubitus (*de-cube-it-us*)	To identify a subpulmonary effusion (a small amount of fluid may be hidden by the diaphragm in the upright position; getting a patient to lie on their side will allow the fluid to redistribute itself so that it can be seen)

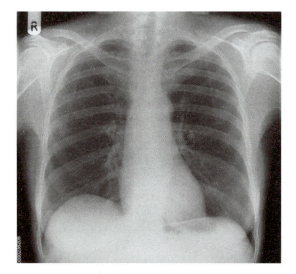

Figure 15.1 A normal chest radiograph.

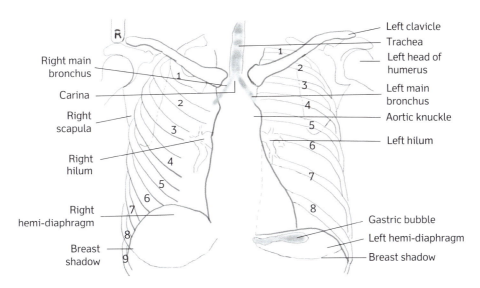

Figure 15.2 Structures shown on a normal chest radiograph. Numbers on the left-hand side of the diagram indicate anterior ribs and numbers on the right-hand side indicate posterior ribs.

How to analyse the chest radiograph (summary)

1 Orientation
2 Patient details
3 Technical factors (optional)
4 Bones
5 Trachea
6 Heart
7 Mediastinum
8 Hilar regions
9 Lungs
10 Fissures
11 Diaphragm
12 Soft tissues
13 Below the diaphragm
14 Hidden areas

How to analyse the chest radiograph (in detail)

There is no single correct method to study a CXR. What matters is how you approach it and whether you follow a routine. An examiner can tell the difference between a candidate who is familiar with a CXR and one who is not, even if they both get the correct diagnosis! You must therefore have a systematic approach and it is probably best to talk as you go along. The scheme below is the one that the author uses.

Getting started

1 Orientation

In an examination situation, the film is likely to be correctly oriented on a light box. It is often the examiner's prize CXR, so it is important that you do not touch it. The easiest way to start off on the wrong foot is to mark the CXR with clammy fingerprints or splodges of ink. If the examiner passes you the CXR, then they will expect you to place it on the light box. Do not hold it up to the light (as you often see done in television dramas).

2 Patient details

First look at the label and identify the patient and the date. Say something like, 'This is a plain PA chest X-ray of Hugh Jart taken on 20 September 2012 at St James's University Hospital.' At this point it is recommended that you tell the examiner that you will be studying the CXR in a systematic order and then stand back and look at the CXR as a whole. This is because if there is a huge lesion in the lung fields that even a mole with cataracts could not miss and you are found to be studying the intricacies of the bone trabeculations (*tra-beck-you-lay-shuns*), the examiner will become frustrated! It is usually prudent to say something like, 'There is an obvious lesion in the left upper zone, which I will come back to study after I have examined the X-ray systematically.'

....

Tip

Watch out for dextrocardia, which is an examination favourite. In this case the heart will lie on the patient's right side. Examiners may be very crafty and put the CXR on the box **the wrong way round** to mimic a normal CXR. The only clue is that the CXR marker will be on the patient's left (on your right-hand side).

....

Technical factors

3 *Technical factors (optional)*

If you are feeling brave, you can mention the alignment of the CXR. If a CXR is central, the medial end of the clavicles will be equidistant from the vertebral spinal processes. If the patient has rotated to the right, then the medial aspect of the right clavicle will be much nearer the vertebral process than the left and if they have rotated to the left the medial aspect of the left clavicle will be closer to the vertebral process. See Fig. 15.3.

The CXR should be correctly exposed. If it is overexposed then the bones will be dark and look transparent (Fig. 15.4). Similarly, if it is underexposed the bones and lung fields will be white (Fig. 15.5). The best way to check is to look at the vertebrae. If you can only just see all the vertebral bodies through the mediastinum (*media-sty-numb*), then it is correctly penetrated (Fig. 15.1).

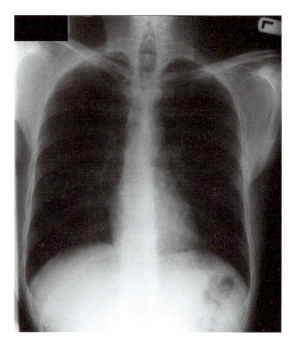

Figure 15.4 Overexposed CXR.

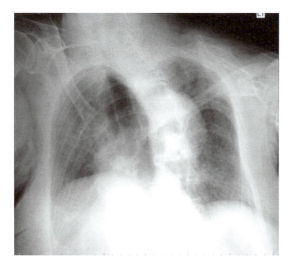

Figure 15.3 Poorly aligned CXR.

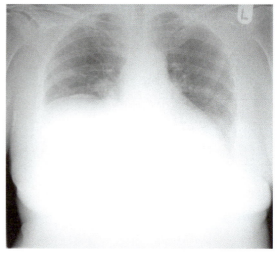

Figure 15.5 Underexposed CXR.

CXRs taken during expiration look different from those that are taken on inspiration (they are normally taken in inspiration) (see Figs. 15.6 and 15.7).

....

Tip

Describing the technical features is optional and not advisable unless you know what you are talking about (it is often best left to the radiologists themselves).

....

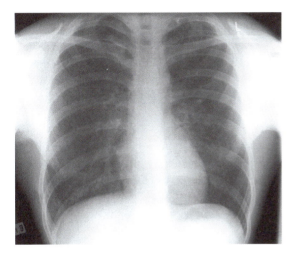

Figure 15.6 CXR on inspiration.

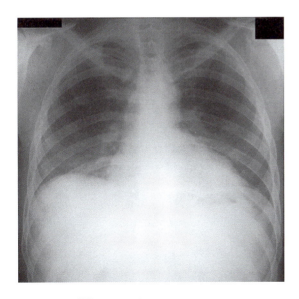

Figure 15.7 CXR on expiration.

Bones

4 Bones

You should carefully survey all the bones. Step closer to the CXR. Start in the periphery with the humeri, the clavicles, and then the scapulae. Progress to the vertebrae and eventually the ribs. Look for fractures, bony metastases (*met-ass-ta-seize*), and osteoporosis. Follow the edges of each bone to look for fractures. Look for areas of blackness within each bone (that might suggest bone metastases) and compare the density of the bones, which should be the same on each side. The CXR shows the ribs as they arch around the thorax. For convention, we therefore divide them into anterior and posterior (see Fig. 15.2).

Trachea

5 Trachea

This is central, with a little deviation to the right around the aortic knuckle. If it is not central, there must be some pathology either pulling or pushing it to one side (see Fig. 15.8). It will be pulled to one side by fibrosis or collapse of a lung segment. It will be pushed away by a superior mediastinal mass, such as retrosternal goitre. The angle of the carina (*ka-reen-a*) is 60–70°. It will be widened by dilatation of the left atrium or lymphadenopathy in this area (see Fig. 15.9).

Heart

6 Heart

Usually only one-third of the heart lies to the right of the mediastinum. The size of the heart should always be determined. We do this by calculating the cardiothoracic ratio. This is the ratio of the transverse cardiac diameter to the transverse internal thoracic diameter and it should be less than 1:2 (see Fig. 15.10). If the cardiothoracic ratio is greater than this, this is called cardiomegaly (see Fig. 15.11). There are at least four important causes that should cross your mind: ischaemic heart disease (IHD), valvular heart disease (VHD), pericardial effusion, and cardiomyopathy. If you are asked to compare the heart on successive CXRs, then any increase in transverse cardiac diameter greater than 1.5 cm is significant. Remember that the heart will look larger on AP films, on supine films, and also on expiration.

The composition of the heart shadow is described in Fig. 15.12 and Table 15.3. If we look at the lateral film then

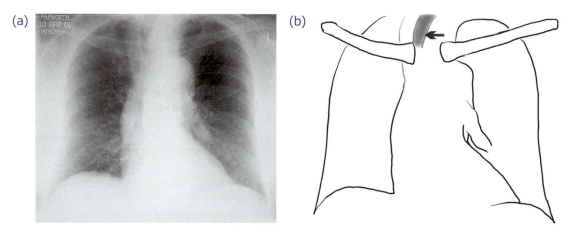

Figure 15.8 Deviation of the trachea (see arrow) due to thyroid cancer.

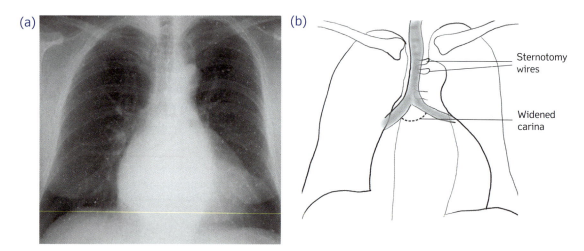

Figure 15.9 Widened carina due to left atrial enlargement. Note sternotomy wires in (b). In this context this would suggest previous cardiac surgery and with left atrial enlargement the likeliest candidate would be the mitral valve.

> **Key point**
>
> The heart will always look larger on AP films, supine films, and also on expiration. Therefore you cannot make an accurate judgement on the size of the heart.

the posterior border of the heart is composed of the left ventricle and the anterior border the right ventricle.

Mediastinum

7 Mediastinum

The edge of the mediastinum should be clear. Some fuzziness is acceptable at the angle between the heart and the diaphragm (the cardiophrenic (*card-ee-owe-fren-ick*) angle), the apices (*ay-pi-seize*), and the right hilum (see Fig. 15.13). A hazy edge to any other parts of the mediastinum suggests a problem with the neighbouring lung (either collapse or consolidation). The mediastinum may be widened: causes include mediastinal tumours, mediatinitis, pleural effusions, and lymphadenopathy.

Hilar regions

8 Hilar regions

These are due to the pulmonary arteries and upper lobe veins. They should be of equal density and size with concave borders. The left hilum (*high-lum*) is usually 1 cm higher than the right (see Figs. 15.1 and 15.2).

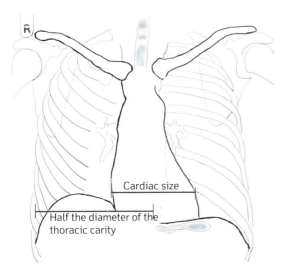

Figure 15.10 How to calculate the cardiothoracic ratio.

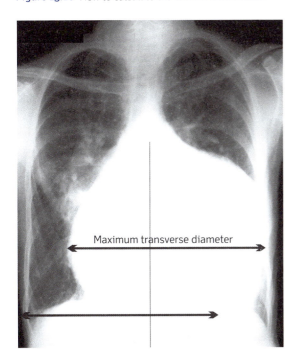

Figure 15.11 CXR showing cardiomegaly. Even with the naked eye it can be seen that the heart dominates the whole thoracic cavity.

Lungs

9 Lungs

Radiologically the lungs are divided into zones. Each lung has three zones:

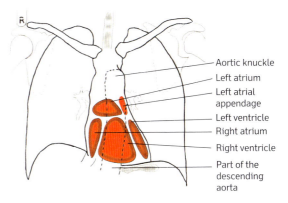

Figure 15.12 Composition of the heart border.

Table 15.3 The composition of the heart border

Heart border	Area	Composition
Right heart border	Right diaphragm to right hilum	Right atrium
Right hilum and above	Superior vena cava	
Left heart border	Left diaphragm to left hilum	Left ventricle
Concavity below left hilum	Left atrial appendage	
Level of left hilum	Left pulmonary artery	
Above left hilum	Aortic knuckle	

- **upper zone**—from apices to anterior rib 2
- **middle zone**—from anterior rib 2 to anterior rib 4
- **lower zone**—from anterior rib 4 to diaphragm.

Remember, anatomically the right lung has three lobes and the left lung only two (see Fig. 5.8). When interpreting the CXR you should talk in terms of zones. The lungs should be of equal translucency. The only structures that can be visualized within the normal lungs are the blood vessels, the interlobar fissures, and the walls of large bronchi seen end on. Blood vessels can be seen because they are relatively opaque when compared with the surrounding air-filled, radiolucent lungs. If the alveoli become filled with fluid, then they will become

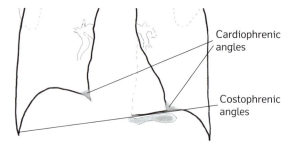

Figure 15.13 Diagram of CXR showing fuzzy areas.

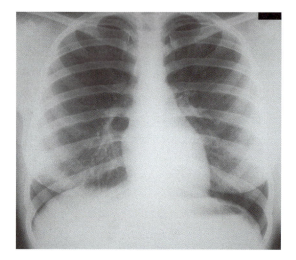

Figure 15.14 CXR showing breast shadowing.

opaque and also any mass lesion will be opaque. Similarly, breast shadows will cause the lower lung zones to appear more opaque (see Figs. 15.14 and 15.15). So, it is important not only to compare one zone with its opposite counterpart, but also to compare zones on the same side.

Fissures

10 Fissures

The interlobar fissures are the anatomical markings of the lobes of the lungs. On the PA view only the right horizontal fissure is seen. It runs from the right hilum to the sixth rib anteriorly in the axillary line. It divides the right upper lobe from the right middle lobe. The oblique fissure is only present on the right side dividing the right middle lobe from the right lower lobe. It tends to be only seen on the lateral CXR. Accessory fissures are

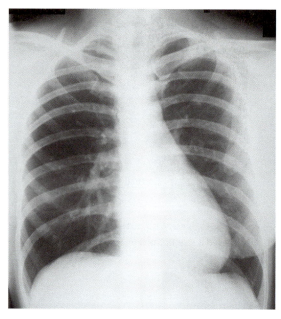

Figure 15.15 Congenital absence of the right breast. Note the darkened lung field on the right compared to the left (and Fig. 15.14).

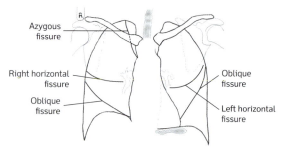

Figure 15.16 Lung fissures.

occasionally seen—the azygus (*as-eye-gus*) and the left horizontal fissure (see Fig. 15.16).

Soft tissues

11 Soft tissues

Look for the normal breast shadowing in women. Watch out for the patient who has had a mastectomy—this is an examination favourite! The soft shadowing will be absent on the side of the mastectomy and is easily missed unless you are actively looking for it (see Fig. 15.24 and compare with Fig. 15.15).

(a)

(b)

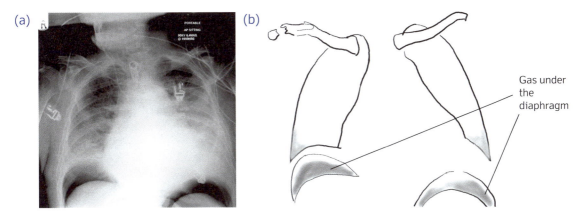

Gas under the diaphragm

Figure 15.17 CXR showing pneumoperitoneum. Note the coincidental fracture of the right clavicle, suggesting that trauma played a role in the genesis of this condition.

Diaphragm

12 Diaphragm

The diaphragm should have a smooth outline and be convex upwards. Loss of the outline implies lower lobe infection. The dome of the right hemidiaphragm is 2 cm higher than the left and on full inspiration lies at the sixth rib anteriorly. The highest point of the right hemidiaphragm is in the middle of the right lung field, the left hemidiaphragm tends to lie more laterally in the left lung field (see Figs. 15.1 and 15.2). There may be a fat pad adjacent to the cardiac border in obese people.

Below the diaphragm

13 Below the diaphragm

Most CXRs will demonstrate gas in the stomach—the gastric bubble (see Figs. 15.1 and 15.2). Only the upper border of the diaphragm is normally seen. If there is air in the abdomen (pneumoperitoneum) (*new-mow-perry-toe-knee-um*) from say a perforation of viscera, then air will be seen below the diaphragm, but only if the film is taken as an erect CXR (see Fig. 15.17). Occasionally, you may see gallstones.

Hidden areas

14 Hidden areas

Areas that are often forgotten are the lung apices and behind the heart. Remember to scan these areas, especially if you have not found any pathology. A fluid level behind the heart could represent a hiatus hernia (see Fig. 15.18), or achalasia (*ay-ka-lazia*) of the oesophagus.

Abnormalities within the chest radiograph

This section takes you through the common and important pathologies that can be identified on a plain CXR. The white lung field, the black lung field, the heart, and the hilum are considered.

White lung field

There are many causes of white lung fields on a CXR. The most common are discussed in this section.

Pleural effusion, collapse, and consolidation

Differentiating between these three pathologies can be difficult. They all cause an area of the lung to become white. See Figs. 15.19–15.21 and Table 15.4. Air bronchograms are useful features. In consolidation, the alveolar (*al-vee-owe-lar*) air spaces become filled with fluid, whereas the airways do not. So, you will see small black airways against a white background (see Fig. 15.22). Because consolidation involves the collection of alveolar fluid, the denser shadowing representing fluid will be found at the bottom of an area of consolidation. Consolidation always requires follow-up CXRs. Radiological resolution always lags behind clinical resolution. Therefore, a follow-up CXR should be done approximately a month later to check if the CXR has

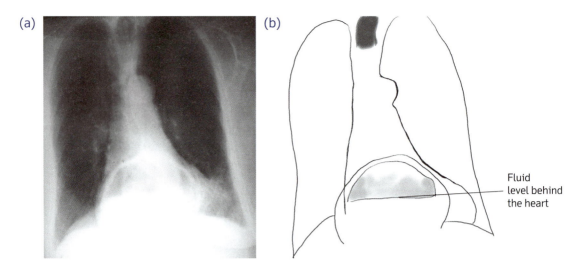

Figure 15.18 CXR showing fluid level behind the heart. This is a hiatus hernia.

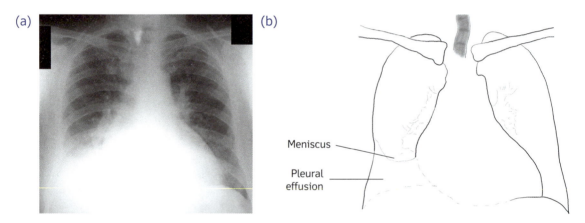

Figure 15.19 Pleural effusion. The right hemidiaphragm is obscured and the clue to the aetiology is the concave meniscus which indicates fluid.

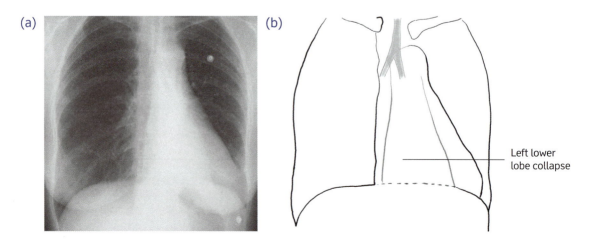

Figure 15.20 Lobar collapse. A triangular shape behind the heart obscures the medial portion of the left hemidiaphragm.

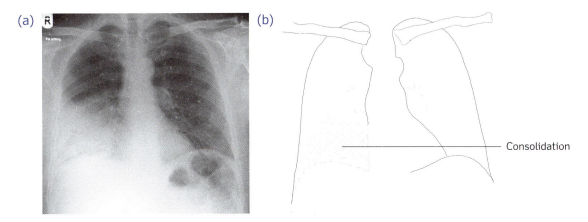

(a)   (b)

Consolidation

Figure 15.21 Consolidation. The right hemidiaphragm is obscured but unlike Fig. 15.19 the superior edge of the opacity is ill-defined (without a meniscus).

Table 15.4 Contrasting the differing characteristics of effusion, collapse, and consolidation

Pathology	Characteristics
Effusion	Homogenous (*hu-mo-jen-us*) shadowing[a], meniscus (especially on lateral CXR), lateral peak (a raised hemidiaphragm will have raised central peak), mediastinal shift away from effusion, look for causes of the effusion (cardiomegaly of heart failure, lung masses/ metastases)
Collapse	Mediastinal shift towards the collapse, distortion of radiological landmarks (movement of fissures, loss of volume of a lung), trachea deviated towards side of collapse, homogeneous shadowing[a]
Consolidation	Heterogeneous (*heh-to-roger-nuss*) shadowing[b], air bronchograms, similar changes on previous CXRs implies fibrosis

[a] In homogenous shadowing the area concerned will look completely white.
[b] In heterogeneous shadowing there will be small areas of blackness.

cleared. If it has not, further investigations are required to rule out an underlying cause such as cancer.

Pneumonectomy

In clinical practice, you will know from the history that a patient has had a pneumonectomy (*new-mow-neck-tummy*). Examinations unfortunately are not always real life! Essentially there will be one white lung field. The remaining lung herniates to the other side, pushing with it both the trachea and the mediastinum. Some of the ribs on the side of the pneumonectomy will have been cut and removed (see Fig. 15.23).

The coin lesion

Coin lesions are exactly what their name suggests. They are large, discrete, often round, white lesions found anywhere in the lung zones. They are significant because they usually represent cancer (either primary lung cancer or metastatic deposits). There are other possible causes:

- **benign tumour**—e.g. benign hamartoma (*hammer-toe-ma*)
- **infection**—causing a focal area of consolidation
- **infarction**—pulmonary embolism (PE)
- **granuloma**—e.g. rheumatoid nodule.

(a)

(b)

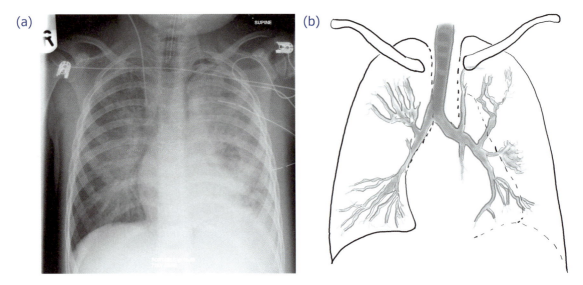

Figure 15.22 Air bronchogram due to extensive consolidation in both lungs.

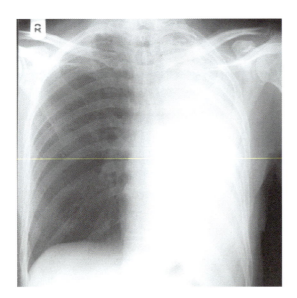

Figure 15.23 Left pneumonectomy. Other possibilities for this appearance include a large left pleural effusion (with associated lung collapse to explain the lack of deviation of the trachea to the right) or extensive consolidation of the left lung.

Metastatic deposits to the lungs are a frequent cause of malignant coin lesions (see Fig. 15.24). Certain radiological characteristics of coin lesions help in determining the cause (but the history and examination are more helpful). For example, consider a young female with a severe symmetrical deforming arthropathy. She is likely to have rheumatoid nodules in the lung, whereas an elderly, cachectic lifelong smoker is likely to have a primary bronchogenic lung carcinoma. The following characteristics suggest the following causes:

- spiculated, irregular, lobulated—**malignancy**
- calcification (dense white within the lesion)—**benign**
- cavitating (darker centre)—**tuberculosis (TB)**
- air bronchogram within the lesion—**consolidation**
- multiple coin lesions—**metastases**
- associated with lymphadenopathy or bony metastases—**malignant**.

The cavitating lesion

These are hollow coin lesions. Essentially you will see a coin lesion with a dark centre representing air/fluid. You may detect a fluid level within the lesion. The causes of cavitating lung lesions are:

- **infection**—abscess, especially *Staphylococcus aureus* (they are sometimes called pneumatoceles) (*new-mat-owe-seals*)
- **true cavitation**—TB
- **tumour**—malignant
- **infarction**—PE, with a central area of necrosis within the coin lesion.

Again look at all the old CXRs to decide the rate of growth. Also, consider the clinical scenario. Patients with staphylococcal lung abscesses are systemically unwell (see Fig. 15.25).

(a) 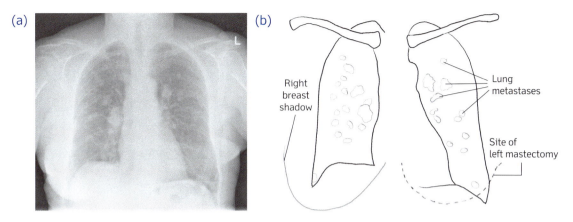 (b)

Figure 15.24 Breast cancer with mastectomy and lung metastases.

(a) 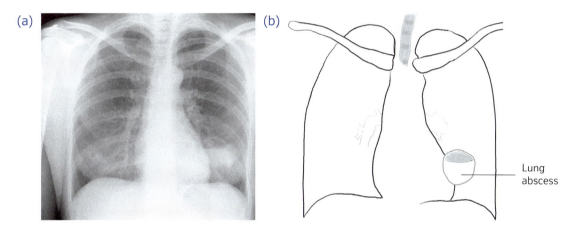 (b)

Figure 15.25 Lung abscess.

Left ventricular failure

The author guarantees that during your first general medical attachment you will admit a patient with acute left ventricular failure. You will have to diagnose and treat it. Often, the patient is too unwell to give a history, so you will rely heavily on the examination and results of investigations. The CXR will be crucial to your diagnosis. Remember left ventricular failure is only one cause of pulmonary oedema. A CXR of left ventricular failure will show the following (see Fig. 15.26).

- **Upper lobe diversion**. Normally, the upper lobe blood vessels are narrower than those of the lower lobe. So, if they are the same width or larger, then this is upper lobe diversion. This only applies if the film is taken erect—upper lobe diversion is normal on supine films. Upper lobe diversion arises because the lower lobe alveoli become hypoxic, thus causing vasoconstriction.

- **Cardiomegaly**. Measure the cardiothoracic ratio as described earlier.

- **Kerley (*curly*) B lines**. (*Peter James Kerley (1900–1978), Irish neurologist with an interest in radiology.*) These are small, horizontal, non-branching white lines seen at the periphery of the lower lung zones (see Fig. 15.27).

- **Bat's wing appearance**. Only in severe left ventricular failure will you see this white wing-shaped appearance spreading from the hilar regions. It represents alveolar oedema.

Lung fibrosis

Lung fibrosis is a less common cause of a white lung. It is a chronic process, so you can see it in a series of CXRs. It causes shrinkage of the lungs. Often the fibrosis is bilateral and basal. It may be unilateral; if so, it will cause the mediastinum to be pulled across to the side of the fibrosis.

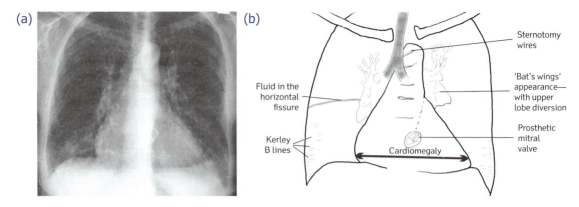

Figure 15.26 Left ventricular failure. Note the prosthetic mitral valve indicating previous VHD.

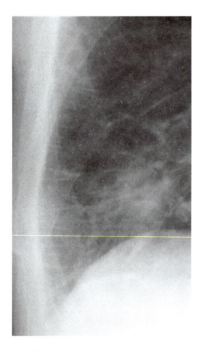

Figure 15.27 Close-up of Kerley B lines.

Radiologically, lung fibrosis is described as being 'reticulonodular'. This really means a meshwork of lines and rings (see Fig. 15.28). The reticular nodular appearance may be very fine, giving a 'ground glass' appearance. In the later stages, the lung becomes 'honeycombed' in appearance (see Fig. 15.29). There are many causes of lung fibrosis. A few are shown in Table 5.16.

Black lung field

You will be pleased to know that there are fewer causes of a black than white lung field. Four causes are discussed

here. An ordinary lung field on a CXR is a dark shade of grey. However, sometimes it is jet black when compared to other zones on the same CXR or to another CXR. When considering how black a lung field is, remember that the penetration of the CXR is important. If the penetration is satisfactory, the most likely cause is chronic obstructive pulmonary disease (COPD). This is bilateral, whereas pneumothoraces (*new-mow-thor-a-seas*) and PE tend to be unilateral.

Tip

Check to see if the patient is rotated (see 'Technical factors'). The rotation can lead to one side of the chest being closer to the CXR source and therefore more penetrated (and hence more black), while the other side is further away, less penetrated (and less black).

Chronic obstructive pulmonary disease

Patients suffering from COPD have hyperexpanded chests (see Fig. 15.30), so if you count the number of ribs anteriorly above the diaphragm there will be more than seven. Similarly, there will be 10 or more above the diaphragm posteriorly. The diaphragms will be flat. If you hold a ruler across one hemidiaphragm, drawing an imaginary line between the costophrenic and cardiophrenic angles, then the highest elevation of the dome of the diaphragm above the line should be no more than 1 cm if the chest is hyperinflated (see Fig. 15.31). The heart will look small and thin in the context of an overexpanded chest. However, if the heart looks normal in size or is enlarged, you should consider heart failure associated with the COPD (cor pulmonale is right ventricular failure secondary to COPD). Bullae (*bully*) may be present on the CXR. These

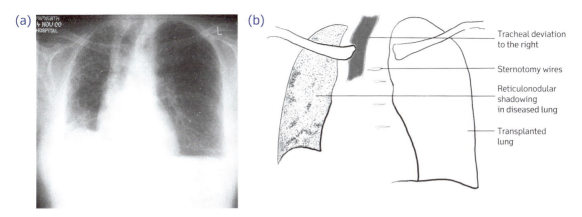

Figure 15.28 Reticular nodular shadowing of the right lung. NB: the patient has had a left lung transplant.

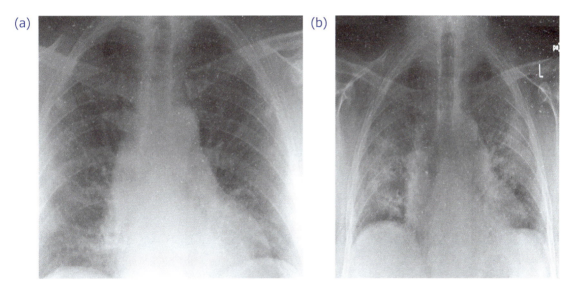

Figure 15.29 Progression of interstitial fibrosis: (a) interstitial lung fibrosis; (b) CXR of patient in Fig 15.28, 7 months later. Note the developing 'honeycombing' of the lung.

are round, dense, black areas surrounded by a thin line representing thin-walled air spaces. If only one is present this is called a bulla.

Pneumothorax

A unilateral black lung field is an important finding. It often indicates a pneumothorax (see Fig. 15.32). Unfortunately, pneumothoraces (*new-mah-thor-a-seas*) can be very small and very difficult to visualize. For this reason, if you suspect a pneumothorax and it is not apparent on the provisional film, then an expiratory film will make it stand out. On expiration the lungs shrink so the pneumothorax becomes more prominent. Check all areas of the lung including the

hidden areas. (It is a good idea to check and then recheck.) A large pneumothorax will be immediately visible. The side with the pneumothorax will have no lung markings. Look for the edge of the collapsed lung. Air producing the pneumothorax will tend to accumulate in the apices first. This produces a vertical white line. Ask the examiner if you may turn the CXR horizontally to search for these vertical lines suggesting a pneumothorax. Sometimes a bulla can mimic a pneumothorax, but there are often lung markings passing through a bulla. Causes of a pneumothorax are:

- spontaneous
- trauma, for example, from central venous line insertion or pleural aspiration

- cystic fibrosis
- Marfan's (*mar-fans*) syndrome (*Antoine Bernard Jean Marfan (1858–1942), French paediatrician*)
- Ehlers–Danlos syndrome.

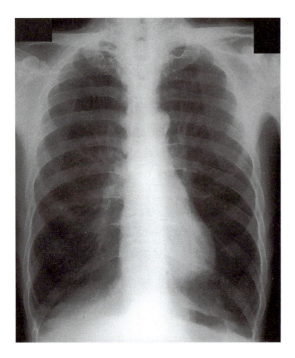

Figure 15.30 Chronic obstructive pulmonary disease.

Pulmonary embolism

The radiological changes associated with a PE are subtle. The CXR is usually normal. Occlusion of a pulmonary artery by a thrombus may result in an oligaemic (poorly perfused) segment of the lung (Westerman's sign). So the black area will be anatomically defined. Try to exclude COPD and a pneumothorax first as these are more common causes of a black lung. Other changes such as acute dilatation of the proximal site of the affected pulmonary artery (Pallas sign), dilatation of the right atrium and ventricle, and a compensatory overperfusion of the rest of the lung should be left to the specialists. Once the PE is established and there is infarction of the lung, secondary changes will occur and are more commonly seen. You may see a small ipsilateral pleural effusion, wedge-shaped shadowing, or a raised hemidiaphragm (see Figs. 15.33 and 15.34).

Heart

Mitral stenosis

Mitral stenosis causes left atrial dilatation (see Fig. 15.9). This can be seen on the CXR as a bulging convex left atrial border and a double right heart border where the left atrium extends across the heart. The carina will become wider and is greater than 90°. If you look closely, within

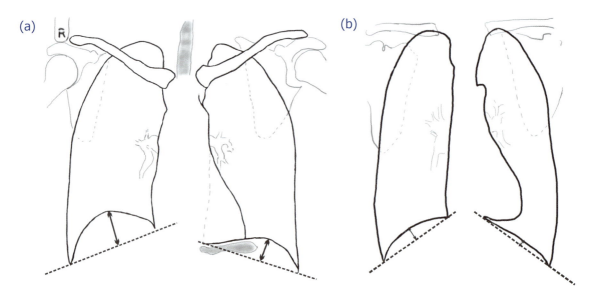

Figure 15.31 Diagram demonstrating imaginary lines used to assess normal and flattened diaphragms: (a) normal diaphragms; (b) flattened diaphragms.

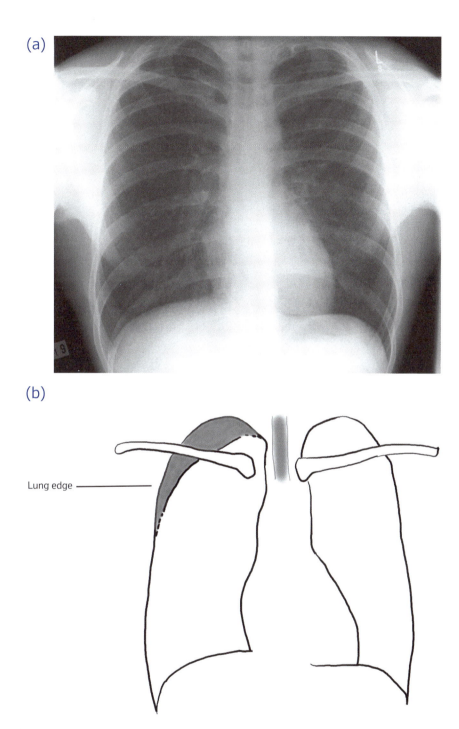

(a)

(b)

Lung edge

Figure 15.32 CXR showing apical pneumothorax. Note that the apex of the right lung is black and lacks lung markings. The lung edge is very subtle and easily missed.

(a) 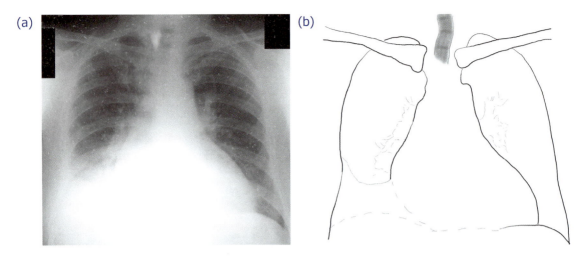 (b)

Figure 15.33 Pulmonary infarction early. Note moderate right pleural effusion and perhaps some increased shadowing just above the meniscus adjacent to the right heart border.

(a) 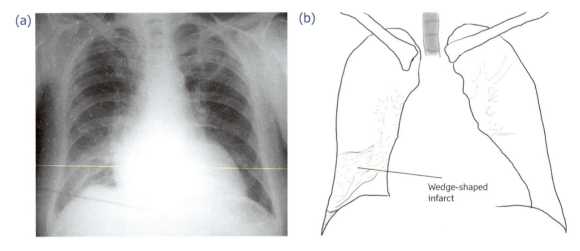 (b)

Wedge-shaped infarct

Figure 15.34 Pulmonary infarction late. Two months later there is a wedge-shaped infarct in the right lower zone (and the suspicion of another infarct in the left upper zone).

the heart shadow you may see the calcified mitral valve. Remember that mitral stenosis can also present with pulmonary oedema.

Left ventricular aneurysm

You should see bulging of the left border of the heart and there may be calcification within it (see Fig. 15.35).

Pericardial effusion

Pericardial effusions surround the heart, so a generalized enlargement (as opposed to a specific area of the heart)

should make you suspicious of a pericardial effusion (see Fig. 15.36). A pericardial effusion develops quickly, so look at old films for comparison.

Hilum

When the hilum is enlarged you should consider:

- bronchogenic lung cancer (see Fig. 15.37)
- hilar lymphadenopathy—due to malignancy, lymphoma, and infection
- vascular shadowing.

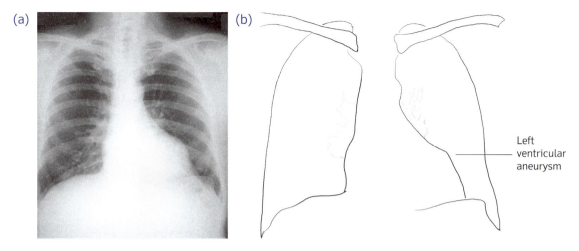

Figure 15.35 Left ventricular aneurysm.

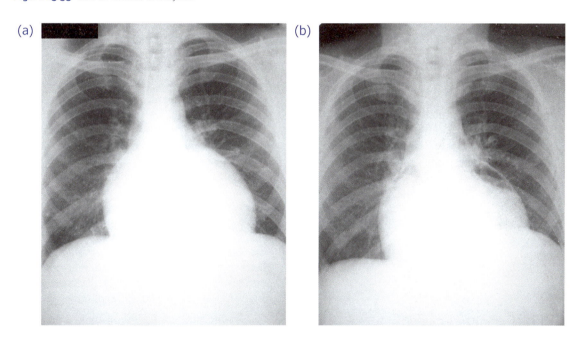

Figure 15.36 Pericardial effusion. (a) Note cardiomegaly with the characteristic globular shape of the heart. (b) Appearance following pericardiocentesis (a pericardial tap). Air has now been introduced into the pericardial sac.

Tip

If a patient is malaligned during a CXR, any rotation will cause the mediastinum to look wide. So, check the technical quality of the film.

The affected hilum will look larger and denser. It will have lost its normal concave shape. However, you may mistake hilar enlargement if the film is rotated, so review the old films. Bilateral hilar enlargement can also be due to vascular markings, cancer, or lymphadenopathy.

Tip

For any lung pathology try and obtain any old CXRs. They will let you know if the abnormality is new or old and how the abnormality is progressing.

(a) 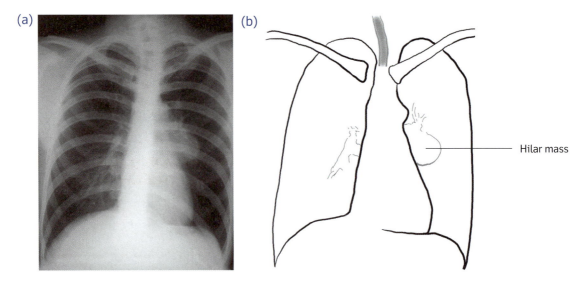 (b)

Hilar mass

Figure 15.37 CXR showing unilateral hilar enlargement, due to malignancy.

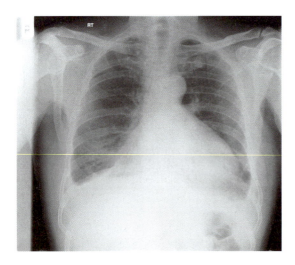

Figure 15.38 CXR for presentation.

Presentation

Presentation is very important. If you were asked to comment on the CXR in Fig. 15.38, you would say the following:

This is a plain, PA chest radiograph of Mr Clause taken on the 25 December at the North Pole General Hospital. The most obvious abnormality is the appearance of cardiomegaly. I will focus on this after I have first studied the radiograph systematically. The radiograph is correctly oriented and the exposure is satisfactory. The patient is not rotated. There are no obvious abnormalities within the bones. The trachea is not deviated. The mediastinum has clearly defined borders and there is no enlargement or change in density of it or the hilar regions. There is no CXR pathology in the lungs and they are expanded normally. The diaphragms are clearly seen although there is blunting at the right costophrenic angle with a meniscus suggesting a small effusion. There are no abnormalities below the diaphragm or within the soft tissues. The cardiothoracic ratio exceeds 1:2. As this is a PA film, this confirms the heart is enlarged. With regard to the cardiomegaly, four causes are IHD, VHD, pericardial effusion, and cardiomyopathy.

References and further reading

Corne J, Pointon K. *CXR made easy*, 3rd edn. Churchill Livingstone, Edinburgh, 2010.

Harvey CJ, Roberts HRS, Shaw RJ. *Radiology casebook for the MRCP*. Oxford University Press, Oxford, 1999.

Ray KK, Ryder REJ, Wellings RM. *An aid to radiology for the MRCP*. Blackwell Science, Oxford, 2000.

Scalley P. *Medical imaging, an Oxford core text*. Oxford University Press, Oxford, 1999.

16 Finals

Introduction

Finals, or the 'end of course quiz', represent the last hurdle to negotiate before reaching the heady heights of foundation doctor. No other exam is surrounded by so much folklore, rumour, and anxiety. However, as with all the examinations that you have successfully navigated before, a methodical and thoughtful approach will ensure success.

If you are reading this chapter with Finals to come in a few years' time, then we applaud your foresight. Many, if not all, of the tips and advice here will carry you through your preliminary clinical years and leave you poised to cruise through Finals when you reach them. If you have Finals in a few months, then it is almost certainly time to start preparation in earnest. A revision group is invaluable, especially for the clinical examinations. Choose your team wisely! Working in a group is a fantastic way to break the tedium of sitting in isolation in the library. It is also a good way to share the burden of a very stressful set of exams. If you have Finals in a few weeks, then we would hope that preparations are well under way. The information below should help refine and streamline the work put in over the last few months. Be careful not to burn out though; make sure that you hit your peak at just the right time. If you have Finals in a few days, then last-minute preparations should be under way. Try to allocate one or two specific topics to the last few days. This helps stop the 'quick look over everything' phenomenon, which never achieves what it seeks to do.

This chapter can be summarized in one word . . . practice! Every component of the Finals examination is to a certain extent predictable. It should always be borne in mind that the exam aims to assess your safety and suitability to progress to the ward. Some medical schools explicitly tailor their examinations to reflect this; other medical schools retain the flavour of the more traditional examinations. However, no matter where you are training, the bottom line remains the same. Are you safe?

It is of course a tired cliché to say that 'the examiners want to pass you', but it is true. This is reflected in the very high pass rate, far higher than all the exams that you will have passed to reach Finals.

Most institutions have a written examination and a clinical examination. This chapter is divided accordingly.

Written examinations

Written examinations vary in format between institutions. You should aim to get details of your written exams at the earliest opportunity and structure your revision to reflect this. Most medical schools use multiple-choice examinations of various formats. They are popular as they allow students to be assessed on a broad curriculum; they are well validated for their purpose and are marked by a computer!

True/false

True/false questions are the older style of multiple-choice question in which students are required to decide whether a statement is true or false. This can be complicated by negative marking whereby a correct answer gains a mark, a wrong answer loses a mark, but a blank answer neither loses nor gains. This introduces the question of 'certainty'. Negatively marked true/false questions are in less widespread use now.

Extended matching questions

Extended matching questions (EMQs) are very popular in medical schools around the UK. Each question usually has a theme, for example, blood gases. Between 10 and 15 appropriate conditions are listed followed by 5 clinical vignettes. In the example below, the 'conditions' are a list of various metabolic abnormalities. According to the question, one must match each vignette with the appropriate metabolic disturbance. The structure of an EMQ is shown in Fig. 16.1.

Each vignette is designed to offer enough information to favour a particular condition. EMQs can be broadly focused into three categories:

- **Diagnostic**. The vignette will contain information on symptoms/signs and a list of possible diagnoses offered. This is often the more straightforward type of question, phrased as 'please select the most likely diagnosis'.

- **Investigation**. The vignette will also give a small amount of clinical information, but the question is often worded in a very specific way: for example, 'Please select the *most diagnostic* investigation'. This requires a very different answer from 'Please select the *next most appropriate* investigation'.

- **Management**. Similar to the investigation questions, but questions may ask for *next immediate* step of management or *definitive* management.

For example in vignette 1 in Fig. 16.1, the first step is to realize that the patient has diabetic ketoacidosis; the next step is to identify which metabolic picture would be expected in this condition. One way to do this type of question is to read the theme first, skip (or even cover up) the stems, read the question, and then work through the vignettes. Once you have thought of an answer for each vignette return to the stems and look for your answers. If they are not there, then reread the question. Look for indirect clues: for example, in vignette 3, the mention of

home oxygen and nebulizers hint at a person with chronic obstructive pulmonary disease (COPD). It is the author's experience that this focuses your attention on the detail in the vignette and helps avoid distraction by a long list of potentially intimidating conditions.

As with true/false questions, there is a 'knack' for EMQs, which is easily acquired with practice. The importance of reading the question is paramount, as a subtle change in wording can change the answer. This is a particular risk in multiple-choice questions where hundreds of questions will be tackled in each paper. Some multiple-choice questions are harder than others. This is intentional and is designed to stratify the final-year students. Your medical school may use a grading system to stratify both the difficulty and importance of a question. For instance, if a question is very difficult but about a rare condition it may be assigned a low mark on the scale. However, if a question is easy and about an important, common condition or emergency then it will be assigned a higher mark on the scale. While this has little bearing on how to answer a particular question, an understanding of how an exam is constructed can help make the whole process seem more transparent.

Essays/short answer questions

These are not widely used in Finals, as it is nearly impossible to assess a large curriculum like medicine in even 10 essays. However, if this is a style of examination used in your medical school then advice about careful reading of a question, planning exam time, and doing practice questions still very much applies. Remember to make sure you set aside a few minutes to plan each of your answers before launching into your essay, as it can be very easy to lose direction of your arguments in the heat of the exam room.

Practice

Multiple-choice questions should be practised regularly. There are a number of resources available in print and on-line. Whichever is chosen, make sure that the question styles used in your Finals are well represented. A good practice resource will have an accompanying explanation for why a particular answer is right or wrong. This can help make revision more directed.

When the exams are close, one or more timed practice examinations are invaluable as a marker of progress. If your confidence is high then it is often helpful to try some practice questions designed for the MRCS or

Theme

A	B	C	D
CO_2 11 O_2 6.2 O_2 saturation 81%	O_2 16 CO_2 3.78 pH 7.48	HCO_3 23 O_2 13.74 CO_2 5.23 pH 7.43	BE –6 HCO_3 12 CO_2 2.9 pH 7.15

E	F	G	H
O_2 saturation 91% HCO_3 35 O_2 7.4 CO_2 9.1 pH 7.345	pH 7.451 HCO_3 38 CO_2 8.2 O_2 13.6 BE +7	pH 7.51 CO_2 3.8 HCO_3 24	pH 6.98 O_2 6.19 CO_2 4.6 HCO_3 8 O_2 saturation 83%

Question

Below are a group of patients that have all had an arterial blood sample taken (on room air). Select the most appropriate ABG result for each patient. Each answer may be used once, more than once or not at all.

(1) A drowsy 25-year-old diabetic man found by his mum. She says he hasn't been taking his usual injections for 2 days because he's got a cold and hasn't been eating.

(2) A 79-year-old woman, 4 days after AP resection for malignancy. She was talking to her daughter and suddenly became short of breath. She clutches her chest and looks very unwell.

(3) A 55-year-old former smoker with home nebulizers and oxygen presents with green sputum, pyrexia, and worsening shortness of breath.

(4) A 26-year-old goalkeeper has an ABG taken at the end of a football match.

(5) An anxious 27-year-old woman presenting with tingling around her mouth saying she just can't get her breath.

Vignette

Ranges

pH	7.35–7.45
pCO_2	4.7–6
pO_2	10.5–14
plasma	HCO_3 22–28

(1) **D.** The history tells you this is a classical case of diabetic ketoacidosis.

(2) **H.** Massive post-operative pulmonary embolism causing metabolic acidosis.

(3) **E.** Infective exacerbation of chronic obstructive pulmonary disease. Note the former smoker, home nebulizers, and oxygen—all clues of a question involving chronic lung disease.

(4) **C.** Normal!

(5) **B.** Tingling lips and anxiety are good clues for the diagnosis of hyperventilation. Respiratory alkalosis.

Answers

Figure 16.1 The structure of an EMQ.

MRCP. However, this should not be done at the expense of comprehensive revision of basic medicine and surgery. Remember you need to demonstrate you are ready to be an F1, not the next professor of surgery.

The big day

Don't forget all the administrative things often required on the exam day. Running back home to collect a forgotten student card is seldom the best way to prepare for a 3-hour written exam. Arrive on time, and avoid like the plague the people who sit talking about how little work they have done, or smugly recite the insertions of tibialis posterior.

Carefully read the instructions. Make sure that enough time is left to transfer answers on to the answer paper (or that it is done as you go along). No extra time will be allocated for this! It is often worth checking that you have put the intended answer in the correct line. There is no worse feeling than noticing with 1 minute to go that you have filled in an answer booklet to 151 when there are only 150 questions.

Clinical examinations

The clinical examinations are arguably the most important and challenging part of medical Finals. The integration of clinical skills represents the culmination of your studies at medical school and experiences as a student doctor. They demand a good working knowledge of medical science and the manifestations of disease, with an inquisitive ear for history-taking and a keen eye for examination. These skills must be complemented by a practical awareness of medical and surgical management, all of which needs to be communicated with kindness and professionalism. Traditionally, the clinical examinations involved a 'short' and 'long' case, but in most medical schools these have been replaced by the Objective Structured Clinical Examination (OSCE).

Long and short cases

The **long case** bears the closest resemblance to the practice of a doctor who is admitting a new patient. You are given 45–60 minutes to take a complete history and examination of a (bona fide) patient, including performing any simple bedside tests (e.g. fundoscopy). At the end of this time you are expected to be able to present a comprehensive presentation of your patient's complaints, the diagnosis, and list of likely differentials, as well as presenting a holistic management plan of the patient's bio-psycho-social needs.

The format of the **short case** usually involves a pair of examiners leading you around a number of patients, whom you are asked to examine. Again the range can be enormous, and there is an inherent lack of standardization in these cases when patients are presented to students who are given any number of different variations of instructions. Some people state that the more cases you see, the greater your chances of success. There is a grain of truth in this; however, you can rush through seven cases, do them badly, and fail, and equally you may see only four in-depth cases, perform well, and pass.

What is required from the traditional short and long cases is not so dissimilar from any other clinical examination, but the task you are given and the discussion with your examiner at the end can be incredibly variable. Examiners differ in what they expect from you; in the long cases, some will sit back and listen to you recite every detail you have unearthed, before asking you straightforward questions about management, whereas others will only ask for a diagnosis before going off at tangents, asking in-depth questions that test your knowledge (and sweat glands!). Furthermore, the degree of involvement from the patient also introduces an unhelpful degree of variability to each examination case. It is this inherent variability in student experience that has led to the charge of unfairness, and a move towards a more structured and objective assessment.

Objective structured clinical examination

The OSCE is a form of clinical assessment which consists of a series of short and highly-focused stations. The emphasis of the OSCE is to assess candidates against the same marking criteria, using patients (who are either actors) with identical (or when examining real individuals, similar) clinical signs and symptoms. Precise instructions are given to the candidate at the beginning of each station, followed by 5–10 minutes in which to complete the task, and then a typically shorter period of 2.5–5 minutes in which to answer a set of predefined questions. Your outcome is not determined by the subjective assessment of your examiner, but rather your ability to satisfy each point in the defined marking scheme.

Format of the OSCE

The OSCE can be used to cover any form of clinical examination, from history-taking or breaking bad news, to examining a patient or performing a procedural skill. They may use actors, particularly in history-taking stations, where the examiners can therefore ensure identical patient responses to each candidate's questions. There are variations on the exact format, and therefore as with all exams you will need to establish the style of OSCEs you will face at your medical school, in order to specifically prepare for them.

For example, one of your OSCEs might consist of eight 15-minute stations, 10 minutes for interaction with the 'patient', and a 5-minute viva for structured questions and answers, per station. Occasionally shorter stations are also used, with 5 minutes for 'patient' interaction and 2.5 minutes for the viva.

Outside each station there is typically a short instruction, which you are usually given 1 minute to read, before beginning the station. There are usually computerized voice-overs during the exam, signalling when you must finish reading the instructions and begin each station; move on to the viva; and leave the station in order to begin reading the instructions for the next station. An examiner (or two) will be present in the corner of each station, and will tend not to interfere with your history-taking or examination, and only interact with you when the signal is given to begin the viva. You are not usually permitted to answer the questions until the designated time for patient interaction (e.g. 10 minutes) is completed, even if you have finished early. So make the most out of the time you have been given. If you have time to spare, use it to gather your thoughts and prepare your answers for the discussion you are likely to face (see 'OSCE viva').

Content of the OSCE

The task you are asked to complete at each OSCE station will differ between medical schools, although will generally cover the same broad content: history-taking and clinical examinations.

History-taking and communication OSCE stations

Your history-taking and communication OSCE stations are likely to test a range of clinical skills, from clinical knowledge and reasoning to a clear and empathetic ability to communicate. These 'simulated encounters' should be treated in exactly the same way as an interaction with a real patient. Although the actors are briefed on how to answer each question, they are able to respond to your comments and behaviour in a realistic way; so unclear or insensitive questioning will be met with less helpful or awkward responses.

Stations will differ in the proportion of marks they allocate for the quality of communication compared with clinical reasoning; in general most stations will award some marks for both. Therefore it is impossible to score well if you fail to communicate professionally, but similarly the kindest history-taker will score poorly if they are unable to focus their questioning and achieve a sensible differential diagnosis.

Examples of history-taking and communication OSCEs that you might expect include:

- You are working as a FY1 in the medical admissions unit; take a history from a 55-year-old man with chest pain.

- You are working as a junior doctor in the neurology outpatients; take a history from a 24-year-old woman with visual disturbance.

- You are the general medical house officer on call. Spend 5 minutes reading the medical notes of a 65-year-old woman admitted with pneumonia, and then phone the intensive care unit (ITU) registrar to negotiate a transfer to ITU.

- You are the house officer on a surgical ward. Speak with the ward sister, who refuses to administer the fentanyl infusion you have prescribed for a patient receiving palliative care.

- You are the surgical house officer on call; you are called to the day surgery unit to speak with a 50-year-old patient who has some questions regarding their scheduled cholecystectomy.

- You are a doctor at a GP surgery; speak with a 48-year-old lorry driver about his new diagnosis of epilepsy.

- You are the FY2 in the emergency department; take a history from the mother of a 2-year-old girl, who has noticed that her child is limping.

Clinical examination OSCE stations

The clinical examination OSCE stations frequently use real patients, although don't be surprised to examine an actor feigning right upper quadrant guarding, or even a 'normal' examination. Your objective in these stations is to safely and professionally examine a patient, identify common obvious signs, and make a reasonable deduction about diagnosis, further investigations and treatment.

Again you are likely to encounter a series of 15-minute and 7.5-minute stations. Some examiners prefer you talking through your clinical examination while you are conducting it, others prefer to hear your summary at the end; most won't mind which you chose, and you should be guided by the examiner if they have a strong preference.

The instructions at your 15-minute stations might include:

- Perform a cardiovascular examination of this patient.
- Perform a respiratory examination of this patient.
- Perform an abdominal examination of this patient.
- Examine this patient's cranial nerves.
- Examine this patient's peripheral nervous system.
- Examine this patient's peripheral vascular system.

The instructions at your 7.5-minute stations might include:

- You are working in the rheumatology clinic: examine this patient's hands.
- Examine this patient who is a regular attender at the endocrinology clinic (e.g. patient with acromegaly).
- Examine this patient who attends the general surgery clinic with a groin lump.
- Examine this patient's hip.
- Examine this patient's skin lesions, commenting on each as you do.
- This station will test your ability to read and interpret common radiological investigations. You will be given instructions relating to a series of radiological images which will be shown to you on a computer.

Rare examinations such as per rectum, fundoscopy, and auriscopy can be included. Real people may not be available or in the case of per rectum, unwilling, but rest assured plastic mock-ups can be brought in. Remember to treat the plastic model as if it were a real patient.

It is worth remembering that most medical schools have a wide selection of patients, to ensure that each cohort of finalists will encounter a different set of patients at different sittings of the 'same' OSCE exam. It is worth bearing this in mind before seeking the advice of your colleagues who have completed their own OSCEs earlier in the day/week.

In medical Finals, you cannot simply go through the process of completing an examination. Instead, you are expected and must be able to observe and identify clinical signs if present, and similarly exclude signs which are not present. In identifying a series of positives and negatives you should be able to clinically deduce a diagnosis and likely differentials. Do not forget to use the alcohol gel on your hands at the beginning of each examination, to introduce yourself and gain consent, and fundamentally to never harm the patient, as this is a guaranteed way to ensure failure at any station.

Marking of the OSCE

The mark sheet for the abdominal examination for example may look something like Fig. 16.2. Medical schools use various methods to obtain their 'pass mark', and you should try to find out which your school employs. In general for medical Finals there is a minimum pass mark which must be obtained. For example using the mark sheet in Fig. 16.2, you may need to obtain 12/20 per station to pass each station (1 mark awarded for good, ½ mark for adequate, 0 marks for inadequate/absent), as well as pass 50% of OSCE stations overall in order to pass the entire exam.

Although applying cut-offs for passing and failing to a 'bell-shaped' distribution of your final year may occasionally be used in some medical schools, it is certainly possible for entire year groups to pass their medical Finals, and there is no fixed percentage of students who must fail each year (by the same token it is indeed possible for an entire year to fail medical Finals, although this has yet to occur!). The aim of medical Finals is to ensure that the successful candidates can practice as safe and competent FY1 doctors.

OSCE viva

The questions you are asked at the end of each OSCE station will differ depending on the type of station. However, in general for typical history-taking and examination stations you will invariably be asked to 'summarize' or 'present your findings'. At the end of your clinical examination station, it is customary to mention how you would complete your examination before presenting your findings. For example, you might complete your abdominal examination by 'looking at the observation chart, examining the external genitalia, and performing a digital rectal examination'.

Remember that you will have a total of 2.5–5 minutes for the entire viva, and therefore you should aim to complete your summary in a timely fashion, and certainly not much longer than 30–40 seconds. You will not be awarded any marks for questions you didn't have time to answer.

The ideal presentation of your findings must include positives and pertinent negatives. The absence of jaundice in a patient with hepatomegaly is far more relevant than the absence of a collapsing pulse in the same patient. In preparing for your OSCEs, it can help to group signs together (e.g. signs of liver failure, or extraintestinal signs of inflammatory bowel disease), in order to produce mental checklists of what to look out for. Practising your presentations is a vital part of revision for OSCEs, and guarantees easy marks in the OSCE viva.

	Good	Adequate	Inadequate/ absent
"Please examine this patient's abdominal system."			
Introduction to patient			
Wash hands			
Asks if the patient is in pain			
Inspects hands looking for stigmata of GI disease			
Inspects face and mouth looking for stigmata of GI disease			
Inspects neck for lymph nodes and chest for GI signs			
Inspects abdomen			
Verify area of maximal tenderness			
Examines at level of patient, palpating superficially then deeply			
Checks for organomegaly and AAA			
Percusses for ascites			
Examines hernial orifices			
Auscultates for bruits and bowel sounds			
Suggests completion with examining external genitalia and rectal examination			
Communicates appropriately			
Examines professionally			
Closure with patient			
"Summarise your findings"			
Presents findings in logical manner			
"What do you think is the most likely diagnosis and why?"			
Logical deduction from signs			
Global Score: Fail, Borderline, Pass, Merit, Distinction.			
Comments:			

Figure 16.2 A sample mark sheet may include these criteria.

After your presentation, if you haven't already said, you will be invited to offer a diagnosis and list of likely differentials. In presenting your *most likely* diagnosis you should aim to make an assessment as to the severity of the disease (e.g. decompensation in liver failure), and whether any complications are manifest (e.g. several different abdominal scars, suggesting multiple operations). When listing your differential diagnoses, use this opportunity to demonstrate your clinical knowledge with a sensible classification of pathologies; it may be appropriate to use an aetiological sieve. Similarly, you should list your differentials in order of most to least common.

You will then be asked about investigations that will help you to distinguish between your list of differentials. Try to structure your answers in a logical manner. It does not make sense to suggest a triple-phase CT chest/abdomen/pelvis before stating that you would perform a urine dipstick and blood tests. As a rule you should therefore present your investigations in order of increasing complexity, beginning with simple bedside investigations, blood tests (haematology, biochemistry, MC&S) before moving on to basic imaging (plain radiograph, CT, MRI, US), and more sophisticated tests (e.g. biopsy).

You can also be sure you will be asked about your management of the patient. Always mention the fact that you would undertake a full history and examination, and if you think that the case warrants emergency treatment do not forget basic and advanced life support.

The management of a patient must also be structured in a sensible order; hence you would not begin your management of a patient with Crohn's disease with a panproctocolectomy and ileostomy. Instead you should answer by beginning with **conservative** measures (e.g. education, diet, counselling, multidisciplinary support); **medical** treatments (e.g. steroids, immunusuppression, biological agents), and finally conclude with **surgical** interventions (e.g. resection, ileostomy). Do not forget to provide a holistic, bio-psycho-social management plan, which treats the patient as an individual as opposed to a scripted list of therapies used in a specific disease. Think about physiotherapy, visual aids, walking aids, home helps, and financial benefits, particularly for the elderly patient.

Succeeding in the OSCE

Practice makes perfect. If this overused cliché could be applied to one situation it would be the OSCE. Each station is timed and so rehearsing obvious scenarios such as history-taking and examinations is vital. Some of these may be core stations, for example, history and examination stations, so not to perfect these is ritual suicide. You should find the clinical examination skills outlined in this textbook are second nature by the time of medical Finals. In doing so, you will be left with the enjoyable task of tying together your clinical findings, rather than worrying about the process of each patient encounter.

It is in this way that you can ensure that you will leave your OSCEs having enjoyed the experience, with a solid foundation on which to enter this exciting and rewarding profession.

Best of luck!

Medical students: distinguished roll of honour

1 Michaela Quinn: *Dr. Quinn, Medicine Woman* (TV series starring Jane Seymour).

2 Leonard McCoy: Dr McCoy, *Star Trek* 'It's life, Jim, but not as we know it.'

3 William Osler: Canadian physician and teacher remembered for eponymous conditions e.g. Osler–Weber–Rendu syndrome and Osler's nodes.

4 Russell Brock: Cardiothoracic surgeon at Guy's Hospital, London and to King George VI who described Brock's Syndrome (Middle lobe syndrome).

5 James Parkinson: English physician who described the condition known as Parkinson's disease.

6 Berkeley Moynihan: English surgeon, Leeds-trained authority on abdominal surgery.

7 Marjory Warren: English surgeon who ironically founded the modern specialty of geriatrics.

8 James Paget: English surgeon with great understanding of pathology who described three separate disease entities: Paget's disease of the nipple, of the skin, and of the bone.

9 Marie Curie: Polish-born French scientist who was a pioneer of radioactivity and won two Nobel prizes.

10 Abraham Colles: Irish surgeon who is famous for the description of the Colles fracture of the wrist.

11 Ernst Moro: Austrian paediatrician who described the Moro reflex.

Index